T0127851

Kinetic Control

The Management of Uncontrolled Movement

REVISED EDITION

Mark Comerford, BPhty, MCSP, MAPA
Technical Director, Comera Movement Science

Sarah Mottram, MSc, MCSP, MMACP
Head, Comera Movement Science

ELSEVIER

ELSEVIER

Elsevier Australia. ACN 001 002 357
(a division of Reed International Books Australia Pty Ltd)
Tower 1, 475 Victoria Avenue, Chatswood, NSW 2067

ISBN: 978-0-7295-4326-2

National Library of Australia Cataloguing-in-Publication Data

A catalogue record for this book is available from the National Library of Australia

Publisher: Melinda McEvoy
Developmental Editor: Rebecca Cornell
Publishing Services Manager: Helena Klijn
Project Coordinators: Natalie Hamad and Karthikeyan Murthy
Content Project Manager: Shravan Kumar
Edited by Stephanie Pickering
Proofread by Forsyth Publishing Services
Cover design by Lisa Petroff
Illustrations by Rod McClean
Index by Robert Swanson
Typeset by Toppan Best-set Premedia Limited
Printed in China by RR Donnelley Asia Printing Solutions Limited

Last digit is the print number: 9 8 7 6 5 4 3 2 1

Contents

Preface

This book presents a comprehensive system for the assessment and retraining of movement control. It has been in evolution for the last 25 years.

Uncontrolled movement has a significant impact on the development of movement disorders and pain. The scientific support for the process of the assessment and retraining of uncontrolled movement has been steadily expanding particularly in the last 10 years. The influence of uncontrolled movement on symptoms, especially pain, movement function, recurrence of symptoms and disability is now well established. We believe that in the next 10 years the literature will support that the presence of uncontrolled movement will also be recognised as a predictor of injury risk and as having an influence on performance.

Uncontrolled movement can be identified by movement control tests. People with pain demonstrate aberrant movement patterns during the performance of these movement control tests. A growing body of evidence supports the use of movement control tests in the assessment and management of chronic and recurrent pain. The identification of uncontrolled movement in terms of the site, direction and threshold of movement impairment is a unique subclassification system of musculoskeletal disorders and pain. The movement testing process proposed enables the classification of uncontrolled movement into diagnostic subgroups that can be used to develop client-specific retraining programs. This process can determine management priorities and optimise the management of musculoskeletal pain and injury recurrence. Subclassification is now recognised as being the cornerstone of movement assessment and the evidence for subclassification of site, direction and threshold is growing. This book details a structured system of testing, clinical reasoning and specific retraining. This system does not preclude other interventions as it is designed to enhance the management of musculoskeletal disorders.

The Kinetic Control process has come a long way in last 25 years. The motivation for the development of the Kinetic Control process was to find a way to blend the new and exciting concepts in movement dysfunction into an integrated clinical process, built on the foundation of a solid clinical reasoning framework. Our aim is to gain a better understanding into the inter-relationship between the restrictions of movement function and movement compensations. The breakthrough came with the realisation that some compensation strategies are normal adaptive coping mechanisms and do not demonstrate uncontrolled movement, while others are maladaptive compensation strategies that present with uncontrolled movement. This led us to develop the structured assessment process detailed in this text including the Movement Control Rating System (Chapter 3). This clinical assessment tool can identify movement control deficiencies and be valuable for reassessing improvements in motor control efficiency.

Recurrent musculoskeletal pain has a significant impact on health care costs, employment productivity and quality of life. Uncontrolled movement can be identified by observation, and corrective retraining of this uncontrolled movement may have an influence on onset and recurrence of symptoms. To date, outcome measures in terms of changes in range and strength, have not influenced the onset and recurrence of injury. The ability to assess for uncontrolled movement and to retrain movement control is an essential skill for all clinicians involved in the management of musculoskeletal pain, rehabilitation, injury prevention, and those working in health promotion, sport and occupational environments. Preventing the recurrence of musculoskeletal pain can both influence quality of life and have an economic impact.

Movement control dysfunction represents multifaceted problems in the movement system. Skills are required to analyse movement, make a clinical diagnosis of movement faults and develop and apply a patient-specific retraining program and management plan to deal with pain, disability, recurrence of pain and dysfunction. The mechanisms of aberrant movement patterns can be complex, so a sound clinical reasoning framework is essential to determine management goals and priorities. We present an assessment framework which will provide the option to consider four key criteria relevant to dysfunctional movement: the diagnosis of movement faults (site and direction of uncontrolled movement), the diagnosis of pain-sensitive tissues (patho-anatomical structure), the diagnosis of pain mechanisms and identifying relevant contextual factors (environmental and personal). This clinical reasoning framework can help identify priorities for rehabilitation, where to start retraining and how to be very specific and effective in exercise prescription to develop individual retaining programs.

Uncontrolled movement can be reliably identified in a clinical environment and related to the presence of musculoskeletal pain, to the recurrence of musculoskeletal pain and to the prediction of musculoskeletal pain. We hope this text will enable clinicians worldwide to effectively identify and retrain uncontrolled movement and help people move better, feel better and do more.

Mark Comerford
Sarah Mottram
2011

Foreword

Comerford and Mottram are to be commended for their extensive and comprehensive presentation of factors involved in movement dysfunctions. This book shares several of my own strong beliefs that have implications for the management of musculoskeletal pain conditions. Those beliefs are: 1) recognising and defining the movement system; 2) identifying and describing pain syndromes based on movement direction; 3) identifying the primary underlying movement dysfunction; 4) describing the various tissue adaptations contributing to the movement dysfunction; and 5) developing a treatment program that is comprehensive and based on the identified contributing tissue adaptations. I also share with the authors a belief that the treatment program requires the patient's active participation, which can range from control of precise, small, low force requiring movements to total body large force requiring movements. Historically – and still prevalent – is the belief that tissues become pathological as an inevitable outcome of trauma, overuse and ageing. The result is a focus on identifying the patho-anatomical structure that is painful rather than on identifying the possible contributing factors, or even how movement faults can be an inducer. We are all aware that movement is necessary to maintain the viability of tissues and bodily systems. Almost daily, studies are demonstrating the essential role of movement, in the form of exercise or activity, in achieving or maintaining health. Yet there is very little recognition that there are optimal ways of moving individual joints and limb segments as well as the total body. Similarly there is little recognition that painful conditions can be treated by correcting the movement rather than resorting to symptom-alleviating modalities, drugs or surgery. Optimal alignment when maintaining prolonged postures, such as sitting, is not considered to be necessary. I believe the situation is analogous to that of diet. For many years, no one worried about the effect on a person's health of the type or amount of food that was consumed. Indeed, more money is still spent on the alignment of the teeth than on the alignment of the body, though the function of the body is more affected by alignment faults than eating is by poor alignment of the teeth.

This book serves to reinforce and define the characteristics of the movement system and how they contribute to movement dysfunctions associated with pain syndromes. The authors have done an extensive review of the relevant literature describing the dysfunctions of the nervous and muscular systems. They have provided a detailed description of a key underlying factor, designated as uncontrolled movement, which then provides a basis for the treatment program. The detailed descriptions of the syndromes, key observations and examination forms should be most helpful in guiding the clinician. Building upon the information taken from the examination, the treatment program is also described in detail. What is particularly noteworthy is the incorporation of most of the perspectives and methods used by the best known approaches to musculoskeletal pain. The authors have organised the rationale and methods from these varying approaches into a comprehensive approach. Comerford and Mottram have done a thorough job of describing all aspects of what could be considered the 'psychobiosocial' model of analysis and treatment of musculoskeletal pain. The timeliness of this book is reflected by the incorporation of their concepts to the International Classification of Functioning, Disability, and Health. As stated previously this book has its particular value in the comprehensiveness and detailed descriptions of possible tissue dysfunctions as reported in the literature, methods of analysis and treatment. The reader will be truly impressed by the many complexities of the movement system and the rigorous analysis that is required to understand, diagnose and treat the dysfunctions that can develop and contribute to pain syndromes. The authors have truly provided an outstanding text in its inclusive and thorough discussion of the topic of movement dysfunction.

Shirley Sahrmann, PT, PhD, FAPTA
Professor Physical Therapy, Neurology, Cell Biology and Physiology
Washington University School of Medicine – St. Louis

Acknowledgements

The content of this book has been a work in progress since 1988. The background to the development of the assessment and retraining of uncontrolled movement has been influenced by the work of Shirley Sahrmann, Vladamir Janda, Gwendolyn Jull, Paul Hodges, Carolyn Richardson and Maria Stokes. Since 1995 many colleagues within Kinetic Control and Performance Stability have helped with the development of the clinical tests and the consolidation of theoretical frameworks. Erik Thoomes contributed to the clinical reasoning process in Chapter 1. We would very much like to thank all these people for their contribution through inspiration, advice, support or feedback. We both appreciate the support of our family and friends and in particular Mark's wife Selina, without whom he would not have found the time to devote to this project.

Reviewers

Technical Reviewer
Prue Morgan M.App.Sc (Research), B.App.Sc (Physio)
Grad Dip Neuroscience
Specialist Neurological Physiotherapist, FACP
Lecturer, Physiotherapy
Monash University

Philippa Tindle BSc. BA. MCSP
Member of Chartered Society of Physiotherapy and Registered with the Health Professions Council (HPC)

Section | 1 |

Chapter | **1** |

Uncontrolled movement

The key to managing movement dysfunction is thorough assessment. This includes the determination of any uncontrolled movement (UCM) and a comprehensive clinical reasoning process by the clinician to evaluate contributing factors which influence the development of UCM. This first chapter details the concept of UCM and the clinical reasoning process which is the framework for assessment and rehabilitation.

UNDERSTANDING MOVEMENT AND FUNCTION

Normal or ideal movement is difficult to define. There is no one correct way to move. It is normal to be able to perform any functional task in a variety of different ways, with a variety of different recruitment strategies. Optimal movement ensures that functional tasks and postural control activities are able to be performed in an efficient way and in a way that minimises and controls physiological stresses. This requires the integration of many elements of neuromuscular control including sensory feedback, central nervous system processing and motor coordination. If this can be achieved, efficient and pain-free postural control and movement function can be maintained during normal activities of daily living (ADL), occupational and leisure activities and in sporting performance throughout many years of a person's life.

The movement system comprises the coordinated interaction of the articular, the myofascial, the neural and the connective tissue systems of the body along with a variety of central nervous system, physiological and psycho-social influences (Figure 1.1). It is essential to assess and correct specific dysfunction in all components of the movement system and to assess the mechanical inter-relationships between the articular, myofascial, neural and connective tissue systems. This chapter will describe a systematic approach to evaluation of the movement system and identification of the relative contributions of individual components to movement dysfunction.

Movement faults

Identifying and classifying movement faults is fast becoming the cornerstone of contemporary rehabilitative neuromusculoskeletal practice (Comerford & Mottram 2011; Fersum et al 2010; Sahrmann 2002). In recent years clinicians and researchers have described movement faults and used many terms to describe these aberrant patterns. These terms include substitution strategies (Richardson et al 2004; Jull et al 2008), compensatory movements (Comerford & Mottram 2001a), muscle imbalance (Comerford & Mottram 2001a; Sahrmann 2002), faulty movement (Sahrmann 2002), abnormal dominance of the mobiliser synergists (Richardson et al 2004; Jull et al 2008), co-contraction rigidity (Comerford & Mottram 2001a), movement impairments

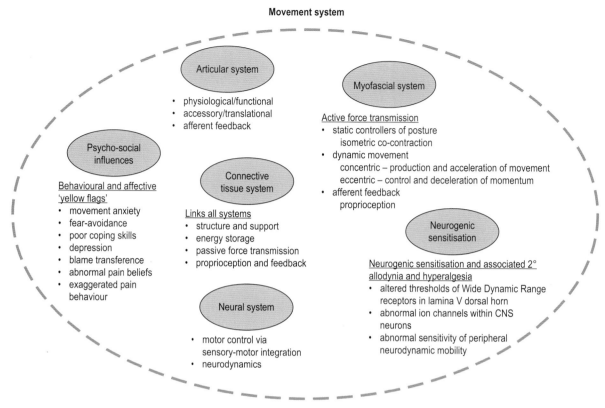

Movement system

Articular system
- physiological/functional
- accessory/translational
- afferent feedback

Myofascial system
Active force transmission
- static controllers of posture
  isometric co-contraction
- dynamic movement
  concentric – production and acceleration of movement
  eccentric – control and deceleration of momentum
- afferent feedback
  proprioception

Psycho-social influences
Behavioural and affective 'yellow flags'
- movement anxiety
- fear-avoidance
- poor coping skills
- depression
- blame transference
- abnormal pain beliefs
- exaggerated pain behaviour

Connective tissue system
Links all systems
- structure and support
- energy storage
- passive force transmission
- proprioception and feedback

Neurogenic sensitisation
Neurogenic sensitisation and associated 2° allodynia and hyperalgesia
- altered thresholds of Wide Dynamic Range receptors in lamina V dorsal horn
- abnormal ion channels within CNS neurons
- abnormal sensitivity of peripheral neurodynamic mobility

Neural system
- motor control via sensory-motor integration
- neurodynamics

Figure 1.1 Inter-related components of the movement system

(Sahrmann 2002; O'Sullivan et al 2005) and control impairments (O'Sullivan et al 2005; Dankaerts et al 2009). All of these terms describe aspects of movement dysfunction, many of which are linked to UCM.

The focus of this text is to describe UCM and explore the relationship of UCM to dysfunction in the movement system (Comerford & Mottram 2011). Movement dysfunction represents multi-faceted problems in the movement system and the therapist needs the tools to relate UCM and faults in the movement system to symptoms, recurrence of symptoms and disability. Skills are required to analyse movement, make a clinical diagnosis of movement faults and apply a patient-specific retraining program and management plan to deal with pain, disability, recurrence of pain and dysfunction.

Sahrmann (2002) has promoted the concept that faulty movement can induce pathology, not just be the result of it; that musculoskeletal pain syndromes are seldom caused by isolated events; and that habitual movements and sustained postures play a major role in the development of movement dysfunction. These statements have been fundamental in the development of the movement dysfunction model. Clinical situations which have a major component of movement dysfunction contributing to pain include: postural pain; pain of insidious onset; static loading or holding pain; overuse pathology (low force repetitive strain or high force and/or impact repetitive strain); recurrent pain patterns; and chronic pain.

It is important to identify UCM in the functional movement system. It is our hypothesis that the uncontrolled segment is the most likely source of pathology and symptoms of mechanical origin. There is a growing body of evidence to support the relationship between UCM and symptoms (Dankaerts 2006a, 2006b; Luomajoki et al 2008; van Dillen et al 2009). The direction of UCM relates to the direction of tissue stress or strain and pain producing movements. Therefore it is important in the assessment to identify the site and the direction of UCM and relate it to the symptoms and pathology. The UCM identifies the *site* and the *direction* of dynamic stability dysfunction and is related to the direction of symptom-producing movement. For example, UCM into lumbar flexion under a flexion load may place abnormal stress or strain on various tissues and result in lumbar flexion-related symptoms. Likewise, uncontrolled lumbar extension under extension load produces extension-related symptoms, while uncontrolled lumbar rotation or side-bend and/or side-shift under unilateral load produces unilateral symptoms.

IDENTIFICATION AND CLASSIFICATION OF UCM

Figure 1.2 illustrates the link between UCM and pain. Abnormal stress or strain that exceeds tissue tolerance can contribute to pain and pathology. The relationship between UCM and pain/pathology will be explored further in Chapter 3.

In this text the identification and classification of movement faults are described in terms of site and direction of UCM. These movement faults will be discussed in Chapter 2 in relation to changes in motor recruitment and strength (Comerford & Mottram 2001b, 2011). Scientific literature and current clinical practice are linking the site and direction of UCM in relation to symptoms, disability, dysfunction, recurrence, risk and performance (Figure 1.3).

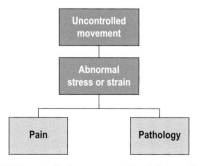

Figure 1.2 Uncontrolled movement: the link to pain and pathology

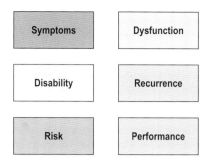

Figure 1.3 Factors relating to the site and direction of uncontrolled movement

Symptoms

Symptoms are what the patient feels and complains of and include pain, paraesthesia, numbness, heaviness, weakness, stiffness, instability, giving way, locking, tension, hot, cold, clammy, nausea and noise. The treatment of symptoms is often the patient's highest priority and is a primary short-term goal of treatment.

Pain is frequently one of the main symptoms that the patient presents with to the therapist and is inherently linked to movement dysfunction. Contemporary research clearly demonstrates that individuals with pain present with aberrant movement patterns (Dankaerts et al 2006a, 2009; Falla et al 2004; Ludewig & Cook 2000; Luoma-joki et al 2008; O'Sullivan et al 1997b, 1998). Research has demonstrated a consistent finding: in the presence of pain, a change occurs in recruitment patterns and the coordination of synergistic muscles. Individuals with pain demonstrate patterns of movements that would normally be used only in the performance of high load or fatiguing tasks (e.g. pushing, pulling, lifting weights) to perform low load non-fatiguing functional tasks (e.g. postural control and non-fatiguing normal movements). Clearly UCM is a feature of many musculoskeletal pain presentations and identifying and classifying these movement faults is essential if therapists are to effectively manage symptoms by controlling movement faults.

Disability

Disability is the experienced difficulty doing activities in any domain of life (typical for one's age and sex group, e.g. job, household management, personal care, hobbies, active recreation) due to a health or physical problem (Verbrugge &

Jette 1994). Movement faults are related to disability. For example, Lin et al (2006) demonstrated that changes in scapular movement patterns (in particular a loss of posterior tilt and upward rotation) correlated significantly with self-report and performance-based functional measures indicating disability. The relationship between disability and movement faults has been identified in many other fields of physical therapy (e.g. neurological and amputee rehabilitation). Indeed, in relation to gait dysfunction, management and retraining of UCM is a key factor in rehabilitation of people with lower limb amputations using a prosthesis (Hirons et al 2007).

Reduction of disability is the primary long-term goal of therapy or rehabilitation. Disability is individual and what one person considers disability another person might consider exceptional function. For example, an elite athlete's disability may be a function that most people do not have the ability to do, do not want to do or need to do. Movement dysfunction, however, can affect a person's ability to function independently and therefore decrease quality of life. The disablement process model in disease as well as in rehabilitation is gaining recognition (Escalante & del Rincon 2002; Verbrugge & Jette 1994) and retraining movement faults has been shown to improve function (O'Sullivan et al 1997a; Stuge et al 2004).

Dysfunction

Dysfunction can imply disturbance, impairment or abnormality in the movement system. It can be objectively measured and quantified and/or compared against a normal or ideal standard or some validated or calculated benchmark. These impairments may present as weakness, stiffness, wasting, sensory–motor changes (including proprioception changes, altered coordination and aberrant patterns or sequencing of muscle recruitment) or combinations of several impairments. Dysfunction measurements include: joint range of motion (physiological or accessory); muscle strength (isometric, concentric, eccentric, isokinetic, power and endurance); muscle length; flexibility; stiffness; speed; motor control (recruitment, inhibition, coordination and skill performance); bulk (girth, volume, cross-sectional area); and alignment.

A baseline measurement of dysfunction, followed by an intervention with some form of treatment or therapy over a variable timeframe and subsequent reassessment of dysfunction provides the basis of evidence-based practice. Reduction of dysfunction is a primary short-term goal of therapeutic intervention, although the patient is frequently symptom free before dysfunction is corrected. Treatment should not cease just because the symptoms have disappeared, but may need to continue until no more dysfunctions are measurable.

The process of identifying and measuring UCM, and linking UCM to musculoskeletal pain, and to changes in muscle function, is a developing area of active research in the field of pain and movement dysfunction (Gombatto et al 2007; Luomajoki et al 2007, 2008; Mottram et al 2009; Morrissey et al 2008; Scholtes et al 2009; Roussel et al 2009a; van Dillen et al 2009). Muscle dysfunction is most clearly apparent in people with pain (Falla & Farina 2008; Hodges & Richardson 1996; Hungerford et al 2003; Lin et al 2005). The changes in muscle function underlying pain can present in two ways: 1) as altered control strategies (van Dillen et al 2009; O'Sullivan 2000); and 2) as physiological peripheral muscle changes (Falla & Farina 2008). Physiological changes associated with muscle dysfunction are discussed further in Chapter 2, and altered control strategies are discussed further in Chapter 3.

Recurrence

The correction or rehabilitation of dysfunction has been shown to decrease the incidence of pain recurrence (Hides et al 1996; Jull et al 2002; O'Sullivan et al 1997a). This reinforces the need for therapy to be aimed at correcting dysfunction in the management of musculoskeletal disorders and not just relieving symptoms.

Risk of injury

Evidence suggests history of injury is a predictive factor for re-injury and therefore outcome measures that are defined in terms of normal range of joint motion and muscle strength are inadequate to prevent recurrence (Mottram & Comerford 2008). Making the link between UCM and pain is not new, but the concept of linking it to injury prevention is.

Some recent research has highlighted the potential for linking UCM to risk of injury. A recent study on dancers identified two movement control tests that may be useful for the identification of dancers at risk of developing musculoskeletal injuries in the lower extremities (Roussel et al 2009a). Athletes with decreased neuromusculoskeletal control of the body's core (core stability) are at an increased risk of knee injury (Zazulak et al 2007). Indeed, there is now growing evidence that motor control and physical fitness training prevent musculoskeletal injuries (Roussel et al 2009b), highlighting the importance for therapists to be more knowledgeable about movement control and function.

Performance

At present there is little published literature to relate UCM to performance. However, anecdotal empirical evidence has shown that retraining movement faults can improve performance in athletes.

The movement dysfunctions associated with pain and disability have been shown to be reversible so there is a developing need to identify UCM in relation to injury risk and performance and to objectively evaluate the outcome of retraining.

A MODEL FOR THE ASSESSMENT AND RETRAINING OF MOVEMENT FAULTS

Many clinicians and researchers have made a significant contribution to the body of evidence relating to movement, movement impairments and corrective retraining. Some have described a particular approach to assessment and retraining and most support each other's philosophies or provide different pieces of the puzzle to enable an understanding of the 'whole picture'. No single approach has all the answers but the therapist who wants to provide 'best practice' for clients can benefit enormously from a synthesis of the different approaches and concepts proposed to date, along with the ongoing development and integration of original ideas and applied principles.

Figure 1.4 illustrates the development of the *movement analysis model*. The movement analysis model identifies UCM in terms of the site (joint), direction (plane of motion) and recruitment threshold (low or high) and further establishes links to pain, disability, dysfunction, recurrence,

risk of injury and performance. This model has been developed through the analysis and synthesis of historical and contemporary research from many sources; however, it is not intended to be a comprehensive summary of the current level of knowledge surrounding movement analysis.

Kendall and colleagues (2005) described muscle function in detail. Their now classic text has been the foundation for assessment of muscle function, especially with reference to the graded testing of muscle strength and analysing the interrelationship of strength and function. Janda (1986) had previously developed the concept of muscle imbalance and patterns of dysfunction by analysing the pattern of movement sequencing. His primary intervention was to increase extensibility of short muscles. Sahrmann (2002) and co-workers further developed the concept of muscle imbalance, again analysing patterns of movement, and have developed a diagnostic framework for movement impairments (direction susceptible to motion).

The 1990s saw a huge advancement in the identification of motor control dysfunction (Jull et al 2008; Richardson et al 2004). Hodges (Hodges & Cholewicki 2007) has developed a large body of evidence linking motor control of deep muscles to spinal stability. O'Sullivan and co-workers have provided objective measurements to support the links between altered muscle recruitment and direction-related musculoskeletal pain (Dankaerts et al 2006a). From this research a classification system based on diagnostic subgroups has been proposed (Vibe Fersum et al 2009).

Vleeming et al (2007) and Lee (2004) have developed the model of form and force closure and have linked this to anatomical fascial slings. McGill's (2002) research has emphasised the importance of training more superficial muscles to stabilise the core during loaded and sporting function and is often referred to as core strengthening. All these clinicians and researchers have contributed important aspects to a comprehensive and integrated model of movement analysis.

Alternative therapies

In the search to identify the defining characteristics of therapeutic exercise, a brief review and analysis of many different approaches and concepts including alternative therapies is appropriate. Some of these approaches are supported by

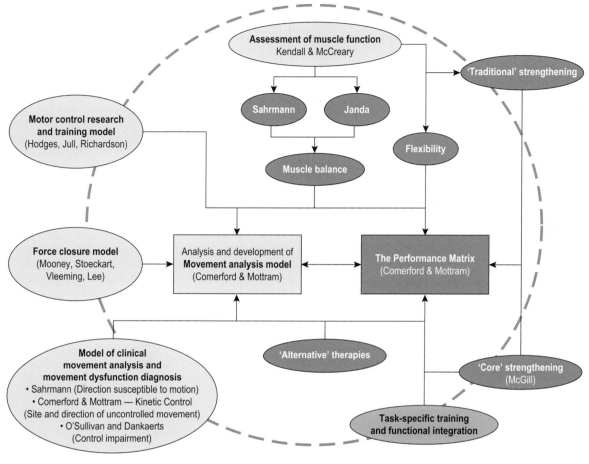

Figure 1.4 The development of the movement analysis model

clinical evidence (Emery et al 2010; Rydeard et al 2006). Box 1.1 lists some useful approaches to pain management and/or movement dysfunction to explore. Many exercise approaches have either stood the test of time or their popularity suggests that people who practise them feel or function better.

Whilst the various exercise concepts feature distinctive elements that characterise their approach, there are features that are common to all approaches (Box 1.2). These common features may contribute to good function and warrant closer inspection and further investigation. Breathing control is a key feature in many of these therapies. The link between respiratory disorders

---

Box 1.1 **Useful alternative therapies in the management of movement dysfunction**

Tai chi
The Alexander technique
Yoga
Pilates
Physio ball (Swiss ball)
Feldenkrais
Martial arts
GYROTONIC®

Box 1.2 **Common features in alternative therapies**

- Multi-joint movements
- Slow movements
- Low force movements
- Large range movements
- Coordination and control of rotation
- Smooth transition of concentric–eccentric movement
- Awareness of gravity
- Concept of a 'core'
- Coordinated breathing
- Awareness of posture
- Intermittent static hold of position
- Control of the centre of mass of one body segment with respect to adjacent segments
- Proximal control for distal movement
- Positive mental attitude

and increased risk of development of back pain has recently been established (Smith et al 2009) and altered breathing patterns have been noted during lumbopelvic motor control tests (Roussel et al 2009c).

THE ASSESSMENT AND MANAGEMENT OF UCM

Effective intervention requires the therapist to have a thorough understanding of the mechanisms of aberrant movement patterns, an ability to confidently diagnose and classify the movement faults and to manage these dysfunctions. Guidelines for a comprehensive *analysis of movement dysfunction* have been described with factors the therapist needs to consider in Box 1.3

Box 1.3 **Procedure for analysis of movement dysfunction**

Uncontrolled movement: assessment and retraining guidelines

1. Assess, diagnose and classify movement in terms of pain and dysfunction from a motor control and a biomechanical perspective.
2. Develop a large range of movement retraining strategies to establish optimal functional control.
3. Use a clinical reasoning framework to prioritise the clinical decision-making challenges experienced in contemporary clinical practice.
4. Develop an assessment framework that addresses the four key criteria relevant to dysfunctional movement:
   a. diagnosis of movement dysfunction
      i. site and direction of uncontrolled movement
      ii. uncontrolled translation
      iii. uncontrolled range of motion
      iv. myofascial and articular restriction
      v. aberrant guarding responses
   b. diagnosis of pain-sensitive tissue(s)
      i. patho-anatomical structure
   c. diagnosis of pain mechanisms
      i. peripheral nociceptive (inflammatory or mechanical)
      ii. neurogenic sensitisation
   d. identification of relevant contextual factors (Verbrugge & Jette 1994)
      i. environmental factors (extra-individual) (e.g. physical and social context)

   ii. personal factors (intra-individual) (e.g. lifestyle and behavioural changes, psychosocial attributes, coping skills).
5. Make links between uncontrolled movement and pain and other symptoms, dysfunction, recurrence, risk of injury and performance.
6. Make a link between uncontrolled movement and disability through the disablement process model.
7. Make links between uncontrolled movement and changes in motor control, strength, joint range of motion, myofascial extensibility and functional activities.
8. Identify the clinical priorities in terms of retraining uncontrolled movement and mobilising restrictions of normal motion.
9. Use a clinical assessment tool to identify deficiencies and reassess improvements in motor control efficiency.
10. Integrate non-functional motor control retraining skills with functionally relevant movement.
11. Use other techniques and strategies (e.g. taping to support uncontrolled movement or facilitate motor relearning and strengthening).
12. Use a clinical reasoning framework to identify priorities for rehabilitation, where to start retraining and how to be specific and effective in exercise prescription to develop individual retaining programs.
13. Know which way and how fast to progress, and know how to tell when retraining has achieved an effective end-point independently of symptoms.

(Comerford & Mottram 2011)

(Comerford & Mottram 2011). An understanding of the inter-relationship of the elements of the movement is needed alongside an understanding of factors relating to normal movement, function and dysfunction (Chapter 2). A sound clinical reasoning process underpins this process to optimise the assessment and retraining strategy. This process is described in the following section.

THE CLINICAL REASONING PROCESS

The efficient and effective management of UCM in relation to symptoms, disability, dysfunction, recurrence, risk of injury and performance is dependent on a comprehensive assessment. This should lead to a specific action plan for the individual patient. Exercise protocols do have a place in the management of musculoskeletal disorders. However, because of differences in presentation and diagnostic subgroups, effective management is dependent on assessment analysis and management planning. Exercise protocols can be effective when dysfunction can be clearly defined into diagnostic subgroups rather than based on pathology. The key to identifying these diagnostic subgroups lies in making the link between movement dysfunction and symptoms (Comerford & Mottram 2001b; Sahrmann 2002; Vibe Fersum 2009).

The following section presents a series of points to direct clinical reasoning for the integration of movement dysfunction assessment and planning of a targeted rehabilitation strategy for movement dysfunction.

The 10 point analysis and clinical reasoning framework for UCM

A clinical reasoning framework can be used to develop an understanding of the relationships between movement, symptoms, dysfunction, and other factors that influence the clinical reasoning process (Comerford & Mottram 2011). Box 1.4 presents 10 key steps to understanding movement and pain. The first five steps relate specifically to the site and direction of UCM. The last five steps relate to other factors necessary to develop a full understanding of the dysfunction, as well as a management plan.

Box 1.4 Ten key steps to understanding movement and pain

1. *Classify the site and direction* of uncontrolled movement.
2. Relate the site and direction of uncontrolled movement to *symptoms*.
3. Relate assessment findings to *disability*.
4. Identify the *uncontrolled movement* in terms of 'uncontrolled translation' and 'uncontrolled range', and *restrictions* in terms of articular restriction and myofascial restrictions.
5. Management plan for uncontrolled movement and restrictions.
6. Relate *pain mechanisms* to presentation.
7. Consider *tissues or structures* that could be contributing to the patient's signs and symptoms.
8. Assess for environmental factors and personal factors (e.g. lifestyle and behavioural changes, psychosocial attributes and coping skills).
9. Integrate other *approaches or modalities* as appropriate.
10. Consider *prognosis*.

---

1 Classify the site and direction of UCM

As indicated above, UCM is labelled in terms of its site and direction. These can be assessed using specific tests and evaluated with a clinical rating system (Chapter 3). Indeed, the assessment may well identify more than one direction of UCM in the same site, or different regions. Some examples of the site and direction of UCM, as well as the appropriate test, are given in Table 1.1. The kinetic medial rotation test has been shown to be valid (Morrissey et al 2008) and the standing bow test is considered reliable (Luomajoki et al 2007; Roussel et al 2009a). These tests are described in detail in following chapters in this text.

Table 1.1 Examples of the site and direction of uncontrolled movement

SITE	DIRECTION	TEST
Scapula	Downward rotation	Kinetic medial rotation test (KMRT) (T60 page 372)
	Forward tilt	
Lumbar spine	Flexion	Standing trunk lean test (T1 page 93)

Chapter 3 of this text will explain the process used to identify the site and direction of UCM using specific tests and evaluation with a systematic clinical rating system.

2 Relate UCMs to symptoms

The link between the site and direction of UCM and the presenting symptoms needs to be established to direct rehabilitation. For example, in the shoulder, less upward rotation and backward tilt (which relates to uncontrolled downward rotation and forward tilt) of the scapula has been identified in people with symptoms related to shoulder impingement (Ludewig & Cook 2000). Uncontrolled lumbar flexion has been identified in people with back pain (Luomajoki et al 2008; Roussel et al 2009a).

Outcome measures commonly used to evaluate pain symptoms include the visual analogue scale (VAS), the numerical rating scale (NRS), the verbal numerical rating scale (VNRS) and the quadruple VAS (Von Korff et al 1993).

3 Relate assessment findings to disability

The link between functional disabilities and movement faults needs to be identified. Functional disabilities as a result of pain or movement dysfunction may relate to reduced ability to participate in work, leisure or relationships. For example, Long et al (2004) showed that subjects with back pain and a direction preference to pain-relieving postures (e.g. flexion provoked lumbar pain relieved by extension movements or postures) who were treated with exercises matched to their direction preference had significant improvements in outcomes of rapidly decreased pain, decreased medication use, reduced disability, reduced depression and decreased work interference.

A standard procedure to record disability is to interview individuals about difficulties by means of self-reports or proxy reports, with simple ordinal or interval scoring of degree of difficulty (Verbrugge & Jette 1994). Examples of commonly used outcome measures are listed in Box 1.5.

4 Identify the UCM and restrictions

UCM can be described in terms of uncontrolled translation (e.g. uncontrolled intersegmental translation) and uncontrolled physiological or functional range of movement (Comerford &

Box 1.5 **Commonly used evaluation measures for disability**

Disability questionnaires

- For the cervical spine:
  - Neck Disability Index (Vernon & Mior 1991)
  - Bournemouth Neck Questionnaire (Bolton & Humphreys 2002).
- For the lumbar spine:
  - Roland-Morris Disability Questionnaire (Roland & Morris 1983)
  - Oswestry Disability Questionnaire (Fairbank et al 1980; Fairbank & Pynsent 2000).
- For the shoulder:
  - Shoulder Pain and Disability Index (Heald et al 1997; Roach 1991)
  - Disabilities of the Arm, Shoulder and Hand Questionnaire (Hudak et al 1996).
- For the hip:
  - Western Ontario and McMaster Universities Osteoarthritis Index (WOMAC) (Bellamy 1988)
  - Hip Outcome Score (Martin & Philippon 2007).

Table 1.2 Uncontrolled movements and restrictions (Comerford & Mottram 2001b)

Uncontrolled movement	Intersegmental translation	Range
	Translation movement at a single motion segment	Physiological or functional range of movement at one or more motion segments
Restriction	**Articular**	**Myofascial**
		+/− neurodynamic influence

Mottram 2001a). This is shown in Table 1.2. Restriction can be described as articular restriction and/or myofascial restriction (Comerford & Mottram 2001a). Neural sensitivity is linked with a neurophysiological response in the myofascial system presenting as a myofascial restriction (Coppieters et al 2001, 2002, 2006; Edgar et al 1994; Elvey 1995).

Table 1.3 gives examples of UCM in terms of translation and range at the shoulder girdle, and joint and myofascial restrictions. Uncontrolled anterior translation can be measured in people

Table 1.3 Example of uncontrolled movement and restrictions at the shoulder girdle

Uncontrolled movement	Intersegmental translation	Range
	Uncontrolled anterior translation at the glenohumeral joint	Uncontrolled scapula forward tilt
Restriction	**Articular**	**Myofascial**
	Posterior translation at glenohumeral joint	Restriction of medial rotation (infraspinatus/ teres minor)

Table 1.4 Example of uncontrolled movement and restrictions at the lumbar spine

Uncontrolled movement	Intersegmental translation	Range
	Uncontrolled intersegmental translation (e.g. at L4 or L5)	Uncontrolled lumbar flexion
Restriction	**Articular**	**Myofascial**
	Restriction of intersegmental translation	Restriction in hip flexion (hamstrings, superficial gluteus maximus)

with shoulder pain (Morrissey 2005), as can uncontrolled range, illustrated with uncontrolled forward tilt (Lin et al 2005, 2006). Interestingly, this uncontrolled forward tilt (and loss of backward tilt) corresponds to a decrease in serratus anterior activity, which confirms the role of serratus in producing backward tilting of the scapula (and controlling forward tilting).

Table 1.4 provides examples of UCM in terms of translation and range at the lumbar spine. UCM in the lumbar spine has been described in terms of uncontrolled lumbar flexion (Dankaerts et al 2006a; Luomajoki et al 2008; Sahrmann 2002; Vibe Fersum et al 2009). Uncontrolled lumbar flexion has been associated with either uncontrolled range of lumbar flexion relative to hip flexion, or abnormal segmental initiation of lumbar motion during forward bending and other flexion-related activities.

5 Management plan for UCM and restrictions

Following the assessment of the UCM and restrictions, a management plan can be established. In this text, we describe the retraining of the site and direction of UCM but specific retraining strategies can also target the local stability muscle systems (to control intersegmental translation) (Comerford & Mottram 2001a) and the global muscle systems (to control range) (Comerford & Mottram 2001a). Restrictions need to be mobilised with appropriate (manual) therapy, to regain extensibility of the myofascial systems (Comerford & Mottram 2001a).

To cover all aspects of motor control assessment and retraining, four principles of assessment and retraining are proposed (Comerford & Mottram 2001a):

1. **Control of direction:** the assessment and retraining of the site and direction of uncontrolled movement (see Chapters 3 and 4).
2. **Control of translation:** specific assessment and retraining strategies to target the local stability muscle system to control translation.
3. **Control through range:** specific assessment and retraining strategies to target the global stability muscle system to control range of movement.
4. **Control of extensibility:** specific assessment and retraining strategies to target the global mobility muscle system to regain extensibility and control the active lengthening of these muscles.

In addition, manual therapy can address any articular restrictions and neural issues that may cause muscle overactivity and restrictions. Elvey (1995) has described how 'muscles protect nerves' so these issues need to be explored in relation to any restrictions (for more detail see Butler 2000; Shacklock 2005).

Figure 1.5 illustrates the management plan outline indicating the targeted interventions applied where uncontrolled translation, uncontrolled range, UCM site or direction, articular or myofascial restriction are identified. An example of a management plan developed for a person presenting with shoulder pain and dysfunction is illustrated in Figure 1.6; and an example of a management plan developed for a person presenting with back pain and lumbar dysfunction is given in Figure 1.7.

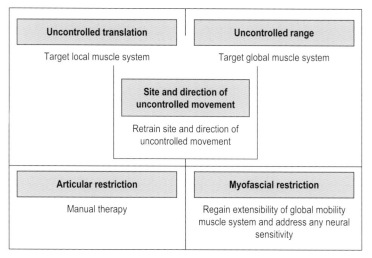

Figure 1.5 The management planning outline

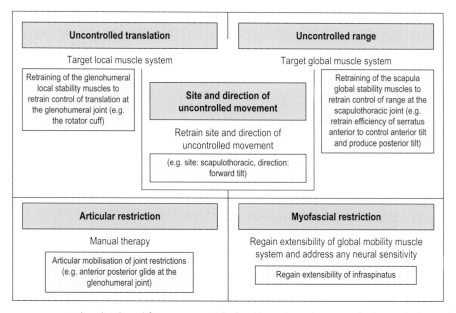

Figure 1.6 The management plan developed for a person with shoulder pain and uncontrolled scapula forward tilt

6 Relate pain mechanisms to presentation

Pain mechanisms can have a significant influence on movement control and consideration of changes within the nervous system is a key component of the clinical reasoning process (for more detail see Breivik & Shipley 2007; Butler & Moseley 2003). It is essential to consider the influence of mechanical nociceptive or inflammatory pain in movement control (e.g. the influence on proprioception, allodynia and motor control). Useful screening tools for neuropathic pain could include the S-LANSS (Bennett et al 2005) or the pain DETECT questionnaire (Freynhagen et al 2006), while the McGill Pain Questionnaire (Melzack 1975; Melzack & Katz 1992) also evaluates the affective aspects of pain for a patient.

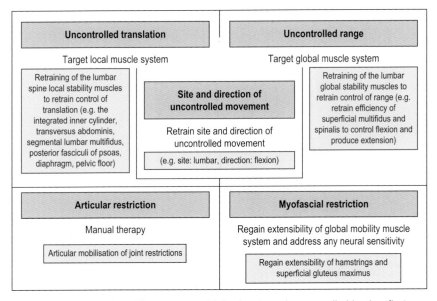

Figure 1.7 The management plan developed for a person with back pain and uncontrolled lumbar flexion

7 Consideration of tissues or structures contributing to symptoms

The site and direction of UCM may match the pathology identified. For example, people with a shoulder impingement demonstrate UCM at the scapula (Morrissey 2005). Abnormal quality of motion in spinal lumbar segments has been demonstrated to be associated with spondylolisthesis pathology (Schneider et al 2005). The link between tissue stress resulting in pathology and abnormal range or quality of movement is becoming more evident. The therapist needs to find a link between the UCM and any presenting pathology.

8 Assess for environmental and personal factors

Personal factors (e.g. lifestyle and behavioural changes, psychosocial attributes, coping and activity accommodations) and environmental factors (e.g. medical care and rehabilitation, medications and other therapeutic regimens, external supports, physical and social environment) should also be assessed. Personal factors commonly assessed within the context of physical therapy include items such as depression, anxiety, coping skills and cognition. These can be

objectively assessed (and reassessed) with valid and reliable questionnaires such as the Pain Coping Inventory (PCI; Kraaimaat & Evers 2003), Tampa Scale of Kinesiophobia (TSK; Swinkels-Meewisse et al 2003; Vlaeyen et al 1995), Fear Avoidance Beliefs Questionnaire (FABQ; Waddell 1998) and the Pain Self-Efficacy Questionnaire (PSEQ; Nicholas 2007; Nicholas et al 2008).

Once the site and direction of UCM have been established, effective rehabilitation should ensure that movement dysfunction is addressed throughout functional tasks. Control of movement during functional activities, and awareness of the UCM during posture, daily activities, sport and training programs should be promoted. For example, a person with uncontrolled scapula downward rotation needs to be aware of this movement fault during daily activities such as reaching for a cup in a cupboard. A person with uncontrolled lumbar flexion needs to be aware of this movement fault when bending forwards to tie up their shoelaces.

9 Integrate other approaches or modalities

There are many other therapeutic modalities that can influence the correction of movement faults. Table 1.5 details some examples. This is not intended to be an exhaustive list but illustrates

Table 1.5 Examples of therapeutic modalities that can influence the correction of movement faults

OTHER THERAPEUTIC APPROACHES	EXAMPLES
Pathophysiological approaches	Ice, heat, electrotherapy, medication
Articular approaches	Joint mobilisation and manipulation (Maitland et al 2005; Cyriax 1980; Kaltenborn et al 2003)
Ergonomic and environmental factors	Work place assessment, postural advice
Neurodynamic approaches	Neurodynamic mobilisation (Butler 2000; Shacklock 2005)
Sensory-motor approaches	Neuromuscular facilitation (Rood in Goff 1972), Bobath 'normal movement' (Bobath 1990), neurofunctional training (Carr & Shepherd 1998), neurosensory approach (Homstøl 2009)
Soft tissue approaches	Massage therapy (Chaitow 2003)
Psychosocial approaches	Behavioural evaluation and therapy (Waddell 1998; Woby et al 2008)
Biomechanical approaches	Taping, orthotics, bracing

useful adjuvant modalities in retraining UCM, managing pain, mobilising restrictions or treating pathology.

10 Consider prognosis

Although the management of symptoms has been the primary aim in the treatment of musculoskeletal disorders, research has also demonstrated links between UCM and dysfunction, disability and the recurrence of symptoms. It is therefore appropriate that dysfunction and disability are also considered, along with symptoms, when providing a prognosis for recovery in the management of musculoskeletal disorders. The timeframe for expected improvement in symptoms should be considered independently of the timeframes for recovery of dysfunction and disability when making prognostic judgments for recovery.

Physiological tissue repair timelines have been well researched and are reasonably well defined. In more acute (less than 6 weeks) conditions, these provide a useful guideline. In more chronic (more than 12 weeks) conditions, other prognostic factors become more important. A systematic review on prognostic factors in whiplash-associated disorders established that factors related to poor recovery included: female gender; a low level of education; high initial neck pain; more severe disability; higher levels of somatisation and sleep difficulties (Hendriks et al 2005; Scholten-Peeters et al 2003). Neck pain intensity

and work disability proved to be the most consistent predictors for poor recovery in these studies.

The relative influence of factors beyond physiological processes is a contemporary research subject and there is a growing body of evidence indicating that socio-demographic, physical and psychological factors strongly affect short- and long-term outcomes. These factors must be taken into consideration when establishing a realistic timeframe for when dysfunction, symptoms and disability could be expected to improve and by how much.

CLINICAL REASONING IN A DIAGNOSTIC FRAMEWORK

As noted in Box 1.3, when a patient presents with neuromusculoskeletal pain and dysfunction, it is good clinical practice to assess and identify four key criteria:

1. diagnosis of movement dysfunction
2. diagnosis of pain-sensitive or pain-generating structures
3. diagnosis of presenting pain mechanisms – peripheral nociceptive and neurogenic sensitisation
4. evaluation and consideration of contextual factors.

1 Diagnosis of movement dysfunction (site and direction of uncontrolled motion)

The initial priority is to identify the site and direction of UCM that best correlates with the patient's presenting mechanical symptoms. In complex presentations, there is frequently more than one site of UCM. When this is the case, it is useful to identify whether one site is the site of primary dysfunction and whether the other site is compensating for the primary one.

If there are obvious restrictions that are causing compensatory UCM, it is very effective for the therapist to work to achieve normal mobility of these restrictions early in the management plan (see Chapter 4).

The therapist should also identify if there is a priority to retrain local stability muscle function early or if this can be retrained later in the rehabilitation process. Similarly, the therapist should identify any contributing muscle imbalance issues related to the dysfunction, such as altered length and recruitment relationships between mono-articular stabiliser muscles and multi-articular mobiliser muscles. If these imbalances are identified, the global stabiliser muscle recruitment efficiency should be retrained to recover active control through the full available range of motion, and the global mobility muscle extensibility should be restored.

2 Clinical diagnosis of pain-sensitive or pain-generating structure(s)

The therapist should identify the structure or tissue that is the source of the symptoms or pain that the patient complains of. Patients who present with a chronic or recurrent condition frequently report more than one tissue contributing to the pain experience. The clinical reasoning process that identifies a variety of pain-sensitive tissues requires a thorough understanding of tissue anatomy and physiology, a knowledge of the mechanism of injury (if there is one) and an understanding of the typical responses of different tissues to stress and strain and injury. All available therapeutic skills, tools or modalities can be utilised to best provide an optimal environment to allow and promote tissue healing and to control or manage the presenting signs and symptoms. Contemporary clinical reasoning in patients with chronic pain suggests it is more appropriate to explore factors affecting impairment of function and participation than to attempt to diagnose specific structures or tissues as a source of nociception.

3 Clinical diagnosis of presenting pain mechanisms

It is essential to have an understanding of the relevant pain mechanisms contributing to any individual's pain presentation. In a person with chronic or recurrent pain it is common to find different mechanisms contributing to their symptoms. Melzack's (1999) neuromatrix theory of pain proposes that pain is a multidimensional experience produced by characteristic 'neurosignature' patterns of nerve impulses generated by a widely distributed neural network in the brain. It proposes that the output patterns of the neuromatrix activate perceptual, homeostatic, and behavioural responses after injury, pathology or chronic stress. The resultant pain experience is produced by the output of a widely distributed neural network in the brain rather than solely by sensory input evoked by injury, inflammation or other pathology (Moseley 2003). Therefore, pain is a multi-system output that is produced when a cortical pain neuromatrix is activated.

Ideally, an attempt should be made to determine the relevant proportions of these mechanisms; that is, the degree to which peripheral nociceptive (mechanical/inflammatory) elements contribute to the pain experience and the degree to which neurogenic sensitisation is present. Behavioural, social and psychosomatic influences further contribute to the multidimensional nature of chronic and recurrent pain. The dominant mechanisms need to be addressed as a priority. A multidisciplinary and multidimensional approach can be more effective in managing symptoms, both in the short and long term.

4 Evaluation and consideration of contextual factors

The therapist should assess for the influence of contextual factors – both personal and environmental – on the patient's signs and symptoms and explore how these might relate to UCM (Figure 1.8).

> **Four key criteria within clinical reasoning framework**
> 1. Diagnosis of movement dysfunction
>   – site and direction of uncontrolled motion.
> 2. Diagnosis of pain-sensitive tissue(s) (linked to pathology).
> 3. Diagnosis of pain mechanisms
>   – peripheral nociceptive
>   – neurogenic sensitisation.
> 4. Evaluation and consideration of contextual factors.

Figure 1.8 Four key criteria within a clinical reasoning framework

THE DISABLEMENT ASSESSMENT MODEL

Researchers and clinicians have become increasingly aware that there is frequently little correlation between pathology and (functional) limitations in activities and participation. This is even more evident for chronic complaints. Contemporary clinical reasoning has seen a paradigm shift from a biomedical to a bio-psychosocial model. For instance, in the analysis of movement dysfunction model presented in Box 1.3, a modified version of a disablement process model (Verbrugge & Jette 1994) is included. Such a disablement assessment model uses the same theoretical construct as a starting point for assessment and treatment (Figure 1.9).

In a disablement process model, the therapist, together with the patient, determines which

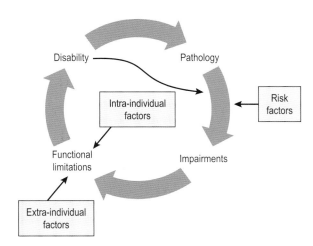

Figure 1.9 Disablement assessment model: modified from Disablement Process Model (Verbrugge & Jette 1994)

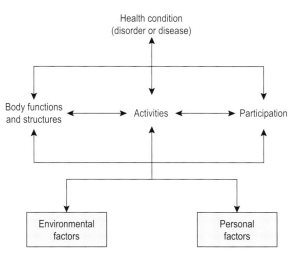

Figure 1.10 Model of functioning and disability, International Classification of Functioning Disability and Health, ICF. World Health Organization, Geneva, 2001

functions and ADL are limited. These are defined as 'disabilities' and can be evaluated by valid and reliable questionnaires and performance tests. This provides the opportunity to reassess the patient in an objective way and evaluate efficacy of interventions. Within the clinical reasoning process the therapist evaluates the four factors in the diagnostic framework criteria (see Figure 1.8), and relates these to the functional limitations. In this partially reversible system, the functional limitations are continuously influenced by extra- and intra-individual factors. These existing and potential risk factors are the reason why pathology presents as or evolves into impairments. Using a clinical decision-making process, the therapist is able to assess and determine if a normal or aberrant course is present.

Different terminology is used in the International Classification of Functioning, Disability, and Health (ICF 2001) model of functioning and disability (Figure 1.10). However, essentially the intra-individual factors in the disablement process model are comparable with the ICF's personal factors and the extra-individual factors are comparable with the environmental factors.

The rehabilitation problem solving (RPS) form (Figure 1.11) was developed to address patients' perspectives and to enhance their participation in the decision-making process during their assessment. The RPS form is based on the ICF model of functioning and disability and

17

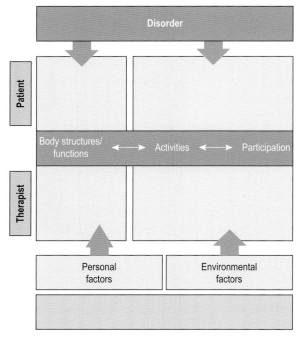

Figure 1.11 The rehabilitation problem solving form, adapted from Steiner et al 2002

facilitates the analysis of patient problems, focusing on specific targets, and relating salient disabilities to relevant and modifiable variables.

This form can include the diagnostic criteria within the clinical reasoning framework described in Figure 1.8 in order to assess the key criteria that relate to the functional limitations. This process identifies links between factors in the diagnostic framework and subsequent functional limitations so that the mechanism behind the dysfunction can be addressed to optimise efficacy of intervention. The form in Figure 1.11 can include the diagnostic framework as described in Figure 1.8.

The essence of both the ICF model of functioning and disability and the RPS form is that an individual's (dys-)functioning or disability represents an interaction between the health condition (e.g. diseases, disorders, injuries, traumas and all factors in the diagnostic framework) and the contextual factors (i.e. 'environmental factors' and 'personal factors'). The interactions of the components in the model are two-way, and interventions in one component can potentially modify one or more other components.

In the ICF model the horizontal dimension of a health status or profile is illustrated as being influenced by elements in the vertical dimension. The ICF model could be considered a method of classification, describing a health condition at a particular moment, such as a picture or 'freeze frame'. In contrast, the disablement process represents constructs within the ICF model under the constant influence of risk factors and hence could be described as more like a 'film'.

To summarise, 'health' can be described in terms of:

- health condition (using ICF terminology)
- course (normal or aberrant)
- prognostic profile
- patient's perspective.

Clinical decision-making should start from the patient's perspective and interventions should be primarily aimed at those aspects of impairment that have a direct bearing on disability and/or functional limitations. In the subjective examination, the patients will define their perspective in terms of disability and functional limitations; for example, the inability (due to low back pain) to bend over from standing to tie shoelaces or the inability (due to shoulder pain) to reach into a cupboard above the shoulders. These self-reported symptoms are explored further within the physical examination to inform the clinical decision-making process. For example, if patients with low back pain are unable to actively control movements of the low back, especially flexion control while performing a waiters' bow (Luomajoki 2008), then clinicians should direct their intervention towards correcting the neuromuscular impairment underpinning this. Similarly, if patients with shoulder pain are unable to actively control the (re-) positioning of the scapula during functional movements (Tate et al 2008; von Eisenhart-Rothe 2005), then clinicians should aim their intervention strategy at regaining this control. Therapists should not solely focus on addressing an isolated pathology, but use frameworks such as the disablement assessment model to facilitate effective intervention. The link between specific movement retraining and improvement in functional tasks is now well supported by evidence (Jull et al 2009; Roussel et al 2009b).

Practitioners need to have the skills to identify and retrain movement faults. These skills should be integrated into current practice and the patient managed in a holistic way with consideration of all aspects of the human motion system, and the influence of both intra- and extra-individual factors. An understanding of how UCM can influence pain is essential in the management of neuromusculoskeletal disorders. To assist in this reasoning process the anatomical and physiological principles are reviewed in Chapter 2 and how pain, dysfunction and pathology can effect UCM is explored in Chapter 3.

REFERENCES

Bellamy, N., Buchanan, W.W., Goldsmith, C.H., Campbell, J., Stitt, L.W., 1988. Validation study of WOMAC: a health status instrument for measuring clinically important patient relevant outcomes to antirheumatic drug therapy in patients with osteoarthritis of the hip or knee. Journal of Rheumatology 15 (12), 1833–1840.

Bennett, M.I., Smith, B.H., Torrance, N., Potter, J., 2005. The S-LANSS score for identifying pain of predominantly neuropathic origin: validation for use in clinical and postal research. Journal of Pain 6 (3), 149–158.

Bobath, B., 1990. Adult hemiplegia: evaluation and treatment. Butterworth-Heinemann, London.

Bolton, J.E., Humphreys, B.K., 2002. The Bournemouth Questionnaire: a short-form comprehensive outcome measure. II. Psychometric properties in neck pain patients. Journal of Manipulative and Physiological Therapeutics 25 (3), 141–148.

Breivik, H., Shipley, M., 2007. Pain. Elsevier, London.

Butler, D., 2000. The sensitive nervous system. NOI Publications, Adelaide, Australia.

Butler, D., Moseley, L., 2003. Explain pain. NOI Publications, Adelaide, Australia.

Carr, J., Shepherd, R., 1998. Neurological rehabilitation – optimizing motor performance. Butterworth Heinemann, Oxford.

Chaitow, L., 2003. Modern neuromuscular techniques – advanced soft tissue techniques. Churchill Livingstone, Edinburgh.

Comerford, M.J., Mottram, S.L., 2001a. Functional stability retraining: principles and strategies for managing mechanical dysfunction. Manual Therapy 6, 3–14.

Comerford, M.J., Mottram, S.L., 2001b. Movement and stability dysfunction. Manual Therapy 6, 15–26.

Comerford, M.J., Mottram, S.L., 2011. Understanding movement and function – assessment and retraining of uncontrolled movement. Course Notes Kinetic Control, UK.

Coppieters, M.W., 2006. Shoulder restraints as a potential cause for stretch neuropathies: biomechanical support for the impact of shoulder girdle depression and arm abduction on nerve strain. Anesthesiology 104 (6), 1351–1352.

Coppieters, M.W., Stappaerts, K.H., Everaert, D.G., Staes, F.F., 2001. Addition of test components during neurodynamic testing: effect on range of motion and sensory responses. Journal of Orthopaedic and Sports Physical Therapy 31 (5), 226–235.

Coppieters, M., Stappaerts, K., Janssens, K., Jull, G., 2002. Reliability of detecting 'onset of pain' and 'submaximal pain' during neural provocation testing of the upper quadrant. Physiotherapy Research International 7 (3), 146–156.

Cyriax, J.H., 1980. Textbook of orthopaedic medicine, vol. 2. Treatment by manipulation, massage and injection. Ballière Tindall, London.

Dankaerts, W., O'Sullivan, P.B., Straker, L.M., Burnett, A.F., Skouen, J.S., 2006a. The inter-examiner reliability of a classification method for non-specific chronic low back pain patients with motor control impairment. Manual Therapy 11 (1), 28–39.

Dankaerts, W., O'Sullivan, P., Burnett, A., Straker, L., 2006b. Altered patterns of superficial trunk muscle activation during sitting in nonspecific chronic low back pain patients: importance of

subclassification. Spine 31 (17), 2017–2023.

Dankaerts, W., O'Sullivan, P., Burnett, A., Straker, L., Davey, P., Gupta, R., 2009. Discriminating healthy controls and two clinical subgroups of nonspecific chronic low back pain patients using trunk muscle activation and lumbosacral kinematics of postures and movements: a statistical classification model. Spine 34 (15), 1610–1618.

Edgar, D., Jull, G., Sutton, S., 1994. The relationship between upper trapezius muscle length and upper quadrant neural tissue extensibility. Australian Journal of Physiotherapy 40, 99–103.

Elvey, R.L., 1995. Peripheral neuropathic disorders and neuromusculoskeletal pain. In: Shacklock M (Ed.), Moving in on pain. Butterworth Heinemann, Sydney.

Emery, K., De Serres, S.J., McMillan, A., Côté, J.N., 2010. The effects of a Pilates training program on arm–trunk posture and movement. Clinical Biomechanics 25 (2), 124–130.

Escalante, A., del Rincon, I., 2002. The disablement process in rheumatoid arthritis. Arthritis and Rheumatism 47 (3), 333–342.

Fairbank, J.C., Couper, J., Davies, J.B., O'Brien, J.P., 1980. The Oswestry low back pain disability questionnaire. Physiotherapy 66 (8), 271–273.

Fairbank, J.C.T., Pynsent, P.B., 2000. The Oswestry disability index. Spine 25 (22), 2940–2953.

Falla, D., Bilenkij, G., Jull, G., 2004. Patients with chronic neck pain demonstrate altered patterns of muscle activation during performance of a functional upper limb task. Spine 29, 1436–1440.

Falla, D., Farina, D., 2008. Neuromuscular adaptation in experimental and clinical neck pain.

Journal of Electromyography and Kinesiology 18 (2), 255–261.

Fersum, K.V., Dankaerts, W., O'Sullivan, P.B., et al., 2010. Integration of subclassification strategies in randomised controlled clinical trials evaluating manual therapy treatment and exercise therapy for non-specific chronic low back pain: a systematic review. British Journal of Sports Medicine 44 (14), 1054–1062.

Freynhagen, R., Baron, R., Gockel, U., Tölle, T.R., 2006. painDETECT: a new screening questionnaire to identify neuropathic components in patients with back pain. Current Medical Research and Opinion 22 (10), 1911–1920.

Goff, B., 1972. The application of recent advances in neurophysiology to Miss R Rood's concept of neuromuscular facilitation. Physiotherapy 58 (2), 409–415.

Gombatto, S.P., Collins, D.R., Sahrmann, S.A., Engsberg, J.R., Van Dillen, L.R., 2007. Patterns of lumbar region movement during trunk lateral bending in 2 subgroups of people with low back pain. Physical Therapy 87 (4), 441–454.

Heald, S.L., Riddle, D.L., Lamb, R.L., 1997. The shoulder pain and disability index: the construct validity and responsiveness of a region-specific disability measure. Physical Therapy 77 (10), 1079–1089.

Hendriks, E.J., Scholten-Peeters, G.G., van der Windt, D.A., Neeleman-van der Steen, C.W., Oostendorp, R.A., Verhagen, A.P., 2005. Prognostic factors for poor recovery in acute whiplash patients. Pain 114 (3), 408–416.

Hides, J.A., Richardson, C.A., Jull, G.A., 1996. Multifidus muscle recovery is not automatic after resolution of acute, first-episode low back pain. Spine 21 (23), 2763–2769.

Hirons, C.A., Mottram, S.L., Tisdale, L., 2007. Controlling the compensation. 12th World Congress of the International Society for Prosthetics and Orthotics Vancouver, Canada, July 29–August 3.

Hodges, P.W., Cholewicki, J., 2007. Functional control of the spine. In: Vleeming, A., Mooney, V., Stoeckart, R. (Eds.), Movement stability and lumbopelvic pain. Churchill

Livingstone, Edinburgh, pp. 489–512.

Hodges, P.W., Richardson, C.A., 1996. Inefficient muscular stabilisation of the lumbar spine associated with low back pain: a motor control evaluation of transversus abdominis. Spine 2 (22), 2640–2650.

Homstøl, G.M., Homstøl, B.O., 2009. Changes in mechanosensitivity due to lumbopelvic and ankle positioning. 3rd International Conference on Movement Dysfunction, Edinburgh, UK. Manual Therapy 14 (1), S38.

Hudak, P.L., Amadio, P.C., Bombardier, C., 1996. Development of an upper extremity outcome measure: the DASH (disabilities of the arm, shoulder and hand) [corrected]. The Upper Extremity Collaborative Group (UECG). American Journal of Industrial Medicine 29 (6), 602–608. Erratum in: American Journal of Industrial Medicine 1996; 30 (3), 372.

Hungerford, B., Gilleard, W., Hodges, P., 2003. Evidence of altered lumbopelvic muscle recruitment in the presence of sacroiliac joint pain. Spine 28 (14), 1593–1600.

International Classification of Functioning, Disability, and Health (ICF), 2001. ICF full version. World Health Organization, Geneva.

Janda, V., 1986. Muscle weakness and inhibition (pseudoparesis) in low back pain. In: Grieve, G.P. (Ed.), Modern manual therapy of the vertebral column. Churchill Livingstone, Edinburgh.

Jull, G., Sterling, M., Falla, D., et al., 2008. Whiplash, headache and neck pain. Elsevier, Edinburgh.

Jull, G., Trott, P., Potter, H., Zito, G., Niere, K., Shirley, D., et al., 2002. Randomized controlled trial of exercise and manipulative therapy for cervicogenic headache. Spine 27 (17), 1835–1843.

Jull, G.A., Falla, D., Vicenzino, B., Hodges, P.W., 2009. The effect of therapeutic exercise on activation of the deep cervical flexor muscles in people with chronic neck pain. Manual Therapy 14 (6), 696–701.

Kaltenborn, F., Evjenth, O., Kaltenborn, T., Morgan, D., Vollowitz, E., 2003. Manual mobilization of the joints:

the spine, 4th edn. OPTP, Minneapolis.

Kendall, F.P., McCreary, E., Provance, P., Rodgers, M., Romanic, W., 2005. Muscle testing and function with posture and pain. Lippincott Williams Wilkins, Baltimore.

Kraaimaat, F.W., Evers, A.W., 2003. Pain-coping strategies in chronic pain patients: psychometric characteristics of the pain-coping inventory (PCI). International Journal of Behavioral Medicine 10 (4), 343–363.

Lee, D., 2004. The pelvic girdle. Elsevier; Edinburgh.

Lin, J.J., Hanten, W.P., Olson, S.L., Roddey, T.S., Soto-quijano, D.A., Lim, H.K., Sherwood, A.M., 2005. Functional activity characteristics of individuals with shoulder dysfunctions. Journal of Electromyography and Kinesiology 15 (6), 576–586.

Lin, J.J., Hanten, W.P., Olson, S.L., Roddey, T.S., Soto-quijano, D.A., Lim, H.K., Sherwood, A.M., 2006. Shoulder dysfunction assessment: self-report and impaired scapular movements. Physical Therapy 86 (8), 1065–1074.

Long, A., Donelson, R., Fung, T., 2004. Does it matter which exercise? A randomized control trial of exercise for low back pain. Spine 29 (23), 2593–2602.

Ludewig, P., Cook, T.M., 2000. Alterations in shoulder kinematics and associated muscle activity in people with symptoms of shoulder impingement. Physical Therapy 80 (3), 276–291.

Luomajoki, H., Kool, J., de Bruin, E.D., Airaksinen, O., 2007. Reliability of movement control tests in the lumbar spine. BMC Musculoskeletal Disorders 8, 90.

Luomajoki, H., Kool, J., D de Bruin, E., Airaksinen, O., 2008. Movement control tests of the low back; evaluation of the difference between patients with low back pain and healthy controls. BMC Musculoskeletal Disorders 9, 170.

McGill, S., 2002. Low back disorders. Evidence-based prevention and rehabilitation. Human Kinetics Europe, Champaign.

Maitland, G., Hengeveld, E., Banks, K., English, K., 2005. Maitland's vertebral manipulation. Butterworth Heinemann, Oxford.

Martin, R.L., Philippon, M.J., 2007. Evidence of validity for the hip outcome score in hip arthroscopy. Arthroscopy 23 (8), 822–826. Erratum in: Arthroscopy 2007;23 (11), 1252.

Melzack, R., 1975. The McGill pain questionnaire: major properties and scoring methods. Pain 1, 277–299.

Melzack, R., 1999. From the gate to the neuromatrix. Pain Suppl 6, S121–S126.

Melzack, R., Katz, J., 1992. The McGill pain questionnaire: appraisal and current status. In: Turk D., Melzack R. (Eds.), Handbook of pain assessment. Guildford Press, New York, pp. 35–52.

Morrissey, D., 2005. Development of the kinetic medial rotation test of the shoulder: a dynamic clinical test of shoulder instability and impingement. PhD thesis, University of London.

Morrissey, D., Morrissey, M.C., Driver, W., King, J.B., Woledge, R.C., 2008. Manual landmark identification and tracking during the medial rotation test of the shoulder: an accuracy study using three dimensional ultrasound and motion analysis measures. Manual Therapy 13 (6), 529–535.

Moseley, G.L., 2003. A pain neuromatrix approach to patients with chronic pain. Manual Therapy 8 (3), 130–140.

Mottram, S.L., Comerford, M., 2008. A new perspective on risk assessment. Physical Therapy in Sport 9 (1), 40–51.

Mottram, S., Warner, M., Chappell, P., Morrissey, D., Stokes, M., 2009. Impaired control of scapular rotation during a clinical dissociation test in people with a history of shoulder pain. 3rd International Conference on Movement Dysfunction Edinburgh, UK. Manual Therapy 14 (1), S20.

Nicholas, M.K., 2007. The pain self-efficacy questionnaire: taking pain into account. European Journal of Pain 11, 153–163.

Nicholas, M.K., Asghari, A., Blyth, F.M., 2008. What do the numbers mean? Normative data in chronic pain measures. Pain 134, 158–173.

O'Sullivan, P.B., 2000. Lumbar segmental 'instability': clinical presentation and specific stabilizing exercise management. Manual Therapy 5 (1), 2–12.

O'Sullivan, P., 2005. Diagnosis and classification of chronic low back pain disorders: maladaptive movement and motor control impairments as underlying mechanism. Manual Therapy 10 (4), 242–255.

O'Sullivan, P.B., Beales, D.J., Beetham, J.A., Cripps, J., 2002. Altered motor control strategies in subjects with sacroiliac joint pain during the active straight leg raise test. Spine 27 (1), E1–E8.

O'Sullivan, P.B., Twomey, L., Allison, G., 1997a. Evaluation of specific stabilising exercises in the treatment of chronic low back pain with radiological diagnosis of spondylosis or spondylolisthesis. Spine 22 (24), 2959–2967.

O'Sullivan, P.B., Twomey, L., Allison, G., Sinclair, J., Miller, K., Knox, J., 1997b. Altered patterns of abdominal muscle activation in patients with chronic low back pain. Australian Journal of Physiotherapy 43 (2), 91–98.

O'Sullivan, P., Twomey, L., Allison, G., 1998. Altered abdominal muscle recruitment in back pain patients following specific exercise intervention. Journal of Orthopaedic and Sports Physical Therapy 27 (2), 114–124.

Richardson, C., Hodges, P., Hides, J., 2004. Therapeutic exercise for lumbopelvic stabilization – a motor control approach for the treatment and prevention of low back pain. Churchill Livingstone, Edinburgh.

Roach, K.E., Budiman-Mak, E., Songsiridej, N., Lertratanakul, Y., 1991. Development of a shoulder pain and disability index. Arthritis Care and Research 4 (4), 143–149.

Roland, M.O., Morris, R.W., 1983. A study of the natural history of back pain. Part 1: Development of a reliable and sensitive measure of disability in low back pain. Spine 8, 141–144.

Roussel, N.A., Daenen, L., Vissers, D., Lambeets, D., Schutt, A., Van Moorsel, A., et al., 2009b. Motor control and physical fitness training to prevent msculoskeletal injuries in professional dancers. 3rd International Conference on Movement Dysfunction, Edinburgh, UK. 30 October–1 November. Manual Therapy 14 (1), S22.

Roussel, N.A., Nijs, J., Mottram, S., van Moorsel, A., Truijen, S., Stassijns, G., 2009a. Altered lumbopelvic movement control but not generalised joint hypermobility is associated with increased injury in dancers. A prospective study. Manual Therapy 14 (6), 630–635.

Roussel, N., Nijs, J., Truijen, S., Vervecken, L., Mottram, S., Stassijns, G., 2009c. Altered breathing patterns during lumbopelvic motor control tests in chronic low back pain: a case-control study. European Spine Journal 18 (7), 1066–1073.

Rydeard, R., Leger, A., Smith, D., 2006. Pilates-based therapeutic exercise: effect on subjects with nonspecific chronic low back pain and functional disability: a randomized controlled trial. Journal of Orthopaedic and Sports Physical Therapy 36 (7), 472–484.

Sahrmann, S.A., 2002. Diagnosis and treatment of movement impairment syndromes. Mosby, St Louis.

Schneider, G., Pearcy, M.J., Bogduk, N., 2005. Abnormal motion in spondylolytic spondylolisthesis. Spine 30 (10), 1159–1164.

Scholten-Peeters, G.G., Verhagen, A.P., Bekkering, G.E., van der Windt, D.A., Barnsley, L., Oostendorp, R.A., et al., 2003. Prognostic factors of whiplash-associated disorders: a systematic review of prospective cohort studies. Pain 104 (1–2), 303–322.

Scholtes, S.A., Gombatto, S.P., Van Dillen, L.R., 2009. Differences in lumbopelvic motion between people with and people without low back pain during two lower limb movement tests. Clinical Biomechanics 24 (1), 7–12.

Shacklock, M., 2005. Clinical neurodynamics: a new system of neuromusculoskeletal treatment. Elsevier Butterworth Heinmann, Edinburgh.

Smith, M.D., Russell, A., Hodges, P.W., 2009. Do incontinence, breathing difficulties, and gastrointestinal symptoms increase the risk of future back pain? Journal of Pain 10 (8), 876–886.

Steiner, W.A., Ryser, L., Huber, E., Uebelhart, D., Aeschlimann, A., Stucki, G., 2002. Use of the ICF model as a clinical problem-solving tool in physical therapy and rehabilitation medicine. Physical Therapy 82 (11), 1098–1107.

Stuge, B., Veierod, M.B., Laerum, E., Vollestad, N., 2004. The efficacy of a treatment program focusing on specific stabilizing exercises for pelvic girdle pain after pregnancy: a two-year follow-up of a randomized clinical trial. Spine 29 (10), E197–E203.

Swinkels-Meewisse, E.J., Swinkels, R.A., Verbeek, A.L., Vlaeyen, J.W., Ostendorp, R.A., 2003. Psychometric properties of the Tampa scale for kinesiophobia and the fear-avoidance beliefs questionnaire in acute low back pain. Manual Therapy 8 (1), 29–36.

Tate, A.R., McClure, P.W., Kareha, S., Irwin, D., 2008. Effect of the scapula reposition test on shoulder impingement symptoms and elevation strength in overhead athletes. Journal of Orthopaedic and Sports Physical Therapy 38 (1), 4–11.

van Dillen, L.R., Maluf, K.S., Sahrmann, S.A., 2009. Further examination of modifying patient-preferred movement and alignment strategies in patients with low back pain during symptomatic tests. Manual Therapy 14 (1), 52–60.

Verbrugge, L.M., Jette, A.M., 1994. The disablement process. Social Science and Medicine 38 (1), 1–14.

Vernon, H., Mior, S., 1991. The neck disability index: a study of reliability and validity. Journal of Manipulative and Physiological Therapeutics 14 (7), 409–415.

Vibe Fersum, K., O'Sullivan, P.B., Kvåle, A., Skouen, J.S., 2009. Inter-examiner reliability of a classification system for patients with non-specific low back pain. Manual Therapy 4 (5), 555–561.

Vlaeyen, J.W., Kole-Snijders, A.M., Boeren, R.G., van Eek, H., 1995. Fear of movement/(re)injury in chronic low back pain and its relation to behavioral performance. Pain 62 (3), 363–372.

Vleeming, A., Mooney, V., Stoeckart, R., 2007. Movement, stability and lumbopelvic pain. Integration of research and therapy. Churchill Livingstone, Edinburgh.

von Eisenhart-Rothe, R., Matsen 3rd., F.A., Eckstein, F., Vogl, T., Graichen, H., 2005. Pathomechanics in a-traumatic shoulder instability: scapular positioning correlates with humeral head centering. Clinical Orthopaedics and Related Research 433, 82–89.

Von Korff, M., Deyo, R.A., Cherkin, D., Barlow, S.F., 1993. Back pain in primary care. Outcomes at 1 year. Spine 18 (7), 855–862.

Waddell, G., 1998. The back pain revolution. Churchill Livingstone, Edinburgh.

Woby, S.R., Roach, N.K., Urmston, M., Watson, P.J., 2008. Outcome following a physiotherapist-led intervention for chronic low back pain: the important role of cognitive processes. Physiotherapy 94 (2), 115–124.

World Health Organization, 2001. ICF: International Classification of Functioning, Disability and Health. WHO, Geneva.

Zazulak, B.T., Hewett, T.E., Reeves, N.P., Goldberg, B., Cholewicki, J., 2007. Deficits in neuromuscular control of the trunk predict knee injury risk: a prospective biomechanical-epidemiologic study. American Journal of Sports Medicine 35 (7), 1123–1130.

Chapter | 2 |

Muscle function and physiology

There has been much interest in and reference to stability of the spine over the last few decades. One of the first texts to explore therapeutic exercise for spinal segmental stabilisation in low back pain was published in 1998 (Richardson et al 1998). These authors referred to Panjabi's model of spinal stabilisation which incorporates a passive subsystem (the osseous and articular structures), the active subsystem (the force generating capacity of muscles which provide mechanical stability) and the neural subsystem (providing control to the muscles) (Panjabi 1992).

The concept of stability, movement control and the process of how it is achieved, has different interpretations depending on the background of the authors (Hodges & Cholewicki 2007; McGill 2007). To date there is still debate as to whether spinal stability exists but there is no debate that the spine must be stable to function (Reeves & Cholewicki 2010). This text considers the control of movement and assessment and retraining of uncontrolled movement (UCM) (as described in Chapters 1, 3 and 4) rather than simply a model of stability.

Aspects of both muscle function and physiology are important when assessing and retraining UCM and will be explored in this chapter.

ANALYSIS OF MUSCLE FUNCTION

All muscles have four broad functions:

1. to concentrically shorten to produce joint range of motion and accelerate body motion segments, which will be termed 'mobility function'
2. to isometrically hold position, which will be termed 'postural control function'
3. to eccentrically lengthen under tension to decelerate motion and control excessive range of motion, which will be termed 'stability function'
4. to provide afferent proprioceptive feedback to the central nervous system (CNS) for coordination and regulation of muscle stiffness and tension.

Stabiliser and mobiliser function

Rood, in Goff (1972), Janda (1996) and Sahrmann (2002) have described and developed functional muscle testing based on stabiliser and mobiliser muscle roles. Table 2.1 describes stabiliser and mobiliser muscle role characteristics.

Some muscles are more efficient at one of these roles and less efficient in the other role. For example: latissimus dorsi is a powerful multi-joint medial rotator of the shoulder to accelerate the arm in the sagittal plane during throwing

Table 2.1 Characteristics of muscles with stabiliser and mobiliser roles

STABILITY MUSCLE ROLE CHARACTERISTICS	MOBILITY MUSCLE ROLE CHARACTERISTICS
• One-joint (monoarticular) • Deep (short lever and short moment arm) • Broad aponeurotic insertions (to distribute and absorb force and load) • Leverage for load maintenance, static holding and joint compression • Postural holding role associated with eccentrically decelerating or resisting momentum (especially in the axial plane – rotation)	• Two-joint (biarticular or multisegmental) • Superficial (longer lever, larger moment arm and greatest bulk) • Unidirectional fibres or tendinous insertions (to direct force to produce movement) • Leverage for range and speed and joint distraction • Repetitive or rapid movement role and high strain/force loading
EXAMPLES OF STABILISER MUSCLES	**EXAMPLES OF MOBILISER MUSCLES**
• External oblique /internal oblique • Semispinalis • Deep gluteus maximus • Subscapularis	• Rectus femoris • Pectoralis major • Levator scapula • Rectus abdominis

actions. Latissimus dorsi is biomechanically suited to large range, high speed, high force movement at the shoulder. This muscle obviously has a power role acting as a *mobiliser* or sagittal plane movement accelerator. Conversely, subscapularis co-activates synergistically but its co-activation force acts to stabilise the humeral head from excessive translation, while the arm is medially rotating in a throwing action. Subscapularis, with its short lever, small moment arm and capsular attachments, is best suited to non-fatiguing, functional movements in postural control tasks. It is also ideally placed to resist or decelerate excessive lateral rotation of the shoulder. This muscle has a greater *stabilisation* role and is less suited biomechanically to a power movement role. A muscle's role must also be customised to its function.

Generating high force may be detrimental in some instances. For example: rectus abdominis is a flexor of the lumbar spine. If it is over-trained and inappropriately strengthened it contributes to pain-related changes in the movement system. It is often over-trained in a misguided belief that it is important to strengthen the abdominals to stabilise and protect the low back or to acquire an abdominal 'six pack'. However, if this muscle becomes excessively dominant in comparison to the lateral abdominal muscles it increases flexion and compression forces on the lumbar spine and rotation stress and strain is inadequately controlled. This imbalance between rectus abdominis and the lateral abdominal stabilisers has been

identified as a common movement-related change in people with low back pain (O'Sullivan et al 1997).

Implications of stabiliser–mobiliser characteristics

1. Muscles with predominantly stability role characteristics (one-joint) *optimally* assist postural holding/anti-gravity/stability and control function. Muscles that have a stability function (one-joint stabiliser) demonstrate a tendency to inhibition, excessive flexibility, laxity and weakness in the presence of dysfunction (Kendall et al 2005). Janda (1983) described these muscles as 'phasic' muscles.

2. Muscles with predominantly mobility role characteristics (multi-joint) *optimally* assist rapid/accelerated movement and produce high force or power. Muscles that have a mobility function (two-joint or multi-joint mobiliser) demonstrate a tendency to overactivity, loss of extensibility and excessive stiffness in the presence of dysfunction (Kendall et al 2005). Janda (1983) described these muscles as 'postural' muscles.

Local and global function

Bergmark (1989) developed a model to describe the muscle control of load transfer across the

Table 2.2 Local and global muscle system characteristics and general features

LOCAL MUSCLE SYSTEM CHARACTERISTICS	GLOBAL MUSCLE SYSTEM CHARACTERISTICS
• Deepest layer of muscles that originate and insert segmentally on lumbar vertebrae • Controls the spinal curvature • Maintains the mechanical stiffness of the spine controlling intersegmental motion • Responds to changes in posture and to changes in low extrinsic load	• Superficial or outer layer of muscles lacking segmental insertions • Large torque producing muscles for range of movement • Global muscles and intra-abdominal pressure transfer load between the thoracic cage and the pelvis • Responds to changes in the line of action and the magnitude of high extrinsic load
GENERAL FEATURES	**GENERAL FEATURES**
• Deepest, one-joint • Minimal force, stiffness • No/min. length change • Does not produce or limit range of motion • Controls translation • Maintains control in all ranges, all directions, all functional activities • Tonic recruitment with low load and high load activities • No antagonists	• Deep one-joint or superficial multi-joint • Force efficient • Concentric shortening to produce range • Eccentric lengthening or isometric holding to control range • No translation control • Direction-specific/antagonist influenced
EXAMPLES OF LOCAL MUSCLES	**EXAMPLES OF GLOBAL MUSCLES**
• Transversus abdominis • Single segment fibres of lumbar multifidus • Longitudinal fibres of longus colli • Vastus medialis obliquus	• Rectus abdominis • Hamstrings • Sternocleidomastoid • Splenius capitis

lumbar spine. He introduced the concept of local and global systems of muscle control. The local and global muscle system characteristics and general features are described in Table 2.2 with examples.

Implications of local and global characteristics

3. *Local muscle 'system'*: the small deep segmental muscles in the local muscle system are responsible for increasing the segmental stiffness across a joint and decreasing excessive intersegmental motion. The relevance of this is that these muscles are ideally situated to control displacement of the path of the instantaneous centre of motion and reduce excessive intersegmental translatatory motion during functional movements. At end range of motion the passive restraints of motion (e.g. ligaments and joint capsules) contribute significantly to controlling translatatory or accessory motion. Local muscles maintain this translatatory control during all functional activities such as postural control tasks, non-fatiguing functional movements, fatiguing high load and high speed activities. Local muscles maintain activity in the background of all functional movements. Their recruitment is independent of the direction of loading or movement and is biased for non-fatiguing low load function, although they maintain the role of controlling intersegmental displacement during fatiguing high load function as well. The local muscles do not significantly change length during normal activation and therefore do not primarily contribute to range of motion. The one-joint (monoarticular) global muscles have a primary stability role, while the multi-joint (biarticular) global muscles have a primary mobility role.

4. *Global muscle 'system'*: the muscles that make up the global muscle system are responsible for the production and control of the range and the direction of movement. The global muscles can change length significantly and therefore are the muscles of range of motion. The global muscles participate in both non-fatiguing low load and fatiguing high load activities.

Both the local and global muscle systems must work together for efficient normal function. Neither system in isolation can control the functional stability of body motion segments.

Functional efficiency

The functional efficiency of a muscle is related to its ability to generate tension. A muscle's tension is not constant throughout a contraction, especially if the muscle is changing length to produce movement. Length and tension properties of a muscle are closely related. The tension or force a muscle produces is the resultant force arising from a combination of both active and passive components of the muscle. The active component of muscle tension is determined by the number of actin–myosin cross-bridges that are linked at any point in time. The passive tension property of muscle is largely due to the elastic

titin filaments which anchor the myosin chain to the Z band. Other connective tissue structures within muscle only contribute partially to passive tension. Figure 2.1 illustrates the actin–myosin filament cross-bridges and titin attachments.

The position in range (usually mid-range) where the active length–tension curve is maximal is known as the muscle's resting length. In this position, the maximum number of actin–myosin cross-bridge links can be established. In a muscle's shortened or inner range position, the passive elastic components do not contribute to muscle tension. Passive tension only begins to play a role after a muscle starts to lengthen or stretch into the muscle's outer range, beyond its resting length or mid-range position. Muscles are most efficient and generate optimal force when they function in a mid-range position near resting length. Muscles are less efficient and appear functionally weak when they are required to contract in a shortened or lengthened range relative to their resting length because of physiological or mechanical insufficiency (Figure 2.2).

Physiological insufficiency occurs when a muscle actively shortens into its inner range where the actin filaments overlap each other, thus reducing the number of cross-bridges that can link to the myosin filament. As the muscle progressively shortens, there are fewer cross-bridges

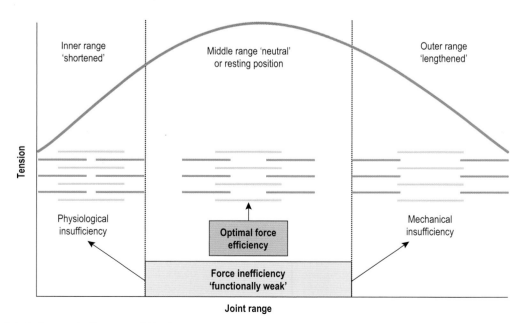

Figure 2.1 Actin–myosin filaments within the sarcomeres

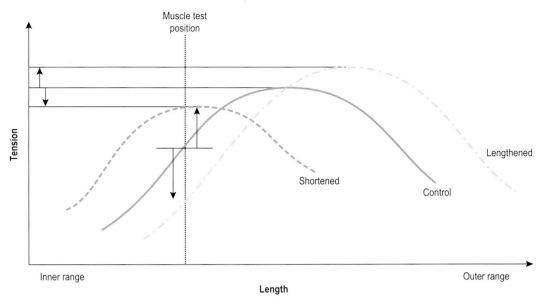

Figure 2.2 Active (contractile) component of a muscle length–tension curve changes when muscles change length: changes in muscle length affect force efficiency in different positions of joint range. Adapted from Goldspink & Williams 1992

able to be linked, and the muscle is unable to generate optimal force. Mechanical insufficiency occurs when a muscle actively contracts in its lengthened or outer range. In this range, the actin filaments do not adequately overlap the myosin filament and again a reduced number of cross-bridges are linked. Consequently the muscle cannot generate optimal force. Mechanical insufficiency during an outer range contraction is offset somewhat by the increase in passive tension from titin filaments.

However, when a muscle habitually functions at an altered length (either lengthened or shortened), its length–tension relationships adapt accordingly. The position in range where it generates optimal force efficiency changes to match the subsequent lengthening or shortening (Goldspink & Williams 1992), as illustrated in Figure 2.2.

When a muscle is persistently elongated or lengthened, it adds sarcomeres in series (the broken line in Figure 2.2). Because the sarcomeres are the force generating units within a muscle, a lengthened or elongated muscle is stronger and is able to generate a higher peak force than normal. This higher peak force, however, is produced in an outer range position and not at its usual resting length, mid-range position. At the

muscle test position (inner to middle range), the lengthened muscle is inefficient due to physiological insufficiency, and consequently tests 'weak' during muscle testing and fatigues more readily in postural control tasks. A persistently shortened muscle, on the other hand, loses sarcomeres in series and increases in connective tissue (the dotted line in Figure 2.2). Because of the reduced number of sarcomeres, the shortened muscle generates less peak force than normal. Interestingly, a shortened muscle's resting length may coincide with the muscle test position. Even though the shortened muscle is weaker than its normal control, muscle testing is performed at the point in range where it is optimally efficient. Consequently, shortened muscles frequently demonstrate good strength during muscle testing (Gossman et al 1982). This explains the clinical observation that 'short muscles test strong and long muscles test weak'.

A muscle's structure also affects its ability to generate force. Muscles that have long lever arms, such as the multi-joint rectus femoris or hamstrings, can contract through a greater range and are biomechanically advantaged to produce range of movement during concentric shortening. These muscles primarily have a mobility role. These multi-joint mobilisers are not particularly efficient at preventing or controlling excessive movement during eccentric lengthening. The smaller one-joint muscles with short lever arms, such as subscapularis or iliacus, are not biomechanically efficient to produce forceful or high speed movement during concentric shortening. However, they are more efficient during eccentric lengthening to control excessive movement and to decelerate momentum and therefore are more able to protect tissues from overstrain. These muscles primarily have a stability role.

When a muscle has such a short lever arm that it produces minimal length change when contracted, it has a greater potential to control intersegmental translation, for example the single segment fibres of lumbar multifidus.

Functional classification of muscle roles

The concepts of local and global muscle systems and stabiliser and mobiliser muscles provide useful frameworks to classify muscle function. However, alone, they have some clinical deficiencies. By interlinking these two concepts a clinically useful model of classification of muscle functional roles has been developed (Comerford & Mottram 2001).

Table 2.3 summarises this classification in terms of function and characteristics and dysfunction.

Postural adjustments are anticipatory and ongoing and all muscles can have an anticipatory timing to address displacement and perturbations to equilibrium. All muscles provide reflex feedback reactions under both low and high threshold recruitment tasks and demonstrate anticipatory feedforward recruitment when appropriate. However, only muscles with a local stability role exhibit anticipatory timing that is independent of the direction of loading or displacement. Muscles recruited in a global range related role are direction-specific in their anticipatory feedforward responses (Hodges & Richardson 1997; Hodges 2001; Hodges & Moseley 2003). Figure 2.3 illustrates an example of the anatomical inter-relationships between the different muscle roles in the lumbar spine.

Muscle characterisation

Although all muscles can perform all basic abilities, some muscles are ideally suited to some roles

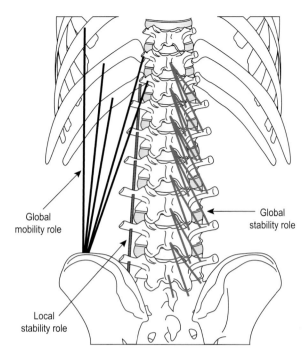

Figure 2.3 Anatomical inter-relationships between the different muscle roles in the lumbar spine

to achieve optimal function better than others. An analysis of a muscle's ideal role should consider the co-relation of the features listed in Table 2.4.

This model of reviewing and analysing muscle function and recruitment provides an opportunity to develop a greater understanding of a muscle's role in functional activities. By analysing the inter-relationships between a muscle's anatomy and histology, its biomechanical potential, its recruitment physiology and consistent changes in the muscle related to pain and pathology (see Table 2.4), we can be more critical of some of the oversimplified roles that have previously been ascribed to some muscles.

If an analysis of all four of these features supports a consistent conclusion, we can be reasonably confident that a particular muscle's primary function or role is understood. Such support is available only for a limited number of the muscles that therapists work with on a regular basis, such as transversus abdominis, external obliquus abdominis, rectus abdominis and hamstrings.

If analysis of these four features provides conflicting conclusions then there may be confusion, misunderstanding or misinterpretation of this

Table 2.3 Classification of muscle functional roles in terms of function, characteristics and dysfunction

LOCAL STABILITY MUSCLE ROLE/STRATEGY	GLOBAL STABILITY MUSCLE ROLE/STRATEGY	GLOBAL MOBILITY MUSCLE ROLE/STRATEGY
Function and characteristics • Increase muscle stiffness to control segmental motion/translation • Controls the *neutral* joint position • Contraction = no/min. length change ∴ does not produce range of movement • Activity is often anticipatory (or at the same instant) to expected displacement or movement to provide protective muscle stiffness prior to motion stress • Recruitment is not anticipatory if the muscle is already active or loaded • ± Muscle activity is independent of direction of movement • ± Continuous activity throughout movement • Proprioceptive input re: joint position, range and rate of movement	**Function and characteristics** • Generates force to *control range* of motion • Contraction = eccentric length change ∴ control throughout range • Functional ability to: i) shorten through the full inner range of joint motion; ii) isometrically hold position; iii) eccentrically control the return against gravity and control hypermobile outer range of joint motion if present • Deceleration of low load/force momentum (especially axial plane: rotation) • Non-continuous activity • Muscle activity is direction dependent ∴ powerfully influenced by muscles with antagonistic actions • High threshold activation under situations of load and speed	**Function and characteristics** • Generates torque to *produce range* of joint movement • Contraction = *concentric* length change ∴ concentric production of movement (rather than eccentric control) • Concentric acceleration of movement (especially sagittal plane: flexion/extension) • Shock absorption of high load • Muscle activity is very direction dependent • Intermittent muscle activity (very on:off phasic patterns of activity – often brief bursts of activity to accelerate the motion segment then momentum maintains movement)
Dysfunction • Motor control deficit associated with delayed timing or recruitment deficiency • Reacts to pain and pathology with inhibition • Decrease muscle stiffness and poor segmental control • Loss of control of joint neutral position	**Dysfunction** • Muscle lacks the ability to: i) shorten through the full inner range of joint motion; ii) isometrically hold position; iii) eccentrically control the return • Inefficient low threshold tonic recruitment • Poor rotation dissociation • If hypermobile – poor control of excessive range • Inhibition by dominant antagonists • Altered recruitment patterns and uncontrolled movement with high threshold recruitment • Strength deficits on high threshold recruitment	**Dysfunction** • Loss of myofascial extensibility – limits physiological and/or accessory motion (which must be compensated for elsewhere) • Overactive low threshold, low load recruitment • Reacts to pain and pathology with spasm • Demonstrate uncontrolled sagittal movement under high threshold recruitment testing

Table 2.4 Features of muscle function used for reviewing muscle roles

FUNCTION	DYSFUNCTION
1. Anatomical location and structure 2. Biomechanical potential 3. Neurophysiology	4. Consistent and characteristic changes in the presence of pain or pathology

muscle's function. Several possibilities exist to explain this apparent conflict:

1. Some discrepancies between biomechanics and neurophysiology need to be explained with some muscles. For example, training latissimus dorsi co-activation with the contralateral gluteal muscles (often referred to as the posterior sacroiliac sling) to stabilise the sacroiliac joint has been

proposed by various authors (Vleeming et al 2007). This training would be appropriate to help manage sacroiliac joint pain associated with high load or high speed activities such as running or throwing because these two muscles are automatically recruited in these activities. However, for patients who have sacroiliac joint pain associated with non-fatiguing functional movements (e.g. normal gait) and postural control activities (e.g. static standing), this training is unlikely to be beneficial. There is often an assumption that the muscles used in strength training will be used in all functional activities. However, this is not the case as there is minimal automatic activation of latissimus dorsi in these low load activities.

Another example of measurement discrepancy occurs following the assumption that psoas major is a hip flexor. Biomechanical modelling of psoas major often assumes that it is a fusiform muscle with a straight line of action from the upper lumbar spine to the femur. This is not the case. Psoas major is a pennate muscle with obliquely orientated fibres. A more detailed mechanical evaluation of its pennate orientation (Gibbons 2007) suggests that its maximum shortening potential is approximately 2.25 cm. This is insufficient to produce the flexion range of motion of the hip. The posterior fascia of psoas major is anchored to the anterior rim of the pelvis (Gibbons 2007). This attachment would produce posterior tilt of the pelvis. Posterior tilt of the pelvis is a conjoined movement with hip flexion, and interestingly the range of movement of the pelvis at the psoas attachment point during posterior tilt perfectly matches the predicted range of shortening of psoas major.

2. There may be misinterpretation of research measurement technology; for example, upper trapezius, lower trapezius, psoas major, vastus medialis obliquus. Upper trapezius has been assumed to elevate the shoulder because it demonstrates high levels of EMG activity during scapular elevation tasks. Johnson et al (1994) demonstrate that 90% of the contractile fibres of upper trapezius insert on the ligamentum nuchae below C6 and are horizontally orientated (the vertical fibres are predominantly fascial and connective tissue).

They state that the upper trapezius muscle cannot elevate the scapula above C6. It is suggested that the reason for the high levels of EMG activation may be to assist the clavicular rotation (necessary for full shoulder elevation), or an attempt to stabilise the cervical spine during arm load activities.

Similarly, vastus medialis obliquus demonstrates high levels of EMG activity in terminal extension of the knee. Lieb & Perry (1968) demonstrated that vastus medialis obliquus has no biomechanical potential to extend the knee in this last 30°. The high level of vastus medialis obliquus recruitment is best explained by its role of maintaining alignment tracking of the patella during the last 30° of full extension.

3. The muscle is designed to participate in more than one primary functional role; for example, Hodges (2003) suggests that a muscle may have three functional roles:
   (i) control of inter-segmental motion
   (ii) control of posture and alignment
   (iii) to produce and control movement.
   Some muscles can effectively perform all three of these functional roles. Gluteus maximus is an example of a muscle that multitasks all three functional roles (Gibbons 2007). Gluteus maximus has deep sacral fibres that run from the inferior lateral corner of the sacrum to the posterior inferior ischial spine. It is believed that these fibres perform a local stability role and have the function of controlling intersegmental translation at the sacroiliac joint. Gluteus maximus also has fibres that run from the medial aspect of the ileum to the gluteal trochanter on the femoral neck. These deep fibres constitute the one-joint part of a muscle that performs a global stability role at the hip joint. The most superficial fibres of gluteus maximus run from the iliac crest and attach into the posterior aspect of the iliotibial band and eventually insert on the anterior aspect of the lateral tibial condyle, below the knee. This multi-joint part of gluteus maximus has a global mobiliser role and produces movement at the hip joint and the knee joint.

For many of the muscles that therapists work with on a regular basis there is currently insufficient information on all four of these features (see Table 2.4) to enable thorough understanding of the primary function or role of these muscles (e.g. serratus anterior, adductor magnus, subscapularis).

MUSCLE FUNCTION: PRIMARY ROLE

Identifying a muscle's primary role is not always simple. Some muscles appear to have a single, very specific primary role (single task/specific muscle) while other muscles appear to be more versatile and contribute to more than one primary role (multitasking muscle).

Single task-specific muscles

Single task muscles have a specific task orientated role associated with having only a local stabiliser role (e.g. transversus abdominis, vastus medialis obliquus), a global stabiliser role (e.g. external obliquus abdominis) or a global mobiliser role (e.g. rectus abdominis, hamstrings, iliocostalis lumborum).

- In the presence of pathology and/or pain, very specific dysfunctions can develop and are associated with the recognised specific primary role. These dysfunctions are consistent and predictable.
- Very specific retraining or correction has been advocated in treatment of this dysfunction (Hodges & Richardson 1996, 1997; Hodges & Richardson 1999; Jull 2000; O'Sullivan 2000; Hides et al 1996, 2001). This specific training or corrective intervention is typically non-functional and as such is designed to correct very specific elements of dysfunction. This specific retraining or correction may or may not integrate into normal functional activity. There is currently no method to predict or clinically measure automatic integration into normal function. In many patients this integration has to be facilitated.

Multitasking muscles

Some muscles appear less specific and seem to participate in a variety of roles without demonstrating dysfunction. They appear to have a multitasking function associated with the potential to perform more than one role. That is, there is good

evidence to support the muscle having both a local role and a global role, or the evidence may support the muscle having a contribution to both stability and mobility roles (e.g. gluteus maximus, infraspinatus and pelvic floor). Such muscles appear to be able to contribute to combinations of local stabiliser, global stabiliser and global mobiliser roles when required in normal function.

- In the presence of pathology and/or pain, a variety of different dysfunctions may develop. These dysfunctions can be identified as being associated with either or all of the multitasking roles and are related to the 'weak links' in an individual's integrated stability system. Because these contribute to more than one functional role, different dysfunctions can present with pain. Therefore, dysfunction in these muscles is not predictable and a more detailed assessment is required with a clinical reasoning process.
- Treatment and retraining has to address the particular dysfunction that presents, usually needs to be multifactorial and should emphasise integration into 'normal' function.

As well as a consideration of the macro function(s) and role(s) of the muscle, the therapist should consider the physiological or micro basis of the muscle with respect to its potential for recruitment in single or multifunction roles.

MOTOR RECRUITMENT

The motor unit

A single motor unit consists of the motor neurone plus the muscle fibres it innervates. All muscle fibres in a single motor unit are of the same fibre type. All skeletal muscle fibres do not have the same mechanical and metabolic characteristics. All human muscles are composed of different motor unit types interspersed with each other. The maximal contraction speed, strength and fatiguability of each muscle depend on the proportions of fibre types (Widmaier et al 2007).

Most muscles are composed predominantly of two different types of motor units (Figure 2.4). There are slow low threshold motor units (SMU) and fast high threshold motor units (FMU). Other

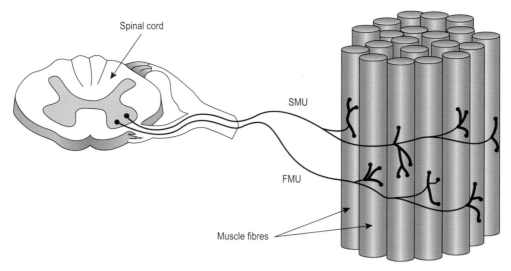

Figure 2.4 Slow and fast motor units (with permission of Comera Movement Science)

Table 2.5 Summary of slow and fast motor unit characteristics		
FUNCTION	**SLOW MOTOR UNITS**	**FAST MOTOR UNITS**
Contraction speed	Slow	Fast
Contraction force	Low	High
Recruitment dominance	Primarily recruited at low % of maximum voluntary contraction (MVC) (<25% MVC)	Increasingly recruited at higher % of maximum voluntary contraction (MVC) (> 40+% MVC) *or* if plan to perform a fast movement
Recruitment threshold	*Low threshold* (sensitive) – easily activated	*High threshold* (insensitive) – requires higher stimulus
Fatiguability	Fatigue resistant	Fast fatiguing
Role	Control of normal non-fatiguing functional movements and unloaded postural control tasks	Rapid or accelerated movement and high load activity

types of motor units have been identified, but this basis classification is useful for rehabilitation purposes (Lieber 2009).

Slow motor units are fatigue resistant with a slow speed of contraction and a low contraction force. Significantly they have a low threshold for activation and as such are predominately recruited in non fatiguing postural control tasks and non fatiguing functional movements. Fast motor units are fast fatiguing when recruited (for example with fast movements or loaded activities). Significantly they have a higher threshold for activation and as such are not recruited to the same extent as slow motor units in non fatiguing function. They are predominantly recruited as load increases, with fatiguing functional activities or if the central nervous system plans to preform a fast movement (Monster 1978).

LOW VERSUS HIGH THRESHOLD RECRUITMENT

Table 2.6 summarises functional activities that stimulate dominant slow and fast motor unit recruitment patterns.

Table 2.6 Functional activities that stimulate dominant slow and fast motor unit recruitment patterns

Low threshold (tonic) recruitment of slow motor units (SMU) (related to low load/force and slow speed)	High threshold (phasic) recruitment of fast motor units (FMU) (related to high load/force and high speed)
• Alignment and postural adjustment • Control of non fatiguing postural activities • Non-fatiguing movements of the unloaded limbs and trunk at a natural comfortable speed	• fatiguing high force or load • bracing co-contraction • initiating fast or accelerated movement

Recruitment is modulated by the higher central nervous system (CNS) and is powerfully influenced by the afferent proprioceptive system along with some behavioural and psychological contextual factors such as fear of pain. Hypertrophy, however, is a peripheral structural adaptation in muscle in response to demand along with CNS adaptation and is the result of overload training (Widmaier et al 2007).

Hodges (2003) argues that high threshold strengthening of the global muscles of range and force potential and low threshold motor control training of deeper (force inefficient) local muscles are two distinctly separate processes, both of which are required to perform to high levels of activity such as competitive sport. One analogy for this is to think of the musculoskeletal system as a computer:

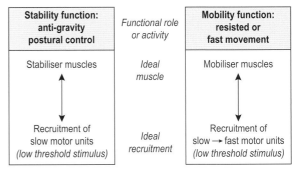

Figure 2.5 The relationship between the biomechanical and physiological characteristics of muscles in stability and mobility function

- High speed or high load strength training changes muscle structure (hypertrophy) and can be likened to upgrading the computer's hardware. This can make the computer work faster and run more complex programs. Upgrading the hardware does not require specific cognitive retraining – the same software is used but more efficiently.
- Low threshold motor control training does not change the peripheral muscle structure to any great extent, but instead improves the central nervous system's recruitment of muscles to fine-tune muscle coordination and improve the efficiency of movement. This can be likened to upgrading the software in a computer to perform its tasks more efficiently and to get the most out of the hardware already present. Upgrading the software, though, always requires cognitive operator training and familiarisation.
- In this analogy, pain is best represented as a computer virus, which primarily affects the software, causing the computer to run slowly and crash more often. In the human body pain has more consistent effects on the motor control aspects of movement rather than directly affecting muscle structure.

In an *ideal or normal* situation, a one-joint muscle performing a non-fatiguing anti-gravity or postural holding function and possessing stabiliser characteristics demonstrates greater recruitment of slow motor units (Figure 2.5). Slow motor units are sensitive to low threshold stimuli and should react efficiently to low force loading situations such as postural sway, maintenance of postural positions and normal functional movements of the unloaded limbs or trunk.

Similarly, for a fast, repetitive movement or power function, muscles with mobiliser characteristics would demonstrate greater recruitment of fast motor units (although the slow motor units are also still recruited). Fast motor units are less sensitive, have higher recruitment thresholds and activate more efficiently in response to high force loading such as accelerated movement, rapid movement, a large or sudden shift of the centre of gravity, high force or heavy loads and conscious maximal contraction.

Functional implications of recruitment within stabiliser and mobiliser roles

Stabiliser roles and slow motor unit recruitment

- Dynamic postural control and normal low load functional movement is primarily a function of slow motor unit (tonic) recruitment.
- Functionally, efficient recruitment of slow motor units will optimise postural holding/anti-gravity and stability function.
- Normal postural control and functional movement of the unloaded limbs and trunk should ideally demonstrate efficient recruitment of deeper, segmentally attaching muscles that provide a stability role.

Mobiliser roles and fast motor unit recruitment

- Functionally, efficient recruitment of fast motor units will optimise rapid/accelerated movement and the production of high force or power.
- High load activity or strength training (endurance or power overload training) is a function of both slow (tonic) and fast (phasic) motor unit recruitment.
- High load or high speed activities normally demonstrate a dominance of recruitment of more superficial, multi-joint muscles that are biomechanically advantaged for high load, large range and high speed.

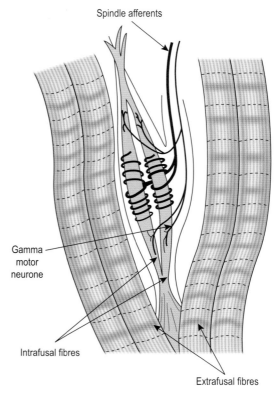

Figure 2.6 Muscle spindle (with permission of Comera Movement Science)

MUSCLE STIFFNESS

Muscle spindles have both sensory and motor functions and are sensitive to changes both in length and in force (Figure 2.6). The information from muscle spindles contributes to proprioception. This allows the central nervous system to be aware of the position of joints, how far they are moving, how fast they are moving, how much force is being used, and relates to the sensation of effort required for particular activities. Muscle spindles play a primary role in proprioception and afferent feedback for motor control but also contribute significantly to the regulation and control of muscle stiffness and therefore segmental stability.

The clinical interpretation of 'stiffness' is often portrayed as a negative outcome. Clinically, 'stiffness' often refers to a loss of motion or function. Biomechanical 'stiffness' on the other hand usually describes a process of providing strength and support. A simple but appropriate way of describing stiffness biomechanically relates to the passive or active tension that may resist a displacing force.

Muscle stiffness (i.e. the ratio of force change to length change) consists of two components: intrinsic muscle stiffness and reflex mediated muscle stiffness (Johansson et al 1991).

1. Intrinsic muscle stiffness is dependent on the viscoelastic properties of muscle and the existing actin–myosin cross-bridges. This can

be affected by hypertrophy or strength training. Hypertrophy, which increases muscle size, muscle fibres in parallel and also increases muscle connective tissue, results in increased muscle stiffness which in turn provides increased resistance to displacement and a mechanism of resisting UCM. This mechanism, however, is largely passive and does not provide dynamic responses to movement challenges.

2. Reflex mediated stiffness is determined by the excitability of the alpha motor neurone pool, which in turn is dependent on descending commands and reflexes which are facilitated by the muscle spindle afferent input (refer again to Figure 2.6). This mechanism is dynamic and provides reflex automatic activation of muscles to provide dynamic responses to postural displacement. For example, in sitting or standing, during activities of leaning forwards at the trunk, the posterior paraspinal stabiliser muscles (multifidus) up-regulate their activation in response to postural loading. During forward leaning, the position of the trunk creates a flexion loading force on the lumbar spine which, in order to maintain spinal neutral alignment, must be resisted by posterior muscles such as multifidus. Likewise, when the trunk returns to an upright position (vertically aligned above the pelvis) the flexion loading force on the lumbar spine is reduced and the posterior muscles down-regulate their activity because they are no longer required to work as hard to resist or stabilise the spine against flexion loading.

Low threshold recruitment and timing

The timing of the automatic reflex activation in response to movement and postural displacement is influenced by the threshold (or sensitivity) of muscle recruitment. For example, during forward weight transfer in normal gait, the multifidus muscle on the rear leg side activates in response to loading. As weight shifts forwards (off the rear leg and towards the front foot) the pelvis on that side has to be supported from dropping down into lateral tilt. Multifidus and the lateral trunk muscles on that side play a role in providing pelvic stabilisation and support while that leg swings through. The activation of multifidus on

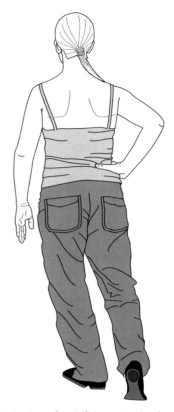

Figure 2.7 Palpation of multifidus activation (rear leg) during weight transfer

the rear leg side during forward weight transfer can be palpated by the therapist or the patient. If multifidus is palpated when full weight is supported on the rear leg, the muscle is unloaded and relaxed. During the transfer of body weight forwards onto the front leg (Figure 2.7) the multifidus muscle on the rear leg side will automatically activate as it is required to support the pelvis from dropping in preparation to lift the rear leg for the swing phase of gait.

The timing of the onset of activation of multifidus is not always consistent. Some people demonstrate automatic activation early in weight transfer, while others demonstrate a delayed activation response. Ideally, the activation of multifidus on the rear leg side should coincide with the initiation of weight transfer, and its onset activation can be palpated as the weight shifts from the heel of the rear foot to the metatarsal heads of that same foot. If multifidus has sufficient low threshold recruitment it should activate before any significant weight is transferred to the front foot. If efficient low threshold recruitment of multifidus is inhibited, multifidus does not palpably activate until body weight is transferred to the front foot and body weight is unloaded from the rear foot. This observed delay in automatic recruitment is associated with altered low threshold activation. It is a very common observation that patients with a history of recurrent low back or pelvic girdle pain consistently demonstrate a timing delay in multifidus activation during forward weight transfer compared to people who have no history of low back pain. This is not an issue of muscle weakness, as it is consistently observed in athletes with back pain who have hypertrophy of the paraspinal muscle groups due to strength and conditioning training programs. This delay may be related to a change in the threshold of automatic activation of low threshold slow motor units.

PAIN AND RECRUITMENT

Recruitment is altered in the presence of pain. Pain affects slow motor unit recruitment more significantly than fast motor unit recruitment. Pain does not appear to significantly limit an athlete's ability to generate power and speed, so long as they can mentally 'put the pain aside'. It has been suggested anecdotally that up to 90% of sporting world records are broken by athletes with a chronic or recurrent musculoskeletal pain problem.

In the pain-free state, research (Hodges & Moseley 2003; Moseley & Hodges 2005) indicates that the brain and the central nervous system (CNS) are able to utilise a variety of motor control strategies to perform functional tasks and maintain control of movement, equilibrium and joint stability. However, in the pain state, the options available to the CNS appear to become limited. These altered (or limited) motor control strategies present as consistent co-contraction patterns usually with exaggerated recruitment of the multi-joint muscles over the deeper segmental muscles.

Recent research on musculoskeletal pain has focused on motor control changes associated with the pain state. This research has provided important new information regarding chronic or recurrent musculoskeletal pain. A large number

of independent research groups are all reporting a common finding (Lee 2011; Jull 2000; Sahrmann 2002; Hodges 2003; Hodges & Moseley 2003; Richardson et al 2004; Falla et al 2004a, b; Sterling et al 2001, 2005; Dankaerts et al 2006; Moseley & Hodges 2006; O'Sullivan et al 2006; O'Leary et al 2001). They have all consistently observed that, in the presence of chronic or recurrent pain, subjects change the patterns or strategies of synergistic recruitment that are normally used to perform low load functional movements or postures. They have demonstrated that these subjects employ strategies or patterns of muscle recruitment that are normally reserved for high load function (e.g. lifting, pushing, pulling, throwing, jumping, running, etc.) for normal postural control and low threshold functional activities. The common observation is that the multi-joint muscles with a primary mobility role for force and speed functions inappropriately become the dominant synergists in non-fatiguing normal functional movements and for low threshold postural control tasks. At the same time, the one-joint muscles that should be dominant in non-fatiguing function and postural control, demonstrate down-regulation of their activation and are less active than controls with no pain history. Figure 2.8 illustrates graphically the differences in recruitment patterns of stabiliser and mobiliser synergists in the pain-free state and the chronic pain state.

These pain-related changes in the patterns or the thresholds of recruitment between one-joint stabilisers and their multi-joint mobiliser synergists can only be demonstrated during unloaded or low threshold testing. Under high load or high threshold function it is normal, in both the pain-free state and in the presence of pain, to demonstrate mobiliser dominance (with respect to stabiliser activation). Therefore, tests based on strength or endurance cannot consistently identify if there is a pain-related change in recruitment thresholds or patterns of recruitment.

These altered strategies or patterns have been described in the research and clinical literature as 'substitution strategies', 'compensatory movements', 'muscle imbalance' between inhibited/lengthened stabilisers and shortened/overactive mobilisers, 'faulty movements', 'abnormal dominance of the mobiliser synergists', 'co-contraction rigidity' and 'control impairments'. The inconsistent terminology used in the clinical and academic literature has contributed to a lack of universal

Pain-free/normal/ideal

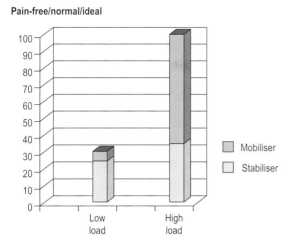

Chronic musculoskeletal pain

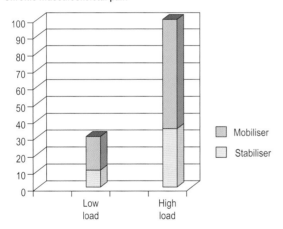

Figure 2.8 Graphical representation of recruitment differences related to chronic or recurrent musculoskeletal pain

recognition of this consistent and almost predictable change related to pain.

RECRUITMENT DYSFUNCTION: INHIBITION AND DYSFACILITATION

Inhibition and dysfacilitation can be identified as abnormal alteration of normal recruitment (Table 2.7). Inhibition relates to a process of neural discharge being actively suppressed by another neural influence. This process is part of normal movement but it may become abnormal in certain situations. Dysfacilitation relates to the utilisation

Table 2.7 Recruitment changes associated with uncontrolled movement

With *uncontrolled movement (UCM)*, inhibition and dysfacilitation present as:

• Poor recruitment under low threshold stimulus – inefficient slow motor unit (SMU) recruitment	Inhibition and dysfacilitation ≠ 'off' ≠ 'weak'
– (evidence in both the local and global muscle systems)	
• Delayed recruitment timing	
– (evidence in the local muscle system)	
• Altered recruitment sequencing	
– (evidence in the global muscle system)	

of altered motor control strategies. These altered strategies contribute to changes in thresholds of facilitation and inefficient pattern of muscle activation.

Example 1: Pain causes active inhibition of SMU recruitment. The pain may resolve and the mechanism of inhibition may be removed, but dysfacilitation may persist.
Example 2: Behavioural and psychological factors such as fear of pain or anxiety of movement also have the potential to contribute to recruitment/inhibition.

ALTERED STRATEGIES IN A DYSFUNCTIONAL SITUATION

Clinically, one-joint stabiliser muscles demonstrate a recruitment problem. They appear to increase their threshold, become less responsive to low load stimulus and respond best when the load becomes greater (Figure 2.9). Therefore the stability muscles respond mainly to higher load activities such as accelerated movement, rapid movement, high force and a large shift of the centre of gravity.

As a consequence, the multi-joint mobilisers take over the stability role. They appear to decrease their threshold and become more reactive to a low load stimulus. Therefore the mobilising muscles appear to respond to low load activities such as postural sway, maintained postural position and slow movement of the unloaded limb (Figure 2.10). The decrease in threshold and

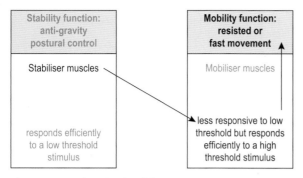

Figure 2.9 Dysfunctional stabiliser recruitment – down-regulation, inhibition and dysfacilitation

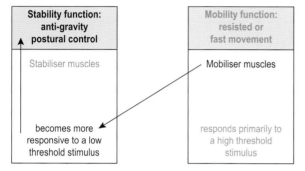

Figure 2.10 Dysfunctional mobiliser recruitment – up-regulation and overactivity

increased tonic activity of SMU recruitment in mobiliser muscles contributes to their observed dominance in postural control (O'Sullivan et al 1998; Jull 2000; Sahrmann 2002).

SENSATION OF EFFORT, AFFERENT INPUT AND RECRUITMENT

The concept of 'sensation of effort' has significant relevance to the clinical assessment of threshold changes in recruitment functions and subsequent implications for the re-assessment of recruitment after exercise interventions. The sense of effort has been defined as a judgment on the effort required to generate a force (Enoka & Stuart 1992). This is processed in higher centres in the central nervous system and relates to the mental challenge required to perform a task in the periphery.

The relative recruitment of slow and fast motor units in sustained voluntary contraction is partly due to the influence of proprioceptive activity

(Grimby & Hannerz 1976). Indeed, proprioceptive information from the primary muscle spindle endings (especially the gamma spindle system loops) is essential for efficient facilitation of tonic or slow motor unit recruitment (Eccles et al 1957; Grimby & Hannerz 1976).

Grimby & Hannerz (1976) reported that when proprioception is diminished, the sense of effort necessary for efficient activation of slow motor units is increased. That is, during *low load activity*, the subject *feels* that they must try harder (even if it *feels* like maximum effort) to achieve tonic recruitment of slow motor units. It *feels* much easier to contract the same muscle against high load or resistance (where fast motor unit recruitment is significant).

> When maximum or high sensation of effort is needed to perform a *low load activity or movement* then it is most likely that there is inefficient facilitation of slow motor unit recruitment and dysfunction of normal spindle responses.
> For the same reasons though, when less sensation of effort is needed to perform that same low load activity or movement (and it feels easier), then it is likely that there is better facilitation of slow motor unit recruitment. This decrease in the sense of effort required is a good indicator of improving motor control stability function.

The sensation of high effort to perform a low load task may be due to:

- recruitment dysfunction (common, with multiple contributing factors), or
- disuse atrophy and weakness (uncommon, but if present, with wasting and functional deficits).

During low threshold motor control stability training it is permissible for the patient to 'feel' or experience the sensation that they are working hard (even maximally) during low load exercise so long as they do not show signs of fatigue of the stability muscle or substitute with a different muscle. It is not appropriate to progress the exercise until that low load exercise feels easy.

- Peripheral fatigue occurs when a muscle can't maintain a level of contraction force for longer because of peripheral factors (e.g. depleted muscle glycogen, phosphagen, and calcium) even though the CNS may be increasing neural discharge to the motor neurone pool. The muscle runs out of fuel. This is best improved by strength training programs.

- Central fatigue relates to alterations in the way that the CNS drives the motor neurone pool. The muscle has the ability (and fuel) to generate more force but an inadequate neural stimulus is provided by the CNS. This is a motor control issue.

Clinical differentiation between central fatigue and peripheral fatigue

When a functional task feels like hard work:
- If added or increased resistive load:
  - → easier = central fatigue (responds to facilitation)
  - → harder = peripheral fatigue or weakness

Implications for training:

When a low load exercise feels or looks like hard work this usually indicates a motor control recruitment dysfunction (*not weakness*) and *needs specific assessment and specific low threshold retraining*.

THE DYSFUNCTION LOOP

Figure 2.11 illustrates some of the inter-related changes in muscle physiology associated with pain and dysfunction. Pain, inflammation and swelling contribute to impaired proprioception which is in turn related to inhibition of SMU recruitment

efficiency and the altered sensation of effort in low load testing. This recruitment inhibition affects both local and global muscle stability function. Articular or myofascial restrictions create compensatory patterns of movement. Pain and the resultant muscle spasm and guarding also contribute to these dysfunctional compensatory movement patterns. Compensation that is efficiently controlled does not appear to contribute to the development of musculoskeletal pain. However, there is abundant evidence to support the link between UCM (uncontrolled intersegmental translation or uncontrolled range of motion) and the development of musculoskeletal pain and degenerative pathology.

This dysfunction loop acts like a 'vicious circle' and contributes to the maintenance of chronicity and insidious recurrence of musculoskeletal pain.

MUSCLE RECRUITMENT TRAINING

Low threshold recruitment dominance

Low threshold motor control training is primarily directed towards restoring normal or ideal recruitment thresholds and strategies. This can be related to upgrading the software in the computer analogy referred to earlier. It is not based on directly restoring function. Improvements in

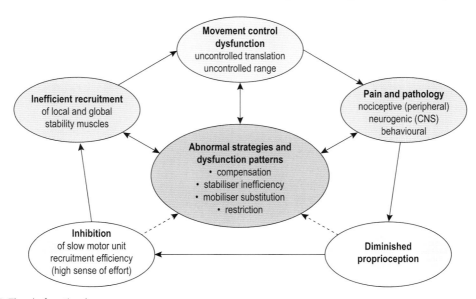

Figure 2.11 The dysfunction loop

function are an indirect consequence of recovering SMU recruitment thresholds and restoring more ideal patterns of recruitment. Low threshold motor control training strategies usually require practising a highly cognitive, very specific, non-functional movement skill until the activation strategy feels more 'familiar' and less 'unnatural' and has a low sensation of effort (feels easy) during its performance. Once this low threshold motor control recruitment skill has been established it can be progressed in several ways:

- While maintaining the cognitive activation, progressively remove or decrease load facilitation (unloading). For example, the multifidus has increased load facilitation in standing with forward leaning of the trunk. Load facilitation is decreased by moving the trunk backwards over the pelvis in sitting and is maximally unloaded by lying supported in prone.
- While maintaining the cognitive activation, impose a low threshold (non-fatiguing) perturbation. This perturbation should consist of small range, low force, non-predictable displacements. For example, this can be achieved while sitting upright on an unstable base (such as an inflatable disc or round balance board) while maintaining the trained cognitive activation.

High threshold recruitment dominance

High threshold strength training affects structure (hardware) of muscle tissue over time. When muscle tissue is loaded and stressed it adapts to stress and hypertrophies and increases the potential to generate force and power. This structural change occurs over a timeframe of 6–8 weeks or more:

- Strength training is progressed by progressively increasing resistive load, using fast alternating movements or progressively increasing holding endurance to the point of fatigue.

CLINICAL GUIDELINE FOR RECRUITMENT TRAINING

Table 2.8 lists the key differences between low and high threshold recruitment retraining strategies.

Table 2.8 Key threshold differences between low and high threshold recruitment strategies

KEY THRESHOLD DIFFERENCES	
Low threshold recruitment	High threshold recruitment
Slow motor unit dominant	**F**ast motor unit dominant
Slow / **S**tatic	**F**ast
and	*or*
Sustained	**F**atiguing
(non-fatiguing, low load)	(high load)

Retraining low threshold recruitment dominance

If the patient is able to perform an exercise or task slowly and consistently for 4 minutes or more without fatigue or needing recovery time, then at least the first 1–2 minutes of that exercise or task will be performed with low threshold recruitment dominance.

Retraining high threshold recruitment dominance

If the load of the exercise or task is such that it cannot be performed continually for 2 minutes because the load is sufficient to cause fatigue then that exercise or task will be performed with high threshold recruitment dominance. If an exercise or task is performed at high speed, then it will be performed with high threshold recruitment dominance (even if it is low load).

In between these two regions there is a 'grey' area that can be significantly influenced by training responses.

These aspects of physiology and muscle recruitment function underpin the processes used in developing assessment principles (Chapter 3). The application of this knowledge to the design and implementation of retraining strategies to address UCM and for the integration of low threshold motor control training into function is further explored and demonstrated in Chapter 4.

REFERENCES

Bergmark, A., 1989. Stability of the lumbar spine. A study in mechanical engineering. Acta Orthopaedica Scandinavica 230 (60), 20–24.

Comerford, M.J., Mottram, S.L., 2001. Movement and stability dysfunction – contemporary developments. Manual Therapy 6, 15–26.

Dankaerts, W., O'Sullivan, P., Burnett, A., Straker, L., 2006. Altered patterns of superficial trunk muscle activation during sitting in nonspecific chronic low back pain patients: importance of subclassification. Spine (Philadelphia Pa 1976) 31 (17), 2017–2023.

Eccles, J.C., Eccles, R.M., Lundberg, A., 1957. The convergence of monosynaptic excitatory afferents onto many different species of alpha motorneurons. Journal of Physiology (London) 137, 22–50.

Enoka, R.M., Stuart, D.G., 1992. Neurobiology of muscle fatigue. Journal of Applied Physiology 72 (5), 1631–1648.

Falla, D., Jull, G., Hodges, P., 2004a. Patients with neck pain demonstrate reduced electromyographic activity of the deep cervical flexor muscles during performance of the craniocervical flexion test. Spine 29, 2108–2114.

Falla, D., Bilenkij, G., Jull, G., 2004b. Patients with chronic neck pain demonstrate altered patters of muscle activation during performance of a functional upper limb task. Spine 29, 1436–1440.

Gibbons, S., 2007. Clinical anatomy and function of psoas major and deep sacral gluteus maximus. In: Vleeming, A., Mooney, V., Stoeckart, R. (Eds.), Movement, stability and lumbopelvic pain. Elsevier, Edinburgh, ch. 6, p. 95.

Goff, B., 1972. The application of recent advances in neurophysiology to Miss R Rood's concept of neuromuscular facilitation. Physiotherapy 58 (2), 409–415.

Goldspink, G., Williams, P.E., 1992. Muscle fibre and connective tissue changes associated with use and disuse. In: Ada, L., Canning, C. (Eds.), Key issues in neurological physiotherapy. Butterworth Heinemann, Oxford.

Gossman, M.R., Sahrmann, S.A., Rose, S.J., 1982. Review of length-associated changes in muscle. Physical Therapy 62 (12), 1799–1808.

Grimby, L., Hannerz, J., 1976. Disturbances in voluntary recruitment order of low and high frequency motor units on blockades of proprioception afferent activity. Acta Physiologica Scandinavica 96, 207–216.

Hides, J.A., Richardson, C.A., Jull, G.A., 1996. Multifidus muscle recovery is not automatic after resolution of acute, first-episode low back pain. Spine 21 (23), 2763–2769.

Hides, J.A., Jull, G.A., Richardson, C.A., 2001. Long term effects of specific stabilizing exercises for first episode low back pain. Spine 26 (11), 243–248.

Hodges, P.W., 2001. Changes in motor planning of feedforward postural responses of the trunk muscles in low back pain. Experimental Brain Research 141, 261–266.

Hodges, P.W., 2003. Core stability exercise in chronic low back pain. Orthopedic Clinics of North America 34 (2), 245–254.

Hodges, P.W., Cholewicki, J., 2007. Functional control of the spine. In: Vleeming, A., Mooney, V., Stoeckart, R. (Eds.), Movement, stability and lumbopelvic pain. Elsevier, Edinburgh, ch. 33.

Hodges, P.W., Moseley, G.L., 2003. Pain and motor control of the lumbo-pelvic region: effect and possible mechanisms. Journal of Electromyography and Kinesiology 13 (4), 361–370.

Hodges, P.W., Richardson, C.A., 1996. Inefficient muscular stabilisation of the lumbar spine associated with low back pain: a motor control evaluation of transversus abdominis. Spine 21 (22), 2640–2650.

Hodges, P.W., Richardson, C.A., 1997. Feedforward contraction of transversus abdominis is not influenced by the direction of arm movement. Experimental Brain Research 114, 362–370.

Hodges, P.W., Richardson, C.A., 1999. Transversus abdominis and the superficial abdominal muscles are controlled independently in a postural task. Neuroscience Letters 265 (2), 91–94.

Horak, F.B., Esselman, P., Anderson, M.E., Lynch, M.K., 1984. The effects of movement velocity, mass displaced, and task certainty on associated postural adjustments made by normal and hemiplegic individuals. Journal of Neurology, Neurosurgery, and Psychiatry 47 (9), 1020–1028.

Janda, V., 1983. On the concept of postural muscles and posture in man. Australian Journal of Physiotherapy 29 (3), 83–84.

Janda, V., 1996. Evaluation of muscle imbalance. In: Liebenson, C. (Ed.), Rehabilitation of the spine. Williams and Wilkins, Baltimore.

Johansson, H., Sjolander, P., Sojka, P., 1991. Receptors in the knee joint ligaments and their role in the biomechanics of the joint. Critical Reviews in Biomedical Engineering 18 (5), 341–368.

Johnson, G., Bogduk, N., Nowitzke, A., House, D., 1994. Anatomy and actions of trapezius muscle. Clinical Biomechanics 9, 44–50.

Jull, G.A., 2000. Deep cervical flexor muscle dysfunction in whiplash. Journal of Musculoskeletal Pain 8 (1/2), 143–154.

Kendall, F.P., McCreary, E., Provance, P., Rodgers, M., Romanic, W., 2005. Muscles: testing and function with posture and pain. Lippincott Williams Wilkins, Baltimore.

Lee, D., 2011. The pelvic girdle: an integration of clinical expertise and research, 4th edn. Churchill Livingstone, Edinburgh.

Lieb, F., Perry, J., 1968. Quadriceps function – an anatomical and mechanical study using amputated limbs. Journal of Bone and Joint Surgery 50A (8), 1535–1548.

Lieber, R.L., 2009. Skeletal muscle structure, function and

plasticity. Lippincott Williams and Wilkins, Baltimore.

McGill, S.M., 2007. The painful and unstable lumbar spine: a foundation and approach for restabilization. In: Vleeming, A., Mooney, V., Stoeckart, R. (Eds.), Movement, stability and lumbopelvic pain. Elsevier, Edinburgh, ch. 35.

Monster, A.W., Chan, H., O'Connor, D., 1978. Activity patterns of human skeletal muscles: relation to muscle fiber type composition. Science 200 (4339), 314–317.

Moseley, G.L., Hodges, P.W., 2005. Are the changes in postural control associated with low back pain caused by pain interference? Clinical Journal of Pain 21 (4), 323–329.

Moseley, G.L., Hodges, P.W., 2006. Reduced variability of postural strategy prevents normalization of motor changes induced by back pain: a risk factor for chronic trouble? Behavioral Neuroscience 120 (2), 474–476.

O'Leary, S., Falla, D., Jull, G., 2011. The relationship between superficial muscle activity during the cranio-cervical flexion test and clinical features in patients with chronic neck pain. Manual Therapy Mar 9 [Epub ahead of print]

O'Sullivan, P.B., 2000. Lumbar segmental 'instability': clinical presentation and specific stabilizing exercise management. Manual Therapy 5 (1), 2–12.

O'Sullivan, P.B., Twomey, L., Allison, G., Sinclair, J., Miller, K., Knox, J., 1997. Altered patterns of abdominal muscle activation in patients with chronic low back pain. Australian Journal of Physiotherapy 43 (2), 91–98.

O'Sullivan, P.B., Twomey, L., Allison, G.T., 1998. Altered abdominal muscle recruitment in patients with chronic back pain following a specific exercise intervention. Journal of Orthopaedic and Sports Physical Therapy.

Panjabi, M.M., 1992. The stabilising system of the spine. Part 1. Function, dysfunction adaption, and enhancement. Journal of Spinal Disorders 5, 383–389.

Reeves, N.P., Cholewicki, J., 2010. Expanding our view of the spine system. European Spine Journal DOI: 10.1007/s00586-009-1220-5.

Richardson, C., Jull, G., Hodges, P., Hides, J., 1998. Therapeutic exercise for spinal segmental stabilization in low back pain. Churchill Livingstone, Edinburgh, pp. 12.

Richardson, C., Hodges, P., Hides, J., 2004. Therapeutic exercise for lumbopelvic stabilization, 2nd edn. Churchill Livingstone, Edinburgh.

Sterling, M., Jull, G., Wright, A., 2001. The effect of musculoskeletal pain on motor activity and control. Journal of Pain 2 (3), 135–145.

Sterling, M., Jull, G., Vicenzino, B., Kenardy, J., Darnell, R., 2005. Physical and psychological factors predict outcome following whiplash injury. Pain 114 (1–2), 141–148.

Sahrmann, S.A., 2002. Diagnosis and treatment of movement impairments syndromes. Mosby, St Louis.

Vleeming, A., Mooney, V., Stoeckart, R., 2007. Movement, stability and lumbopelvic pain. Integration of research and therapy. Churchill Livingstone, Edinburgh.

Widmaier, E., Raff, H., Strang, K., 2007. Vander's human physiology: the mechanisms of body function. McGraw Hill, Boston.

Chapter | 3 |

Assessment and classification of uncontrolled movement

The development of valid classification methods to assist therapists in the management of neuro-musculoskeletal disorders has been recognised as a clinical priority (Fritz & Brennan 2007; Fritz et al 2007). Identifying and classifying movement faults is fast becoming an essential tool in contemporary rehabilitative neuromusculo-skeletal practice (Comerford & Mottram 2001a; Sahrmann 2002; O'Sullivan 2005). Traditionally, assessment of musculoskeletal problems is based on the clinical history, mechanism of injury and symptom responses to examination procedures. Symptoms are assessed during active movements (Cyriax 1980; McKenzie & May 2003; Maitland et al 2005), passive movements (Kaltenborn 2003; Maitland et al 2005), combined movements (Edwards 1999) or sustained positions (McKenzie & May 2003). A mechanism-based approach has now been proposed (Schafer et al 2007) with contemporary assessment moving away from individual symptom responses to exploring movement impairments and how these relate to symptoms (Comerford & Mottram 2001a; Sahrmann 2002; Burnett et al 2004; Dankaerts et al 2006b; Comerford & Mottram 2011, Van Dillen et al 2009).

Given the complexity of neuromuscular dysfunction, therapists have continued to search for a systematic framework to assist clinical assessment and management. One focus is on identifying clinical prediction rules (CPR) that determine subgroups within patient presentations that may respond to certain treatments (Hicks et al 2005);

however, it has yet to be established if CPR can change symptoms as well as function and dysfunction or correlate to changes in muscular recruitment. The following section explores issues relating to the classification of subgroups in neuromusculoskeletal pain management.

CLASSIFICATION OF SUBGROUPS IN NEUROMUSCULOSKELETAL PAIN

Non-specific musculoskeletal pain often has a history of chronicity or recurrence along with multiple tissues being diagnosed as contributory elements to the pain presentation. Significant pain mechanisms are often present (Chapter 1) and there may or may not be identifiable elements of behavioural adaptation. If mechanical subgroups can be identified within the broad group known as non-specific neuromusculoskel-etal pain, then manual therapy and therapeutic exercise interventions have a better rationale for predicting positive outcomes.

Classification and categorisation of subgroups can be based on a variety of systems of analysis, for example:

- *Non-specific musculoskeletal pain*: no single anatomical based pathology can account for the presenting symptoms. The evaluation of movement-related dysfunction can be used to explain some of the symptoms presenting in multiple tissues. These movement-based

Box 3.1 **Classification of subgroups based on non-specific mechanical pain related to movement dysfunction**

Subgroups within non-specific musculoskeletal pain

1. Site and direction of uncontrolled movement

(a) Site and direction of uncontrolled motion (Comerford & Mottram 2001a).

(b) Direction susceptible to motion (Sahrmann 2002).

(c) Control impairments and movement impairments (O'Sullivan 2005).

2. Recruitment efficiency of local muscle stability system

(a) Changes in feedforward mechanism, for example:

(i) transversus abdominis, multifidus, pelvic floor, diaphragm (Richardson et al 2004)

(ii) deep neck flex (Jull et al 2008)

(iii) upper trapezius (Wadsworth & Bullock-Saxton 1997).

(b) Recruitment efficiency changes:

(i) deep neck flex (Jull et al 2008)

(ii) psoas, subscapularis, upper trapezius, lower trapezius, posterior neck ext. (Gibbons 2007; Comerford & Mottram 2010)

(iii) deep sacral glut. max. (Gibbons 2007)

(iv) clinical rating system (Comerford & Mottram 2011).

(c) Ultrasound changes:

(i) transversus abdominis (Richardson et al 2004)

(ii) multifidus (Stokes et al 1992; Hides et al 2008)

(iii) psoas (Gibbons 2005; Comerford & Mottram 2011)

(iv) pelvic floor (Peng et al 2007; Whittaker 2007).

3. Muscle imbalance

(a) Sahrmann (relative flexibility) (Sahrmann 2002).

(b) Kinetic Control (restriction and compensation) (Comerford & Mottram 2011).

(c) Janda (recruitment sequencing) (Janda 1986).

4. Patterns of movement provocation and relief with postural positioning

(a) McKenzie (derangement patterns) (McKenzie & May 2006).

(b) Jones positional release (strain–counterstrain) (Jones et al 1995).

5. Positional diagnosis

(a) Osteopathic process (muscle energy technique).

6. Patterns of symptom relief associated with manual mobilisation

(a) Mulligan (Nags, Snags, MWM) (Mulligan 2003).

(b) DonTigny (pelvic dysfunction) (DonTigny 1997).

(c) Cyriax (1980), Maitland et al (2005), Kaltenborn (2003).

(d) Patterns of symptom relief with manual mobilisation (Fritz et al 2005).

dysfunctions include the evaluation of the site and direction of uncontrolled movement (UCM), recruitment efficiency of local muscle stability system, muscle imbalance, patterns of movement provocation and relief with postural positioning, positional diagnosis, patterns of symptom relief associated with manual mobilisation. Box 3.1 illustrates some of these subgroups.

- *Specific musculoskeletal pain – classification by implying a patho-anatomical source*: definite pathology is identified that accounts for the presenting signs and symptoms, for example: spondylolisthesis, disc herniation and nerve root compression, spinal stenosis, bony injury/fracture, articular derangement (meniscal/labral tear, chondral defect), muscle haematoma and osteoligamentous damage (ligament sprain).

- *Classification by pain mechanisms* in particular identifying components of inflammatory/ biochemical sensitisation, neurogenic sensitisation and behavioural or psychosomatic issues (Watson & Kendall 2000; Butler & Moseley 2003; Sterling et al 2003, 2004; Waddell 2004).

Classification based on movement dysfunction

In the absence of reliable diagnostic tests for musculoskeletal disorders, classifying movement control faults is gaining recognition and acceptance (Comerford & Mottram 2001a; Sahrmann 2002; Dankaerts et al 2006b; Mottram & Comerford 2008). For example, identifying subcategories of movement faults to guide interventions has been applied to the lumbar spine and the reliability of some tests has been established (Luomajoki et al 2007; Trudelle-Jackson et al 2008). Comerford & Mottram (2001a, 2011) contend that the observation of aberrant movement in itself may not be the most critical factor influencing pain and dysfunction. It could be argued that some observations of excessive or reduced range of movement may just be variations within the normal distribution of the population. People who have no pain and no history of previous symptoms may present with range of motion that may be considered excessive or hypermobile. It is possible that this 'excessive' range of movement is controlled well by automatic and cognitive recruitment mechanisms during movement and postural tasks (Roussel et al 2009). The ability to cognitively recruit appropriate movement control strategies may be a better indicator of whether there is UCM or whether the aberrant movement is merely a bad habit at one extreme of the normal distribution curve. Not only is the observation of aberrant movement important but it is important to be able to test for the ability to control it.

The identification of aberrant movement and the evaluation of the control of movement is complex. The following section will discuss a range of elements that should be considered during the observation and quantification of aberrant movement. These include the assessment of relative stiffness/relative flexibility, movement control dysfunction, movement system impairments and motor control impairments.

Relative stiffness – relative flexibility

Sahrmann (2002) proposes the concept of 'relative flexibility' or 'relative stiffness'. If one-joint muscles become excessively lengthened and strained or are 'weak' and lack the ability to adequately shorten, they demonstrate increased flexibility. This increased flexibility can contribute to uncontrolled or excessive motion at that joint. Similarly, if multi-joint muscles lack extensibility or generate excessive tension they develop increased stiffness. This increased stiffness then has the potential to limit or restrict normal motion at that joint. When increased stiffness limits motion at a joint, then in order to maintain normal function, the restriction must be compensated for elsewhere in the movement system. If these muscles are linked in functional movements then excessive or uncontrolled motion develops at the joint that is inadequately controlled by the one-joint muscles relative to the adjacent restriction. Relatively more flexible structures compensate for relatively stiffer structures in function, creating direction-specific stress and strain. During functional movements direction-specific hypermobility is re-enforced and if repetitively loaded, tissue pathology results (Comerford & Mottram 2001a).

An example of this concept can be observed in the active prone knee extension test (Woolsey et al 1988). If the rectus femoris is relatively stiffer than the abdominals, then in order to achieve 120° of knee flexion, the pelvis tilts anteriorly, and the spine extends. Sahrmann (2002) suggests that the abdominals are relatively more flexible than the rectus femoris, which is relatively stiffer, creating uncontrolled or abnormal spinal extension, which in turn contributes to mechanical back pain (Figure 3.1).

Sahrmann (2002) also identified a similar pattern during forward bending manoeuvres. If the hamstrings are relatively stiffer than the back extensors (which are relatively more flexible), then during forward bending the hip lacks

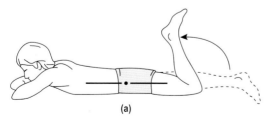 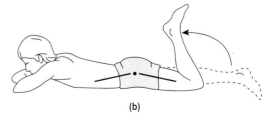

(a)   (b)

Prone knee flexion. (a) Ideally, there should be approximately 120° knee flexion without significant lumbopelvic motion. (b) To achieve 120° knee flexion with a relatively stiffer rectus femoris, the pelvis will anteriorly tilt and the relatively flexible lumbar spine will extend.

Figure 3.1 Relative stiffness and relative flexibility influencing lumbar extension

sufficient flexion but the spine hyperflexes to compensate. This may predispose to mechanical back pain. Esola et al (1996) reported that subjects with a history of low back pain, in early forward bending, flex more at their lumbar spine and have stiffer hamstrings than do subjects with no history of low back pain. This is supported by Hamilton & Richardson (1998) who show that subjects who have no low back pain can actively maintain spinal neutral alignment through 30° of forward leaning (hip flexion) in sitting, but subjects with low back pain cannot. The low back pain subjects lost neutral alignment earlier and to a greater extent, indicating that the spine was relatively more flexible than the hips in low back pain subjects.

Similar evidence has been reported in cervical spine dysfunction. The normal ranges of segmental flexion–extension range of motion for C5–6 is 18° and 17° for C4–5 with 3.2 mm of intersegmental translation at both levels (Bhalla & Simmons 1969; Dvorak et al 1988). Singer et al (1993) reported that subjects with neck pain and discogenic pathology demonstrated changes in range of segmental motion and intersegmental translation. The C5–6 motion segment became relatively stiff. It demonstrated reduced range of flexion–extension from 18° to 8° and intersegmental translation reduced from 3.2 mm to 1 mm. In order to maintain functional range of motion of the head and neck, the C4–5 motion segment increased flexibility. It demonstrated increased range of flexion–extension from 17° to 23° and intersegmental translation increase from 3.2 mm to 6 mm. This paper demonstrated that a significant restriction of motion at one vertebral level could be compensated for by relatively increasing range at an adjacent level.

Norlander & Nordgren (1998) suggest that deviation from synchronous distribution of normal mobility between motion segments might be a factor causing provocation of joint mechanoreceptors and subsequent pain. They measured segmental relative flexion mobility between C5 and T7 and identified that hypomobility of C7–T1 with hypermobility of T1–2 significantly predicted neck–shoulder pain.

Relative stiffness/flexibility changes have also been measured at the shoulder girdle. Sahrmann (1992, 2002) identifies several clinical patterns of dysfunction. Increased glenohumeral motion compensates for insufficient upward rotation of the scapula during shoulder flexion or abduction.

Increased forward tilt of the scapula compensates for shortness or stiffness of the lateral rotator muscles during shoulder medial rotation. Increased anterior translation of the humeral head compensates for restriction of glenohumeral medial rotation. She further suggests that these compensations are associated with the development of pathology.

A test of shoulder girdle relative stiffness/flexibility (the kinetic medial rotation test – Chapter 8) identifies a restriction of shoulder medial rotation, which is compensated for by relatively increasing scapular forward tilt or glenohumeral translation to maintain a functional range of arm rotation. It is suggested that the compensatory motion at the scapula correlates with impingement pathology, while glenohumeral compensatory motion correlates with instability pathology. This test has been further validated and quantified by Morrissey (2005) and Morrissey et al (2008).

The clinical implication is that in ideal or 'normal' function, complex motor control processes exist. These processes regulate muscle relative stiffness or relative flexibility in linked multi-joint movements. The movement system has a remarkable ability to adapt to change. Minor variations are acceptable and tolerated by the tissues involved. However, when significant restriction of motion occurs at a joint, the body adapts and in the attempt to maintain function, some other joint or muscle must compensate by increasing relative mobility. The cost of compensating with uncontrolled movement is often insidious pathology.

Movement control dysfunction

A common feature of movement control faults is reduced control of active movements, or movement control dysfunction, termed MCD by Luomajoki et al (2007). The MCD is identified by a series of clinical tests. These tests have been shown to be reliable in the lumbar spine (Luomajoki et al 2007; Roussel et al 2009) and have been promoted in clinical practice (Mottram 2003; Comerford & Mottram 2011). The tests are based on the concept known as dissociation, defined as the ability to control motion at one segment while concurrently producing an active movement at another joint segment (Comerford & Mottram 2001a; Sahrmann 2002). A dissociation test evaluates the ability to actively control movement and demonstrates MCD.

Once a MCD has been identified it can guide the choice of therapeutic exercise (Comerford & Mottram 2001b; Mottram 2003). In the case of shoulder dysfunction, muscles around the shoulder girdle may be unable to control the scapula during arm function. In the lumbar spine, trunk muscles may be unable to control lumbar alignment during movements of the hip or thoracic spine. The distinctive features of these tests start with the positioning of the spine or segment in its 'neutral position' by the therapist, which is then actively controlled by the patient while they move the joint region either above or below the joint system being tested. These clinical dissociation tests can identify the site (e.g. scapula or lumbar spine) and direction (e.g. downward rotation/forward tilt, and flexion) of movement control faults (Luomajoki et al 2008; Barr & Burden 2009; Mottram et al 2009). Adapting the principles associated with dissociation testing, UCM can be identified and classified by the therapist using palpation and visual observation. These clinical tests are described in Chapters 5–9.

Movement impairments

A standardised clinical examination, based on Sahrmann's conceptual model of movement impairment, has been described for the lumbar spine (Scholtes & Van Dillen 2007; Van Dillen et al 2009), the knee (Harris-Hayes & Van Dillen 2009) and the shoulder (Caldwell et al 2007). The underlying assumption is that movement faults and abnormal resting postures are associated with musculoskeletal tissue changes (Sahrmann 2002). For example, muscle dysfunction in relation to: i) muscle length changes; ii) altered recruitment patterns between synergistic or antagonistic muscles; and iii) direction specific increased motion which arises as compensation for relative restrictions of motion at adjacent joints may be determined. Movement system impairments (MSI) may present as abnormal alignment and impaired movement during testing or functional activities (Sahrmann 2002; Trudelle-Jackson et al 2008; van Dillen et al 2009).

The lumbar spine examination includes a number of clinical tests of trunk, limb or combined trunk and limb movements to ascertain movement impairments (Van Dillen et al 1998,

2009). The MSI diagnosis is based on identifying, firstly, a consistent pattern of movement which is associated with the patient's symptoms and, secondly, a decrease in pain when the MSI is corrected. For the lumbar region the clinician makes a judgment as to whether the patient moves his or her lumbopelvic region early in the test. For example, in a forward bending movement it may be observed that the lumbar spine initiates the forward bending movement, with hip flexion contributing to the forward bending much later. The person usually notes that their symptoms are provoked by and are linked to the lumbar flexion phase of the movement. The therapist also observes whether a significant reduction in the symptoms is achieved if the person can learn to initiate forward bending with hip flexion, while actively preventing the lumbar spine flexion. On this basis a diagnosis of lumbar flexion movement impairment is made.

People with low back pain (LBP) demonstrate early lumbopelvic movement with clinical tests (Scholte et al 2000; Gombatto et al 2007; van Dillen et al 2001 2009). The inter-rater reliability between two physical therapists classifying patients with chronic LBP into lumbar spine movement impairment strategies has substantial agreement (Trudelle-Jackson et al 2008). The suggestion is that this links to the pattern of movement during everyday activities and relates to LBP. The hypothesis here is that early lumbopelvic movement during everyday activities suggests an increase in frequency of movement of a specific region which may contribute to increased stress on tissue resulting in pain (Mueller & Maluf 2002). This becomes the diagnosis of movement impairment.

Motor control impairments (MCI)

O'Sullivan (2000) proposed a classification system based on motor control impairments (MCI). His classification system of clinical subgroups is based on altered strategies for postural and movement control. The inter-tester reliably of this classification system has been established (Vibe Fersum et al 2009). O'Sullivan describes a subgroup of patients presenting with impairments in control of spinal segments in the direction of pain which are associated with deficits in motor control (O'Sullivan et al 2006). Interestingly, Dankaerts (2006a), in applying this system, did not identify differences in superficial trunk muscle activation between a group of healthy controls and non-specific chronic LBP subjects in sitting. The authors stressed the importance of the 'washout effect' when interpreting this finding. When results from all subjects with chronic LBP were pooled the findings in one subgroup of patients were 'washed out' by the others. However, once subjects were grouped by flexion and extension control impairment patterns, clear differences in muscle activation patterns were identified.

The classification of a flexion control impairment pattern, for example, is based on linking several clinical observations: i) patients relate their symptoms to flexion activities or postures; ii) they are unable to maintain a neutral lumbar lordosis and habitually position their lumbar spine in postures of increased flexion and posterior pelvic tilt; iii) they initiate forward bending or flexion activities with movement at their symptomatic segments; iv) specific muscle testing identifies an inability to activate lumbar multifidus appropriately at the symptomatic segments (bracing or co-contraction strategies are utilised instead); v) palpation examination reveals increased flexion mobility at the symptomatic segments. The research in this area highlights the usefulness and importance of sub-classification models in chronic LBP and suggests that therapeutic management may be different between groups.

Uncontrolled movement (UCM) and pain

The identification of UCM should be made in terms of site and direction based on the ability to cognitively control the movement, not just on observation of altered range of motion. The consideration that a significant amount of pain in the neuromusculoskeletal system is a result of cumulative microtrauma caused by uncontrolled movement is gaining credibility (Sahrmann 2002; Luomajoki et al 2007; Van Dillen et al 2009). The uncontrolled motion leads to increased loading and pain (Cholewicki & McGill 1996; Mueller & Maluf 2002). UCM is not identified by merely noting hypermobile range of motion or relative flexibility. Furthermore, UCM is not solely identified by habitual postures or initiation of function with movement at one segment. UCM is identified by a lack of the

ability to actively control or prevent movement (or lack of ability to learn how to control movement) in a particular direction at a particular joint or motion segment. The UCM can be identified in the presence or in the absence of a symptomatic episode. The UCM is independent of hypermobile or hypomobile range of motion. That is, some people may demonstrate UCM even in situations of reduced functional range, while other people with hypermobile range of motion may demonstrate good active control of their excessive range of motion. The presence of UCM is a powerful indicator of symptomatic function associated with recurrence and chronicity of musculoskeletal pain.

The development of motion restrictions in function

The development of restrictions within normal motion is common. The body acquires restrictions over time for a variety of reasons, as described in Box 3.2. Motion restrictions may be passive or active, affecting either the accessory translation or the physiological range available to a joint. Passive restrictions may involve: i) a loss of extensibility of normal contractile structures (e.g. muscle shortening); ii) connective tissue structures (e.g. capsule shortening); iii) the development of abnormal connective tissue (e.g. fibrotic adhesions); or iv) bony changes (osteophytes or spurs) that contribute to a reduction of available passive joint motion. Active restrictions may involve neurally mediated changes in

---

Box 3.2 **Common causes of acquired movement restriction**

- Injury and increased scar tissue.
- Protective or guarding responses.
- Postural shortening associated with habitual positioning and a lack of movement.
- Degenerative changes over time.
- Overuse.
- Hypertrophy and excessive increases in intrinsic muscle stiffness.
- Recruitment dominance (often associated with habitual overuse).
- Behavioural and psychological contextual factors.
- Environment and occupational contextual factors.

contractile (muscle) tissues. This may occur as a result of: i) muscle guarding or spasm in response to pain sensitive movement; or ii) increased muscle tension/stiffness due to altered patterns (strategies) of muscle recruitment between synergistic muscle groups or increased muscle tension in response to emotional, behavioural or environmental stressors. These altered patterns of muscle recruitment may in turn be reinforced due to overuse, overtraining, postural loading or maladaptive responses to pain, stress and psychosocial factors.

Because restrictions of normal motion are common, the body normally compensates for these restrictions by increasing motion elsewhere to maintain function. In normal functional movement, the central nervous system (CNS) has a variety of strategies available to perform any functional task or movement and, ideally, the CNS determines the most appropriate strategy for the demands of the functional task. So long as the trajectory or path of motion is well controlled by the coordination of forces in the local and global synergists, the movement system appears to cope well (Hodges 2003).

Compensation that demonstrates effective active control is a normal adaptive process and does not constitute a stability dysfunction, and is usually non-symptomatic. However, inefficient active control (uncontrolled movement) identifies a dynamic stability dysfunction and has greater potential to accumulate microtrauma within a variety of tissues and if this exceeds tissue tolerance may contribute to the development of pathology and pain (Comerford & Mottram 2001a) (Figure 3.2).

A proposition for the aetiology of UCM

UCM is defined as a lack of efficient active recruitment of the local or global muscle's ability to control motion at a particular motion segment in a specific direction (Comerford & Mottram 2001a). For example, uncontrolled lumbar flexion demonstrates a lack of efficient active recruitment of spinal muscles to control or prevent movement of the lumbar spine into flexion when attempting to do so.

The development of UCM may have several contributing factors:

1. *Compensation for restriction to maintain function.* The UCM most commonly develops insidiously to compensate for an articular or myofascial restriction in order to maintain normal function. This is commonly observed as lack of control of hypermobile range; however, it can also present as a lack of control of normal range. For example, uncontrolled lumbar flexion *compensates* for a restriction of hip flexion (hamstrings) to maintain the normal function of forward bending. The back extensor stabiliser muscles lack efficient control of the lumbar spine during flexion loading. Therefore, the UCM is in the *lumbar* spine in the direction of *flexion.*

Restriction → Compensation → UCM → Pathology → Pain

2. *Direct overfacilitation.* Occasionally the UCM develops because excessive range of movement is habitually performed (without compensating for restrictions). A particular muscle pulls too hard on a joint in a particular direction due to dominant recruitment, active shortening or overtraining. This develops slowly as a progressive insidious process. This is due to an active process of overuse and shortening of a particular muscle that holds a joint towards its end-range position (away from neutral or mid-range positions). For example, uncontrolled lumbar flexion develops due to overtraining of rectus abdominis with repetitive trunk curls. Rectus abdominis *actively* holds the lumbar spine excessively flexed at rest and during flexion

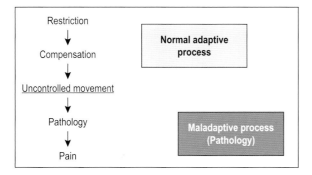

Figure 3.2 The restricted segment may be a cause of compensatory uncontrolled movement

load activities and postures. The back extensor stabiliser muscles lack efficient control of the lumbar spine during flexion loading. Therefore, the UCM is in the *lumbar* spine in the direction of *flexion*.

Overpull vs underpull → Compensation → UCM → Pathology → Pain

3. *Sustained passive postural positioning*. The UCM may also be a result of a passive process where sustained postural positioning habitually maintains the joint or region towards its end-range position (away from neutral or mid-range positions). This usually results in a lengthening strain of the controlling stabiliser muscles and passive postural or positional shortening of the underused but unstretched mobiliser muscles. Body weight and gravity combine to create a sustained, direction-specific loading mechanism. This process is passive and mainly insidious. For example, uncontrolled lumbar flexion is the result of *passive*, habitual or sustained sitting in a slouched (flexed) posture. The back extensor stabiliser muscles lack efficient control of the lumbar spine during flexion loading. Therefore, the UCM is in the *lumbar* spine in the direction of *flexion*.

Postural strain → UCM → Pathology → Pain

4. *Trauma*. The functional stability of the movement system may be very efficient but an injury may occur where load or strain exceeds the tolerance of normal tissues and damage to the normal restraints of motion results. Hence the UCM may be unrelated to habitual movements and postures or compensation for restriction, and be the sole result of trauma due to normal tissue being overloaded. For example, uncontrolled lumbar flexion may be the result of a forced flexion *injury* to the lumbar spine such as may occur in a collapsing rugby scrum or a motor vehicle accident. The back extensor stabilisers lack efficient control of the lumbar spine during flexion loading. Therefore, the UCM is in the *lumbar* spine in the direction of *flexion*.

Trauma → UCM → Pathology → Pain

The UCM can be present within normal ranges of functional motion, hypermobile range or even within a segment with reduced range. It may be identified in the physiological or functional movements of joint range, or it may be identified in the accessory segmental translational gliding movements of a joint.

Movement dysfunction may present as a disorder of translation movements at a single motion segment; for example, abnormal segmental translational motion and/or a range disorder in the functional movements across one or more motion segments, abnormal myofascial length and recruitment or as a response to neural mechanosensitivity (Comerford & Mottram 2001b). These two components of the movement system are inter-related and consequently translation and range UCM dysfunctions often occur concurrently.

UCM often develops to compensate for a loss of motion or restriction and this relationship is illustrated in Table 3.1. The restriction may be associated with limitation of articular translation and a lack of extensibility of the connective tissue (intra-articular or periarticular) at a motion segment. This presents with a loss of translational motion at a joint and is confirmed with manual palpation assessment (Maitland et al 2005). The restriction may be associated with a lack of extensibility of contractile myofascial tissue or neural tissue. The muscles may lose extensibility: i) because of increased low threshold recruitment (overactivity) (Janda 1985; Sahrmann 2002); ii)

Table 3.1 Key elements of UCMs and restrictions		
	Translation	**Range**
Uncontrolled movement	Uncontrolled intra-articular and interarticular joint hypermobility	Uncontrolled range of motion (in myofascial system)
	Articular	**Myofascial**
Restriction	Intra-articular and interarticular joint hypomobility	Lack of myofascial extensibility restricting range of motion

due to a lack of range because of length-associated changes (Gossman et al 1982; Goldspink & Williams 1992); or iii) due to a lack of normal neural compliance and a protective response associated with abnormal neural mechanosensitivity. This restriction is confirmed with myofascial extensibility tests.

If the UCM is translation related, it may be associated with laxity of articular connective tissue and a lack of local muscle control. Panjabi (1992) defined spinal instability in terms of laxity around the neutral position of a spinal segment called the neutral zone. Maitland et al (2005) have described joint hypermobility. The end result of this process is abnormal development of UCM and a loss of functional or dynamic stability. Uncontrolled translation can compensate for three mechanisms of restriction (Table 3.2): i) articular restriction in the same joint (restriction and UCM at an intra-articular level); ii) articular restriction in an adjacent joint (restriction and UCM at an interarticular level); or iii) myofascial restriction (restriction and UCM at a regional level).

If the UCM is range related, it may be associated with elongation or a change in recruitment sequencing of global muscles resulting in a lack of myofascial coordination or a lack of force efficiency of myofascial tissue to control range of motion. This uncontrolled range of movement is a potential compensation for three mechanisms of restriction (Table 3.2): i) myofascial restriction at an adjacent region (restriction and UCM at a regional level); ii) abnormal mechanosensitivity at an adjacent region (restriction and UCM at a regional level); or iii) segmental articular translation restriction at an adjacent joint (restriction and UCM at an interarticular level).

The complex inter-relationships between restrictions and potential compensation strategies can be observed presenting in three distinct ways. These three compensations are detailed in Table 3.2.

1. **Intra-articular UCM**

   The UCM and the restriction may both be in the same joint segment. A loss of translational movement in one direction may be compensated for by increased uncontrolled translation in another direction in the *same joint*. As a result the restriction, the UCM and the pain may all be in the same joint.

   Example 1: the shoulder may have limited A-P (posterior) translation and posterior restriction and compensate with excessive

UCM	CHARACTERISTICS	
	Intra-articular	**Interarticular**
Translational/articular dysfunction	• Occurs within the same joint • In different or opposing directions • Associated with abnormal accessory or translational movement • UCM and restriction primarily involve connective tissue changes *Relates to a displaced path of the instantaneous centre of motion and uncontrolled translation* (Can confirm the articular or translation UCM and restriction by manual palpation assessment and muscle recruitment tests)	• Occurs between adjacent joints • Usually in the same direction
	Regional	
Range/myofascial dysfunction	• Occurs between adjacent regions • In the same direction • Associated with abnormal physiological or functional range • UCM and restriction primarily involve myofascial tissue changes *Relates to relative flexibility – relative stiffness and uncontrolled range* (Can confirm the myofascial/range UCM and restriction with movement analysis and muscle length and recruitment tests)	

Table 3.2 Restriction and compensation relationships that present as UCM

P-A (anterior) translation and anterior overstrain to keep function.

Example 2: C3–4 may have limited A-P (posterior) translation while the same joint segment may have excessive P-A (anterior) translation.

Example 3: the sacroiliac joint that tests positive for motion restriction may have a restriction of anterior glide along the long arm and may have uncontrolled posterior glide along the long arm.

2. **Interarticular UCM**

The UCM may have adjacent joint articular stiffness. A loss of physiological range or translational movement at one joint (in any *one direction*) may be compensated for by increased uncontrolled physiological range or uncontrolled translation at an adjacent joint in the *same direction*. As a result the restriction may be in one joint and the UCM and the pain may all be in an adjacent joint.

Example 1: L4–5 may be restricted in extension or P-A (anterior) direction while L5–S1 may compensate by increasing extension or P-A (anterior) movement.

Example 2: C5–6 may have a restriction of extension and P-A (anterior) translation, which may be compensated for by increased extension and P-A (anterior) translation at C4–5.

Example 3: the left sacroiliac joint may test positive for motion restriction while the right sacroiliac joint may compensate and as a result become the painful side.

3. **Regional UCM**

The UCM may have adjacent joint soft tissue restriction. A loss of physiological range (due to a lack of extensibility or reactivity of myofascial or neural tissue) at one joint region in any *particular direction* may be compensated for by increased physiological range (due to excessive myofascial length or a lack of dynamic control) in an adjacent joint region in the *same direction*. As a result the restriction may be in one joint and the UCM and the pain may all be in an adjacent joint.

Example 1: a lack of extensibility of hamstring muscles contributes to limiting hip flexion range during forward bending. However, function is maintained by excessively increasing lumbar spine flexion range to compensate with resultant

lengthening or overstrain of the spinal extensor muscles (lumbar spinalis and superficial multifidus).

Example 2: a lack of extensibility of glenohumeral lateral rotator muscles (infraspinatus and teres minor) contributes to limiting glenohumeral medial rotation range. However, function is maintained by excessively increasing scapular motion (forward tilt and downward rotation) to compensate with resultant lengthening or overstrain of the scapular stabiliser muscles (middle and lower trapezius).

Example 3: a lack of extensibility of hip flexor muscles (tensor fasciae latae and rectus femoris) contributes to limiting hip extension range. However, function is maintained by excessively increasing lumbar spine extension range to compensate with resultant lengthening or overstrain of the abdominal muscles (oblique abdominis).

Example 4: a lack of extensibility of anterior scalene muscles contributes to limiting lower cervical extension range. However, function is maintained by excessively increasing upper or middle cervical spine extension range to compensate with resultant lengthening or overstrain of the longus colli muscles.

It is possible for translational or range UCM to present in isolation without restriction. Examples of this type of presentation are: i) a traumatic incident (capsular/ligamentous laxity or instability); ii) inhibition associated with pain and pathology; or iii) sustained postural strain positioning.

Integrated model of mechanical movement dysfunction

In a pyramid model of musculoskeletal pain there are several factors that require consideration (Figure 3.3).

The mechanical components of restriction and compensation form the base of the pyramid and the foundation of movement assessment. These mechanical components of the dysfunction need to be evaluated. This includes identifying and understanding the relationships between articular and myofascial restrictions and the compensations that develop to maintain good function. The compensations require more detailed assessment and the ability to actively control

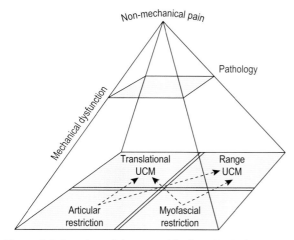

Figure 3.3 Overview of the 'pyramid' of mechanical movement dysfunction

compensations needs to be identified in terms of the site and direction of UCM. The UCM can present as uncontrolled translation which is best controlled by local muscle retraining or uncontrolled range which is best controlled by global muscle retraining. The top of the pyramid involves diagnosing the pain-sensitive tissues that develop in response to being overloaded with compression stresses of tensile strain. If the dysfunction is longstanding (chronic or recurrent), then 'yellow flag' issues also need consideration. 'Yellow flag' issues may include peripheral and central neurogenic sensitisation and behavioural or psychosocial contextual factors that can affect both the perception of pain and the prognosis for symptom change. It is important to relate the site and direction of UCM to symptoms and pathology and to the mechanisms of provocation of symptoms. The dysfunctions can be labelled and classified by the site and direction of UCM and are described in Section 2.

PRINCIPLES OF ASSESSMENT OF UCM

As described earlier in this chapter, tests to identify UCM are based on the concept of dissociation, defined as the ability to control motion at one joint segment while concurrently producing an active movement at another joint segment

(Comerford & Mottram 2001a). The MSI and MCI classification systems rely on observations of aberrant movements during spinal and limb activities and functional tasks. A typical feature of impaired motor control is reduced control of active movement (Luomajoki et al 2007). The assumption is this loss of active control causes physical stress on tissue and leads to pain (Mueller & Maluf 2002).

Neutral training region

Establishment of the neutral training region is a key requirement of the assessment process. The neutral training region is not a single specific point within range. It is a relative region within joint mid-range, within Panjabi's conceptual 'neutral zone', where there is minimal support or restraint of motion from the passive restraints (Panjabi 1992). It may be more appropriate to call this the 'neutral training region' rather than neutral joint position. The 'anatomical or postural ideal' joint position or 'loose pack' joint position is often arbitrarily chosen as the reference for 'neutral'. There is currently debate and lack of consensus as to precisely where this point is. The control of a single static position or point in range is not the answer to normal function where stability is required dynamically at variable points within the whole of the available range of motion. There may be too much emphasis on a single static position when function requires control of more than one isolated point and is never so specific.

The defining characteristic of a motor control test of dissociation that identifies UCM, is the repositioning of the region to be tested in its 'neutral position' by the therapist, which is then maintained as the patient moves the relevant joint either above or below or a joint in the same region in a different direction. The neutral position is controlled by myofascial support (from the interaction of the local and global muscle system – Chapter 2), with minimal support from the passive osteoligamentous system. The passive osteoligamentous system provides considerable support and control of motion at end range when those passive restraints are loaded. Neutral cannot be end of range, just as the neutral position of the lumbar spine is a region between anterior and posterior tilt (Dankaerts et al 2006a). It is crucial for the assessment *and* retraining of motor control that the spine be initially positioned in the neutral training region (O'Sullivan et al 2002; O'Sullivan et al 2006). This supports the concept of the stabilising muscle system working within the neutral zone to support the spine (Panjabi 1992).

Most exercises for retraining movement control, whether performed isometrically or dynamically through range, usually use a recommended starting position. The suggested 'neutral' starting position is best defined as somewhere within the neutral training region, as close as possible to the anatomical or postural ideal alignment. However, if a joint system has significant loss of normal functional range, the 'anatomical ideal' joint position may also be that person's end-range position. In this situation the 'neutral' joint starting position for assessment and retraining of UCM is modified to a place within the region of that person's mid-range where end-range restraints are no longer providing stiffness to support or restrain motion and preferably close to the anatomical or postural ideal alignment.

CLINICAL ASSESSMENT OF UCM

Dysfunction can be evaluated, quantified and compared against a normal measure, ideal standard or some validated benchmark. The measurement of dysfunction, followed by intervention with some form of treatment or therapy over an appropriate timeframe and the reassessment of dysfunction to demonstrate a positive outcome of intervention, provides the framework of good clinical practice. Dysfunction is indirectly related to pathology but as the pathology heals and the symptoms subside, the dysfunction does not always automatically return to a normal baseline.

To date, measurement of motor control-related stability dysfunction has required complex measurement tools (EMG and imaging ultrasound) and highly specific training to use and interpret the results. There has been a need to develop a 'clinic friendly' measurement system that is simple, easy to learn, quick and can be used to assist clinical decision-making about when to progress and when there is no longer a need to continue training a particular exercise or muscle. A rating system for assessment and reassessment of UCM and motor control-related stability dysfunction has been developed to

address this need. This rating system is described in the following section.

Movement control rating system (MCRS)

This MCRS does not rate or measure inhibition of muscle function. A certain amount of inhibition or dysfunction due to pain and pathology is consistent and predictable. These changes are reliable and can be assumed to be present when the pain or pathology are present (Hodges & Richardson 1996; Hodges 2001; Hodges & Moseley 2003; Richardson et al 2004; Falla et al 2004a, b; Jull et al 2004, 2008). Instead, this MCRS evaluates low threshold voluntary recruitment efficiency. It is probable that if low threshold voluntary recruitment efficiency is effective in the presence of pain inhibition, then, when the pain or pathology resolves, the muscle recruitment patterns and thresholds may automatically return to normal (ideal) function. The observation that when some people recover from pathology and their symptoms resolve they return to ideal function and normal physiology without any specific retraining supports this contention. However, if the evaluation of low threshold voluntary recruitment efficiency is poor, then when the pain or pathology resolves, the dysfunction in the muscle physiology is more likely to persist. An assessment of recruitment efficiency would help to determine priorities of clinical management while reassessment helps guide progression.

Two parameters are evaluated in the application of the MCRS. The first parameter tests the ability to correctly perform a specific motor control recruitment pattern or movement. The second parameter assesses the efficiency of low threshold recruitment in the performance of that motor control skill. It is essential that the patient understand the test movement or activation required. To pass the test (✓✓) the subject needs to demonstrate the correct recruitment pattern or movement without substitution (for the first ✓) and demonstrate that it can be easily controlled to benchmark standards without fatigue or high sensation of effort (for the second ✓). Because many of these tests are not habitual or 'familiar' movement skills there needs to be a short learning or familiarisation process before rating the test movement. If the patient fails a test (i.e. rates ✓✗ or ✗✗), it is important that this is because they cannot perform the test, not because they are not sure what to do. Verbal description, visual demonstration, hands-on facilitation and visual or tactile self-feedback should be used to ensure that the patient understands and has experienced the movement or activation required before rating the efficiency of low threshold voluntary recruitment.

> The correction or rehabilitation of motor control dysfunction has been shown to decrease the incidence of recurrence of pain (Hides et al 1996; O'Sullivan et al 1997; Jull et al 2002). Along with symptom management this is a primary short-term goal of therapeutic intervention. The patient frequently becomes symptom-free before dysfunction is fully corrected. Treatment should not necessarily cease just because the symptoms have disappeared if measurable dysfunction persists. A rating system (such as the MCRS) for the assessment and reassessment of dysfunction is necessary to justify this in clinical practice.

Testing for the site and direction of UCM

During all normal functional activities, the muscles that have global stability and local stability roles co-activate in integrated patterns to maintain stability. All functional activities impose stress and strain forces on the movement system in varying loads and in all three planes or directions of motion. Normal functional movements rarely eliminate motion from one joint system while others move through range. Functional movement rarely occurs in only one plane. However, everybody has the ability to perform patterns of movement that are not habitually used in 'normal function' (e.g. pat the head and rub the stomach). Some of these patterns of movement are unfamiliar and feel 'unnatural' precisely because they are not habitual patterns of recruitment.

Low threshold recruitment patterns should be efficient, when stability muscles are recruited to control motion or to produce movement within normal, non-fatiguing functional loads. Normal functional loading includes static holding of postures and dynamic movement through available range of the unloaded limbs and trunk (even in unfamiliar or non-habitual movements). If low threshold recruitment is efficient then there should be a perceived low sensation of effort to perform these normal, non-fatiguing activities.

Performance of some of these unfamiliar movements is a test of motor control (recruitment skill and coordination). The ability to activate muscles to isometrically hold a position or prevent motion at one joint system, while concurrently actively producing a movement at another joint system in a specific direction, is a test of motor recruitment skill. The process of dissociating movement at one joint from movement at another joint, or controlling the pattern or path of movement about the same joint, has potential benefits for retraining the stability muscles to enhance their recruitment efficiency to control direction-specific stress and strain. The global and the local stability muscle systems can be trained to recruit in co-activation patterns to prevent movement in a specific direction at a vulnerable (or unstable) joint while an adjacent joint is loaded in that direction. In this way the stability system can be trained to control a specific UCM (site and direction). Box 3.3 summarises some key points to consider when using dissociation movements to test for UCM or to retrain control of the UCM.

Example of dissociation in 'series'

If the hamstrings lack extensibility and restrict the hips from normal flexion, the lumbar spine can 'give' into increased flexion to compensate during functional forward bending movements. This eventually results in the back extensor stability muscles losing the ability to protect the back from flexion loading stresses. A movement pattern or recruitment skill of keeping the back straight and hinging forwards at the hips is a motor control exercise for the back extensor muscles. By using the back extensor stabiliser muscles to hold the back in a more neutral (mid-range) position and prevent the back from flexing while independent isolated hip flexion is performed, the back extensor muscles are trained to become more efficient at stabilising the spine against flexion stress and strain. This pattern of movement dissociation initially feels unfamiliar for most people and is not part of normal or natural forward bending function, but it is a pattern of movement that everybody has the ability to perform (or learn to perform).

Example of dissociation in 'parallel'

If the tensor fasciae latae exhibits recruitment dominance over posterior gluteus medius at the

Box 3.3 **Key points of dissociation tests and retraining exercises**

- Direction control or 'dissociation' exercises are not usually normal functional movements. These exercises and movements are tests of ability and efficiency of recruitment and motor control. Even though it is accepted that they are not 'normal' functional movements, they are, however, movement skills and motor patterns that everybody should normally be able to perform so long as they are taught and understand the movement pattern.
- Range of movement (even hypermobile range) or a compensation that can be easily controlled actively during a dissociation test is normal and does not highlight UCM or stability dysfunction. However, this could be considered to be hypermobility with good functional control and stability.
- UCM may be present in one or more directions (or planes) of movement at any given joint. That is, any particular site may have UCM in more than one direction.
- The UCM is not always proximal to the restriction. The restriction can be at the trunk or girdle and the compensation or the UCM can be distal.
- Direction control tests and movements are not stretches or strengthening exercises.
- Direction control (dissociation) tests are low threshold (low force and non-fatiguing) and there should be no pain.

hip, instead of flexing in the path of neutral hip alignment, the hip will be pulled into medial rotation, for example during the descending of stairs. This eventually results in the posterior gluteus medius losing the ability to protect the hip from flexion–medial rotation loading stresses. This can result in a hip impingement dysfunction. By using the posterior gluteal muscles to hold the hip in a more neutral (mid-range) alignment during the swing phase hip and knee flexion movements, they can resist the uncontrolled deviation into hip medial rotation. The posterior gluteal muscles are trained to become more efficient at stabilising the hip against flexion–medial rotation stress and strain.

Indications to test for UCM

Observe or palpate for:

1. symptoms (pain, discomfort, strain) associated with specific movement direction

2. hypermobile or excessive range of movement
3. hypermobile or excessive translation during primary movement
4. excessive initiation of compensation during primary movement
5. discrepancies of range in different positions of function.

UCM presents as a lack of ability to perform these dissociation patterns of movement (motor control tests) to benchmark standards. A dissociation test that cannot be actively controlled through appropriate dissociation range (rating ✗✗), or can only be controlled with difficulty (e.g. high perceived or actual effort) (rating ✓✗), is considered to demonstrate UCM and present as a significant stability dysfunction.

During the assessment of the site and direction of UCM there are two steps that can help the clinician with the diagnosis.

1. Observation of natural functional movement to identify:
   (a) restrictions within function – note a loss of range of motion, either segmentally or multisegmentally, during the movement
   (b) hypermobile range – note excessive range of movement at the site that the patient complains of symptoms
   (c) compensatory movement strategies – note abnormal initiation of movement at the site that the patient complains of symptoms
   (d) symptoms (pain, discomfort, strain, etc.) associated with the functional movement.

2. Test for site and direction of UCM. Start with the joint in a neutral or mid-range position and *prevent movement or 'uncontrolled movement'* into the test direction and: (a) move the adjacent joint (above or below) in the same direction; or (b) move the test joint in a different direction. Assess the person's ability to actively control movement in the specified direction (control the UCM) and move independently at the adjacent joint in the direction of the specific stability dysfunction. That is, dissociate movement at one joint from movement at another. This is the aspect that is rated as assessment of recruitment efficiency.

For example, during functional forward bending excessive lumbar flexion is observed as compensation for restricted hip flexion (hamstrings) and lumbar pain is provoked as the lumbar flexion increases. A dissociation test would involve actively keeping the spine straight and preventing lumbar flexion (with active recruitment of the lumbar extensor stabiliser muscles) while bending forwards with isolated and independent hip flexion.

Movement control test procedure

- **Start position.** Position in the person's neutral (mid-range) training region.
- **Teaching the test movement.** The dissociation tests are not natural movements. Consequently, the person needs to be taught the test movement before assessing the quality of active control. The therapist instructs the person in the test dissociation movement, the principle being to control the uncontrolled movement and move the adjacent joint. Teaching skills are key here and include visual, auditory and kinaesthetic cues. For example:
  - visually demonstrate the test movement or action, or help the person visualise the task with the use of imagery
  - verbally explain and describe the test movement or action
  - manually facilitate or 'hands on' guide the person through the test movement or action.
  The therapist facilitates the test action and guides the elimination substitution strategies.
- **Assessment of passive or available range.** The therapist passively stabilises the test region and assesses the passive available range of the test movement.
- **Active learning**. The person actively practises the movement with the necessary cues; for example, visual and palpation feedback, unloading (if required), therapist support ('hands on' facilitation) and verbal correction. Usually, 3–8 repetitions are sufficient for teaching, learning and familiarisation with the test movement. If a person fails the test, it should be because they cannot perform the movement skill to

the benchmark standard, not because they do not understand or have not learnt what to do.
- **Test.** When the therapist is confident that the person understands the test movement or action and knows what is expected, the person is required to perform the test without visual or tactile feedback, verbal facilitation or corrective instruction.
- **Rating.** The therapist then rates the performance of the test. A failure to adequately perform the test movement identifies the site and direction of UCM.
- **Relate dysfunction to symptoms to identify clinical priorities.** Look for a link between the direction of UCM and the direction of symptom provocation:
  - Does the site of UCM relate to the site or joint that the person complains of as the source of symptoms?
  - Does the direction of movement or load testing relate to the direction or position of provocation of symptoms? This identifies clinical priorities.

Using the MCRS

UCM can be present, even if there is no obvious excessive or hypermobile range, if active recruitment of the muscle stability system cannot control movement to the benchmark range. UCM may be non-symptomatic. Even if there is obvious hypermobile range, so long as the control of the benchmark range is efficient there is no significant stability dysfunction. So long as the direction being tested has good control it can achieve a 'pass' (✓✓) rating. (The ability to efficiently control hypermobile range is evaluated during the assessment of 'control of range'.)

If the ability to dissociate and control the UCM throughout the *available* range appears to be efficient but the range available is significantly restricted, then to maintain normal function, stability is sacrificed and compensation for the restriction is required. Note what structure lacks extensibility (if the restriction is obvious) so that direct intervention to regain normal mobility can be commenced. If the restriction is structural and therefore permanent, then there must be compensation elsewhere to maintain function. If the compensation has poor control (UCM) this obviously has implications for ongoing risk of recurrence.

If the available range is excessive (significantly more than the benchmark standard), the dissociation requirements for control of direction are achieved if the subject can demonstrate good motor control of dissociation throughout the benchmark range only. This demonstrates efficient coordination of motor control strategies related to the recruitment pattern required to control direction-specific stress and strain. Control throughout the full hypermobile range is not assessed at this level. That is dealt with by the principles of 'control of range'.

A ✓✗ rating or ✗✗ rating labels or diagnoses the UCM or stability dysfunction. The diagnosis of UCM should label both the **SITE** and the **DIRECTION** of movement that is uncontrolled.

✓✓ = the person demonstrates the correct dissociation movement pattern to the benchmark range and efficient low threshold recruitment

- If **all** requirements for the first ✓ and **all** requirements for the second ✓ are demonstrated, then rate the test as ✓✓.

✓✗ = the person demonstrates the correct dissociation movement pattern to the benchmark range, but inefficient low threshold recruitment

- If the test demonstrates **all** the requirements for the first ✓ but fails **any** of the requirements for the second ✓, then rate the test as ✓✗. Note the reason for the ✗.

✗✗ = the person is unable to demonstrate the correct dissociation movement pattern to the benchmark range

- If there is failure to achieve **all** of the requirements of the first ✓, then rate the test as ✗✗. Note what proportion of benchmark range can be controlled.

Each direction is assessed separately. If during a test of *one specific direction*, UCM into *another direction* is observed, then the stability dysfunction (i.e. site and direction) is at the site of poor control and in the *direction of actual UCM*. For example, if during a test of control of lumbar flexion, the lumbar spine loses control into extension, there is likely to be a problem with stability function for lumbar extension. The ability to control this apparent stability dysfunction should be specifically assessed with extension-related tests. If there was no UCM into flexion, then flexion is not the primary direction of dysfunction.

For clarification purposes, the scoring or rating of each test can be detailed in a rating table (Table 3.3).

Rating interpretation

The first (left) column ✓ relates to correct *pattern* of voluntary dissociation.

The second (right) column ✓ relates to the *efficiency* of low threshold recruitment.

(Always qualify a ✗ rating with the reason for that ✗.)

Clarification of a 'grey' area of interpretation. If movement is observed in the opposite direction and presents only through partial range, for example, a small range of extension is observed while testing flexion control, the flexion control test should be rated as ✓✓. However, if movement in the opposite direction consistently uses end-range positioning to prevent movement in the test direction, for example, if end-range extension is used to prevent flexion, this indicates inefficient control of flexion and poor afferent feedback. This should be rated as ✓✗ for inefficient flexion control.

The therapist should monitor the person's symptom responses to testing for UCM. If symptom provocation can be noticeably reduced by performing movement dissociation, then retraining active movement control with the retraining strategies suggested in this text is likely to have a positive effect on symptom reduction. This response, that is, actively controlling or preventing movement in the provocative direction and achieving symptom relief, further supports the hypothesis that UCM is a significant mechanism in the production of tissue pathology.

Clinical priorities for retraining are determined by identifying the link between the direction of movement provocation and an inability to pass a test of movement control for that direction. For

Table 3.3 Movement control rating system table (Comerford & Mottram 2011)

Control point:
- Prevent: *[site and direction]*
  Movement challenge: *[movement]*
  Benchmark range: *[range]*

RATING OF LOW THRESHOLD RECRUITMENT EFFICIENCY

	✓ or ✗		✓ or ✗
• Able to prevent UCM into the test direction. Correct dissociation pattern of movement Prevent *[site]* of UCM into: *[direction]* and move *adjacent region*	☐	• Looks easy, and in the opinion of the assessor, is performed with confidence • Feels easy, and the subject has sufficient awareness of the movement pattern that they confidently prevent UCM into the test direction	☐ ☐
• Dissociate movement through the benchmark range of *[benchmark]* *(If there is more available range than the benchmark standard, only the benchmark range needs to be actively controlled)*	☐	• The pattern of dissociation is smooth during concentric and eccentric movement • Does not (consistently) use *end-range* movement into the opposite direction to prevent the UCM	☐ ☐
• Without holding breath (though it is acceptable to use an alternate breathing strategy)	☐	• No extra feedback needed *(tactile, visual or verbal cuing)* • Without external support or unloading	☐ ☐
• Control during eccentric phase • Control during concentric phase	☐ ☐	• Relaxed natural breathing *(even if not ideal – so long as natural pattern does not change)* • No fatigue	☐ ☐
CORRECT DISSOCIATION PATTERN		**RECRUITMENT EFFICIENCY**	

example, if lumbar symptoms are provoked by bending forwards and prolonged sitting in a posterior tilted or flexed back posture and if that person also lacks the ability to prevent lumbar flexion while actively flexing the hips, then retraining this movement dissociation becomes a clinical priority for symptom management and for changing recruitment patterns to manage recurrence.

The MCRS is used to diagnose the site and direction of UCM. This will support the clinical reasoning framework and the development of the management plan (Chapter 1). A checklist summarising the complete process from testing UCM through to clinical analysis and rehabilitation is shown in Box 3.4.

The next chapter (Chapter 4) details the application of key principles in the design of therapeutic exercise interventions for the retraining of UCM.

Box 3.4 **Checklist for testing UCM**

Checklist for testing of UCM

Observe the natural or normal pattern of movement. Note relative stiffness: relative flexibility issues or restrictions and compensation.

Teach the test movement or action using visual, auditory and kinaesthetic cues with feedback and support.

Test the person's ability to reproduce the test movement or action without cuing, feedback or support.

Rate the performance of the test in terms of voluntary low threshold recruitment efficiency (✓✓ = good motor control, while ✓✗ or ✗✗ = stability dysfunction) then …

Relate poor performance (✓✗ or ✗✗) to the symptomatic area (high clinical priority).

Rehab is required for stability dysfunction that relates to symptoms or pathology.

REFERENCES

Barr, A., Burden, A., 2009. A comparison of two styles of the football instep kick and their relationship to lumbopelvic stability. 2009 3rd International Conference on Movement Dysfunction in Edinburgh, UK, pp. S33.

Bhalla, S.K., Simmons, E.H., 1969. Normal ranges of intervertebral-joint motion of the cervical spine. Canadian Journal of Surgery 12 (2), 181–187.

Burnett, A.F., Cornelius, M.W., Dankaerts, W., O'Sullivan, P.B., 2004. Spinal kinematics and trunk muscle activity in cyclists: a comparison between healthy controls and non-specific chronic low back pain subjects – a pilot investigation. Manual Therapy 9 (4), 211–219.

Butler, D., Moseley, L., 2003. Explain pain. NOI, Adelaide.

Caldwell, C., Sahrmann, S., Van, D.L., 2007. Use of a movement system impairment diagnosis for physical therapy in the management of a patient with shoulder pain. Journal of Orthopaedic and Sports Physical Therapy 37 (9), 551–563.

Cholewicki, J., McGill, S.M., 1996. Mechanical stability of the in vivo lumbar spine: implications for injury and chronic low back pain. Clinical Biomechanics 11 (1), 11.

Comerford, M., Mottram, S.L., 2001a. Movement and stability dysfunction – contemporary developments. Manual Therapy 6 (1), 15–26.

Comerford, M.J., Mottram, S.L., 2001b. Functional stability re-training: principles and strategies for managing mechanical dysfunction. Manual Therapy 6 (1), 3–14.

Comerford, M.J., Mottram, S.L., 2011. Understanding movement and function – assessment and retraining of uncontrolled movement. Course Notes, Kinetic Control, UK.

Cyriax, J.H., 1980. Textbook of orthopaedic medicine. Volume II. Treatment by manipulation, massage and injection, 10th edn. Ballière Tindall, London.

Dankaerts, W., O'Sullivan, P., Burnett, A., Straker, L., 2006a. Altered patterns of superficial trunk muscle activation during sitting in nonspecific chronic low back pain patients: importance of subclassification. Spine 31 (17), 2017–2023.

Dankaerts, W., O'Sullivan, P.B., Straker. L.M., Burnett. A.F., Skouen, J.S., 2006b. The inter-examiner reliability of a classification method for non-specific chronic low back pain patients with motor control impairment. Manual Therapy 11 (1), 28–39.

DonTigny, R.L., 1997. Mechanics and treatment of the SIJ joint. In: Vleeming, A., Mooney, V., Snijders, C.J., Dorman, T.A., Stoekart, R. (Eds.), Movement, stability and low back pain. Churchill Livingstone, Edinburgh, ch 38.

Dvorak, J., Dvorak, V., 1990. Manual medicine: diagnostics, 2nd edn. Thieme, Stuttgart.

Dvorak, J., Froelich, D., Penning, L., Baumgartner, H., Panjabi, M., 1988. Functional radiographic diagnosis of the cervical spine: flexion/extension. Spine 13 (7), 748–755.

Edwards, B., 1999. Manual of combined movements: their use in the examination and treatment of mechanical vertebral column disorders. Butterworth-Heinemann, Oxford.

Esola, M.A., McClure, P.W., Fitzgerald, G.K., Siegler, S., 1996. Analysis of lumbar spine and hip motion during forward bending in subjects with and without a history of low back pain. Spine 21 (1), 71–78.

Falla, D., Bilenkij, G., Jull, G., 2004b. Patients with chronic neck pain demonstrate altered patterns of muscle activation during performance of a functional upper limb task. Spine 29, 1436–1440.

Falla, D., Jull, G., Hodges, P., 2004a. Patients with neck pain demonstrate reduced electromyographic activity of the deep cervical flexor muscles during performance of the craniocervical flexion test. Spine 29, 2108–2114.

Fritz, J.M., Brennan, G.P., 2007. Preliminary examination of a proposed treatment-based classification system for patients receiving physical therapy interventions for neck pain. Physical Therapy 87 (5), 513–524.

Fritz, J.M., Childs, J.D., Flynn, T.W., 2005. Pragmatic application of a clinical prediction rule in primary care to identify patients with low back pain with a good prognosis following a brief spinal manipulation intervention. BMC Family Practice 6 (1), 29.

Fritz, J.M., Cleland, J.A., Childs, J.D., 2007. Subgrouping patients with low back pain: evolution of a classification approach to physical therapy. Journal of Orthopaediac and Sports Physical Therapy 37 (6), 290–302.

Gibbons, S.G.T., 2005. Muscle function and a critical evaluation. KC MACP, 2nd International Conference on Movement Dysfunction, Edinburgh, UK.

Gibbons, S.G.T., 2007. Clinical anatomy and function of psoas major and deep sacral gluteus maximus. In: Vleeming, A., Mooney, V., Stoeckart, R. (Eds.), Movement, stability and lumbopelvic pain: integration of research and therapy. Elsevier, Edinburgh, part 1, section 1, ch 6.

Goldspink, G., Williams, P.E., 1992. Muscle fibre and connective tissue changes associated with use and disuse. In: Ada, L., Canning, C. (Eds.), Key issues in neurological physiotherapy. Butterworth Heinemann, Oxford, ch 8, pp. 197–218.

Gombatto, S.P., Collins, D.R., Sahrmann, S.A., Engsberg, J.R., Van Dillen, L.R., 2007. Patterns of lumbar region movement during trunk lateral bending in two subgroups of people with low back pain. Physical Therapy 87 (4), 441–454.

Gossman, M.R., Sahrmann, S.A., Rose, S.J., 1982. Review of length-associated changes in muscle. Physical Therapy 62 (12), 1799–1808.

Hamilton, C., Richardson, C., 1998. Active control of the neural lumbopelvic posture; a comparison between back pain and non back pain subjects. In: Vleeming, A., Mooney, V., Tilsher, H., Dorman, T., Snijders, C. (Eds.), 3rd Interdisciplinary World Congress on Low Back Pain and Pelvic Pain, Vienna, Austria.

Harris-Hayes, M., Van Dillen, L.R., 2009. The inter-tester reliability of physical therapists classifying low back pain problems based on the movement system impairment classification system. PM & R 1 (2), 117–126.

Hicks, G.E., Fritz, J.M., Delitto, A., McGill, S.M., 2005. Preliminary development of a clinical prediction rule for determining which patients with low back pain will respond to a stabilization exercise program. Archives of Physical Medicine and Rehabilitation 86 (9), 1753–1762.

Hides, J.A., Richardson, C.A., Jull, G.A., 1996. Multifidus muscle recovery is not automatic after resolution of acute, first-episode low back pain. Spine 21 (23), 2763–2769.

Hides, J., Gilmore, C., Stanton, W., Bohlscheid, E., 2008. Multifidus size and symmetry among chronic LBP and healthy asymptomatic subjects. Manual Therapy 13 (1), 43–49.

Hodges, P.W., 2001. Changes in motor planning of feedforward postural responses of the trunk muscles in low back pain. Experimental Brain Research 141, 261–266.

Hodges, P.W., 2003. Core stability exercise in chronic low back pain. Orthopedic Clinics of North America 34 (2), 245–254.

Hodges, P.W., Moseley, G.L., 2003. Pain and motor control of the lumbopelvic region: effect and possible mechanisms. Journal of Electromyography and Kinesiology 13 (4), 361–370.

Hodges, P.W., Richardson, C.A., 1996. Inefficient muscular stabilisation of the lumbar spine associated with low back pain: a motor control evaluation of transversus abdominis. Spine 21 (22), 2640–2650.

Janda, V., 1985. Pain in the locomotor system – a broad approach. In: Glasgow, E.F. (Ed.), Aspects of manipulative therapy. Churchill Livingstone, Edinburgh, pp. 148–151.

Janda, V., 1986. Muscle weakness and inhibition (pseudoparesis) in low back pain. In: Grieve, G.P. (Ed.), Modern manual therapy of the vertebral column. Churchill Livingston, Edinburgh.

Jones, L.H., Kusunose, R., Goering, E., 1995. Jones strain-counterstrain. Jones Strain-CounterStrain Inc. Boise, ID.

Jull, G.A., 2000. Deep cervical flexor muscle dysfunction in whiplash. Journal of Musculoskeletal Pain 8 (1/2), 143–154.

Jull, G., Kristjansson, E., Dall'Alba, P., 2004. Impairment in the cervical flexors: a comparison of whiplash and insidious onset neck pain patients. Manual Therapy 9, 89–94.

Jull, G., Sterling, M., Falla, D., Treleaven, J., O'Leary, S., 2008. Whiplash, headache and neck pain. Elsevier, Edinburgh.

Jull, G., Trott, P., Potter, H., Zito, G., Niere, K., Shirley, D., et al., 2002. A randomized controlled trial of exercise and manipulative therapy for cervicogenic headache. Spine 27 (17), 1835–1843.

Kaltenborn, F.M., 2003. Orthopedic manual therapy for physical therapists Nordic System: OMT Kaltenborn-Evjenth concept. Journal of Manual and Manipulative Therapy 1 (2), 47–51.

Luomajoki, H., Kool, J., de Bruin, E.D., Airaksinen, O., 2007. Reliability of movement control tests in the lumbar spine. BMC Musculoskeletal Disorders 8, 90.

Luomajoki, H., Kool, J., de Bruin, E.D., Airaksinen, O., 2008. Movement control tests of the low back: evaluation of the difference between patients with low back pain and healthy controls. BMC Musculoskeletal Disorders 9, 170.

McKenzie, R., May, S., 2003. The lumbar spine: mechanical diagnosis and therapy, 2nd edn. Spinal Publications New Zealand, Wellington, New Zealand.

Maitland, G., Hengeveld, E., Banks, K., English, K., 2005. Maitland's vertebral manipulation, 7th edn. Butterworth-Heinemann, Oxford.

Morrissey, D., 2005. Development of the kinetic medial rotation test of the shoulder: a dynamic clinical test

of shoulder instability and impingement. PhD thesis, University of London.

Morrissey, D., Morrissey, M.C., Driver, W., King, J.B., Woledge, R.C., 2008. Manual landmark identification and tracking during the medial rotation test of the shoulder: an accuracy study using three dimensional ultrasound and motion analysis measures. Manual Therapy 13 (6), 529–535.

Mottram, S.L., 2003. Dynamic stability of the scapula. In: Beeton, K.S. (Ed.), Manual therapy masterclasses – the peripheral joints. Churchill Livingstone, Edinburgh, pp. 1–17.

Mottram, S.L., Comerford, M., 2008. A new perspective on risk assessment. Physical Therapy in Sport 9 (1), 40–51.

Mottram, S., Warner, M., Chappell, P., Morrissey, D., Stokes, M., 2009. Impaired control of scapular rotation during a clinical dissociation test in people with a history of shoulder pain. 3rd International Conference on Movement Dysfunction, Edinburgh, UK. Manual Therapy 14 (1), S20.

Mueller, M.J., Maluf, K.S., 2002. Tissue adaptation to physical stress: a proposed 'physical stress theory' to guide physical therapist practice, education, and research. Physical Therapy 82 (4), 383–403.

Mulligan, B.R., 2003. Manual therapy NAGS SNAGS MWMS, etc. Plane View Services, Wellington, New Zealand.

Norlander, S., Nordgren, B., 1998. Clinical symptoms related to musculoskeletal neck-shoulder pain and mobility in the cervico-thoracic spine. Scandinavian Journal of Rehabilitation Medicine 30 (4), 243–251.

O'Sullivan, P.B., 2000. Lumbar segmental instability': clinical presentation and specific stabilizing exercise management. Manual Therapy 5 (1), 2–12.

O'Sullivan, P., 2005. Diagnosis and classification of chronic low back pain disorders: maladaptive movement and motor control impairments as underlying mechanism. Manual Therapy 10 (4), 242–255.

O'Sullivan, P., Dankaerts, W., Burnett, A., Chen, D., Booth, R., Carlsen, C., et al., 2006. Evaluation of the flexion relaxation phenomenon of the trunk muscles in sitting. Spine 31 (17), 2009–2016.

O'Sullivan, P.B., Grahamslaw, K.M., Kendell, M., Lapenskie, S.C., Moller, N.E., Richards, K.V., 2002. The effect of different standing and sitting postures on trunk muscle activity in a pain-free population. Spine 27 (11), 1238–1244.

O'Sullivan, P.B., Twomey, L., Allison, G., 1997. Evaluation of specific stabilising exercises in the treatment of chronic low back pain with radiological diagnosis of spondylosis or spondylolisthesis. Spine 22 (24), 2959–2967.

Panjabi, M.M., 1992. The stabilising system of the spine. Part II. Neutral zone and instability hypothesis. Journal of Spinal Disorders 5 (4), 390–397.

Peng, Q., Jones, R., Shishido, K., Constantinou, C.E., 2007. Ultrasound evaluation of dynamic responses of female pelvic floor muscles. Ultrasound in Medicine and Biology 33 (3), 342–352.

Richardson, C., Hodges, P., Hides, J., 2004. Therapeutic exercise for lumbopelvic stabilization – a motor control approach for the treatment and prevention of low back pain. Churchill Livingstone, Edinburgh.

Roussel, N.A., Nijs, J., Mottram, S., van Moorsel, A., Truijen, S., Stassijns, G., 2009. Altered lumbopelvic movement control but not generalised joint hypermobility is associated with increased injury in dancers. A prospective study. Manual Therapy 14 (6), 630–635.

Sahrmann, S.A., 1992. Posture and muscle imbalance: faulty lumbar-pelvic alignment and associated musculoskeletal pain syndromes. Orthopaedic Division Review Nov/Dec, 13–20.

Sahrmann, S.A., 2002. Diagnosis and treatment of movement impairment syndromes. Mosby, St Louis.

Schafer, A., Hall, T., Briffa, K., 2007. Classification of low back-related leg pain – a proposed patho-mechanism-based approach. Manual Therapy 14 (2), 222–230.

Scholtes, S.A., Gombatto, S.P., Van Dillen, L.R., 2008. Differences in lumbopelvic motion between people with and people without low back pain during two lower limb movement tests. Clinical Biomechics 24 (1), 7–12.

Scholtes, S.A., Van Dillen, L.R., 2007. Gender-related differences in prevalence of lumbopelvic region movement impairments in people with low back pain. Journal of Orthopaedic and Sports Physical Therapy 37 (12), 744–753.

Singer, K.P., Fitzgerald, D., Milne, N., 1993. Neck retraction exercises and cervical disk disease. MPAA Conference Proceedings, Australia.

Sterling, M., Jull, G., Vicenzino, B., Kenardy, J., 2003. Sensory hypersensitivity occurs soon after whiplash injury and is associated with poor recovery. Pain 104 (3), 509–517.

Sterling, M., Jull, G., Vicenzino, B., Kenardy, J., 2004. Characterization of acute whiplash-associated disorders. Spine (Phila Pa 1976) 29 (2), 182–188.

Stokes, M.A., Cooper, R., Morris, G., Jayson, M.I.V., 1992. Selective changes in multifidus dimensions in patients with chronic low back pain. European Spine Journal 1 (1), 38–42.

Torstensen, T.A., Ljunggren, A.E., Meen, H.D., Odland, E., Mowinckel, P., Geijerstam, S., 1998. Efficiency and costs of medical exercise therapy, conventional physiotherapy, and self-exercise in patients with chronic low back pain. A pragmatic, randomized, single-blinded, controlled trial with 1-year follow-up. Spine 23 (23), 2616–2624.

Trudelle-Jackson, E., Sarvaiya-Shah, S.A., Wang, S.S., 2008. Interrater reliability of a movement impairment-based classification system for lumbar spine syndromes in patients with chronic low back pain. Journal of Orthopaedic and Sports Physical Therapy 38 (6), 371–376.

Van Dillen, L.R., Bloom, N.J., Gombatto, S.P., Susco, T.M., 2008. Hip rotation range of motion in people with and without low back pain who participate in rotation-related sports. Physical Therapy in Sport 9, 72–81.

Van Dillen, L.R., Maluf, K.S., Sahrmann, S.A., 2009. Further examination of modifying patient-preferred movement and alignment strategies in patients with low back pain during symptomatic tests. Manual Therapy 14 (1), 52–60.

Van Dillen, L.R., Sahrmann, S.A., Norton, B.J., Caldwell, C.A., Fleming, D.A., McDonnell, M.K., et al., 1998. Reliability of physical examination items used for classification of patients with low back pain. Physical Therapy 78 (9), 979–988.

Van Dillen, L.R., Sahrmann, S.A., Norton, B.J., Caldwell, C.A., Fleming, D., McDonnell, M.K., et al., 2001. Effect of active limb movements on symptoms in patients with low back pain. Journal of Orthopaedic and Sports Physical Therapy 31 (8), 402–413.

Vibe Fersum, K., O'Sullivan, P.B., Kvåle, A., Skouen, J.S., 2009. Inter-examiner reliability of a classification system for patients with non-specific low back pain. Manual Therapy 4 (5), 555–561.

Waddell, G., 2004. The back pain revolution. Churchill Livingstone, Edinburgh.

Watson, P., Kendall, N., 2000. Assessing psychosocial yellow flags. In: Gifford, L. (Ed.), Topical issues in pain 2. Physiotherapy Pain Association. CNS Press, Falmouth, pp. 111–129.

Whittaker, J.L., 2007. Ultrasound imaging for rehabilitation of the lumbo-pelvic region – a clinical approach. Churchill Livingstone Elsevier, Edinburgh.

Woolsey, N.B., Sahrmann, S.A., Dixon, L., 1988. Triaxial movement of the pelvis during prone knee flexion. Physical Therapy 68, 827.

Chapter 4

Retraining strategies for uncontrolled movement

REHABILITATION MANAGEMENT AND RETRAINING

The retraining of efficient control of uncontrolled movement (UCM) will depend on the pattern of the dysfunction and the site and direction of the UCM. From the assessment (as outlined in Chapter 3) the translation and range of UCM and restriction will have been identified. Correcting aberrant motor control and recruitment patterns is the priority in the rehabilitation of the local stability system. Correcting length and recruitment dysfunction is the priority of the global system. Addressing the UCM and restriction is the key to rehabilitation and this principle is covered throughout this text.

As well as dealing with mechanical components of movement dysfunction the pathology must be addressed and non-mechanical issues identified and managed. Dependent upon reported signs and symptoms, local tissues should be assessed to identify the pain-producing or most damaged structure(s). Intervention may include treatment of the pain mechanisms, inflammation and pathology with techniques such as large amplitude manual mobilisations, cryotherapy, heat, active exercise, electrophysiological modalities, neurodynamic techniques, acupuncture, trigger point release, positional release and appropriate medication. These interventions should be supplemented with fitness and exercise programs which are effective approaches for the management of chronic low back pain (Frost et al 1998;

Torstensen et al 1998). Consideration and management of psychosocial factors is also essential in the management of chronic low back pain and other chronic musculoskeletal conditions. Cognitive behavioural approaches have a significant role to play for optimal outcomes in chronic low back pain (Waddell 2004). The more multifactorial the patient's pain presentation is, the more likely a multidisciplinary approach will be required. The clinical reasoning framework to encompass these factors has previously been described in Chapter 1.

Management overview

In the integrated management of musculoskeletal pain there are several factors that require consideration (Figure 4.1).

Firstly, the mechanical components of the dysfunction need to be addressed. These include identifying and understanding the relationships between articular and myofascial restrictions and the compensations that develop to maintain good function. The compensations require more detailed assessment and UCM needs to be identified in terms of the site and direction of UCM. The UCM can present as uncontrolled translation which is best controlled by local muscle retraining or uncontrolled range which is best controlled by global muscle retraining. These restrictions and uncontrolled compensations make up the base of the 'pyramid' of mechanical movement dysfunction. The top of the pyramid involves treating the pain-sensitive tissues to optimise the

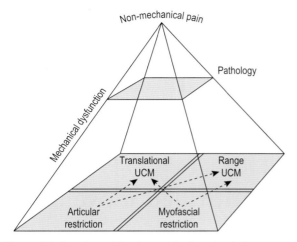

Figure 4.1 Overview of the 'pyramid' of mechanical movement dysfunction

resolution of inflammatory pathology and to promote an optimal healing environment. Finally, if the dysfunction is longstanding (chronic or recurrent), then 'yellow flag' issues also need consideration. Yellow flag issues may include peripheral and central neurogenic sensitisation and contextual factors such as behavioural or psychosocial factors that can affect both the perception of pain and the prognosis for symptom change.

It is important to relate the site and direction of UCM to symptoms and pathology and to the mechanisms of provocation of symptoms. Management of the dysfunction that relates to the symptoms and pathology becomes the clinical priority. UCM that may be evident, but does not relate to symptoms, is not a priority of pathology management. However, it may indicate a potential risk for the future (Mottram & Comerford 2008; Roussel et al 2009). The movement control dysfunction can be labelled and classified by the site and direction of UCM and is described in following chapters.

THERAPEUTIC EXERCISE

Therapeutic exercise within clinical practice is beneficial (Taylor et al 2007). There is evidence that different types of therapeutic exercise are beneficial to many different groups of patients,

including those with osteoarthritis of the knee (Brosseau et al 2003; Pelland et al 2004), chronic low back pain (Hayden et al 2005), shoulder pain (Green et al 2003) and chronic neck pain (Kay et al 2005). Different patients appear to need different therapeutic exercises to manage different therapeutic goals. There are indications that specifically targeted and individualised exercise programs are more beneficial than standardised programs (Stuge et al 2004; Taylor et al 2007). The development of rehabilitation strategies directed at correcting the movement faults, identified by evidence-based assessment, rather than developing rehabilitation strategies based on diagnosis of pathology alone, is gaining recognition and acceptance because patients may present with a similar diagnosis of pathology but differing kinematic mechanisms. However, there remain many examples of exercise programs being developed with the 'one size fits all' ideology. Most of these programs become 'protocols' for 'core stability' training or a particular injury such as patellar malalignment, shoulder instability or a post-surgical protocol.

Protocol-based training regimens can be designed with clear goals, performance targets and structured timeframes and the 'protocol' can be readily disseminated to a large number of people. The developers of these protocols have the unenviable task of producing a program that must be simple yet at the same time comprehensive enough to deal with a wide range of variability in patient presentation and complications. However, it is difficult for one protocol to cover the timeframe from injury to return to high level function (e.g. elite sport).

An inherent weakness with protocol-based training programs is an assumption that all people who use the protocol have, to a large extent, the same problem. Most protocols are designed along a linear framework. That is, there are a series of linear progressions from one skill or stage to the next. Consequently, in the attempt to account for individual differences in presentation (especially if injury and pathology are involved) many protocols are modified or adapted, often many times over. The primary problem then with protocol-based training programs is that they are forced to become 'recipes'. The recipe works well for one particular goal or a 'textbook' presentation of a problem. However, therapists and trainers who regularly work with injured athletes know that they rarely present

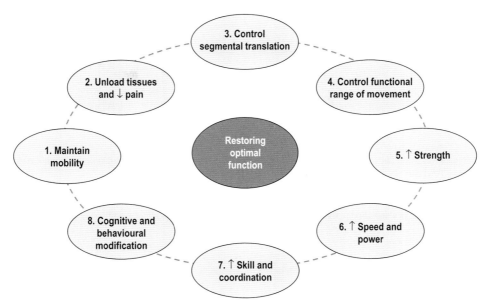

Figure 4.2 A paradigm of therapeutic exercise goals

as the 'textbook case'. Each patient has his or her own variations, complications and differing expectations.

Thus, a paradigm shift is needed towards a process of systematic assessment and analysis that can be used to guide the rehabilitation of dysfunction and retraining of performance deficits. Based on a comprehensive assessment of an individual's deficits, the development of individualised and specific retraining programs to better manage real priorities in injury rehabilitation and performance training can be developed. The subsequent retraining program is designed along a multidimensional and parallel framework, rather than a linear recipe.

When a clinical reasoning process is used in the application of exercise for a therapeutic purpose, several distinct goals can be identified.

Therapeutic exercise can be used to:

1. maintain mobility/flexibility and mobilise restrictions (especially after manual therapy mobilisation or myofascial stretching)
2. manage pain and symptoms (unload or support pain sensitive tissues)
3. control segmental translatatory motion (local muscle system motor control)
4. control aberrant motion – uncontrolled direction or range (global muscle system motor control)
5. recondition and recover from atrophy and tolerate load (increase strength and endurance)
6. cope with speed (produce acceleration and control momentum)
7. train and re-enforce sport-specific skills (skill and coordination)
8. influence mood and sense of wellbeing to assist in the management of behavioural/affective issues.

Figure 4.2 incorporates these goals into a non-linear therapeutic exercise paradigm.

In a clinical situation, a patient may be prescribed an exercise program to achieve one or several goals at the same time. As the condition changes the exercise prescription should progress to match the changing nature of the condition and the goals themselves will change as the condition improves and resolves. Some of the exercise goals may also be incorporated into either a short-term or a long-term maintenance program. These goals should not be prescribed in rigid linear progressions; that is, start with one, then as its aims are achieved, progress to the next one. There seems to be an assumption that the skills acquired with one goal are a necessary prerequisite before starting the next one. This assumption does not have any real evidence base.

Box 4.1 Clinical reasoning steps in therapeutic exercise prescription

- Identify general aim of an exercise process – look at the process (i.e. what the exercise can make a difference to).
- Identify key therapeutic goals that may be helped by exercise (these goals will continually change and evolve as the patient's condition changes).
- Match an exercise process to the immediate therapeutic goals.
- Keep it simple – do not over-complicate the application.
- Where appropriate, work on more than one goal at the same time – integrate and progress along parallel paths.
- Do not use recipes – ensure a clear reason for giving any particular exercise and make sure there is a clear understanding of when the exercise can be stopped or progressed.

Box 4.2 Key factors to be explained with the therapeutic exercise plan

- What is the reason for giving this exercise?
- Is this exercise appropriate for this patient, having considered their presenting symptoms and dysfunction?
- Should the exercise be started now or later?
- What is the exercise dosage? (e.g. For how long? How many repetitions? How often?)
- When can it be progressed?
- When can it be stopped?
- How do I know it is working? What changes should I look for?
- Over what timeframe should I expect to see some change?
- Are there any risks? Can the exercise be provocative or increase symptoms? If so, what is acceptable and what is not?

It is more appropriate and more functional to prescribe therapeutic exercise in parallel combinations based on a clinical assessment and then decide what rehabilitative changes are required and how and when those changes can be implemented. Therapeutic exercise uses movement as a tool to decrease pain, increase joint range and muscle extensibility, to enhance movement performance and to improve wellbeing. The best way to approach therapeutic exercise is to use a clinical reasoning approach. The steps involved in this approach are outlined in Box 4.1. Box 4.2 highlights some key questions that the therapist should be able to answer and justify. These factors should be understood by the therapist prescribing therapeutic exercise and can be explained and supported with the therapeutic exercise plan.

Therapeutic exercise can use movement as a tool to decrease pain, to increase joint range and muscle extensibility, to enhance muscle performance and to promote wellbeing. This and other chapters in this text detail the concept and strategy to 'look at movement'; to be able to make mechanical subclassifications according to site and direction of UCM; relate UCM to symptoms, disability, dysfunction, recurrence, risk and performance; make a clinical diagnosis in terms of site and direction of uncontrolled motion, complaining tissue and presenting pain mechanisms. Rehabilitation will focus on re-establishing control of the site and direction of UCM including functional integration. The key to delivering effective treatment is to understand the principles behind assessment and sound clinical reasoning.

The therapist's clinical decision-making should consider the patient's perspective and interventions should be primarily aimed at those aspects of impairments that have a direct bearing on disability and/or functional limitations. In the subjective examination, patients define their perspective in terms of pain, disability and dysfunction. These factors will be further influenced by contextual factors such as fear of pain/provocation, their coping ability, their work and social requirements, their belief systems, etc.

Therapeutic exercise needs to address real everyday functional limitations; for example, the inability to bend over when tying shoelaces (due to low back pain or the fear of provoking low back pain), or the inability (due to shoulder pain) to reach up to a cupboard. If a patient with low back pain is unable to actively control movements of the low back, especially flexion control while performing a 'waiter's bow' (Luomajoki 2008), then clinicians should aim an intervention at the neuromuscular impairment underpinning this. Likewise, if a patient with shoulder pain is unable to actively control the scapula during functional movements of reaching with the arm (von Eisenhart-Rothe et al 2005; Tate et al 2008), then clinicians should aim an intervention strategy at regaining this control. There is evidence to support the use of movement retraining to gain an improvement in function (Jull et al 2009; Roussel et al 2009b).

Altering movement patterns via exercise can influence clinical signs (Tate et al 2008). However, it is important to establish a clear diagnosis of the movement faults and from this diagnosis develop an appropriate rehabilitation strategy. The therapist requires a sound knowledge of exercise concepts so a patient-specific retraining program can be developed. This is dependent on expertise in the assessment of movement disorders as described in Chapters 1 and 3, and effective clinical reasoning.

THE SITE AND DIRECTION OF UCM

Chapter 3 has detailed the assessment of the site and direction of UCM. The next stage is regaining control of the UCM and integrating this new movement pattern into normal movement and function.

The key goal to effective retraining is to re-establish control of the UCM and regain normal mobility of motion restrictions. The dissociation tests, as described in Chapter 3, are tests of motor control and these establish the site and direction of UCM. If this UCM is related to symptoms, disability, recurrence, risk of injury and performance, a key focus of rehabilitation is regaining the control of movement and changing motor control patterns. The aim is to change the recruitment pattern and actively control movement at the site and in the direction of stability dysfunction. This is a process of sensory-motor reprogramming.

Retraining in control of the site and direction of UCM

- Firstly, position the site of UCM within its neutral training region (as described in Chapter 3) and teach the person how to recruit the appropriate muscles to control a specific direction of movement at this site, while concurrently moving an adjacent joint (above or below) in the same direction (or moving the same segment in a different direction). For example, if the site of the UCM is the lumbar spine, position it in a long shallow mid-range lordosis. If the direction of the UCM is uncontrolled flexion, the therapist instructs the person to control or prevent lumbar flexion while the person flexes forwards independently at the hips, or flexes the thoracic spine independently of any lumbar movement. The person is taught to use whatever feedback helps to monitor and ensure that the lumbar spine does not increase flexion during the retraining exercise.

- The motor control retraining emphasis is focused at the joint and in the direction that movement is isometrically controlled (not where the movement is actively performed). That is, for the lumbar flexion UCM control exercise described above, the lumbar extensor stabiliser muscles are actively recruited to isometrically control lumbar flexion during repetitions of the retraining exercise. The flexion movement at the hip or the thoracic spine creates a flexion loading challenge that the lumbar extensor stabiliser muscles have to work against. Throughout the dissociation retraining movements, local and global stability muscles are continually active to control the UCM.

- The person is taught to move an adjacent joint above or below in the same direction as the UCM, or same joint (in a different direction of the UCM) only as far as:
  - movement is *independent* of the UCM
  - control can be maintained at the site of the UCM
  - any joint or myofascial restriction permits.

- A variety of feedback tools can be employed to teach and facilitate the required retraining movement. These can involve visual feedback (watch the movement), visualisation (including imagery), palpation feedback (with the person's own hands), kinaesthetic feedback (with adhesive tape and skin tension), verbal instruction and verbal correction, and motion monitoring equipment (e.g. pressure biofeedback). Effective cueing is essential for effective retraining.

- Repetitions are required to change motor control patterns. Slow, low effort repetitions are encouraged and movement takes place through the range that the UCM can be actively controlled. A general guide is to perform 20–30 slow repetitions or up to 2 minutes of slow repetitions. Occasionally, the body or limb weight has to be unloaded (supported) so that the stability muscles can control the UCM. As unloaded control gets easier, the training is progressed to controlling the normal functional load of the unsupported limbs or trunk. For example, if lumbar flexion is the UCM and it is difficult to retrain, an early retraining option could be to stand with both hands on a chair or bench top and take partial body weight through the hands. Then, with the weight of the trunk partially supported through the hands, the person is instructed to push the hips away from the bench or chair and try to keep the lumbar spine straight and control lumbar flexion (Figure 4.3). When the ability to perform this retraining exercise is well established, it can be progressed to performing the same strategy without any partial support of the trunk through the hands (Figure 4.4)

- The focus is on the quality of control. Substitution strategies or UCM must be avoided. Again, patient awareness is paramount. Retraining is focused on training motor control of inefficient muscle groups and establishing efficiency of a corrective movement pattern, not on strengthening the dominant muscles.
- The efficiency of control at the UCM is more important initially than the range of motion at the adjacent joint. This movement is practised until it feels familiar and natural. Initially, when these low load exercises 'feel' difficult or a high sensation of effort is perceived, then it is likely that slow motor unit or tonic recruitment is inefficient (see Chapter 2). However, when the same low load exercise starts to feel easy and less unnatural, then it is likely that there is better facilitation of slow motor unit recruitment and improved proprioceptive feedback is becoming established. This is a good clinical indicator of improving stability function and motor control efficiency.
- The aim of this dissociation retraining is to facilitate the active and eventually automatic recruitment of the local and global stability

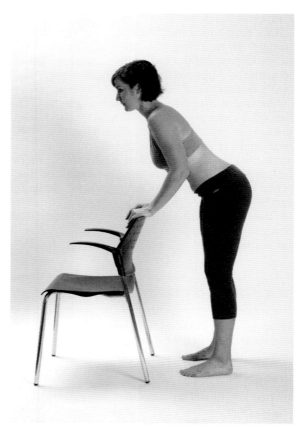

Figure 4.3 Retraining lumbar flexion control with partial support

muscle systems to control movement and by restoring the appropriate use of muscle stiffness to control movement.

- With retraining the person should regain awareness of:
  - alignment and postural position
  - movement precision
  - muscle tension and effort
  - the sensation of 'easy' low load holding
  - multi-joint motion differences.
- This is also linked to improving proprioceptive responses and low threshold recruitment efficiency.
- Encourage normal breathing patterns. People with chronic non-specific low back pain may exhibit altered breathing patterns during tests for UCM (Roussel et al 2009c).
- The therapist needs to educate the person about the concept of movement retraining

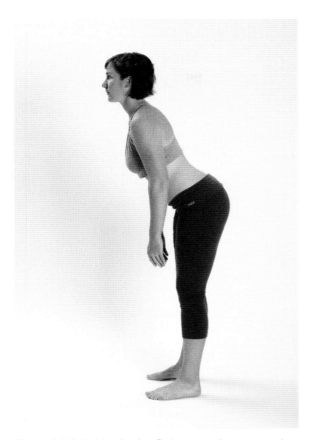

Figure 4.4 Retraining lumbar flexion control unsupported

and emphasise the importance of cognitive input into the retraining process. This promotes a concept of 'mindful' movement. Awareness and concentration is essential. The focus is on retraining the coordination of movement patterns and not the range of movement or the strength of muscle activation. Dissociation exercise is one of many strategies that can be employed in the retraining of movement. The goal is to be mindful of movements during pain-provoking activities.

- None of the corrective exercises to improve dynamic stability should produce or provoke any symptoms at all.
- The speed of progression and prognosis will depend on many factors, including changes in proprioceptive input, chronic pain patterns with sensitisation and behavioural issues and pathology.

- Patients with proprioceptive deficits often:
  - need more supervision and correction to ensure retraining exercises are performed properly
  - experience a high sensation of effort with low load skills
  - are less aware of substitution strategies ('cheating') – they need to rely heavily on 'external' feedback
  - progress through movement control training more slowly
  - do not integrate into automatic unconscious function as easily
  - have a higher incidence of recurrence
  - are more likely to require a long-term maintenance program to stay symptom free.

The key retraining processes and principles are summarised in Box 4.3.

Progression of training the site and direction of UCM

Initially training may begin in an unloaded and supported position but progressed to normal low functional load and unsupported positions. Progression is often challenged by reducing load facilitation (unloading) or by adding a proprioceptive challenge to the stability of the base of support. Balance boards, inflatable discs, Pilates reformer, gym balls and other small equipment can be used to train these movement control patterns by exercising on an unstable base, thereby adding a proprioceptive challenge. Retraining can be further progressed into functional and task-specific situations, discussed later in this chapter.

Management of symptoms using retraining control of the UCM

The therapist should ensure that the person performing the exercise understands the link between the UCM and symptoms/disability so they can use the control strategies to decrease symptoms and improve disability. Regaining the control of movement, which is dependent on a patient-specific exercise program, can be used as a pain control strategy.

Retraining exercises need to be prescriptive, that is, modality-sensitive and dose-specific.

Retraining the motor control patterns to control the site and direction of UCM aims to unload mechanical stress and strain which exceeds tissue tolerance and subsequently has a provocative effect on pain-sensitive structures. This can be seen to have a direct effect on symptoms. Direction control movements can also be used to unload pathology, decrease mechanical provocation of pathology and assist in symptom management. Regaining control of the UCM may be very useful for early symptom control, particularly when UCM has been established as a contributing factor to the development of symptoms. The aim is for the patient to take control of their symptoms, to manage the pain by controlling the UCM themselves and therefore be less dependent on the therapist.

KEY PRINCIPLES IN THE RETRAINING OF MOTOR CONTROL PATTERNS

Motor unit recruitment

Some of the key physiological principles relevant to motor control retraining were described in Chapter 2. From these principles, clinical strategies to facilitate slow motor unit recruitment can be developed. Situations where slow motor unit (SMU) recruitment is preferential to fast motor unit (FMU) recruitment can be utilised in retraining strategies. Conversely, there are situations where FMU recruitment becomes preferential to SMU recruitment. Awareness of these situations allows the therapist to avoid them if they are linked with aberrant movement patterns. These situations are illustrated in Table 4.1.

Retraining strategies to facilitate more efficient SMU recruitment may be beneficial in recovering the detrimental changes to SMU recruitment

---

Box 4.3 **Key features and principles of retraining control of the UCM**

- Position the site of the UCM within the *neutral training region*.
- Train the person to use the stability muscles to control a specific direction of movement at this site and move the adjacent joint (above or below), or move the same site in a different direction.
- Use appropriate visual, auditory and kinaesthetic cues.
- Movement occurs only through the range that:
  - movement is *independent* of the *UCM*
  - stability can be maintained at the *UCM* (isometric control)
  - any joint restriction allows.
- Quality is more important.
- Slow, low effort repetitive movement.
- Perform 20–30 or up to 2 minutes of slow repetitions.
- Unload body or limb weight as necessary to gain control.
- Progress to normal functional load of the unsupported limbs or trunk.
- Practised until it *feels* familiar and natural.
- Retrain awareness of:
  - alignment and postural position
  - movement
  - muscle tension and effort
  - the sensation of 'easy' low load holding
  - multi-joint motion differences.
- Encourage normal breathing patterns.
- It is mindful movement and requires cognitive retraining.
- No pain provocation.
- No co-contraction rigidity, i.e. dominance of the global mobility muscle.

Table 4.1 **Situations of preferential slow or fast motor unit recruitment**

CONDITIONS CONTRIBUTING TO DOMINANT SLOW MOTOR UNIT RECRUITMENT
• Performance of slow non fatiguing movement
• Low force static muscle holding
• Maintain consistency of non fatiguing muscle contraction
• Manage the symptoms of pain and swelling to minimise their inhibitory influence
• Stimulate afferent proprioceptors to facilitate recruitment

CONDITIONS CONTRIBUTING TO DOMINANT FAST MOTOR UNIT RECRUITMENT
• increasing load to the point of fatigue
• fatiguing eccentric exercise
• exercising with a length tension disadvantage (e.g. maximum inner or outer range)
• conscious initiation of fast movements

Box 4.4 **Additional recruitment strategies to facilitate SMU recruitment**

- Increasing or decreasing base of support.
- Adding non-fatiguing low load or facilitatory resistance to stimulate recruitment.
- Co-contraction of other stability muscles.
- Awareness of sensation of effort.
- Change position.
- Unload restriction.
- Increase proprioceptive input.
- Passive support of the UCM.

---

that have been demonstrated to be associated with chronic and recurrent pain (see Chapter 2 for details). A number of these strategies may be incorporated into the retraining program as the patient progresses. Some examples for facilitating SMU recruitment are described in Box 4.4.

Cognitive awareness

Understanding how the site and direction of UCM relates to pain provocation is the initial step in gaining cognitive awareness of how movement can influence pain. Patient education should include information to promote awareness of their own UCM and:

- develop an understanding of the retraining movement strategy and why it will help symptoms and recurrence
- demonstrate an ability to perform the retraining movement strategy
- learn to judge when they are controlling the UCM and when they lose control.

This knowledge can lead directly into developing strategies for increasing proprioception and awareness and retraining more appropriate movement patterns.

The effect of posture on retraining

Clinically maintaining a position of neutral alignment will enhance the outcome of movement fault retraining (Comerford & Mottram 2011). There has been some evaluation of this in the literature. For example, Falla et al (2007) noted an increase in activity of the deep cervical flexors when sitting in a posture which facilitated a position of neutral spinal orientation. O'Sullivan (2002) also reported that passive postures (e.g.

slump sitting and sway back) inhibit muscle function that provides spinal stabilisation.

The integration of specific recruitment retraining into function is discussed in the following section.

CHALLENGES IN RETRAINING NEUROMUSCULOSKELETAL DYSFUNCTION

It is frequently observed that patients with chronic or recurrent musculoskeletal conditions are often labelled as having 'non-specific' low back, neck or hip pain. This label is used in many systematic reviews and meta-analyses. The label 'non-specific' pain, is used when no single particular patho-anatomical process can account for the patient's symptoms. These patients frequently become frustrated and disillusioned with the search for a diagnosis and complain that 'no one knows what's wrong with them'. They may have seen many different health care practitioners who have, between them, diagnosed (usually correctly) many different tissues as a cause of their symptoms. This should not be surprising if someone has UCM contributing to their symptoms. UCM can increase compression or impingement of tissues on one side of a joint while concurrently increasing tensile strain within tissues on the other side of a joint. If this UCM is not managed and the related tissue stress and strain is sustained or repeated beyond the limits of tissue tolerance, multiple tissues eventually develop pathological changes and a combination of symptoms develop. These patients have usually already experienced that the model of treating one symptom-producing tissue (of the multiple involved) does not resolve the problem.

If presented with the opportunity to take a different approach to the model that has consistently failed them in the past, patients with chronic pain may appear more motivated to explore the possibility of a different treatment model. If they are educated about the link between UCM and their symptoms, and if they can learn to regain control of the site and direction of the UCM, then the tissues that have been undergoing provocative stress and strain are now unloaded and are allowed a chance to heal and recover. The body has a remarkable ability to heal itself if it is given the opportunity. This model is a paradigm shift for many therapists – by managing the dysfunction and regaining control of the UCM, the symptoms are affected in a positive way.

Once the site and direction of UCM has been identified, and is considered a significant factor in the presentation, then correction of the faulty movement strategy (site and direction of UCM) is the focus of rehabilitation (Roussel et al 2009). This is not easy, but a clinical reasoning approach, as described in Chapter 1 and earlier in this chapter, is essential if a good outcome is to be achieved. Box 1.4 in Chapter 1 described the analysis and clinical reasoning of movement faults with 10 key points to understanding the relationship between movement and pain. Figure 4.1 illustrates a paradigm of therapeutic exercise goals and Box 4.1 outlines the clinical reasoning steps in therapeutic exercise prescription.

The main focus should be on addressing the four criteria of pain and dysfunction – as detailed in 'clinical reasoning in a diagnostic framework' (Chapter 1). UCM may or may not be a significant component. If UCM is a significant component, then retraining control of the dysfunction/impairment should be the key focus rather than administering a non-specific rehabilitation protocol. Motor control dysfunction has been identified in elite, highly trained individuals highlighting the need to be able to identify this dysfunction (Hides et al 2008) rather than non-specific retraining. Chapter 3 described the assessment of UCM and this chapter has outlined retraining principles and strategies (i.e. retraining control of the site and direction of UCM). This is often started in a supported and non-functional position. This non-functional retraining is often necessary to establish recovery of efficient low threshold recruitment. Once this is achieved, progression into functional postures and positions is essential.

INTEGRATION INTO FUNCTIONAL TASKS AND ACTIVITIES

Functionally orientated exercises should be incorporated as early as possible to ensure both the feedforward and feedback mechanisms can be integrated with the appropriate motor pattern. It is important to vary the task being carried out to ensure cortical connections are developed – for example control of direction retraining in functional situations – as patients presenting with musculoskeletal problems may have altered cortical maps and practice may be able to reverse these changes, reinforcing the need to take rehabilitation into function (Van Vliet & Hennigan 2006). Habitual movement patterns and postures have facilitatory influences on the central nervous system (CNS) and re-enforcement of these patterns of recruitment produces long-lasting neuroplastic changes. These patterns become so efficient that we unconsciously use them automatically in normal function. Likewise the absence or the loss of certain movement patterns or postures results in adverse neuroplastic change and the CNS appears to virtually 'forget' them so that we are unable to use them efficiently in automatic or normal function unless we cognitively think about what we are doing.

Other clinicians and researchers advocate the integration of movement retraining into functional tasks (O'Sullivan et al 1997; Jull et al 2002; Stuge et al 2004; O'Sullivan & Beales 2007) and have demonstrated the clinical effectiveness and importance of the integration of the retraining movement control and specific stability muscle activation into functional movements, activities of daily living and even to high load activity and provocative positions.

Evidence suggests that postural habits can change automatic muscle activation patterns in unsupported sitting (Dankaerts et al 2006) and this supports the belief that movement patterns need to be established in daily function and habits. This is particularly important in standing as sway postures have been shown to inhibit the automatic recruitment of stability muscles (O'Sullivan et al 2002). Falla et al (2008) have demonstrated that retraining specific recruitment of the deep neck flexors does not automatically change muscle activity in sternocleidomastoid (SCM) in an untrained functional task, suggesting retraining needs to take place in functional positions with modification through retraining of functional activities.

The first goal should be establishing the correct movement pattern or recruitment strategy; that is, regaining control of the UCM and then progression by integrating the control of movement into functional activity. As a general rule, retraining should take place in functional positions but if this demonstrates unwanted substitution strategies then specific retraining is required as detailed earlier in this chapter. It has been shown that 'non-functional' retraining can affect dysfunction; for example, a persistent improvement in the feedforward activation of transversus abdominis can be achieved with training of isolated voluntary contraction (Tsao et al 2008). This study suggests that motor learning had occurred and changes been made within the CNS established, which can then be accessed during a functional task.

Figure 4.5 illustrates the progression of retraining *the site and direction* of UCM. If a patient is unable to demonstrate efficient active control of the UCM then rehabilitation needs to be directed towards training, highly specific, non-functional movement patterns and strategies (such as dissociation exercise) to regain control of the site and the direction of the UCM. Training the ability to demonstrate efficient active control of the site and the direction of the UCM ideally should be present before progressing into functional integration. Functional movements use the strategies and movement patterns that are currently automatically used. If these current strategies and movement patterns are already associated with pain and dysfunction, then functional integration, if emphasised too soon in a rehabilitation program, may contribute to maintaining these aberrant patterns of movement. Alternatively, if the patient can demonstrate efficient active control of the site and direction of the UCM (or

has retrained this control), then rehabilitation can be progressed earlier and fast-tracked into functional integration.

The process of stability retraining involves elements of motor learning, movement awareness and proprioception, skill acquisition and neural plasticity. Figure 4.6 illustrates the pathway of correcting UCM with clinical assessment and retraining and finally integration into function.

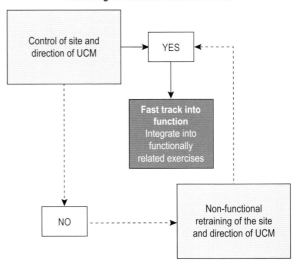

Retraining the site and direction of UCM

Figure 4.5 Flow diagram for the integration of UCM retraining into function

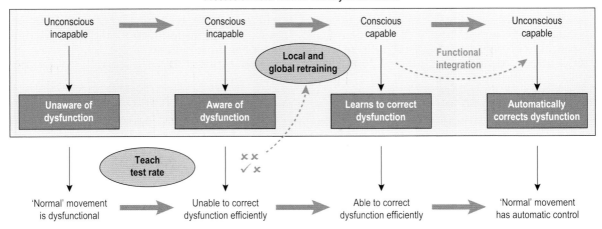

Process of motor control stability rehabilitation

Figure 4.6 The process of regaining conscious and eventual automatic control of the site and direction of uncontrolled movement (adapted Strassl)

Initially, the person with chronic or recurrent musculoskeletal pain, who has aberrant patterns of recruitment, is unaware that they have UCM contributing to their pain. The way they move feels 'normal' to them, even thought it hurts. Their 'normal' movement is dysfunctional. They lack conscious awareness of the problem and they are unable to recruit a corrective strategy. On clinical assessment of the UCM using the movement control rating system (see Chapter 3) they achieve a score of ✗✗.

After clinical assessment of the UCM the person is now aware of the dysfunctional pattern of movement, but is still often unable to correct the aberrant movement pattern. However, with some time spent retraining the aberrant movement, the person learns to correct the dysfunction. They are now conscious of the UCM but are now able to correct the movement efficiently. They can tell the difference between good control and poor control of the UCM. On clinical assessment of the UCM using the movement control rating system they achieve a score of ✓✓.

Although cognitive control of the UCM may be effective while the person is actively thinking about how to perform the corrective exercise, it does not necessarily mean that this correction automatically integrates into normal functional movement. For some people this integration does occur automatically, but for many people this integration is not automatic and requires some functional integration training. The ideal end result is that their normal functional movement has automatic control. By this time, they do not have to consciously think about correcting the UCM.

Motor control retraining can be effective in altering specific motor control deficits identified in people with low back pain (O'Sullivan et al 1997a, 1998), cervical pain (Jull et al 2000), sacroiliac joint pain (O'Sullivan et al 2007), headaches (McDonnell et al 2005; Van Ettekoven & Lucas 2006; Amiri et al 2007), knee pain (Cowan et al 2002), and can positively influence symptoms (Cowan et al 2002) and disability (Stuge et al 2004; McDonnell et al 2005; Jull et al 2009).

Personality and behavioural traits for motivation and compliance

One of the greatest challenges facing the therapist is the integration of specific training regimens into functional activities and automating recruitment. Of the four key criteria highlighted within the clinical reasoning framework described in Chapter 1, the assessment and management of contextual factors is critical here. Because of individual behavioural traits and psychosocial factors there is no single strategy that is appropriate for everyone. We have attempted to categorise various approaches in order to identify a processes that can accommodate individual differences in motivation and compliance.

Some patients benefit from a very structured process with very clear goals and progressions. Other patients, however, do better with a non-structured, more flexible process with an end goal but without a rigid step-by-step pathway. Some patients respond to specific motor control retraining where they think about, try to feel or visualise a specific muscle activating. Other patients do not seem to be able to do this but appear to get the correct recruitment when they do not think about a specific muscle. Instead they seem to use non-specific motor control strategies such as correcting alignment or posture, controlling the site and direction of UCM, achieving a certain position or moving in a certain way to get the recruitment required.

Various combinations of structured or non-structured approaches with specific or non-specific processes (Figure 4.7) can be used to optimise motivation and compliance in the performance of therapeutic exercise and movement retraining.

By finding the right combination of structured or non-structured and specific or non-specific motor control retraining strategies, the therapist has many options available to find a combination that will maintain motivation and achieve compliance for most patients.

Several applications of these options are presented below.

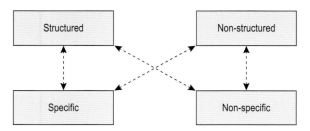

Figure 4.7 Strategies to enhance motor control retraining

Red dot functional integration

Rothstein (1982) has suggested that to integrate an activity or skill into normal, automatic or unconscious function many repetitions must be performed under diverse functional situations. To do this, some form of 'reminder' is needed. He has proposed that small 'red dots' placed so that they are frequently seen will 'remind' the subject to perform a specific task each time they are observed.

When the red dot is sighted, the subject is reminded to actively control the site and direction of UCM (or to perform a specific muscle activation strategy). This process is repeated each time that a red dot is sighted. Place red dots in appropriate positions (e.g. wristwatch, clock, telephone, coffee/tea making area, office drawer, bathroom mirror, red traffic light). Auditory (e.g. phone ringing), time-specific or activity-related reminders may be similarly appropriate.

Low load (facilitatory) proprioceptive stimulus

Providing a proprioceptive challenge can be a useful facilitation and progression strategy. The aim here is to facilitate stability muscle recruitment around neutral joint positions with automatic postural reflex responses and use unstable bases of support. The eyes are open for initial training but as control improves the eyes can be closed to rely on the muscle system for proprioception. A balance board, the 'Pilates reformer' and the 'physio ball' are also appropriate and useful tools.

Integrative dissociation

Once the basic recruitment skill to actively control the site and direction of UCM has been established, this strategy of controlling the region of dysfunction is incorporated with functionally orientated exercises where, so long as the problem region is controlled, any other movement is appropriate. This can be built into an exercise program or just simply control the UCM while performing functional tasks.

Other approaches

Many other approaches used in clinical practice have great potential to assist the control of the

Box 4.5 Alternative approaches useful in the retraining of UCM

Tai chi
Alexander technique
Pilates
Yoga
Physio ball
Feldenkrais
Gyrotonic

site and direction of the UCM once the basic motor control recruitment has been established. Box 4.5 lists some of these approaches.

The Pilates method was initially popularised by the dance community. It is a unique method incorporating body awareness and movement control and is based on established principles (Isacowitz 2006). These are integrated with the repertoire and recent literature has demonstrated evidence supporting the value of many of these principles. Table 4.2 illustrates evidence to support some of them.

Therapists can develop skills in motor control retraining and core stability training by understanding and applying the principles, repertoire and adaptations of Pilates; for example:

- Language is client friendly and facilitatory; for example, 'tuck your chin in' may be less effective than the thought of 'lengthening through the back of the neck'.
- Cues that target the auditory, kinaesthetic and visual learning.
- Cues can work on the somatic mind–body integration (e.g. 'float, soften, and lengthen'). These cues encourage the 'letting go' of the global mobility muscles. In the literature these muscles have been shown to be dominant and overactive under low threshold (functional) loading (Hungerford et al 2003; Falla et al 2004; Richardson et al 2004).
- Eccentric control is emphasised and this is a requirement for good postural control.
- Maintaining control of the 'centre' is the key for controlled movement. Joseph Pilates called it the 'powerhouse' and advocated bracing – this is appropriate for high loads but a modified activation of the abdominals is more appropriate for low load activity.

Table 4.2 Consistencies between Pilates principles and neuromusculoskeletal research	
Concentration	Moseley (2004) has demonstrated a link between pain cognition and physical performance. A higher sensation of effort (concentration) is required in subjects with proprioceptive deficits for efficient activation of slow motor units (Grimby & Hannerz 1976).
Breath	O'Sullivan et al (2002) have identified altered motor control strategies and alteration of respiratory function in subjects with sacroiliac joint pain. Roussel et al (2009c) have demonstrated low back pain patients exhibit altered breathing patterns during performances in which trunk stability muscles are challenged.
Alignment	O'Sullivan et al (2002) have demonstrated that the lumbopelvic stabilising musculature is active in maintaining optimally aligned erect postures, and these muscle are less active during passive postures (slump sitting and sway standing).
Centre/control	Van Dillen et al (2009) examined the effect on symptoms of altering the patient's habitual movements and alignments of the lumbar spine. There was a significant reduction in symptoms when the lumbar spine is supported in neutral during direction-specific tests.

- Maintaining appropriate alignment during movement facilitates appropriate recruitment.
- A focus on breath control can help encourage slow motor unit recruitment and retrain dysfunction.
- Flowing movements require efficient motor control.
- A 'repertoire' of linked multi-joint movements influences the whole body rather than just one segment.
- Concentration encourages the mind–body connection.
- The mind–body connection can influence pain (Moseley 2004).

- Joseph Pilates promoted the influence of 'mind, body and spirit'. 'It's the mind that builds the body.'
- Motor control learning is mindful exercise, requiring the development of awareness through concentration and focus.
- Its popularity may influence compliance.

The Pilates method traditionally focused on high load retraining, but in recent years this has been modified to include low threshold motor control training for the rehabilitation environment. Effectiveness of this approach has been demonstrated by Rydeard et al (2006).

Use of training tools/equipment

The objective of training is to retrain the UCM to effect symptoms, disability and dysfunction. The use of tools and equipment to enhance the control of movement is of great value to clinicians (e.g. body blade, Pilates reformer, and gym ball). However, the appropriate use of these tools is paramount and they should only be used to enhance the retraining process. Close observation of technique and control of movement are essential if these tools are to be an effective adjunct to retraining with the elimination of substitution strategies (Moreside et al 2007). One key point to remember is when retraining UCM, low load (low threshold slow motor unit dominant recruitment) is paramount and although it seems that the easy progression is to add load or resistance to the exercise, this may not be an optimal progression initially for retraining control of the UCM. Low load retraining is best progressed by challenging low threshold recruitment (taking away load), not by adding load or by cognitive activation in the presence of a proprioceptive challenge.

Manual therapy

The value of integrating manual therapy techniques into the management of movement dysfunction must not be overlooked. Jull et al (2002) have demonstrated the value of manual therapy in the management of headaches. There is some evidence that spinal manipulative therapy (SMT) can change the functional activity of trunk muscles in people with low back pain (LBP), suggesting that SMT can have an effect on motor neurone excitability (Ferreira et al 2007). The mechanism of how this may happen is unclear but could be a useful clinical tool assisting in helping change motor recruitment patterns. Indeed this research supports the need for a multimodal effect.

Mulligan's Mobilisations with Movement (MWM) is a manual therapy treatment technique in which a manual force, usually in the form of a joint glide, is applied to a motion segment and sustained while a previously impaired action (e.g. painful movement) is performed (Vicenzino et al 2009). These techniques may well assist in restoring normal movement patterns and have been shown to have an effect on the management of musculoskeletal conditions (Vicenzino 1993; Exelby 2001; Folk 2001; Vicenzino et al 2009) but the mechanisms to date are poorly understood.

Skin taping (e.g. adhesive sports tape, kinesio tape) can be a useful tool to facilitate recruitment or control UCM (Constantinou & Brown 2010).

How long does training take?

The literature suggests that a training period of 8–20 weeks is necessary to change automatic 'unconscious' motor control patterns (Stuge et al 2004; O'Sullivan & Beales 2007) and have a long-term effect on automatic or unconscious 'normal' function (Jull et al 2002; Stuge et al 2004). The therapist is reminded that the training period will also be influenced by interactions between the patient's health condition and contextual (environmental and personal) factors (Chapter 1).

Movement control retraining

The movement control rating system (MCRS) is used to diagnose the site and direction of UCM. This will support the clinical reasoning framework and the development of the management plan (Chapter 1).

There are three key processes involved in managing UCM (Table 4.3):

1. retrain control of the site and direction of the UCM
2. retrain control of translation associated with the UCM
3. correct recruitment and length imbalances associated with the UCM.

CONCLUSION

It is clear that there is a need to identify subgroups within our patients who present with pain, dysfunction, disability and contextual

Table 4.3 Three key processes for the retraining of UCM		
Control of the site and direction of UCM		Retrain control of the stability dysfunction in the direction of symptom-producing movements. Use the low load integration of local and global stabiliser recruitment to control and limit motion at the segment or region of UCM and then actively move the adjacent restriction. Only move through as much range as the restriction allows or as far as the UCM is dynamically controlled.
Control of translation		Retrain tonic, low threshold activation of the local stability system to increase muscle stiffness and train the functional low load integration of the local and global stabiliser muscles to control the neutral joint position.
Control of imbalance	Retrain global stabiliser control through range	Retrain the global stability system to actively control the full available range of joint motion. These muscles are required to be able to actively shorten and control limb load through to the full passive inner range of joint motion. They must also be able to control any hypermobile outer range. The ability to control rotational forces is an especially important role of global stabilisers. Eccentric control of range is more important for stability function than concentric work. This is optimised by low effort, sustained holds in the muscle's shortened position with controlled eccentric lowering.
	Regain extensibility and inhibit excessive dominance of the global mobilisers	When the two-joint global mobility muscles demonstrate a lack of extensibility due to overuse or adaptive shortening, compensatory overstrain or UCM occurs elsewhere in the kinetic chain in an attempt to maintain function. It becomes necessary to lengthen or inhibit overactivity in the global mobiliser muscles to eliminate the need for compensation to keep function.

Box 4.6 **Key factors to help the therapist retrain UCM in practice**

- Use clinical reasoning to help you with the decision-making process (Chapter 1).
- Work on your observation skills and review again once you have established the site and direction test results – this will help you confirm what you see.
- Be specific with your training and exercise prescription.
- Ensure your patient understands the link between UCM and their presenting signs and symptoms.
- Discuss the diagnostic framework with them and how each component relates to their symptoms:
  - site and direction of UCM
  - presenting pathology and symptomatic tissues
  - pain mechanisms
  - contextual factors.

- Use this knowledge to empower the patient to better manage their own condition.
- Consider how the local and global muscle function contributes to the control of movement.
- Consider carefully how you prioritise your management – symptoms, disability and dysfunction need to be addressed at the same time.
- Use the same principles to address risk of injury and performance issues related to movement dysfunction (Mottram & Comerford 2008).
- Remember facilitating and retraining movement is a skill and needs practice! … and gaining compliance is an art as much as a science.
- Consider how you can adapt the retraining to suit the patient with tools and other retraining approaches (e.g. Pilates).

psychosocial factors that influence their function and lifestyle. If UCM is a feature in presentation of the symptoms, dysfunction, disability, recurrence, risk of injury and performance issues, then an appropriate assessment and retraining is appropriate. Box 4.6 highlights some key practical guidelines.

The following section (Chapters 5–9) details a comprehensive assessment of UCM for the lumbar spine, cervical spine, thoracic spine shoulder and hip. These chapters have been written to be used as clinical reference guides as well as for academic study and for use on movement analysis and training courses. To this end, there is a certain amount of repetition in the description of each movement test and retraining. This repetition maintains consistency and completeness while allowing the user to quickly refer to any movement test and its retraining options and access all of the relevant information without having to search for background information at the beginning of each chapter.

REFERENCES

Amiri, M., Jull, G., Bullock-Saxton, J., Darnell, R., Lander, C., 2007. Cervical musculoskeletal impairment in frequent intermittent headache. Part 2: subjects with concurrent headache types. Cephalalgia 27 (8), 891–898.

Brosseau, L., Macleay, L., Welch, V., Tugwell, P., Wells, G.A., 2003. Intensity of exercise for the treatment of osteoarthritis. Cochrane Library Issue 2, Update Software, Oxford.

Comerford, M.J., Mottram, S.L., 2010. Understanding movement and function – assessment and retraining of uncontrolled movement. Course Notes, Kinetic Control, UK.

Constantinou, M., Brown, M., 2010. Therapeutic taping for musculoskeletal conditions. Churchill Livingstone, Edinburgh.

Cowan, S.M., Bennell, K.L., Crossley, K.M., Hodges, P.W., McConnell, J., 2002. Physical therapy alters recruitment of the vasti in patellofemoral pain syndrome. Medicine and Science in Sports and Exercise 34 (12), 1879–1885.

Dankaerts, W., O'Sullivan, P., Burnett, A., Straker, L., 2006. Differences in sitting postures are associated with nonspecific chronic low back pain disorders when patients are subclassified. Spine 31 (6), 698–704.

Exelby, L., 2001. The locked lumbar facet joint intervention using mobilisations with movement. Manual Therapy 6 (2), 116–121.

Falla, D., Bilenkij, G., Jull, G., 2004. Patients with chronic neck pain demonstrate altered patterns of muscle activation during performance of a functional upper limb task. Spine 29 (13), 1436–1440.

Falla, D., O'Leary, S., Fagan, A., Jull, G., 2007. Recruitment of the deep cervical flexor muscles during a postural-correction exercise performed in sitting. Manual Therapy 12 (2), 139–143.

Falla, D., Jull, G., Hodges, P., 2008. Training the cervical muscles with prescribed motor tasks does not change muscle activation during a functional activity. Manual Therapy 13 (6), 507–512.

Ferreira, M.L., Ferreira, P.H., Hodges, P.W., 2007 Changes in postural activity of the trunk muscles following spinal manipulative therapy. Manual Therapy 12 (3), 240–248.

Folk, B., 2001. Traumatic thumb injury management using mobilization with movement. Manual Therapy 6 (3), 178–182.

Frost, H., 1998. Exercise for patients with low back pain. Spine 23 (4), 508.

Green, S., Buchbinder, R., Hetrick, S., 2003. Physiotherapy intervention for shoulder pain. Cochrane Library Issue 2, Update Software, Oxford.

Grimby, L., Hannerz, J., 1976. Disturbances in voluntary recruitment order of low and high frequency motor units on blockades of proprioception afferent activity. Acta Physiologica Scandinavica 96, 207–216.

Hayden, J.A., van Tulder, M.W., Tomlinson, G., 2005. Systematic review: strategies for using exercise therapy to improve outcomes in chronic low back pain. Annals of Internal Medicine 142 (9), 776–785.

Hides, J.A., Stanton, W.R., McMahon, S., Sims Richardson, C.A., 2008. Effect of stabilization training on multifidus muscle cross-sectional area among young elite cricketers with low back pain. J Orthop Sports Phys Ther 38 (3), 101–108.

Hungerford, B., Gilleard, W., Hodges, P., 2003. Evidence of altered lumbopelvic muscle recruitment in the presence of sacroiliac joint pain. Spine 28 (14), 1593–1600.

Isacowitz, R., 2006. Pilates. Champaign, IL: Human Kinetics, pp. 1–42.

Jull, G., Trott, P., Potter, H., Zito, G., Niere, K., Shirley, D., et al., 2002. A randomized controlled trial of exercise and manipulative therapy for cervicogenic headache. Spine 27 (17), 1835–1843.

Jull, G.A., Falla, D., Vicenzino, B., Hodges, P.W., 2009. The effect of therapeutic exercise on activation of

the deep cervical flexor muscles in people with chronic neck pain. Manual Therapy 14 (6), 696–701.

Kay, T.M., Gross, A., Goldsmith, C., Santaguida, P.L., Hoving, J., Bronfort, G., 2005. Exercises for mechanical neck disorders. Cervical Overview Group. Cochrane Database Systematic Review July 20 (3), CD004250.

Luomajoki, H., Kool, J., de Bruin, E.D., Airaksinen, O., 2008. Movement control tests of the low back: evaluation of the difference between patients with low back pain and healthy controls. BMC Musculoskeletal Disorders 9, 170.

McDonnell, M.K., Sahrmann, S.A., Van, D.L., 2005. A specific exercise program and modification of postural alignment for treatment of cervicogenic headache: a case report. Journal of Orthopaedic and Sports Physical Therapy 35 (1), 3–15.

Moreside, J.M., Vera-Garcia, F.J., McGill, S.M., 2007. Trunk muscle activation patterns, lumbar compressive forces, and spine stability when using the bodyblade. Physical Therapy 87 (2), 153–163.

Moseley, G.L., 2004. Evidence for a direct relationship between cognitive and physical change during an education intervention in people with chronic low back pain. European Journal of Pain 8 (1), 39–45.

Mottram, S.L., Comerford, M., 2008. A new perspective on risk assessment. Physical Therapy in Sport 9 (1), 40–51.

O'Sullivan, P.B., Twomey, L., Allison, G., 1997. Evaluation of specific stabilising exercises in the treatment of chronic low back pain with radiological diagnosis of spondylosis or spondylolisthesis. Spine 22 (24), 2959–2967.

O'Sullivan, P., Twomey, L., Allison, G., 1998. Altered abdominal muscle recruitment in back pain patients following specific exercise intervention. Journal of Orthopaedic and Sports Physical Therapy 27(2): 114–124

O'Sullivan, P.B., Grahamslaw, K.M., Kendell, M., Lapenskie, S.C., Moller, N.E., Richards, K.V., 2002. The effect of different standing and sitting

postures on trunk muscle activity in a pain-free population. Spine 27 (11), 1238–1244.

O'Sullivan, P.B., Beales D.J., 2007. Changes in pelvic floor and diaphragm kinematics and respiratory patterns in subjects with sacroiliac joint pain following a motor learning intervention: a case series. Manual Therapy 12 (3), 209–218.

Pelland, L., Brosseau, L., Wells, G., Maclearly, L., Lambert, J., Lamonthe, C., et al., 2004. Efficacy of strengthening exercises for osteoarthritis (part 1) a meta-analysis. Physical Therapy Reviews 9, 77–108.

Richardson, C., Hodges, P., Hides, J., 2004. Therapeutic exercise for lumbopelvic stabilization. Churchill Livingstone, Edinburgh.

Rothstein, J.M.1982. Muscle biology clinical considerations. Physical Therapy 62 (12), 1823–1830.

Roussel, N.A., Nijs, J., Mottram, S., Van Moorsel, A., Truijen, S., Stassijns, G., 2009a. Altered lumbopelvic movement control but not generalised joint hypermobility is associated with increased injury in dancers. A prospective study. Manual Therapy 14 (6), 630–635.

Roussel, N.A., Daenen, L., Vissers, D., Lambeets, D., Schutt, A., Van Moorsel, A., et al., 2009b. Motor control and physical fitness training to prevent musculoskeletal injuries in professional dancers. 3rd International Conference on Movement Dysfunction, Edinburgh, UK. 30 October–1 November. Manual Therapy 14, 1 pS22.

Roussel, N., Nijs, J., Truijen, S., Vervecken, L., Mottram, S., Stassijns, G., 2009c. Altered breathing patterns during lumbopelvic motor control tests in chronic low back pain: a case-control study. European Spine Journal 18 (7), 1066–1073.

Rydeard, R., Leger, A., Smith, D., 2006. Pilates-based therapeutic exercise: effect on subjects with nonspecific chronic low back pain and functional disability: a randomized controlled trial. Journal of Orthopaedic and Sports Physical Therapy 36 (7), 472–484.

Stuge, B., Veierod, M.B., Laerum, E., Vollestad, N., 2004. The efficacy of a treatment program focusing on specific stabilizing exercises for pelvic girdle pain after pregnancy: a two-year follow-up of a randomized clinical trial. Spine 29 (10), E197–E203.

Tate, A.R., McClure, P., Kareha, S., Irwin, D., 2008. Effect of the scapula reposition test on shoulder impingement symptoms and elevation in overhead athletes. Journal of Orthopaedic and Sports Physical Therapy 38 (1), 4–11.

Taylor, N.F., Dodd, K.J., Shields, N., Bruder, A., 2007. Therapeutic exercise in physiotherapy practice is beneficial: a summary of systematic reviews 2002–2005. Australian Journal of Physiotherapy 53 (1), 7–16.

Torstensen, T.A., Ljunggren, A.E., Meen, H.D., Odland, E., Mowinckel, P., Geijerstam, S., 1998. Efficiency and costs of medical exercise therapy, conventional physiotherapy, and self-exercise in patients with chronic low back pain. A pragmatic, randomized, single-blinded, controlled trial with 1-year follow-up. Spine 23 (23), 2616–2624.

Tsao, H., Hodges, P.W., 2008. Persistence of improvements in postural strategies following motor control training in people with recurrent low back pain. Journal of Electromyography and Kinesiology 18 (4), 559–567.

Van Dillen, L.R., Maluf, K.S., Sahrmann, S.A., 2009. Further examination of modifying patient-preferred movement and alignment strategies in patients with low back pain during symptomatic tests. Manual Therapy 14 (1), 52–60.

van Ettekoven, H., Lucas, C., 2006. Efficacy of physiotherapy including a craniocervical training programme for tension-type headache; a randomized clinical trial. Cephalalgia 26 (8), 983–991.

Van Vliet, P.M., Heneghan, N.R., 2006. Motor control and the management of musculoskeletal dysfunction. Manual Therapy 11 (3), 208–213.

Vicenzino, B., 2003. Lateral epicondylalgia: a musculoskeletal physiotherapy perspective. Manual Therapy 8 (2), 66–79.

Vicenzino, B., Smith, D., Cleland, J., Bisset, L., 2009. Development of a clinical prediction rule to identify initial responders to mobilisation with movement and exercise for lateral epicondylalgia. Manual Therapy 14 (5), 550–554.

von Eisenhart-Rothe, R., Matsen 3rd., F.A., Eckstein, F., Vogl, T., Graichen, H., 2005. Pathomechanics in a-traumatic shoulder instability: scapular positioning correlates with humeral head centering. Clinical Orthopaedics and Related Research (433), 82–89.

Waddell, G., 2004. The back pain revolution. Churchill Livingstone, Edinburgh.

Section | 2 |

Chapter | 5 |

The lumbopelvic region

INTRODUCTION

There is rapidly growing acceptance among clinicians and researchers that the development of movement-based diagnostic frameworks is the way forwards in managing chronic and recurrent low back pain (LBP). The systems most supported by evidence are those that examine interrelationships between altered patterns of muscle recruitment and motor control strategies and establish a direction-based mechanism of provocation or relief of symptoms (Sahrmann 2002; Dankaerts et al 2006; Luomajoki et al 2008; Van Dillen et al 2009; Vibe Fersum et al 2009). In the lumbar spine, this approach is now well established. In the management of non-specific low back pain, the subgrouping and classification of patients' symptoms based on the assessment of movement and motor control has become more important than trying to identify a pathology-based diagnosis (Sahrmann 2002; Fritz et al 2007; Gombatto et al 2007). The influence of movement faults on pain has been illustrated (Van Dillen et al 2009) and a link between the direction of uncontrolled motion in low threshold motor control testing and pain provocative movements identified (Sahrmann 2002; O'Sullivan 2005; Dankaerts et al 2006; Luomajoki et al 2008; Vibe Fersum et al 2009). Research to date highlights the poor to moderate treatment effects with current intervention strategies for chronic specific low back pain, highlighting the need for further research and clinical developments (Airaksinen et al 2006).

This chapter sets out to explore the assessment and retraining of uncontrolled movement (UCM) in the lumbopelvic region. Understanding the development of lumbopelvic UCM and the process of assessment and diagnostic classification of lumbopelvic UCM are integral steps in retraining control of lumbopelvic pain provocative movements and postures. Before details of the assessment and retraining of UCM in the lumbopelvic region are explained, a brief review of changes in movement and postural control in the region is presented.

Changes in movement and postural control in the lumbopelvic region

Different postural positions have been shown to alter trunk muscle activation (O'Sullivan et al 2002a; O'Sullivan et al 2006). In particular a lumbopelvic upright posture (with a maintained lumbar lordosis and some anterior pelvic tilt) recruits more of the internal oblique and superficial multifidus muscles than does an upright posture of thoracic extension, where there is less lumbar extension and anterior pelvic tilt, less superficial multifidus and internal oblique recruitment and more erector spinae activation. Similarly, sway standing postures and slump sitting postures decrease activity in the internal oblique and multifidus muscles and sway standing increases the activity in rectus abdominis. These

83

changes in muscle recruitment patterns have been linked to the presence of lumbopelvic pain (Sahrmann, 2002; O'Sullivan 2005; Dankaerts et al 2006; O'Sullivan et al 2002b, 2003, 2006).

Changes in the alignment of the lumbar spine have been noted in subjects with flexion-related lumbar pain (O'Sullivan et al 2006). These people sit with their lumbar spines closer towards the end of flexion range and with more posterior pelvic tilt than healthy pain-free controls. Interestingly they also had reduced back muscle endurance compared to the controls, suggesting a link between changes in muscle function and changes in postural position. Differences in sitting postures and control of the lumbar neutral position have been identified in patients with back pain (Trudelle-Jackson et al 2008).

Segmental dysfunction has been identified in low back pain subjects with uncontrolled segmental movement noted around the neutral zone, as described by Panjabi (1992), during lumbar flexion (Teyhen et al 2007). The dysfunctional movement occurs during the early part of movement when the motion should be under neuromuscular control and not at end of range where the passive osteoligamentous system contributes to stability. These changes illustrate alterations in control of segmental motion.

Gombatto et al (2007) have identified different patterns of lumbar region movement during trunk lateral bending in two subgroups in people with LBP. In people with patterns of uncontrolled extension and rotation, the lumbar region demonstrated asymmetry in movement and contributed more to trunk lateral bend particularly in the early stages of lateral bending on one side. They suggest that this lumbar region movement will unilaterally load one or more lumbar segments and repeated stress on the tissues during functional movements which involve side-bend, will cause cumulative stress of the lumbar region and eventually result in pain.

Van Dillen et al (2009) demonstrated that movement tests can provoke symptoms in people with LBP. These researchers explored the effect of modifying, or 'correcting', symptomatic alignment or movement in people with LBP. This was done by correcting the spinal alignment or movement that occurred when symptoms were provoked. The modifications involved: i) restricting movement of the lumbar spine while encouraging movement elsewhere (e.g. thoracic spine or hip); and ii) positioning and maintaining the lumbar spine in a neutral position during movement similar to the principles discussed in Chapters 3 and 4. The modifications resulted in a decrease in symptoms in the majority of patients. This illustrates a classification system of subjects with LBP based on the direction(s) of alignment and movement consistently associated with a change in symptoms.

Luomajoki et al (2008) demonstrated significant differences between healthy people without back pain and back pain subjects in their ability to control movement in the lumbar spine using a battery of six movement control tests (Luomajoki et al 2008). These six tests (all of which are described later in this chapter), are based on cognitively controlling lumbar flexion, lumbar extension and lumbopelvic rotation. The back pain subjects failed a significantly greater proportion of these tests than the healthy people. The ability to perform these six movement control tests can reveal differences between subjects with chronic low back pain and subjects with acute or subacute pain (Luomajoki et al 2008).

Reliability of movement observation

The reliability of therapist observation to identify UCM and to make consistent clinical judgements based on movement observation has significant support. Van Dillen et al (2009), Dankaerts et al (2006), Luomajoki et al (2007), Vibe Fersum et al (2009) and Roussel et al (2009) have all demonstrated good intra-tester and inter-tester reliability for observational assessment of a patient's ability to perform cognitively learned movement patterns or motor control tests of movement control. Van Dillen et al (2009) and Morrissey et al (2008) have further demonstrated that therapist observation correlates closely with 3D motion analysis.

Efficacy of treatment to retrain control of lumbopelvic UCM

The efficacy of retraining the activation of muscles that contribute to lumbopelvic stability is well supported (Hides et al 2001; Hodges 2003; O'Sullivan 2005; Tsao & Hodges 2008; Luomajoki et al 2010). More recently there is evidence from randomised clinical trials (RCTs) that retraining programs which focus on motor control are beneficial (Macedo et al 2009). Stabilising exercises have been shown to have an effect on pain and disability (O'Sullivan et al 1997; Moseley 2002; Stuge et al 2004) and can effectively reduce recurrence of back pain at long term follow-up (Hides et al 2001). Specific recruitment of these deep stability muscles seems to be an important part of retraining (Hall et al 2007).

Motor control impairment during functional movement tasks can change following a motor learning intervention (Dankaerts et al 2007; O'Sullivan & Beales 2007a). Once the site and direction of UCM have been identified specific muscle retraining can be used to retrain control of the dysfunction. For example, 'drawing in' the abdominal wall, to activate the deep abdominal muscles, has been shown to decrease erector spinae activity and increase gluteus maximus activity in prone hip extension lift test (Oh et al 2007).

In subjects with spondylosis and spondylolisthesis, lumbopelvic stability training has resulted in decreased pain intensity and pain descriptor scores and improvements in functional disability levels (O'Sullivan et al 1997). Exercise interventions have been described based on the evaluation of spinal alignment with postures and during active movements of both the spine and the extremities (Maluf et al 2000; Van Dillen et al 2009). Their treatment approach is to teach the patient specific strategies to reduce the symptoms associated with movements to enable them to perform activities they would otherwise avoid.

Aberrant motor control strategies have also been identified in people with sacroiliac joint (SIJ) and pelvic girdle pain. O'Sullivan et al (2002b) observed abnormal kinematics of the diaphragm and pelvic floor during an active straight leg raise test in subjects with SIJ pain, and noted that these aberrant motor control strategies could be eliminated with manual compression during the test. In addition these people demonstrated bracing strategies in the abdominal wall not seen in the non-pain group. Transversus abdominis recruitment has been shown to increase sacroiliac joint stiffness to a significantly greater degree than the general abdominal exercise pattern illustrating the stability role that this muscle has on the SIJ (Richardson et al 2002).

People with musculoskeletal pain demonstrate consistent changes in muscle recruitment patterns during the performance of functional movements and postural control tasks. There is evidence to support that assessment and classification of these aberrant uncontrolled movement patterns

can identify subgroups within the non-specific musculoskeletal pain population. These UCM can be retrained and correction of these aberrant movement patterns has been advocated as an effective treatment intervention. This chapter details the assessment of UCM at the lumbopelvic region and describes relevant retraining strategies.

DIAGNOSIS OF THE SITE AND DIRECTION OF UCM IN THE LUMBAR SPINE

The diagnosis of the site and direction of UCM in the lumbar spine can be identified in terms of the *site* (being lumbar) and the *direction* of flexion, extension and rotation/side-bend (asymmetry) (Table 5.1). As with all UCM, the motor control deficit can present as uncontrolled translational movement (e.g. spondylolisthesis at L5–S1) or uncontrolled range of functional movement (e.g. lumbar flexion) (Sahrmann 2002; O'Sullivan 2005).

A diagnosis of UCM requires evaluation of its clinical priority. This is based on the relationship between the UCM and the presenting symptoms. The therapist should look for a link between the direction of UCM ('give') and the direction of symptom provocation: a) Does the site of UCM relate to the site or joint that the patient complains of as the source of symptoms? b) Does the direction of movement or load testing relate to the direction or position of provocation of symptoms? This identifies the clinical priorities.

The site and direction of UCM at the lumbar spine can be linked with different clinical presentations, postures and activities aggravating symptoms. The typical assessment findings in the lumbar spine are identified in Table 5.2.

Table 5.1 Site and direction of UCM in the lumbar spine	
SITE	**DIRECTION**
Lumbar	• Flexion • Extension • Rotation/side-bend

Table 5.2 The link between the site and direction of UCM and different clinical presentations

SITE AND DIRECTION OF UCM	SYMPTOM PRESENTATION	PROVOCATIVE MOVEMENTS, POSTURES AND ACTIVITIES
LUMBAR FLEXION UCM Can present as: • segmental flexion hinge (usually at L5–S1, occasionally at L4–5 or L3–4) • multisegmental hyperflexion (involving all lumbar levels)	• Presents with symptoms in the lumbar spine • May present with a segmental localised pain pattern • ±Radicular pain from myofascial and articular structures • ±Referral from neural tissue	Symptoms provoked by flexion movements and postures (especially if repetitive or sustained) For example, sustained sitting, bending forwards, driving, lifting, sleeping supine on a soft bed
LUMBAR EXTENSION UCM Can present as: • segmental extension hinge (usually at L5–S1, occasionally at L4–5 or L3–4) • multisegmental hyperextension (involving all lumbar levels)	• Presents with symptoms in lumbar spine • May present with a segmental localised pain pattern • ±Radicular pain from myofascial and articular structures • ±Referral from neural tissue	Symptoms provoked by extension movements and postures (especially if repetitive or sustained) For example, walking (especially downhill), looking up, reaching overhead, sustained standing, lying prone
LUMBOPELVIC ROTATION/ SIDE-BEND UCM (asymmetry superimposed on any of the above flexion or extension UCM) Can present as: • uncontrolled rotation or side-bend in the lumbar spine. The rotation or side-bend UCM is usually unilateral (i.e. more pronounced to either the right or left side) • can present bilaterally	• Presents with unilateral symptoms ± unilateral radicular symptoms • Coupled with any of the above flexion or extension uncontrolled movements • Symptoms can be localised to either a single segment or generalised across the whole multisegmental lumbar region	Unilateral symptoms provoked by movements or sustained postures away from the midline For example, rotation or side-bend with symptoms usually worse in one direction more than another Unilateral symptoms provoked by either flexion or extension activities or sustained postures linked to the above UCM

IDENTIFYING SITE AND DIRECTION OF UCM AT THE LUMBAR SPINE

The key principles for assessment and classification of UCM have previously been described in Chapter 3. All dissociation tests are performed with the lumbar spine in the neutral training region.

Segmental and multi-segmental uncontrolled motion in the sagittal plane

When direction-specific, uncontrolled sagittal motion (flexion or extension) is observed in the spine, it can present in two ways. The uncontrolled motion can present as either a segmental UCM or a multisegmental UCM.

Segmental UCM

A single segment UCM may appear to 'hinge' into excessive translatory displacement associated with the flexion (segmental 'flexion hinge') or extension (segmental 'extension hinge'). This is observed as either a 'hinge' or 'pivot point' or excessive translational shear during motion testing. Identification of segmental UCM phenomena is described below.

A segmental *flexion hinge* (which opens posteriorly and translates backwards) can be identified in motion testing in the following ways:

1. Place a short piece of adhesive strapping tape across the primary hinging segment. The skin is tensioned from the adjacent segment below to the adjacent segment above. If the subject cannot prevent flexion across this segment, the tape pulls off the skin when uncontrolled flexion is produced.

2. Place one finger tip on the spinous process of the primary hinging segment and another finger tip on the spinous process of each adjacent segment (above and below). If the subject is unable to prevent flexion at this segment the therapist palpates uncontrolled opening (spinous processes moving apart).

A segmental *extension hinge* (which closes poster-iorly and translates forwards) can be identified in motion testing in the following ways:

1. Place one finger tip on the spinous process of the primary hinging segment. During normal extension the spinous process can be palpated moving slightly forwards (as the articular surfaces close and compress), then the spinous process is palpated moving backwards and down as the articular surface of the upper segment glides backwards on the lower segment. If the subject is unable to prevent extension or translation shear at this segment the therapist palpates uncontrolled and excessive forward displacement of the spinous process during active extension (spinous process moving forwards too far) and a lack of sufficient backward glide.

2. Place one finger tip on the spinous process of the primary hinging segment and another finger tip on the spinous process of each adjacent segment (above and below). If the subject is unable to prevent extension at this segment the therapist palpates uncontrolled closing (spinous processes moving together) during lumbar spine extension.

Multisegmental UCM

A multisegmental UCM demonstrates hypermobile motion into flexion (multisegmental 'hyper-flexion') or into extension (multisegmental 'hyperextension') across a group of adjacent vertebral levels. This is observed as either an exaggeration of the spinal curve or hypermobile range.

A multisegmental *hyperflexion* can be identified in motion testing in the following ways:

1. Observe or palpate the multisegmental group of spinal segments (e.g. whole lumbar lordosis L1–S1). The therapist relies on visual observation or manual palpation to identify if the subject cannot maintain a neutral lordosis and prevent flexion during the test movement. The subject demonstrates a decrease in the depth or flattening or reversal of the lordosis curve when instructed to prevent flexion.

2. Place a long piece of adhesive strapping tape across the entire group of spinal segments (e.g. whole lumbar lordosis L1–S1). The skin is tensioned from the lowermost segment (below) to the uppermost segment. If the subject cannot prevent flexion across this multisegmental group, the tape pulls off the skin when uncontrolled flexion motion is produced.

A multisegmental *hyperextension* can be identified in motion testing in the following ways:

1. Observe or palpate the multisegmental group of spinal segments (e.g. whole lumbar lordosis L1–S1). The therapist relies on visual observation or manual palpation to identify if the subject cannot maintain a neutral lordosis and prevent extension during the test movement. The subject demonstrates an increase in the depth or exaggeration of the lordosis curve when instructed to prevent extension.

2. Place a long piece of adhesive strapping tape across the anterior abdomen (e.g. from the ASIS (anterior superior iliac spine) to the lower anterolateral ribcage or along the rectus abdominis muscle). The skin is tensioned from the lowermost attachment (below) to the uppermost attachment. If the subject cannot prevent spinal extension or anterior pelvic tilt across this multisegmental group, the tape pulls off the skin when uncontrolled extension motion is produced.

Occasionally, both single segment and multisegmental dysfunctions can present together.

CLINICAL EXAMPLES

Lumbar extension UCM

The patient complains of extension-related symptoms in the lumbar spine. The lumbar spine demonstrates UCM *into extension* relative to the hips or thoracic spine under extension load. During a motor control test of active hip or thoracic extension where the instruction is to prevent lumbar extension (dissociation), the lumbopelvic region demonstrates UCM into either:

• segmental extension hinge – uncontrolled segmental extension and translational shear at a pivot point (primarily at L5–S1, but potentially also at L3–4–5)

or

• multisegmental hyperextension – uncontrolled lumbar hyperextension and exaggerated anterior tilt.

During the attempt to dissociate the lumbar spine from independent hip or thoracic extension, the subject either cannot control the lumbar extension UCM or has to concentrate and try too hard.

Lumbar flexion UCM

The patient complains of flexion related symptoms in the lumbar spine. The lumbar spine demonstrates UCM *into flexion* relative to the hips or thoracic spine under flexion load. During a motor control test of active hip or thoracic flexion where the instruction is to prevent lumbar flexion (dissociation), the lumbopelvic region demonstrates UCM into either:

• segmental flexion hinge – uncontrolled segmental flexion and translational shear at a pivot point (primarily at L5–S1)

or

• multisegmental hyperflexion – uncontrolled lumbar hyperflexion and exaggerated posterior tilt.

During the attempt to dissociate the lumbar spine from independent hip or thoracic flexion, the subject either cannot control the lumbar flexion UCM or has to concentrate and try too hard.

MOVEMENT AND POSTURAL CONTROL AT THE SACROILIAC JOINT (SIJ) AND PELVIS

The relationship between SIJ or pelvic girdle pain and insufficiencies in the stability of the lumbopelvic region is currently an active area of research (Hungerford et al 2003; Stuge et al 2004; O'Sullivan & Beales 2007b). The classification of UCM in terms of site and direction at the SIJ and pelvis is gaining recognition and reports of labelling movement and positional faults can be seen in the literature (Cibulka 2002).

The range of motion that is available to the SIJ is very small in terms of translation and rotation between the sacrum and the innominates. Reports vary, but it is generally accepted that there are approximately 2–6° of rotation and 2 mm of translation (Sturesson et al 1989; Bogduk 1997; Lee 2004). These small ranges of motion are only able to be measured with specialised radiographic techniques (Sturesson et al 1989). Consequently, it is not possible to visually measure this range of motion and therefore not reliable to evaluate the site and direction of sacroiliac motion visually.

However, the muscles that provide movement control and functional stability for the lumbar spine and the hip also appear to be effective in controlling movement and stability of the SIJ and pelvis. Aberrant motor control strategies involving these muscles also have the potential to contribute to pelvic girdle pain and dysfunction, hence strategies to promote movement control and functional stability in the lumbar spine may have a positive effect on reducing sacroiliac and pelvic girdle pain.

Identifying UCM at the SIJ and pelvis

Aberrant motor control strategies have been identified in people with SIJ and pelvic pain. O'Sullivan et al (2002b) observed abnormal kinematics of the diaphragm and pelvic floor during an active straight leg raise test in subjects with SIJ pain, and noted that these aberrant motor control strategies could be eliminated with manual compression during the test. In addition, these people demonstrated bracing strategies in the abdominal wall not seen in the non-pain group. Transversus abdominis recruitment has been shown to increase SIJ stiffness to a significantly greater degree than the general abdominal exercise pattern, illustrating the stability role that this muscle has on the SIJ (Richardson et al 2002).

Evaluation of the presence of SIJ dysfunction has historically been difficult to evaluate (Riddle & Freburger 2002). Laslett et al (2005) have demonstrated that composites of provocation tests are of value in clinical diagnosis of the symptomatic SIJ but do not evaluate movement faults or guide diagnosis. Some authors have reconsidered the influence on force closure but not detailed specific assessment of movement faults (Pool-Goudzwaard 1998). O'Sullivan & Beales (2007a) have recognised that movement faults can be a part of SIJ dysfunction but do not detail the site and direction of UCM. Altered motor control strategies and alteration of respiratory function have been identified in subjects with sacroiliac pain (O'Sullivan & Beales 2007a). Hungerford et al (2003) have indentified delayed onset of internal oblique, multifidus and gluteus maximus on the supporting leg during hip flexion in subjects with SIJ changes, which they consider evidence of altered lumbopelvic control. Muscle recruitment dysfunction has been shown to be reversible: an individualised specific exercise training program has been shown to be more effective than physical therapy for women with pelvic girdle pain after pregnancy (Stuge et al 2004).

Although research has demonstrated the presence of movement faults in subjects with SIJ or pelvic girdle pain (Mens et al 2002; Hungerford et al 2004) reliability and validity of clinical tests are lacking. However, Hungerford et al (2007) have shown that physical therapists can reliably palpate and recognise altered patterns of intra-pelvic motion with a weight shift from bilateral stance to unilateral hip flexion.

The range of movement within the SIJ is so small that it is not possible to observe normal movement at the articulation between the sacrum and innominate. Consequently, we are unable to diagnose either the site or direction of UCM of the SIJ using movement observation. It may be possible to palpate motion between the sacrum and innominate during functional movement testing. However, there are almost no studies that demonstrate good intra-tester or inter-tester reliability for palpation of SIJ movement.

The osteopathic process of positional diagnosis, as advocated by Mitchell et al (1979) and Greenman (2003), uses manual palpation of the pelvis during functional movement testing to determine motion restriction of the SIJ. There is a lack of consensus among the clinicians who use this approach as to which motion tests identify restriction in function and as to precisely where to palpate the pelvis to interpret the positional change of adaptation. Once the restriction is determined as being related to abnormal motion of the sacrum, the right innominate or the left innominate, palpation of pelvic landmarks is then used to determine the position of adaptive change.

This process of positional diagnosis attempts to identify and label the site and direction of

adaptive compensatory motion of the pelvis. The site and direction of adaptive compensatory motion appears to be related to the site and direction of UCM. The process of positional diagnosis currently labels three separate sites of pelvic girdle adaptation: i) the sacrum; ii) the innominate; and iii) the pubis. These three sites also demonstrate specific directions of adaptive compensation or UCM (Table 5.3).

If the process of manual palpation to determine the positional adaptation of segmental motion within the SIJ eventually becomes validated, then clinicians will have an indirect method of diagnosing the site and direction of uncontrolled motion in the sacroiliac complex. When these diagnoses are made using manual palpation assessment, restrictions can be mobilised by movement of the segment in the opposite direction to compensation. Likewise, the UCM can be stabilised by training myofascial recruitment strategies to prevent or resist movement in the direction of adaptation at those sites (sacrum, innominate or pubis).

In the absence of being able to easily observe the site and direction of UCM within the sacroiliac complex, this process of positional diagnosis using manual palpation is potentially an alternative method of identifying site and direction of

Table 5.3 Potential site and direction of UCM in the pelvic girdle

SITE	DIRECTION
	Forward torsion
Sacrum	Backward torsion
	Nutated and side-bent (unilateral flexion)
	Counternutated and side-bent (unilateral extension)
	Anterior rotation
Innominate	Posterior rotation
	Superior shear (upslip)
	Inferior shear (downslip)
	Inflare
	Outflare
	Superior shear
Pubis	Inferior shear
	Anterior shear
	Posterior shear

sacroiliac uncontrolled motion. Primary SIJ UCM usually demonstrates good lumbar flexion control even though the patient usually complains of flexion-related symptoms. Movement control dysfunctions of the SIJ and pelvic girdle are consistently unilateral in nature and always demonstrate significant open chain or closed chain rotation UCMs.

A suggestion for early management of primary sacroiliac and pelvic girdle pain is to assess for and retrain uncontrolled rotation as a primary intervention. Secondly, if a positional diagnosis of the site and direction of pelvic girdle UCM can be made then specific movement correction can be implemented. However, because of the lack of reliability and validity for using palpation to determine motion restriction or the positional change of adaptation, specific diagnosis of the site and direction of UCM of the SIJ is not specifically covered in this text.

Each direction is assessed separately! If during a test of *one specific direction* (e.g. flexion), a movement into *another direction* (e.g. extension) is observed, it is possible to score a ✓✓ rating for the test. For example, if during a test of control of lumbar flexion control, the lumbar spine moves into extension, there is a possibility of a problem with lumbar extension control. The ability to control this potential UCM should be specifically assessed with extension related tests. However, if there was no UCM into flexion, then flexion is not the direction of UCM and the flexion control test should be rated as ✓✓.

Exception: if the movement in another direction consistently reaches end range the control of the primary test direction is deemed to be inefficient. For example, if, during a test of control of lumbar flexion control, the lumbar spine consistently uses full end-range extension to prevent flexion, then the efficiency of flexion control is inadequate, and the flexion control test should be rated as ✓✗.

TESTING FOR UCM – REVIEW OF PRINCIPLES

Identifying the site and the direction of UCM uses a cognitive motor control test demonstrating the efficiency of learning and performing a movement skill of dissociated movement. That is, to actively prevent a particular movement at one site (the provocative movement direction at the painful joint system while actively moving in the same direction at an adjacent joint). When the therapist is confident that the person understands the test movement and knows what is expected of the test, the person is required to perform the test without visual or tactile feedback, verbal facilitation, or corrective instruction. The therapist then rates the performance of the test as:

- ✓✓ (good control of site and direction)
- ✓✗ (inefficient control of site and direction)
- ✗✗ (uncontrolled site and direction).

To achieve a ✓✓ rating, the person must demonstrate good control to the benchmark standard and the test movement must look and feel easy and does not require any specific movement retraining. An assessment rating of ✓✗ or ✗✗ for any particular test identifies the presence of UCM.

The UCM is always qualified by a diagnostic label of its site and direction.

A ✓✗ rating or ✗✗ rating labels or diagnoses the stability dysfunction. The diagnosis should label both the **SITE** and the **DIRECTION** of give that is uncontrolled.

The following section will demonstrate the specific procedures for testing for UCM in the lumbar spine.

LUMBOPELVIC TESTS FOR UNCONTROLLED MOVEMENT

Lumbar flexion control

FLEXION CONTROL TESTS AND FLEXION CONTROL REHABILITATION

These flexion control tests assess the extent of flexion UCM in the lumbar spine and assess the ability of the dynamic stability system to adequately control flexion load or strain. It is a priority to assess for flexion UCM if the patient complains of or demonstrates flexion-related symptoms or disability.

OBSERVATION AND ANALYSIS OF LUMBAR FLEXION AND FORWARD BENDING

Description of ideal pattern

The subject is instructed to stand with the feet in a natural stance and bend forwards in a normal relaxed pattern. Ideally, there should be even flexion throughout the lumbar and thoracic regions with the hips flexing to approximately 70°. The spinal flexion and hip flexion should occur concurrently. The finger tips should reach the floor without the need to bend the knees (Figure 5.1). There should be good symmetry of movement without any lateral deviation, tilt or rotation of the trunk or pelvis. The pelvis and hips should lead the return to standing with the spine unrolling on the way back to the upright posture.

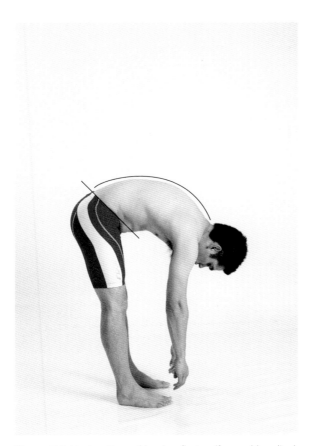

Figure 5.1 Ideal pattern of lumbar flexion (forward bending)

Movement faults associated with lumbar flexion

Relative stiffness (restrictions)

- *Hamstrings restriction of hip flexion* – the hips lack 70° of normal range in standing forward bending. The lumbar spine frequently increases flexion to compensate for the lack of hip mobility. Hamstring extensibility can be tested passively and dynamically with manual muscle extensibility examination.
- *Thoracic restriction of flexion* – mid and upper thoracic flexion restriction may also contribute to compensatory increases in lumbar flexion range. This is confirmed with manual segmental assessment (e.g. Maitland passive physiological intervertebral movements or passive accessory intervertebral movements) (Maitland et al 2005).

Relative flexibility (potential UCM)

- *Lumbar flexion* – the lumbar spine may initiate the movement into flexion and contribute more to producing forward bending while the hips and thoracic contributions start later and contribute less. At the limit of forward bending, excessive or hypermobile range of lumbar flexion may be observed. During the return to neutral the lumbar flexion and posterior pelvic tilt persists and unrolls late.

During the assessment of flexion control, the uncontrolled movement can be identified as either a segmental or a multisegmental UCM.

- *Segmental flexion hinge.* If only one spinous process is observed as prominent and protruding 'out of line' compared to the other vertebrae then the UCM is interpreted as a *segmental flexion hinge*. The specific hinging segment should be noted and recorded. This commonly occurs at the L5–S1 segment. Ideally, when lumbar flexion control is assessed, the positional alignment between the low lumbar spine and the pelvis should be maintained during hip flexion or thoracic flexion challenges. If lumbopelvic stability and control is inadequate, L5 alignment with the sacrum cannot be maintained and during flexion control tests the L5 and S1 segments appear to 'open' (the spinous processes move apart) as the pelvis posteriorly tilts instead of moving forwards with the spinal position. The upper lumbar lordosis can be maintained well and the failure of control is demonstrated only at the lumbopelvic junction.

- *Multisegmental hyperflexion*. If, on the other hand, excessive or hypermobile lumbar flexion is observed, but no one particular spinous process is prominent from the adjacent vertebrae then the UCM is interpreted as a *multisegmental hyperflexion*. This is commonly observed as excessive reversal of the lumbar lordosis and hypermobile flexion of the whole lumbar region. Instead of maintaining positional control of the lumbar lordosis and the pelvis during hip flexion or thoracic flexion

challenges, uncontrolled lumbar flexion and posterior pelvic tilt are observed.

Indications to test for lumbar flexion UCM

Observe or palpate for:

1. hypermobile lumbar flexion range
2. excessive initiation of forward bending with lumbar flexion
3. symptoms (pain, discomfort, strain) associated with flexion.

The person complains of flexion-related symptoms in the lumbar spine. Under flexion load, the lumbar spine has greater give *into flexion* relative to the hips or relative to the thoracic spine. The dysfunction is confirmed with motor control tests of flexion dissociation.

Tests of lumbar flexion control

T1 STANDING: TRUNK LEAN TEST (tests for lumbar flexion UCM)

This dissociation test assesses the ability to actively dissociate and control lumbar flexion and posterior pelvic tilt then lean forwards by moving the hips through flexion while standing.

Test procedure

The person should have the ability to actively lean forwards by flexing at the hips while controlling the lumbar spine and pelvis. The person stands tall with legs straight and the lumbar spine and pelvis positioned in neutral (Figure 5.2). Lumbopelvic motion is monitored by the therapist.

The therapist monitors the lumbosacral neutral position by palpating the spinous process of L2, L5, and S2 with their finger tips (Figure 5.3). During testing, if the palpating fingers do not move, the lumbosacral region is able to maintain neutral (Figure 5.4). If the palpating fingers move

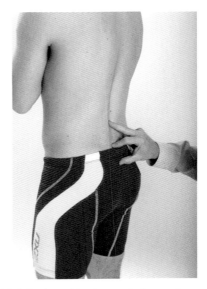

Figure 5.3 Palpation of lumbosacral alignment

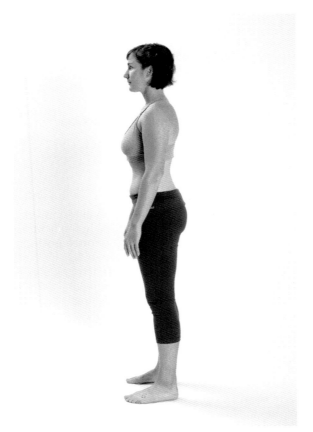

Figure 5.2 Start position for trunk lean test

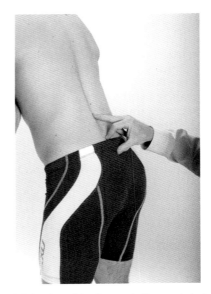

Figure 5.4 Palpation of lumbosacral alignment during movement

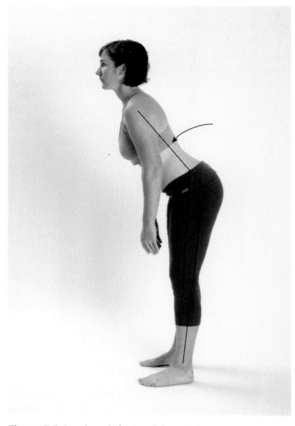

spine starts to flex before achieving 50° forward lean. During the attempt to dissociate the lumbar spine from independent hip flexion the person either cannot control the UCM or has to concentrate and try hard.

- If only one spinous process is observed as prominent and protruding 'out of line' compared to the other vertebrae then the UCM is interpreted as a *segmental flexion hinge*. The specific hinging segment should be noted and recorded.
- If excessive lumbopelvic flexion is observed, but no one particular spinous process is prominent from the adjacent vertebrae, then the UCM is interpreted as a *multisegmental hyperflexion*.

Clinical assessment note for direction-specific motor control testing

If some other movement (e.g. a small amount of extension or rotation) is observed during a motor control (dissociation) test of flexion control, *do not* score this as uncontrolled flexion. The extension and rotation motor control tests will identify if the observed movement is uncontrolled. A test for lumbar flexion UCM is only positive if uncontrolled lumbar flexion is demonstrated.

Figure 5.5 Benchmark for trunk lean test

further apart, uncontrolled segmental lumbar flexion is identified.

The person is instructed to stand tall and to 'bow' or lean the trunk forwards from the hips, keeping the back straight (neutral spine). Ideally, the subject should have the ability to dissociate the lumbar spine from hip flexion as evidenced by 50° forward lean while preventing lumbar flexion or posterior pelvic tilt (Figure 5.5). This test should be performed without any feedback (self-palpation, vision, tape, etc.) or cueing for correction.

Lumbar flexion UCM

The person complains of flexion-related symptoms in the lumbar spine. The lumbar spine has UCM into flexion relative to the hips under flexion load. During active hip flexion, the lumbar

Rating and diagnosis of lumbar flexion UCM

(T1.1 and T1.2)

Correction

The person stands tall with legs straight and the lumbar spine and pelvis positioned in the neutral. They monitor the lumbosacral neutral position by palpating the spinous process of L2, L5, and S2 with their fingers (Figure 5.6). The person is instructed to stand tall and to 'bow' or lean the trunk forwards from the hips, keeping the back straight (neutral spine). If the palpating fingers do not move further apart, lumbar flexion is being controlled (Figure 5.7).

The person should self-monitor the lumbopelvic alignment and control with a variety of feedback options (T1.3). In some cases it may be useful to tension a strip of adhesive sports strapping tape to the skin across the uncontrolled segments. This will provide sensory feedback and some degree of mechanical support to the control of flexion.

T1.1 Assessment and rating of low threshold recruitment efficiency of the Trunk Lean Test

ASSESSMENT

Control point:
- prevent multisegmental lumbar flexion and posterior pelvic tilt
- prevent segmental flexion hinge and posterior tilt

Movement challenge: hip flexion (standing)

Benchmark range: 50° forward lean of trunk with independent hip flexion

RATING OF LOW THRESHOLD RECRUITMENT EFFICIENCY FOR CONTROL OF DIRECTION

	✓ or ✗		✓ or ✗

• Able to prevent 'UCM' into the test direction. Correct dissociation pattern of movement
Prevent lumbar UCM into:
  posterior pelvic tilt and hyperflexion (multi-segment)
  posterior pelvic tilt and flexion hinge (single segment)
and move hip flexion
	☐	• Looks easy, and in the opinion of the assessor, is performed with confidence	☐

		• Feels easy, and the subject has sufficient awareness of the movement pattern that they confidently prevent 'UCM' into the test direction	☐
• Dissociate movement through the benchmark range of: 50° forward lean of trunk with independent hip flexion *If there is more available range than the benchmark standard, only the benchmark range needs to be actively controlled*	☐	• The pattern of dissociation is smooth during concentric and eccentric movement	☐
		• Does not (consistently) use *end range* movement into the opposite direction to prevent the UCM	☐
		• No extra feedback needed *(tactile, visual or verbal cueing)*	☐
• Without holding breath (though it is acceptable to use an alternate breathing strategy)	☐	• Without external support or unloading	☐
		• Relaxed natural breathing *(even if not ideal – so long as natural pattern does not change)*	☐
• Control during eccentric phase	☐	• No fatigue	☐
• Control during concentric phase	☐		☐

CORRECT DISSOCIATION PATTERN   **RECRUITMENT EFFICIENCY**

T1.2 Diagnosis of the site and direction of UCM from the Trunk Lean Test

TRUNK LEAN TEST – STANDING

Site	Direction	Segmental/ multisegmental	✗✗ or ✓✗
Lumbar	Flexion	Segmental flexion hinge (indicate level)	☐
		Multisegmental hyperflexion	☐

T1.3 Feedback tools to monitor retraining

FEEDBACK TOOL	PROCESS
Self-palpation	Palpation monitoring of joint position
Visual observation	Observe in a mirror or directly watch the movement
Adhesive tape	Skin tension for tactile feedback
Cueing and verbal correction	Listen to feedback from another observer

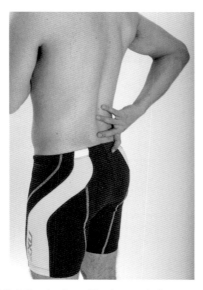

Figure 5.6 Self-palpation of lumbosacral alignment

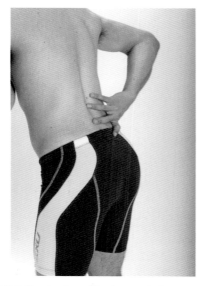

Figure 5.7 Self-palpation of lumbosacral alignment during correction

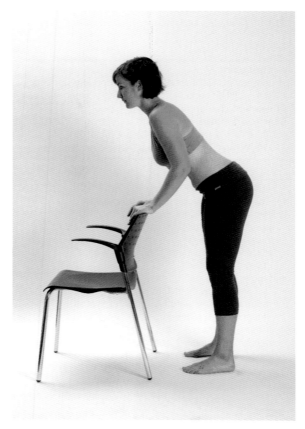

Figure 5.8 Retraining lumbar flexion control with partial support

Visual feedback (e.g. observation in a mirror) is also a useful retraining tool. Ideally, the subject should have the ability to dissociate the lumbar spine from hip flexion as evidenced by 50° forward lean while preventing lumbar flexion or posterior pelvic tilt. There should be no provocation of any symptoms under flexion load, within the range that the flexion UCM can be controlled.

If control is poor, the pattern of forward leaning with a straight back and independent hip flexion should be performed *only* as far as lumbar flexion and posterior pelvic tilt can be actively controlled or prevented. Also, the upper body and trunk weight can be supported by weight bearing through the arms to decrease the load that must be controlled by the local and global stabiliser muscles (Figure 5.8). As the ability to control the UCM gets easier and the pattern of dissociation feels less unnatural, the exercise can be progressed to the unsupported position. This exercise can also be performed with the knees bent to decrease the influence of the hamstrings and to encourage the gluteal muscles to eccentrically control the hip. Once the pattern of dissociation is efficient and feels familiar it should be integrated into various functional postures and positions.

T2 4 POINT: BACKWARD PUSH TEST (tests for lumbar flexion UCM)

This dissociation test assesses the ability to actively dissociate and control lumbar flexion/posterior pelvic tilt and push the body backwards with the hands by moving the hips backwards through flexion while in 4 point kneeling (hands and knees) position.

Test procedure

The person should have the ability to actively push the body away with the hands while leaning forwards by flexing at the hips and controlling the lumbar spine and pelvis. The person positions themselves in 4 point kneeling (hands and knees) with the lumbar spine and pelvis in neutral alignment (Figure 5.9). Lumbopelvic motion is monitored by the therapist. The therapist monitors the lumbosacral neutral position by palpating the spinous process of L2, L5, and S2 with their fingertips (Figure 5.10).

During testing, if the palpating fingers do not move, the lumbosacral region is able to maintain neutral. If the palpating fingers move further apart, uncontrolled segmental lumbar flexion is identified.

The person is instructed to push with the hands to rock backwards from the hips towards their heels, keeping the back straight (neutral spine). Ideally, the neutral lumbar lordosis should be maintained until about 120° of hip flexion as the pelvis moves backwards (half way back towards the heels).

Ideally, the person should have the ability to dissociate the lumbar spine and pelvis from hip flexion as evidenced by 120° of hip flexion during the backward push while preventing lumbar flexion or posterior pelvic tilt (Figure 5.11). After 120° hip flexion the pelvis should start to tilt posteriorly and the spine should start to flex as the pelvis moves towards the heels. The lumbar spine and pelvis should return to a neutral position as the subject rocks forwards, back to the starting position. The pelvis should have good symmetry. That is, no lateral tilt or rotation. This test should be performed without any feedback (self-palpation, vision, tape, etc.) or cueing for correction.

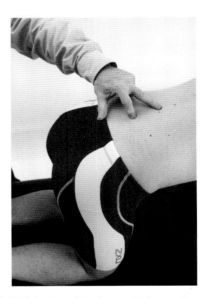

Figure 5.10 Palpation of lumbosacral alignment

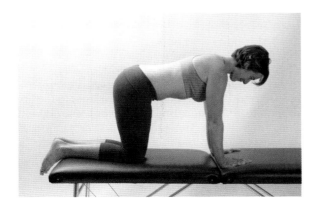

Figure 5.9 Start position for backward push test

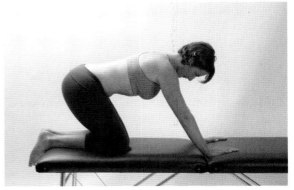

Figure 5.11 Benchmark for backward push test

Lumbar flexion UCM

The person complains of flexion-related symptoms in the lumbar spine. The lumbar spine has UCM into flexion relative to the hips under flexion load. During a backward push from the hands, in a hands and knees position that produces hip flexion, the lumbar spine starts to flex before achieving 120° of hip flexion. During the attempt to dissociate the lumbar spine and pelvis from independent hip flexion, the person either cannot control the UCM or has to concentrate and try hard.

- If only one spinous process is observed as prominent and protruding 'out of line' compared to the other vertebrae then the UCM is interpreted as a *segmental flexion hinge*. The specific hinging segment should be noted and recorded.
- If excessive lumbopelvic flexion is observed, but no one particular spinous process is prominent from the adjacent vertebrae then the UCM is interpreted as a *multisegmental hyperflexion*.

Clinical assessment note for direction-specific motor control testing

If some other movement (e.g. a small amount of extension or rotation) is observed during a motor control (dissociation) test of flexion control, *do not* score this as uncontrolled flexion. The extension and rotation motor control tests will identify if the observed movement is uncontrolled. A test for lumbar flexion UCM is only positive if uncontrolled lumbar flexion is demonstrated.

Rating and diagnosis of lumbar flexion UCM

(T2.1 and T2.2)

Correction

The person positions themselves in 4 point kneeling (hands and knees) with the lumbar spine and pelvis in neutral alignment. The person rocks backwards from the pelvis towards their heels by

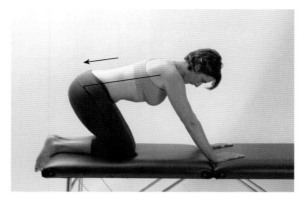

Figure 5.12 Retraining lumbar flexion control

pushing with the hands. The goal is to push the pelvis backwards with independent hip flexion, but only as far as the neutral lumbopelvic position can be maintained. Ideally, the person should have the ability to dissociate the lumbopelvic region from hip flexion as evidenced by 120° of hip flexion as the pelvis moves backwards (half way back towards the heels) (Figure 5.12) while preventing lumbar flexion or posterior pelvic tilt.

The person should self-monitor the lumbopelvic alignment and control with a variety of feedback options (T2.3). It is very useful to tension a strip of adhesive sports strapping tape to the skin across the uncontrolled segments. This will provide sensory feedback and some degree of mechanical support to the control of flexion. Visual feedback (e.g. observation in a mirror) is also a useful retraining tool.

If control is poor, the pattern of pushing the pelvis backwards from the hands with a straight back and independent hip flexion should be performed *only* as far as lumbar flexion and posterior pelvic tilt can be actively controlled or prevented. There should be no provocation of any symptoms, so long as the flexion give can be controlled. Progress until good control through half range (120° hip flexion) is easy, but not beyond this range. Once the pattern of dissociation is efficient and feels familiar it should be integrated into various functional postures and positions.

T2.1 Assessment and rating of low threshold recruitment efficiency of the Backward Push Test

BACKWARD PUSH TEST – 4 POINT KNEELING

ASSESSMENT

Control point:
- prevent multisegmental lumbar flexion and posterior pelvic tilt
- prevent segmental flexion hinge and posterior tilt

Movement challenge: hip flexion (4 point kneeling)

Benchmark range: 120° backward rocking of pelvis with independent hip flexion

RATING OF LOW THRESHOLD RECRUITMENT EFFICIENCY FOR CONTROL OF DIRECTION

	✓ or ✗		✓ or ✗

• Able to prevent 'UCM' into the test direction. Correct dissociation pattern of movement
Prevent lumbar UCM into:
   posterior pelvic tilt and hyperflexion
   (multisegment)
   posterior pelvic tilt and flexion hinge (single
   segment)
and move hip flexion
	☐	• Looks easy, and in the opinion of the assessor, is performed with confidence	☐

		• Feels easy, and the subject has sufficient awareness of the movement pattern that they confidently prevent 'UCM' into the test direction	☐
• Dissociate movement through the benchmark range of: 120° backward rocking at pelvis with independent hip flexion *(If there is more available range than the benchmark standard, only the benchmark range needs to be actively controlled)*	☐	• The pattern of dissociation is smooth during concentric and eccentric movement	☐
		• Does not (consistently) use *end range* movement into the opposite direction to prevent the UCM	☐
• Without holding breath (though it is acceptable to use an alternate breathing strategy)	☐	• No extra feedback needed *(tactile, visual or verbal cueing)*	☐
• Control during eccentric phase	☐	• Without external support or unloading	☐
• Control during concentric phase	☐	• Relaxed natural breathing *(even if not ideal – so long as natural pattern does not change)*	☐
		• No fatigue	☐

CORRECT DISSOCIATION PATTERN   **RECRUITMENT EFFICIENCY**

T2.2 Diagnosis of the site and direction of UCM from the Backward Push Test

BACKWARD PUSH TEST – 4 POINT KNEELING

Site	Direction	Segmental/multisegmental	✗✗ or ✓✗
Lumbar	Flexion	Segmental flexion hinge (indicate level)	☐
		Multisegmental hyperflexion	☐

T2.3 Feedback tools to monitor retraining

FEEDBACK TOOL	PROCESS
Self-palpation	Palpation monitoring of joint position
Visual observation	Observe in a mirror or directly watch the movement
Adhesive tape	Skin tension for tactile feedback
Cueing and verbal correction	Listen to feedback from another observer

T3 CROOK: DOUBLE BENT LEG LIFT TEST (tests for lumbar flexion UCM)

This dissociation test assesses the ability to actively dissociate and control lumbar flexion and posterior pelvic tilt when lifting both feet off the floor by actively flexing the hips in a crook lying position.

Test procedure

The person should have the ability to lift both feet off the floor (in crook lying) by flexing at the hips and controlling the lumbar spine and pelvis. The person lies on the back in crook lying (hips and knees bent and feet resting on the floor) with the lumbar spine and pelvis relaxed in neutral alignment (Figure 5.13). Lumbopelvic motion is monitored by the placement of a Pressure Biofeedback Unit (PBU) (Stabilizer – Chattanooga) under the back, centred at L3 in the middle of the lumbar lordosis (Figures 5.14 and 5.15). During limb load tests and exercises the PBU can objectively monitor the functional stability of the trunk (Richardson et al 1992, Jull et al 1993). In crook lying the PBU is inflated to a base pressure of 40 mmHg (Figure 5.16). This pressure is used to position and support the lumbar spine in neutral alignment. Under functional limb load or movement, no pressure change = no loss of neutral position = good control. If the lumbar spine flexes beyond the neutral starting position an increase in pressure is registered by the PBU. If the lumbar spine extends beyond the neutral starting position a decrease in pressure is registered by the PBU.

The person is instructed to slowly lift both feet off the floor (*both at the same time*) until both hips are flexed to 90°. They are instructed to keep the knees bent and the lumbar spine neutral (no pressure change) while they flex the hips to 90° by lifting the feet from the floor. They are required to hold this position (Figure 5.17) and keep the back stable (no pressure change) for at least 5 seconds. Ideally, the person should have the ability to dissociate the lumbar spine and pelvis from hip flexion as evidenced by 90° of bilateral hip flexion during the double leg lift while preventing lumbar flexion or posterior pelvic tilt.

The person is permitted to watch the PBU to monitor the accuracy of their ability to control

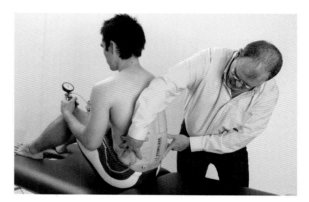

Figure 5.14 Therapist positioning the PBU in the lumbar lordosis

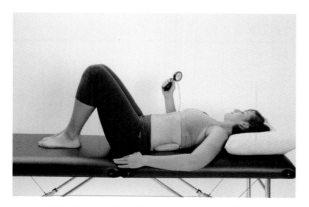

Figure 5.13 Start position for double bent leg lift test

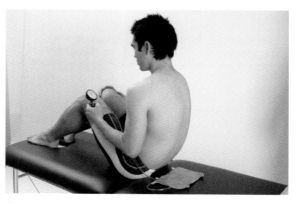

Figure 5.15 Self-positioning the PBU in the lumbar lordosis

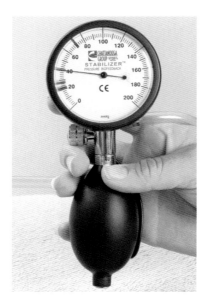

Figure 5.16 Inflating the PBU to a base pressure of 40 mmHg

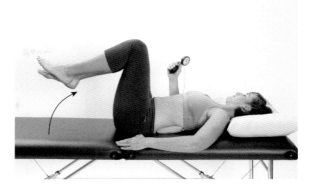

Figure 5.17 Benchmark for double bent leg lift test

the lumbar spine and prevent lumbar flexion. The PBU is initially inflated to a base pressure of 40 mmHg while the lumbar spine is relaxed and supported in a neutral resting position. During the double leg lift some small movement of the pelvis is normal. This is accounted for in the test by allowing a small tolerance of pressure change during the leg movement phase. Therefore, a pressure *increase* or *decrease* of 10 mmHg either side of the base pressure of 40 mmHg is acceptable. However, when the hips are flexed to 90° the lumbar spine should be maintained in the original resting neutral position with the pressure held constantly at 40 mmHg for at least 5 seconds.

If no PBU is available the therapist should place a hand under the lumbar lordosis instead of inserting the PBU. It has been anecdotally claimed that the hand is sensitive to a pressure change roughly equivalent to a pressure change of 40 mmHg. So if no pressure increase is detected by the hand, the control would seem to be within the limits as determined by the PBU.

Lumbar flexion UCM

The person complains of flexion-related symptoms in the lumbar spine. The lumbar spine has UCM into flexion relative to the hips under

flexion load. During a double leg lift from crook lying that produces hip flexion, the lumbar spine starts to flex before achieving 90° of hip flexion. During the attempt to dissociate the lumbar spine and pelvis from independent hip flexion, the person either cannot control the UCM or has to concentrate and try hard.

In the process of trying to keep the back neutral, the pelvis must not tilt posteriorly and flex the lumbar spine. The anterior abdominal wall should stay hollow or flat. Excessive recruitment (dominance) of rectus abdominis causes the anterior abdominal wall to 'bulge' out or 'crunch', flexing the trunk and increasing the flattening pressure. A pressure increase of more than 10 mmHg (increase to more than 50 mmHg) indicates gross posterior tilt and a loss of stability into spinal flexion due to overactivation of rectus abdominis or a lack of posterior counterbalance from the back extensor stabilisers (e.g. superficial lumbar multifidus).

As soon as any pressure increase (beyond 50 mmHg) is registered, the leg movement must stop and the feet lower back to the start position. If control is poor, a series of graduated progressions using relatively less load and specific facilitation of the oblique abdominals can be used.

- If excessive lumbopelvic flexion occurs, a significant increase in pressure is registered by the PBU (pressure increase by more than 10 mmHg to >50 mmHg), then the UCM is interpreted as a *multisegmental hyperflexion*.

Clinical assessment note for direction-specific motor control testing

If some other movement (e.g. a small amount of extension or rotation) is observed during a motor control (dissociation) test of flexion control, *do not* score this as uncontrolled flexion. The extension and rotation motor control tests will identify if the observed movement is uncontrolled. A test for lumbar flexion UCM is only positive if uncontrolled lumbar flexion is demonstrated.

Rating and diagnosis of lumbar flexion UCM

(T3.1 and T3.2)

Correction

The person lies in crook lying with the lumbar spine and pelvis relaxed in neutral alignment. The person is permitted to watch the PBU to monitor the accuracy of their ability to control the lumbar spine and prevent lumbar flexion. During all retraining of uncontrolled lumbar flexion a pressure increase of 10 mmHg is acceptable during unsupported leg movements. That is, if the start pressure is 40 mmHg, a pressure increase of 10 mmHg (up to 50 mmHg) is acceptable during leg movement. Likewise, if the start pressure is 35 mmHg (with multifidus facilitation), a pressure increase of 10 mmHg (up to 45 mmHg) is acceptable during leg movement. However, when leg movement stops the pressure must be maintained at the original start pressure.

Multifidus facilitation

If uncontrolled lumbar flexion is identified, facilitation of superficial lumbar multifidus is encouraged. Take a relaxed breath in and breathe out and consciously hold the sternum and ribcage down towards the bed. Try to visualise pulling the sacrum horizontally up along the bed towards the shoulders. The lumbar lordosis should increase slightly and the pressure should decrease. Do not use thoracic extension to decrease the pressure (no lifting of the chest). Ideally, with efficient superficial lumbar multifidus activation, the pressure should decrease by 5–10 mmHg (from 40 mmHg to approximately 35–30 mmHg) (Figure 5.18). This pressure decrease should be able to be consistently maintained.

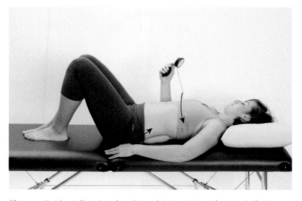

Figure 5.18 Adjusting lumbopelvic position for multifidus facilitation

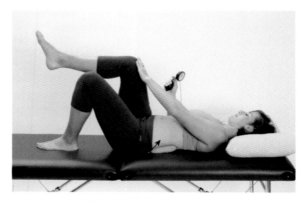

Figure 5.19 Facilitation with opposite knee to hand push

Static diagonal: isometric opposite knee to hand push

First facilitate superficial lumbar multifidus (PBU held at 30–35 mmHg or other hand to monitor that no pressure change = spinal control), slowly lift one knee towards the opposite hand and push them isometrically against each other on a diagonal line (Figure 5.19). Push for 10 seconds and repeat 10 times so long as stability is maintained (no pressure change). As soon as any pressure increase or decrease is registered the movement must stop and return to the start position. Do not stabilise with the opposite foot or allow substitution or fatigue.

Static diagonal heel lift: isometric knee to hand push + 2nd heel lift

First facilitate superficial lumbar multifidus (PBU held at 30–35 mmHg or other hand to monitor that no pressure change = spinal stability), slowly lift one knee towards the opposite hand and push them isometrically against each other on a diagonal line. While keeping this pressure slowly lift the second heel off the floor and bring it up beside the first leg (Figure 5.20). Hold this position for 10 seconds and repeat 10 times so long as stability is maintained (no pressure change). As soon as any pressure increase or decrease is registered the movement must stop and return to the start position. The point of greatest risk of losing stability is when the second heel leaves the floor. Do not allow substitution or fatigue.

Alternate single leg heel touch: (Sahrmann level 1)

First facilitate superficial lumbar multifidus (PBU held at 30–35 mmHg or other hand to monitor that no pressure change = spinal control), slowly lift one foot off the floor (Figure 5.21) and then lift the second foot off the floor and bring it up beside the first leg (Figure 5.22). Crook lying with hips flexed to 90° and *both* feet off the floor is the starting position.

Hold this position and keeping the back stable (no pressure change) slowly lower one heel to the floor (Figure 5.23) and lift it back to the start position. Repeat this movement, slowly alternating legs, for 10 seconds so long as stability is maintained (no pressure change), and then return both feet to the floor. Repeat the whole process 10 times.

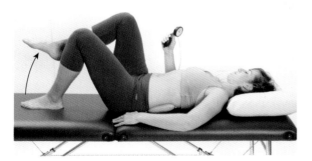

Figure 5.20 Facilitation with second leg lift

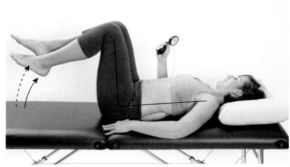

Figure 5.22 Progression: second leg lift

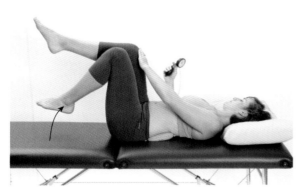

Figure 5.21 Progression: first leg lift

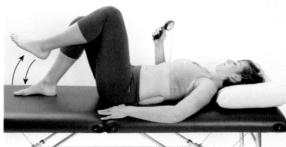

Figure 5.23 Progression: first leg lower

As soon as any pressure increase (or decrease) is registered the movement must stop and return to the start position. The point of greatest risk of losing stability is when the heel is lowering to the floor. Do not allow substitution or fatigue.

The person should self-monitor the lumbopelvic alignment and control with a variety of feedback options (T3.3). It is very useful to use a PBU for precise monitoring of lumbar position. Taping will also provide sensory feedback and some degree of mechanical support to the control of flexion. Visual feedback (e.g. observation in a mirror) is also a useful retraining tool.

If control is poor, the leg lift with a controlled back and independent hip flexion should be performed *only* as far as lumbar flexion and posterior pelvic tilt can be actively controlled or prevented. There should be no provocation of any symptoms, so long as the lumbar flexion can be controlled. Once the pattern of dissociation is efficient and feels familiar it should be integrated into various functional postures and positions.

T3.1 Assessment and rating of low threshold recruitment efficiency of the Double Bent Leg Lift Test

DOUBLE BENT LEG LIFT TEST – CROOK LYING

ASSESSMENT

Control point:
- prevent multisegmental lumbar flexion and posterior pelvic tilt

Movement challenge: hip flexion (crook lying)

Benchmark range: 90° bilateral hip flexion with independent hip flexion

RATING OF LOW THRESHOLD RECRUITMENT EFFICIENCY FOR CONTROL OF DIRECTION

	✓ or ✗		✓ or ✗

• Able to prevent 'UCM' into the test direction. Correct dissociation pattern of movement
Prevent lumbar UCM into:
   posterior pelvic tilt and hyperflexion
    (multisegment)
and move hip flexion
	☐	• Looks easy, and in the opinion of the assessor, is performed with confidence	☐

		• Feels easy, and the subject has sufficient awareness of the movement pattern that they confidently prevent 'UCM' into the test direction	☐

• Dissociate movement through the benchmark range of: 90° bilateral independent hip flexion and:
   maintain the PBU at 40 mmHg ± 10 mmHg
    while the legs are moving
   Hold the PBU at 40 mmHg for 5 seconds
    with hips flexed at 90°
If there is more available range than the benchmark standard, only the benchmark range needs to be actively controlled
	☐	• The pattern of dissociation is smooth during concentric and eccentric movement	☐

		• Does not (consistently) use *end range* movement into the opposite direction to prevent the UCM	☐
		• No extra feedback needed *(tactile, visual or verbal cueing)*	☐
		• Without external support or unloading	☐
		• Relaxed natural breathing *(even if not ideal – so long as natural pattern does not change)*	☐
• Without holding breath (though it is acceptable to use an alternate breathing strategy)	☐	• No fatigue	☐
• Control during eccentric phase	☐		
• Control during concentric phase	☐		

CORRECT DISSOCIATION PATTERN   **RECRUITMENT EFFICIENCY**

T3.2 Diagnosis of the site and direction of UCM from the Double Bent Leg Lift Test

DOUBLE BENT LEG LIFT TEST – CROOK LYING

Site	Direction	Segmental/ multisegmental	✗✗ or ✓✗
Lumbar	Flexion	Multisegmental hyperflexion	☐

T3.3 Feedback tools to monitor retraining

FEEDBACK TOOL	PROCESS
Self-palpation	Palpation monitoring of joint position
Visual observation	Observe in a mirror or directly watch the movement
Adhesive tape	Skin tension for tactile feedback
Pressure biofeedback	Visual confirmation of the control of position
Cueing and verbal correction	Listen to feedback from another observer

T4 SITTING: FORWARD LEAN TEST (tests for lumbar flexion UCM)

This dissociation test assesses the ability to actively dissociate and control lumbar flexion and posterior pelvic tilt then lean forwards by moving the hips through flexion while sitting.

Test procedure

The person should have the ability to actively lean forwards by flexing at the hips while controlling the lumbar spine and pelvis. The person sits tall with the feet on the floor and with the lumbar spine and pelvis positioned in neutral (Figure 5.24). Lumbopelvic motion is monitored by the therapist. The therapist monitors the lumbosacral neutral position by palpating the spinous process of L2, L5, and S2 with their finger tips (Figure 5.25).

During testing, if the palpating fingers do not move, the lumbosacral region is able to maintain neutral. If the palpating fingers move further apart, uncontrolled lumbar flexion is identified.

The person is instructed to sit tall and to lean the trunk forwards from the hips, keeping the back straight (neutral spine). Ideally, the subject should have the ability to dissociate the lumbar spine from hip flexion as evidenced by 30° forward lean (Hamilton & Richardson 1998) while preventing lumbar flexion or posterior pelvic tilt (Figure 5.26). This test should be performed without any feedback (self-palpation, vision, tape, etc.) or cueing for correction.

Lumbar flexion UCM

The person complains of flexion-related symptoms in the lumbar spine. The lumbar spine has UCM into flexion relative to the hips under flexion load. During active hip flexion in sitting, the lumbar spine starts to flex before achieving 30° forward lean. During the attempt to dissociate the lumbar spine from independent hip flexion the person either cannot control the UCM or has to concentrate and try hard.

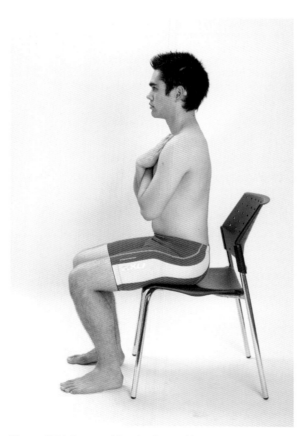

Figure 5.24 Start position for forward lean test

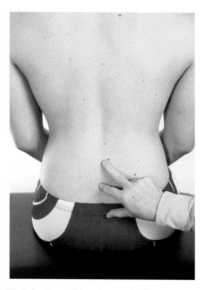

Figure 5.25 Palpation of lumbosacral alignment

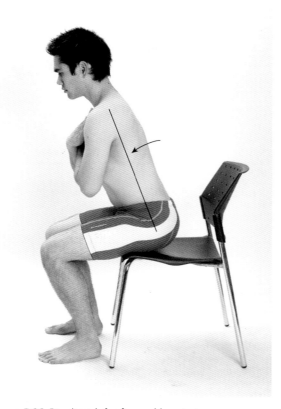

Figure 5.26 Benchmark for forward lean test

- If only one spinous process is observed as prominent and protruding 'out of line' compared to the other vertebrae then the UCM is interpreted as a *segmental flexion hinge*. The specific hinging segment should be noted and recorded.
- If excessive lumbopelvic flexion is observed, but no one particular spinous process is prominent from the adjacent vertebrae then the UCM is interpreted as a *multisegmental hyperflexion*.

Clinical assessment note for direction-specific motor control testing

If some other movement (e.g. a small amount of extension or rotation) is observed during a motor control (dissociation) test of flexion control, *do not* score this as uncontrolled flexion. The extension and rotation motor control tests will identify if the observed movement is uncontrolled. A test for lumbar flexion UCM is only positive if uncontrolled lumbar flexion is demonstrated.

Rating and diagnosis of lumbar flexion UCM

(T4.1 and T4.2)

Correction

The person sits tall with the feet on the floor and with the lumbar spine and pelvis positioned in the neutral. The person should monitor the lumbar alignment and control with a variety of feedback options (T4.3). They monitor the lumbosacral neutral position by palpating the spinous process of L2, L5 and S2 with their fingers. The person is instructed to sit tall and to lean the trunk forwards from the hips, keeping the back straight (neutral spine). If the palpating fingers do not move further apart, lumbar flexion is being controlled.

In some cases it may be useful to tension a strip of adhesive sports strapping tape to the skin across the uncontrolled segments. This will provide sensory feedback and some degree of mechanical support to the control of flexion. Visual feedback (e.g. observation in a mirror) is also a useful retraining tool. Ideally, the subject should have the ability to dissociate the lumbar spine from hip flexion as evidenced by 30° forward lean while preventing lumbar flexion or posterior pelvic tilt. There should be no provocation of any symptoms under flexion load, within the range that the flexion UCM can be controlled.

If control is poor, the pattern of forward leaning with a straight back and independent hip flexion should be performed *only* as far as lumbar flexion and posterior pelvic tilt can be actively controlled or prevented. Also, the upper body and trunk weight can be supported by weight bearing through the arms to decrease the load that must be controlled by the local and global stabiliser muscles. As the ability to control the UCM gets easier and the pattern of dissociation feels less unnatural the exercise can be progressed to the unsupported position. Once the pattern of dissociation is efficient and feels familiar it should be integrated into various functional postures and positions.

T4.1 Assessment and rating of low threshold recruitment efficiency of the Forward Lean Test

FORWARD LEAN TEST – SITTING

ASSESSMENT

Control point:
- prevent multisegmental lumbar flexion and posterior pelvic tilt
- prevent segmental flexion hinge and posterior tilt

Movement challenge: hip flexion (sitting)

Benchmark range: 30° forward lean of trunk with independent hip flexion

RATING OF LOW THRESHOLD RECRUITMENT EFFICIENCY FOR CONTROL OF DIRECTION

	✓ or ✗		✓ or ✗
• Able to prevent 'UCM' into the test direction. Correct dissociation pattern of movement Prevent lumbar UCM into: posterior pelvic tilt and hyperflexion (multisegment) posterior pelvic tilt and flexion hinge (single segment) and move hip flexion	☐	• Looks easy, and in the opinion of the assessor, is performed with confidence	☐
		• Feels easy, and the subject has sufficient awareness of the movement pattern that they confidently prevent 'UCM' into the test direction	☐
• Dissociate movement through the benchmark range of: 30° forward lean of trunk with independent hip flexion *If there is more available range than the benchmark standard, only the benchmark range needs to be actively controlled*	☐	• The pattern of dissociation is smooth during concentric and eccentric movement	☐
		• Does not (consistently) use *end range* movement into the opposite direction to prevent the UCM	☐
		• No extra feedback needed *(tactile, visual or verbal cueing)*	☐
• Without holding breath (though it is acceptable to use an alternate breathing strategy)	☐	• Without external support or unloading	☐
		• Relaxed natural breathing *(even if not ideal – so long as natural pattern does not change)*	☐
• Control during eccentric phase	☐	• No fatigue	☐
• Control during concentric phase	☐		

CORRECT DISSOCIATION PATTERN   **RECRUITMENT EFFICIENCY**

T4.2 Diagnosis of the site and direction of UCM from the Forward Lean Test

FORWARD LEAN TEST – SITTING

Site	Direction	Segmental/multisegmental	✗✗ or ✓✗
Lumbar	Flexion	Segmental flexion hinge (indicate level)	☐
		Multisegmental hyperflexion	☐

T4.3 Feedback tools to monitor retraining

FEEDBACK TOOL	PROCESS
Self-palpation	Palpation monitoring of joint position
Visual observation	Observe in a mirror or directly watch the movement
Adhesive tape	Skin tension for tactile feedback
Cueing and verbal correction	Listen to feedback from another observer

T5 SITTING: CHEST DROP TEST
(tests for lumbar flexion UCM)

This dissociation test assesses the ability to actively dissociate and control lumbar flexion and posterior pelvic tilt then actively flex the thoracic spine while sitting.

Test procedure

The person should have the ability to actively lower the sternum towards the pelvis by flexing the thoracic spine while controlling the lumbar spine and pelvis. The person sits tall with the feet off the floor and with the lumbar spine and pelvis positioned in the neutral. Make the spine as tall or as long as possible to position the normal curves in an elongated 'S' without leaning

backwards. Position the head directly over the shoulders without chin poke. Monitor thoracolumbar motion by placing one hand on the sternum. Monitor lumbopelvic motion by placing the other hand on the sacrum (Figure 5.27) (alternative lumbopelvic monitoring: place one finger on the pubic bone). Without letting the lumbopelvic region move (pelvis and sacral hand does not move), allow the sternum to lower (drop) towards the stationary pelvis. This is independent thoracic flexion.

Ideally, the person should have the ability to keep the lumbopelvic region neutral while independently flexing the thoracic region from a position of extension through to full thoracic flexion, without any movement of the pelvis (Figure 5.28). This test should be performed without any feedback (self-palpation, vision, tape, etc.) or cueing for correction.

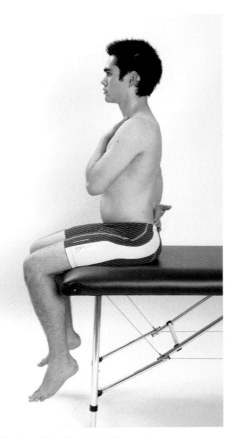

Figure 5.27 Start position for chest drop test

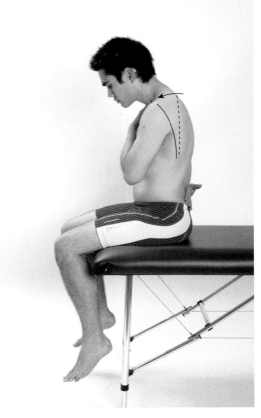

Figure 5.28 Benchmark for chest drop test

Lumbar flexion UCM

The person complains of flexion-related symptoms in the lumbar spine. The lumbar spine has UCM into flexion relative to the thorax under flexion load. The lumbar spine starts to flex before full thoracic flexion is achieved. The person either cannot control the UCM or has to concentrate and try hard to dissociate the lumbar spine from independent thoracic flexion.

- If only one spinous process is observed as prominent and protruding 'out of line' compared to the other vertebrae then the UCM is interpreted as a *segmental flexion hinge*. The specific hinging segment should be noted and recorded.
- If excessive lumbopelvic flexion is observed, but no one particular spinous process is prominent from the adjacent vertebrae then the UCM is interpreted as a *multisegmental hyperflexion*.

When rectus abdominis (global mobiliser) is the dominant trunk flexor, it produces concurrent thoracolumbar flexion and lumbopelvic flexion. If the lumbopelvic region can actively resist flexion (with segmental extensor stabiliser activation) while the thoracolumbar region actively flexes the thorax, the rectus abdominis must be inhibited to some extent. The oblique abdominals (global stabilisers) will probably contribute more to the thoracolumbar flexion component because they are less directly inhibited by the thoracic flexion.

Clinical assessment note for direction-specific motor control testing

If some other movement (e.g. a small amount of extension or rotation) is observed during a motor control (dissociation) test of flexion control, *do not* score this as uncontrolled flexion. The extension and rotation motor control tests will identify if the observed movement is uncontrolled. A test for lumbar flexion UCM is only positive if uncontrolled lumbar flexion is demonstrated.

Rating and diagnosis of lumbar flexion UCM

(T5.1 and T5.2)

Correction

The person sits tall with the feet on the floor and with the lumbar spine and pelvis positioned in neutral. The person should monitor the lumbar alignment and control with a variety of feedback options (T5.3). They monitor the lumbosacral neutral position by palpating the spinous process of L2, L5 and S2 with their fingers. If the palpating fingers do not move further apart and the pelvis does not roll back into posterior tilt, lumbar flexion is being controlled.

In some cases it may be useful to tension a strip of adhesive sports strapping tape to the skin across the uncontrolled segments. This will provide sensory feedback and some degree of mechanical support to the control of flexion. Visual feedback (e.g. observation in a mirror) is also a useful retraining tool.

Ideally, the subject should have the ability to dissociate the lumbar spine from thoracic flexion as evidenced by the ability to keep the lumbopelvic region neutral while independently flexing the thoracic region from a position of extension through flexion. Move the thoracic spine into flexion, but only as far as the neutral lumbopelvic position can be maintained. There must be no loss of neutral or UCM into lumbar flexion or posterior pelvic tilt. There should be no provocation of any symptoms under flexion load, so long as the flexion give can be controlled.

As the ability to independently control movement of the thoracic spine and lumbopelvic region gets easier and the pattern of dissociation feels less unnatural, the exercise can be progressed to performing concurrent thoracic flexion with lumbopelvic extension.

If control is poor, the upper body and trunk weight can be supported on hands and knees. Position the pelvis over the knees and the shoulders over the hands with the knees and hands comfortably apart. Rock the pelvis backwards and forwards from the sacrum (posterior and anterior tilt) until the lumbar spine is in a long *shallow* lordosis. Then, push the body gently away from the hands without flexing the thoracic spine or lowering the head. Then lift the head (without chin poke) so that the back of the head touches an imaginary line connecting the sacrum and mid-thoracic spine. Use minimal effort to maintain this neutral spine position (Figure 5.29).

When control is poor, rather than specific dissociation, for some patients, it is easier to use a recruitment reversal exercise to start with:

- Actively flex the thoracic spine and then extend the lumbar spine and anterior tilt the pelvis (Figure 5.30).
- The reverse order of this same pattern may also be used. That is, actively extend the

T5.1 Assessment and rating of low threshold recruitment efficiency of the Chest Drop Test

CHEST DROP TEST – SITTING

ASSESSMENT

Control point:
- prevent multisegmental lumbar flexion and posterior pelvic tilt
- prevent segmental flexion hinge and posterior tilt

Movement challenge: thoracic flexion (sitting)

Benchmark range: full available independent thoracic flexion

RATING OF LOW THRESHOLD RECRUITMENT EFFICIENCY FOR CONTROL OF DIRECTION

	✓ or ✗		✓ or ✗

• Able to prevent 'UCM' into the test direction. Correct dissociation pattern of movement
Prevent lumbar UCM into:
  posterior pelvic tilt and hyperflexion (multisegment)
  posterior pelvic tilt and flexion hinge (single segment)
and move hip flexion
	☐	• Looks easy, and in the opinion of the assessor, is performed with confidence	☐

		• Feels easy, and the subject has sufficient awareness of the movement pattern that they confidently prevent 'UCM' into the test direction	☐
• Dissociate movement through the benchmark range of: full available independent thoracic flexion *If there is more available range than the benchmark standard, only the benchmark range needs to be actively controlled*	☐	• The pattern of dissociation is smooth during concentric and eccentric movement	☐
		• Does not (consistently) use *end range* movement into the opposite direction to prevent the UCM	☐
		• No extra feedback needed *(tactile, visual or verbal cueing)*	☐
• Without holding breath (though it is acceptable to use an alternate breathing strategy)	☐	• Without external support or unloading	☐
		• Relaxed natural breathing *(even if not ideal – so long as natural pattern does not change)*	☐
• Control during eccentric phase	☐	• No fatigue	☐
• Control during concentric phase	☐		

CORRECT DISSOCIATION PATTERN   **RECRUITMENT EFFICIENCY**

T5.2 Diagnosis of the site and direction of UCM from the Chest Drop Test

CHEST DROP TEST – SITTING

Site	Direction	Segmental/ multisegmental	✗✗ or ✓✗
Lumbar	Flexion	Segmental flexion hinge (indicate level)	☐
		Multisegmental hyperflexion	☐

T5.3 Feedback tools to monitor retraining

FEEDBACK TOOL	PROCESS
Self-palpation	Palpation monitoring of joint position
Visual observation	Observe in a mirror or directly watch the movement
Adhesive tape	Skin tension for tactile feedback
Cueing and verbal correction	Listen to feedback from another observer

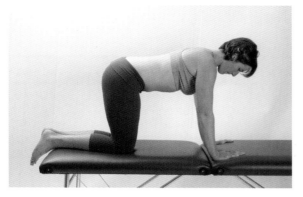

Figure 5.29 Correction (neutral start position)

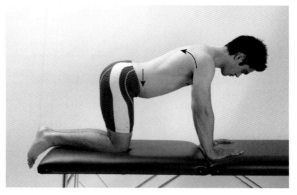

Figure 5.31 Correction (lumbar extension followed by thoracic flexion)

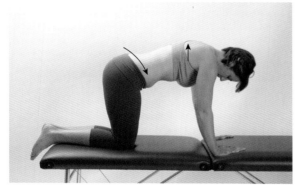

Figure 5.30 Correction (thoracic flexion followed by lumbar extension)

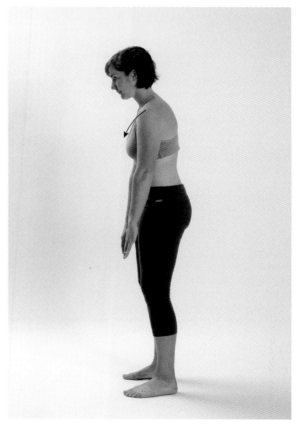

Figure 5.32 Progression: standing thoracic flexion

lumbar spine and anterior tilt the pelvis and then flex the thoracic spine (Figure 5.31).

When the pattern of this recruitment reversal feels easy, then progress back to the sitting dissociation.

As the ability to independently control movement of the thoracic spine and lumbopelvic region gets easier and the pattern of dissociation feels less unnatural, the exercise can be progressed to standing. Stand upright with the knees and hips slightly flexed (unlocked) to prevent hip flexor tightness influencing the pelvis). Without letting the lumbopelvic region move (pelvis and sacrum do not move) lower the sternum (thoracic flexion) towards the stationary pelvis (Figure 5.32).

Once the pattern of dissociation is efficient and feels familiar it should be integrated into various functional postures and positions.

T6 SITTING: DOUBLE KNEE EXTENSION TEST
(tests for lumbar flexion UCM)

This dissociation test assesses the ability to actively dissociate and control lumbar flexion and posterior pelvic tilt while sitting, then actively extend both knees to engage the point where hamstring tension starts to pull the pelvis into posterior tilt.

Test procedure

The person sits tall with both feet off the floor and with the lumbar spine and pelvis positioned in neutral. Make the spine as tall or as long as possible to position the normal curves in an elongated 'S' with the acromions vertical over the ischiums (do not lean backwards) (Figure 5.33). Without letting the lumbopelvic region move they should then straighten both knees simultaneously to within 10–15° of full extension, keeping the back straight (neutral spine) and without leaning back or allowing the pelvis to posteriorly tilt (Figure 5.34). Ideally, the person should have the ability to keep the lumbopelvic region neutral and prevent the hamstrings pulling the pelvis into posterior tilt and lumbar flexion. This test should be performed without any feedback (self-palpation, vision, tape, etc.) or cueing for correction.

Lumbar flexion UCM

The person complains of flexion-related symptoms in the lumbar spine. The lumbar spine has UCM into flexion relative to the pelvis under hamstrings tension and posterior tilt load. The pelvis posteriorly tilts or the lumbar spine starts to flex before the knees reach 10–15° from full

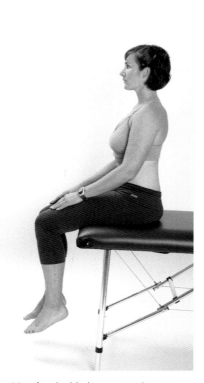

Figure 5.33 Start position for double knee extension test

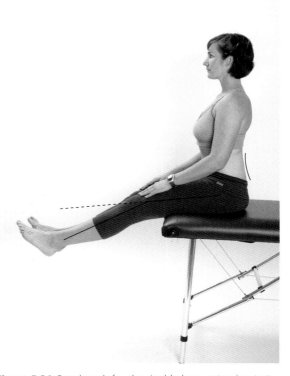

Figure 5.34 Benchmark for the double knee extension test

extension. The subject either cannot control the UCM or has to concentrate and try hard to dissociate the lumbar spine from independent hamstrings tension.

- If only one spinous process is observed as prominent and protruding 'out of line' compared to the other vertebrae then the UCM is interpreted as a *segmental flexion hinge*. The specific hinging segment should be noted and recorded.
- If excessive lumbopelvic flexion is observed, but no one particular spinous process is prominent from the adjacent vertebrae then the UCM is interpreted as a *multisegmental hyperflexion*.

Clinical assessment note for direction-specific motor control testing

If some other movement (e.g. a small amount of extension or rotation) is observed during a motor control (dissociation) test of flexion control, *do not* score this as uncontrolled flexion. The extension and rotation motor control tests will identify if the observed movement is uncontrolled. A test for lumbar flexion UCM is only positive if uncontrolled lumbar flexion is demonstrated.

Rating and diagnosis of lumbar flexion UCM

(T6.1 and T6.2)

Correction

The person sits tall with the feet on the floor and with the lumbar spine and pelvis positioned in the neutral. The person should monitor the lumbar alignment and control with a variety of feedback options (T6.3). They monitor the lumbosacral neutral position by palpating the spinous process of L2, L5 and S2 with their fingers. The person is instructed to slowly straighten both knees simultaneously to within 10–15° of full extension, keeping the back straight (neutral spine) and without leaning back or allowing the pelvis to posteriorly tilt. If the palpating fingers do not move further apart, lumbar flexion and posterior tilt are being controlled.

In some cases it may be useful to tension a strip of adhesive sports strapping tape to the skin across the uncontrolled segments. This will provide sensory feedback and some degree of mechanical support to the control of flexion. Visual feedback (e.g. observation in a mirror) is also a useful retraining tool. There should be no provocation of any symptoms under flexion load, so long as the flexion give can be controlled. Only straighten the knees as far as the neutral lumbopelvic position (monitored with feedback) can be maintained. There must be no loss of neutral or UCM into flexion or posterior tilt.

If control is poor it is acceptable to start with unilateral (then progress to bilateral) knee extension with a straight back, but only as far as the neutral lumbopelvic position can be maintained. There must be no loss of neutral or give into flexion. There should be no provocation of any symptoms under flexion load, so long as the flexion give can be controlled. Beware neurodynamic symptoms associated with positive slump responses. Unload the neural system with ankle plantarflexion or cervical extension. Once the pattern of dissociation is efficient and feels familiar it should be integrated into various functional postures and positions.

T6.1 Assessment and rating of low threshold recruitment efficiency of the Double Knee Extension Test

DOUBLE KNEE EXTENSION TEST – SITTING

ASSESSMENT

Control point:
- prevent multisegmental lumbar flexion and posterior pelvic tilt
- prevent segmental flexion hinge and posterior tilt

Movement challenge: posterior tilt force from hamstring tension (sitting)

Benchmark range: 10–15° from full knee extension (bilateral)

RATING OF LOW THRESHOLD RECRUITMENT EFFICIENCY FOR CONTROL OF DIRECTION

	✓ or ✗		✓ or ✗

• Able to prevent 'UCM' into the test direction. Correct dissociation pattern of movement
Prevent lumbar UCM into:
   posterior pelvic tilt and hyperflexion (multisegment)
   posterior pelvic tilt and flexion hinge (single segment)
and move bilateral knee extension
	☐	• Looks easy, and in the opinion of the assessor, is performed with confidence	☐

		• Feels easy, and the subject has sufficient awareness of the movement pattern that they confidently prevent 'UCM' into the test direction	☐
• Dissociate movement through the benchmark range of: 10–15° from full knee extension *If there is more available range than the benchmark standard, only the benchmark range needs to be actively controlled*	☐	• The pattern of dissociation is smooth during concentric and eccentric movement	☐
		• Does not (consistently) use *end range* movement into the opposite direction to prevent the UCM	☐
• Without holding breath (though it is acceptable to use an alternate breathing strategy)	☐	• No extra feedback needed *(tactile, visual or verbal cueing)*	☐
		• Without external support or unloading	☐
• Control during eccentric phase	☐	• Relaxed natural breathing *(even if not ideal – so long as natural pattern does not change)*	☐
• Control during concentric phase	☐	• No fatigue	☐

CORRECT DISSOCIATION PATTERN   **RECRUITMENT EFFICIENCY**

T6.2 Diagnosis of the site and direction of UCM from the Double Knee Extension Test

DOUBLE KNEE EXTENSION TEST – SITTING

Site	Direction	Segmental/multisegmental	✗✗ or ✓✗
Lumbar	Flexion	Segmental flexion hinge (indicate level)	☐
		Multisegmental hyperflexion	☐

T6.3 Feedback tools to monitor retraining

FEEDBACK TOOL	PROCESS
Self-palpation	Palpation monitoring of joint position
Visual observation	Observe in a mirror or directly watch the movement
Adhesive tape	Skin tension for tactile feedback
Cueing and verbal correction	Listen to feedback from another observer

T7 STAND TO SIT: ISCHIAL WEIGHT BEARING TEST
(tests for lumbar flexion UCM)

This dissociation test assesses the ability to actively dissociate and control lumbar flexion and posterior pelvic tilt while moving from standing to sitting.

Test procedure

The chair seat height should be adjusted so that when seated the hips are slightly higher (about 10°) than the knees. The feet should be positioned where they feel natural to stand up from sitting (Figure 5.35). The person is instructed to stand tall with the lumbar spine and pelvis positioned in neutral and to keep the lumbopelvic region neutral as they sit down on a chair. Then, *slowly* sit down on the chair by leaning forwards

and bending at the hips and knees, and not using the hands for support. Keeping the spine straight, the person should flex forwards at the hips as the pelvis is lowered onto the chair. The heels do *not* have to stay on the floor. The critical control point occurs when the ischiums contact the chair and weight bearing load is transferred to the ischiums (Figure 5.36).

Ideally, the person should have the ability to maintain lumbopelvic neutral and prevent lumbar flexion or posterior pelvic tilt as the hips flex and the pelvis lowers to the chair and weight is transferred to the ischiums. This test should be performed without any feedback (self-palpation, vision, tape, etc.) or cueing for correction.

Lumbar flexion UCM

The person complains of flexion-related symptoms in the lumbar spine. The lumbar spine has UCM into flexion relative to the hips. The pelvis

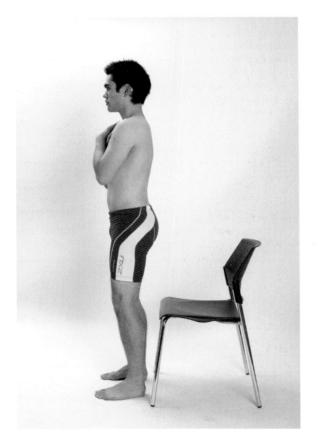

Figure 5.35 Start position for ischial weight bearing test

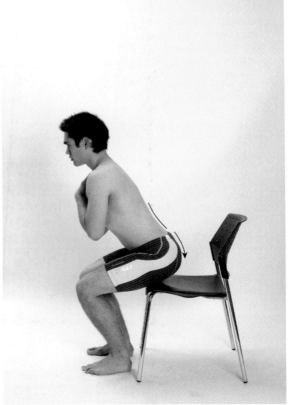

Figure 5.36 Benchmark for ischial weight bearing test

posteriorly tilts and the lumbar spine starts to flex as weight bearing load is transferred to the ischiums. The subject either cannot control the UCM or has to concentrate and try hard to dissociate the lumbar spine from independent thoracic flexion.

- If only one spinous process is observed as prominent and protruding 'out of line' compared to the other vertebrae then the UCM is interpreted as a *segmental flexion hinge*. The specific hinging segment should be noted and recorded.
- If excessive lumbopelvic flexion is observed, but no one particular spinous process is prominent from the adjacent vertebrae then the UCM is interpreted as a *multisegmental hyperflexion*.

Clinical assessment note for direction-specific motor control testing

If some other movement (e.g. a small amount of extension or rotation) is observed during a motor control (dissociation) test of flexion control, *do not* score this as uncontrolled flexion. The extension and rotation motor control tests will identify if the observed movement is uncontrolled. A test for lumbar flexion UCM is only positive if uncontrolled lumbar flexion is demonstrated.

Rating and diagnosis of lumbar flexion UCM

(T7.1 and T7.2)

Correction

The person stands with the feet positioned where they feel natural to stand up from sitting. They are instructed to *slowly* begin to sit down on the chair by leaning forwards and bending at the hips and knees, not using the hands for support. The person should monitor the lumbar alignment and control with a variety of feedback options (T7.3). Keeping the spine straight, the person should flex forwards at the hips as the pelvis is lowered onto the chair. The heels do *not* have to stay on the floor. Only move backwards towards sitting as far as the neutral lumbopelvic position (monitored with feedback) can be maintained. Initially, it may be easier to just touch the chair with the ischiums (and not transfer any weight

from the feet to the pelvis), then immediately return to standing.

There must be no loss of neutral or UCM into flexion or posterior tilt. There should be no provocation of any symptoms under flexion load, so long as the flexion UCM can be controlled. In some cases it may be useful to tension a strip of adhesive sports strapping tape to the skin across the uncontrolled segments. This will provide sensory feedback and some degree of mechanical support to the control of flexion. Visual feedback (e.g. observation in a mirror) is also a useful retraining tool.

If control is poor it is acceptable to start by increasing the chair seat height (or use a stool or table) so that less hip flexion is required before ischial weight bearing is loaded (Figure 5.37). There must be no loss of neutral or UCM into flexion. As control improves, lower the chair

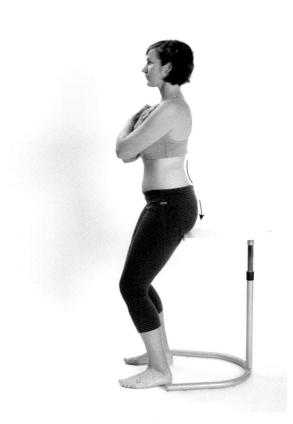

Figure 5.37 Correction through less range

T7.1 Assessment and rating of low threshold recruitment efficiency of the Ischial Weight Bearing Test

ISCHIAL WEIGHT BEARING TEST – STANDING TO SITTING

ASSESSMENT

Control point:
- prevent multisegmental lumbar flexion and posterior pelvic tilt
- prevent segmental flexion hinge and posterior tilt

Movement challenge: hip flexion (standing to sitting)

Benchmark range: weight bearing transfer to the ischiums while sitting down onto a chair height adjusted so that the hips are slightly higher (about 10°) than the knees

RATING OF LOW THRESHOLD RECRUITMENT EFFICIENCY FOR CONTROL OF DIRECTION

	✓ or ✗		✓ or ✗
• Able to prevent 'UCM' into the test direction. Correct dissociation pattern of movement Prevent lumbar UCM into: 　posterior pelvic tilt and hyperflexion 　　(multisegment) 　posterior pelvic tilt and flexion hinge (single 　　segment) and move hip flexion	☐	• Looks easy, and in the opinion of the assessor, is performed with confidence	☐
		• Feels easy, and the subject has sufficient awareness of the movement pattern that they confidently prevent 'UCM' into the test direction	☐
• Dissociate movement through the benchmark range of: hip flexion from standing to sitting (chair height) and weight bearing transfer to the ischiums *If there is more available range than the benchmark standard, only the benchmark range needs to be actively controlled*	☐	• The pattern of dissociation is smooth during concentric and eccentric movement	☐
		• Does not (consistently) use *end range* movement into the opposite direction to prevent the UCM	☐
		• No extra feedback needed *(tactile, visual or verbal cueing)*	☐
• Without holding breath (though it is acceptable to use an alternate breathing strategy)	☐	• Without external support or unloading	☐
		• Relaxed natural breathing *(even if not ideal – so long as natural pattern does not change)*	☐
• Control during eccentric phase	☐	• No fatigue	☐
• Control during concentric phase	☐		

CORRECT DISSOCIATION PATTERN　　　　　　**RECRUITMENT EFFICIENCY**

T7.2 Diagnosis of the site and direction of UCM from the Ischial Weight Bearing Test

ISCHIAL WEIGHT BEARING TEST – STANDING TO SITTING

Site	Direction	Segmental/ multisegmental	✗✗ or ✓✗
Lumbar	Flexion	Segmental flexion hinge (indicate level)	☐
		Multisegmental hyperflexion	☐

T7.3 Feedback tools to monitor retraining

FEEDBACK TOOL	PROCESS
Self-palpation	Palpation monitoring of joint position
Visual observation	Observe in a mirror or directly watch the movement
Adhesive tape	Skin tension for tactile feedback
Cueing and verbal correction	Listen to feedback from another observer

Table 5.4 Summary and rating of lumbar flexion tests		
UCM DIAGNOSIS AND TESTING		
SITE: LUMBAR	DIRECTION: FLEXION	CLINICAL PRIORITY ☐
TEST	RATING (✓✓ or ✓✗ or ✗✗) and rationale	
Standing: trunk lean		
4 point: backward push		
Crook: double bent leg lift		
Sitting: forward lean		
Sitting: chest drop		
Sitting: double knee extension		
Stand to sit: ischial weight bearing		

height slightly and first practise moving forwards from sitting to standing while monitoring the control of lumbar flexion and posterior pelvic tilt. Progress until control is efficient on a chair with the height adjusted so that the hips are slightly higher (about 10°) than the knees. Once the pattern of dissociation is efficient and feels familiar it should be integrated into various functional postures and positions.

Lumbar flexion UCM summary

(Table 5.4)

Tests of lumbar extension control

EXTENSION CONTROL TESTS AND EXTENSION CONTROL REHABILITATION

These extension control tests assess the extent of extension UCM in the lumbar spine and assess the ability of the dynamic stability system to adequately control extension load or strain. It is a priority to assess for extension UCM if the patient complains of or demonstrates extension-related symptoms or disability.

OBSERVATION AND ANALYSIS OF LUMBAR EXTENSION AND BACKWARD ARCHING

Description of ideal pattern

The subject is instructed to extend and arch backwards as they normally would. Ideally, there should be even extension throughout the spine as the patient actively extends, with the pelvis contributing slight to moderate *concurrent* anterior tilt and finishing with the hips in 10–15° of extension. The whole lumbar and lower thoracic spine should contribute to the spinal extension. The pelvis should not sway forwards any further than approximately 10 cm and there should be good symmetry of movement without any deviation, tilt or rotation of the trunk or pelvis (Figure 5.38).

Movement faults associated with lumbar extension

Relative stiffness (restrictions)

- *Hip flexor muscles (tensor fasciae latae and iliotibial band) restriction of hip extension* – the hips lack 10–15° of normal range in standing backward arching. The lumbar spine frequently increases extension to compensate for the lack of hip mobility. tensor fasciae latae-iliotibial band extensibility can be tested passively and dynamically with manual muscle extensibility examination.
- *Thoracic restriction of extension* – the middle and lower thoracic spine (posturally

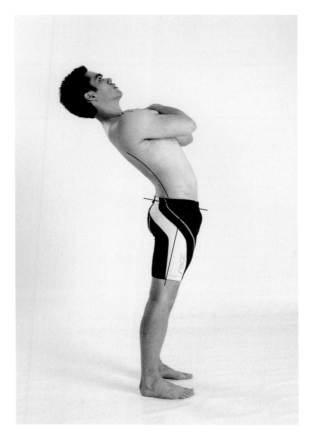

Figure 5.38 Ideal pattern of lumbar extension (backward arching)

kyphotic) has an extension restriction that may also contribute to compensatory increases in lumbar extension range. This is confirmed with manual segmental assessment (e.g. Maitland PPIVMs or PAIVMs).

Relative flexibility (potential UCM)

- *Lumbar extension.* There are two dominant mechanisms of uncontrolled extension. The first involves extension being initiated with excessive forward pelvic sway and uncontrolled extension occurring segmentally at the lumbosacral junction with the upper lumbar and lower thoracic spine contributing relatively less. The second involves extension being initiated by excessive anterior pelvic tilt and lumbar hyperextension so that uncontrolled extension occurs across the whole of the lumbar region. The lumbar spine may initiate the movement into extension, contribute more to producing backward arching, while the hips and thoracic contributions start later and contribute less. At the limit of backward arching, excessive or hypermobile range of lumbar extension may be observed. During the return to neutral the lumbar extension and anterior pelvic tilt persists and recovers later.

In the assessment of extension movement, the UCM can be identified as either segmental or multisegmental.

- *Segmental extension hinge*. If forward pelvic sway (with hip extension) initiates backward arching, the anterior pelvic tilt required for ideal extension is inadequate. The concurrent upper lumbar and lower thoracic extension contribution is late or absent. Consequently, instead of at least nine vertebral levels (T9–L1) contributing to (and sharing the load stresses) of spinal extension, only three segments appear to contribute significantly (L3–5). Of these, the segment at the pelvic junction (L5–S1) appears to translate forwards excessively, producing a skin crease as it hinges backwards into extension against the posteriorly tilted pelvis. If this segment is observed as hinging into translation 'out of line' compared to the other vertebrae then the UCM is interpreted as a *segmental extension hinge*. The specific hinging segment should be noted and recorded. This commonly occurs at the L5–S1 segment. Ideally, when lumbar extension control is assessed, the positional alignment between the low lumbar spine and the pelvis should be maintained during hip extension or thoracic extension challenges. If lumbopelvic stability and control is inadequate, L5 alignment with the sacrum cannot be maintained and during extension control tests the L5 and S1 segments appear to 'hinge' (observe a deep skin crease) as the pelvis sways forwards instead of anteriorly tilting and matching the alignment with the spinal movement. The upper lumbar and lower thoracic vertebral contribution is either late or absent.

- *Multisegmental hyperextension*. If, on the other hand, excessive or hypermobile lumbar extension and anterior pelvic tilt are observed, but no one particular vertebral level is dominant from the adjacent vertebrae then the UCM is interpreted as a *multisegmental hyperextension*. This is commonly observed as an excessive (deep) lumbar lordosis and hypermobile extension of the whole lumbar region. This excessive hyperlordosis is commonly initiated with exaggerated anterior pelvic tilt or occasionally it may be initiated with excessive thoracolumbar extension. Instead of maintaining positional control of the lumbar lordosis and the pelvis during hip extension or thoracic extension challenges, uncontrolled lumbar extension and anterior pelvic tilt are observed.

Indications to test for lumbar extension UCM

Observe or palpate for:

1. hypermobile lumbar extension range
2. excessive initiation of backward arching with forward pelvic sway and a lumbosacral hinge
3. excessive initiation of backward arching with hyperlordosis
4. symptoms (pain, discomfort, strain) associated with extension.

The person complains of extension-related symptoms in the lumbar spine. Under extension load, the lumbar spine has UCM *into extension* relative to the hips or relative to the thoracic spine. The dysfunction is confirmed with motor control tests of extension dissociation.

EXTENSION LOAD TESTING PREREQUISITES

These are not tests of extension stability function, but are considered a basic prerequisite for such tests. Back flattening on the wall is especially relevant for extension control between the thoracic and lumbar regions. It is important to be able to move the lumbar spine out of extension to at least the flat back position. Lateral abdominal–gluteal co-activation is especially relevant for extension control between the lumbar–pelvic region and

121

the hips. It is important to be able to co-activate the major stability muscle groups that can control excessive lumbopelvic extension strain.

BACK FLATTENING ON WALL – STANDING (PREREQUISITE)

Ideal

The person is instructed to stand with the feet 5–10 cm from the wall, with the feet wide apart (at least shoulder width apart) and with the knees slightly bent. This is to take the hip flexors off tension. Ideally, with the hip flexors off load and with the sacrum and thoracic spine on the wall, the person should be able to contract the abdominal and gluteal muscles to flatten the lumbar spine onto the wall and hold it there (Figure 5.39).

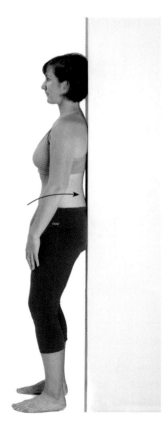

Figure 5.39 Extension control prerequisite: back flattening on wall

Dysfunction

Recruitment dysfunction

There is a lack of abdominal and gluteal co-activation. The flattening action is performed only with the abdominals and the gluteals do not participate or the flattening action is performed only with the gluteals and the abdominals do not participate.

Mobility dysfunction

The lumbar spine cannot flatten the lordosis sufficiently to get out of extension. This is not particularly common, but may occur with the longstanding lordotic posture where the back extensors have lost extensibility.

Correction

With the hip flexors unloaded and the sacrum and thoracic spine on the wall, actively flatten the low back towards the wall. Do not allow the thoracic spine to move or force so hard that thoracic pain is provoked. Hold this position for 10 seconds and repeat 10 times. Progression is achieved by increasing the holding time until it feels easy to get a confident low effort co-activation while maintaining the back flat against the wall continually for 2–3 minutes.

CO-ACTIVATION OF LATERAL ABDOMINALS AND GLUTEALS – PRONE (PREREQUISITE)

Ideal

The subject is instructed to actively 'hollow' or pull in the abdominal wall by activating and holding a contraction of the lateral abdominal muscles (transversus and the oblique abdominals). While this contraction is being held the subject is instructed to also contract the gluteal muscles. Ideally, the gluteals should confidently and strongly switch on with good symmetry and maintain this contraction without losing the abdominal contraction (Figure 5.40). These muscle groups are the muscles which can control extension strain at the lumbopelvic region under hip extension load.

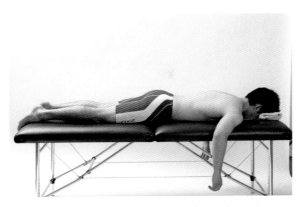

Figure 5.40 Extension control prerequisite: abdominal gluteal co-activation

Dysfunction

Recruitment dysfunction

The gluteal muscles have difficulty co-activating with the abdominal muscles. They either cannot activate or can only activate in a sluggish or asymmetrical way (similar to a quadriceps lag).

Correction

Activate the abdominals (hollowing contraction) and, while maintaining this contraction, consciously contract the gluteals. Hold this co-activation for 10 seconds and repeat 10 times. Progression is achieved by increasing the holding time until it feels easy to get a confident low effort co-activation while maintaining the co-activation continually for 2–3 minutes.

Note: if the person fails any of these extension prerequisites tests, care should be taken during the subsequent extension control tests. Monitor for any increase in symptoms while performing the extension control tests. If the person cannot adequately co-activate the stability muscles to control extension or cannot move out of extension sufficiently then the attempt to control extension may result in a substitution overload. If the extension control test cannot be performed without provocation of symptoms, start with the prerequisites as the entry level retraining option.

Tests of lumbar extension control

T8 STANDING: THORACIC EXTENSION (SWAY) TEST
(tests for lumbar extension UCM)

This dissociation test assesses the ability to actively control pelvic forward sway and lumbar segmental hinging into extension translation while actively lifting the sternum up and forwards into thoracic extension in standing.

Test procedure

The person initially stands tall with the upper thighs against the edge of a plinth, bench or table and with the feet as far under the table as balance can be maintained. Position the head directly over the shoulders without chin poke. Demonstrate or manually assist the movement of thoracic extension. The sternum, clavicles and acromions should all move up and *forwards* (Figure 5.41). There should be no forward sway of the pelvis (the table/bench provides feedback and support). The normal anterior pelvic should be present (with slight concurrent hip flexion) and all of the lumbar spine and the lower thoracic vertebrae should contribute to the spinal extension initiated from the thoracic region. There should be no segmental skin crease at the lumbosacral junction. There should be no scapular retraction (acromions moving backwards). The thoracic extension should be performed by spinal muscles, not the rhomboids. Allow the person to practise the test movement using feedback and support and with verbal and manual correction.

For testing, feedback and the support of the table are taken away. The person stands tall and unsupported with legs straight and the lumbar spine and pelvis positioned in the neutral. The head is positioned directly over the shoulders without chin poke (Figure 5.42). Without letting the lumbopelvic region move into forward sway, the person should have the ability to actively lift the sternum and chest up and *forwards* through the full available range of extension of the thoracic spine.

Ideally, the person should have the ability to prevent segmental hinging of the lumbar spine and forward sway of the pelvis while independently extending the thoracic region from a

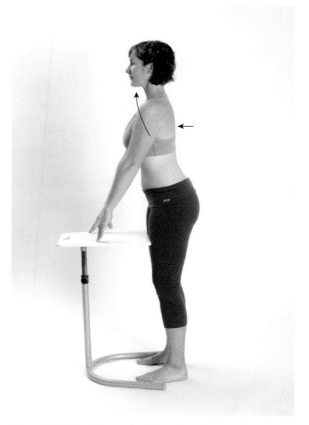

Figure 5.41 Teaching and training thoracic extension with sway control

position of relaxed flexion through to full extension (Figure 5.43). The available range of dissociated thoracolumbar extension is small. This test should be performed without any feedback (self-palpation, vision, tape, etc.) or cueing for correction.

Lumbar extension UCM

The person complains of extension-related symptoms in the lumbar spine. The lumbar spine has UCM into forward pelvic sway and lumbar segmental extension translational shear relative to the thoracic spine under extension load. During active thoracic extension, the pelvis starts to sway forwards or the upper body sways backwards and the low lumbar spine hinges into segmental extension before achieving end-range thoracic extension. A significant skin crease is observed at

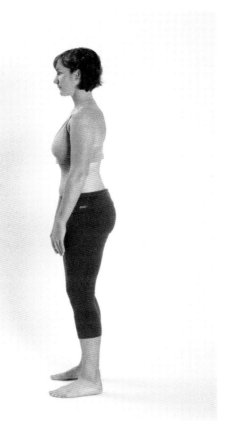

Figure 5.42 Start position for thoracic extension – sway test

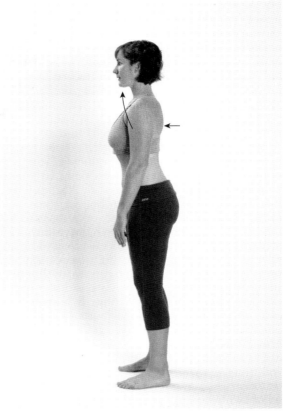

Figure 5.43 Benchmark for thoracic extension – sway test

the 'pivot point' of uncontrolled extension translation. The hinge occurs primarily at L5–S1, but can potentially also occur at L3–4 or L4–5. The upper lumbar spine and thoracic spine may only contribute (if at all) to extension at the completion of pelvic 'sway'. The pelvis essentially stays in relative posterior tilt. During the attempt to dissociate the pelvic sway and segmental lumbar hinge from independent thoracic extension (while allowing normal slight anterior pelvic tilt) the person either cannot control the UCM or has to concentrate and try hard.

- Note if one vertebral level appears to translate forwards excessively, producing a skin crease as it hinges backwards into extension. If this segment is observed as hinging into translation 'out of line' compared to the other vertebrae then the UCM is interpreted as a *segmental extension hinge*. The specific hinging segment should be noted and recorded.

Clinical assessment note for direction-specific motor control testing

If some other movement (e.g. a small amount of flexion or rotation) is observed during a motor control (dissociation) test of extension control, *do not* score this as uncontrolled extension. The flexion and rotation motor control tests will identify if the observed movement is uncontrolled. A test for lumbar extension UCM is only positive if uncontrolled lumbar extension is demonstrated.

Rating and diagnosis of lumbar extension UCM

(T8.1 and T8.2)

Correction

The person stands tall and unsupported with legs straight and the lumbar spine and pelvis positioned in the neutral. Without letting the lumbopelvic region move into forward sway, the person actively lifts the sternum and chest up and forwards *only* as far as the forward sway of the pelvis can be actively controlled or prevented and without swaying the upper body or shoulders backwards. The normal anterior pelvic should be present (with slight concurrent hip flexion) and all of the lumbar spine and the lower thoracic vertebrae should contribute to the spinal extension initiated from the thoracic region.

The person should monitor the lumbopelvic alignment and control with a variety of feedback options (T8.3). It may be especially useful to palpate the spinous process of the primary hinging segment for uncontrolled and excessive forward displacement of the spinous process during active extension. This will provide sensory feedback for the control of the segmental extension hinge. Visual feedback (e.g. observation in a mirror) is also a useful retraining tool. There should be no provocation of any symptoms under extension load, within the range that the extension UCM can be controlled.

If control is poor, start retraining with additional feedback. The person stands with the upper thighs against the edge of a bench or table and with the feet as far under the table as balance can be maintained. With the table preventing forward sway of the pelvis, the sternum, clavicles and acromions should all move up and *forwards*. Also, the upper body and trunk weight can be supported by weight bearing through the arms to decrease the load that must be controlled (Figure 5.44). Train by moving into thoracic extension only as far as the forward sway of the pelvis can be prevented and without swaying the upper body or shoulders backwards. As the ability to control the UCM gets easier, and the pattern of dissociation feels less unnatural, the exercise can be progressed to the unsupported position without a bench or table and then it should be integrated into various functional postures and positions.

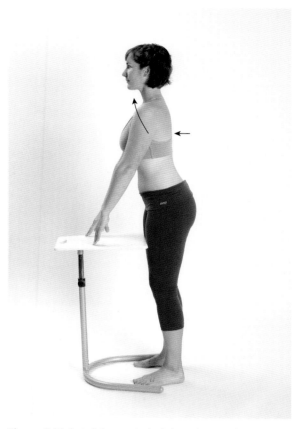

Figure 5.44 Retraining control of thoracic extension – sway with thighs against table for feedback and support

T8.1 Assessment and rating of low threshold recruitment efficiency of the Thoracic Extension – Sway Test

THORACIC EXTENSION – SWAY TEST – STANDING

ASSESSMENT

Control point:
• prevent forward pelvic sway into segmental hinging into extension translation
Movement challenge: thoracic extension (standing)
Benchmark range: full available dissociated thoracic extension (sternum upwards and forwards) without compensation

RATING OF LOW THRESHOLD RECRUITMENT EFFICIENCY FOR CONTROL OF DIRECTION

	✓ or ✗		✓ or ✗

• Able to prevent 'UCM' into the test direction. Correct dissociation pattern of movement
Prevent lumbar UCM into:
    forward pelvic sway and extension hinge
      (single segment)
and move thoracic extension
	☐	• Looks easy, and in the opinion of the assessor, is performed with confidence	☐

		• Feels easy, and the subject has sufficient awareness of the movement pattern that they confidently prevent 'UCM' into the test direction	☐
• Dissociate movement through the benchmark range of: full available thoracic extension *If there is more available range than the benchmark standard, only the benchmark range needs to be actively controlled*	☐	• The pattern of dissociation is smooth during concentric and eccentric movement	☐
		• Does not (consistently) use *end range* movement into the opposite direction to prevent the UCM	☐
• Without holding breath (though it is acceptable to use an alternate breathing strategy)	☐	• No extra feedback needed *(tactile, visual or verbal cueing)*	☐
		• Without external support or unloading	☐
• Control during eccentric phase	☐	• Relaxed natural breathing *(even if not ideal – so long as natural pattern does not change)*	☐
• Control during concentric phase	☐	• No fatigue	☐

CORRECT DISSOCIATION PATTERN　　　　　**RECRUITMENT EFFICIENCY**

T8.2 Diagnosis of the site and direction of UCM from the Thoracic Extension – Sway Test

THORACIC EXTENSION (SWAY) TEST – STANDING

Site	Direction	Segmental/ multisegmental	✗✗ or ✓✗
Lumbar	Extension	Segmental extension hinge (indicate level)	☐

T8.3 Feedback tools to monitor retraining

FEEDBACK TOOL	PROCESS
Self-palpation	Palpation monitoring of joint position
Visual observation	Observe in a mirror or directly watch the movement
Adhesive tape	Skin tension for tactile feedback
Cueing and verbal correction	Listen to feedback from another observer

T9 STANDING: THORACIC EXTENSION (TILT) TEST
(tests for lumbar extension UCM)

This dissociation test assesses the ability to actively control pelvic anterior tilt and lumbar extension while actively lifting the sternum up and forwards into thoracic extension in standing.

Test procedure

To teach the person the test movement, the person stands tall and unsupported with legs straight and the lumbar spine and pelvis positioned in the neutral. The head is positioned directly over the shoulders without chin poke (Figure 5.45).

Demonstrate or manually assist the movement of thoracic extension. The sternum, clavicles and acromions should all move up and *forwards*. Allow the person to practise the test movement using feedback and support and with verbal and manual correction.

For testing, feedback and the support of the table are taken away. Without letting the pelvis anteriorly tilt or the lower lumbar lordosis increase, the person should have the ability to actively lift the sternum and chest up and *forwards* through the full available range of extension of the thoracic spine (Figure 5.46). The gluteals should activate to prevent anterior pelvic tilt. The available range of dissociated thoracolumbar extension is small. This test should be performed without any feedback (self-palpation, vision, tape, etc.) or cueing for correction.

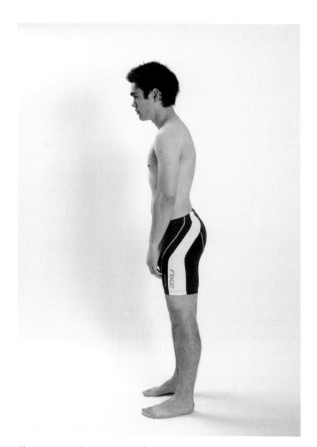

Figure 5.45 Start position for thoracic extension – tilt test

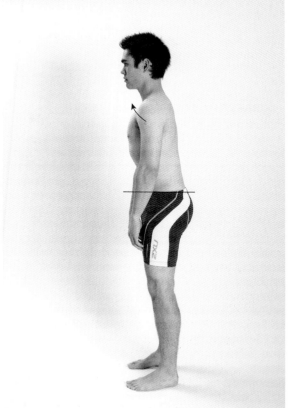

Figure 5.46 Benchmark for thoracic extension – tilt test

Lumbar extension UCM

The person complains of extension-related symptoms in the lumbar spine. The lumbar spine has UCM into anterior pelvic tilt and lumbar multisegmental hyperextension relative to the thoracic spine under extension load. During active thoracic extension, the pelvis starts to anteriorly tilt and the lumbar spine increases extension (increased lordosis) before achieving end-range thoracic extension. During the attempt to dissociate the pelvic tilt and lumbar extension from independent thoracic extension, the person either cannot control the UCM or has to concentrate and try hard.

- If increased extension (increased lumbar lordosis) of the whole lumbar region and increased anterior pelvic tilt are observed, but no one particular vertebral level is dominant from the adjacent vertebrae, then the UCM is interpreted as a *multisegmental hyperextension*.

Clinical assessment note for direction-specific motor control testing

If some other movement (e.g. a small amount of flexion or rotation) is observed during a motor control (dissociation) test of extension control, *do not* score this as uncontrolled extension. The flexion and rotation motor control tests will identify if the observed movement is uncontrolled. A test for lumbar extension UCM is only positive if uncontrolled lumbar extension is demonstrated.

Rating and diagnosis of lumbar extension UCM

(T9.1 and T9.2)

Correction

The person stands tall and unsupported with legs straight and the lumbar spine and pelvis positioned in the neutral. Without letting the lumbar spine extend or the pelvis anteriorly tilt, the person actively lifts the sternum and chest up and forwards *only* as far as the lumbar extension and anterior tilt can be actively controlled or prevented.

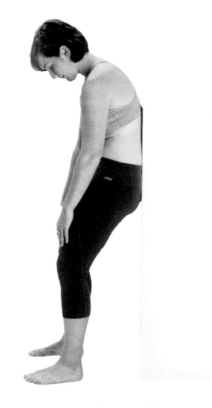

Figure 5.47 Correction: posterior tilt onto wall

The person should monitor the lumbopelvic alignment and control with a variety of feedback options (T9.3). It may be especially useful to palpate the pelvis for uncontrolled and anterior tilt or palpate the lumbar lordosis for any increase in lumbar extension during active thoracic extension. This will provide sensory feedback for the control of the lumbar extension tilt. Visual feedback (e.g. observation in a mirror) is also a useful retraining tool. There should be no provocation of any symptoms under extension load, within the range that the extension UCM can be controlled.

If control is poor, start standing against a wall with the feet apart, the knees unlocked and the thoracic spine slumped forwards into flexion so that the lumbar spine is flattened onto the wall (Figure 5.47). Monitor the pelvic tilt and slowly

T9.1 Assessment and rating of low threshold recruitment efficiency of the Thoracic Extension – Tilt Test

THORACIC EXTENSION – TILT TEST – STANDING

ASSESSMENT

Control point:
• prevent anterior pelvic tilt and lumbar extension
Movement challenge: thoracic extension (standing)
Benchmark range: full available dissociated thoracic extension (sternum upwards and forwards) without compensation

RATING OF LOW THRESHOLD RECRUITMENT EFFICIENCY FOR CONTROL OF DIRECTION

	✓ or ✗		✓ or ✗
• Able to prevent 'UCM' into the test direction. Correct dissociation pattern of movement Prevent lumbar UCM into: hyperextension (multisegment) and anterior pelvic tilt and move thoracic extension	☐	• Looks easy, and in the opinion of the assessor, is performed with confidence	☐
		• Feels easy, and the subject has sufficient awareness of the movement pattern that they confidently prevent 'UCM' into the test direction	☐
• Dissociate movement through the benchmark range of: full available thoracic extension *If there is more available range than the benchmark standard, only the benchmark range needs to be actively controlled*	☐	• The pattern of dissociation is smooth during concentric and eccentric movement	☐
		• Does not (consistently) use *end range* movement into the opposite direction to prevent the UCM	☐
• Without holding breath (though it is acceptable to use an alternate breathing strategy)	☐	• No extra feedback needed (*tactile, visual or verbal cueing*)	☐
		• Without external support or unloading	☐
• Control during eccentric phase	☐	• Relaxed natural breathing (*even if not ideal – so long as natural pattern does not change*)	☐
• Control during concentric phase	☐	• No fatigue	☐

CORRECT DISSOCIATION PATTERN

RECRUITMENT EFFICIENCY

T9.2 Diagnosis of the site and direction of UCM from the Thoracic Extension – Tilt Test

THORACIC EXTENSION (TILT) TEST – STANDING

Site	Direction	Segmental/ multisegmental	✗✗ or ✓✗
Lumbar	Extension	Multisegmental hyperextension	☐

T9.3 Feedback tools to monitor retraining

FEEDBACK TOOL	PROCESS
Self-palpation	Palpation monitoring of joint position
Visual observation	Observe in a mirror or directly watch the movement
Adhesive tape	Skin tension for tactile feedback
Cueing and verbal correction	Listen to feedback from another observer

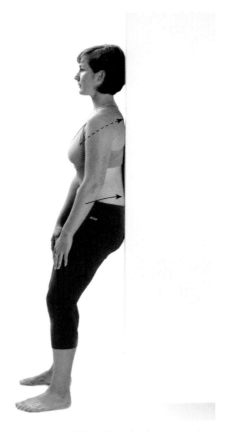

Figure 5.48 Progression: unroll thoracic spine into extension

'unroll' the thoracic spine up the wall. Only unroll the thoracic spine into extension as far as the lumbar spine can be stabilised on the wall (Figure 5.48). Using the wall for feedback and support, do not allow the lumbar spine to extend off the wall at all.

Retraining with additional feedback is also a good option. Tension a piece of adhesive strapping tape across the anterior abdomen (e.g. from the ASIS to the lower anterolateral ribcage or along the rectus abdominis muscle). If the person cannot prevent spinal extension or anterior pelvic tilt across this multisegmental group, the tape pulls the skin to provide sensory feedback about the UCM. Also, the upper body and trunk weight can be supported by weight bearing through the arms to decrease the load that must be controlled. Train by controlling lumbar extension and pelvic tilt while moving into thoracic extension *only* as far as the UCM can be prevented. As the ability to control the UCM gets easier and the pattern of dissociation feels less unnatural it should be integrated into various functional postures and positions.

T10 SITTING: CHEST LIFT (TILT) TEST (tests for lumbar extension UCM)

This dissociation test assesses the ability to actively control pelvic anterior tilt and lumbar extension while actively lifting the sternum up into thoracic extension in sitting.

Test procedure

To teach the person the test movement, the person sits tall with the feet off the floor and with the lumbar spine and pelvis positioned in the neutral. Make the spine as tall or as long as possible to position the normal curves in an elongated 'S' without leaning backwards. Position the head directly over the shoulders without chin poke (Figure 5.49). Demonstrate or manually assist the movement of thoracic extension. Monitor thoracolumbar motion by placing one hand on the sternum. Monitor lumbopelvic motion by placing the other hand on the sacrum (alternative lumbopelvic monitoring: place one finger on the pubic bone). Without letting the lumbopelvic region move (pelvis and sacral hand does not move) lift the sternum up. This is independent thoracic extension. The sternum, clavicles and acromions should all move up (Figure 5.50). Allow the person to practise the test movement using feedback and support and with verbal and manual correction.

For testing, feedback and the support of the table are taken away. Ideally, the person should have the ability to keep the lumbopelvic region neutral while independently extending the thoracic region (chest lift) from a position of flexion through to full thoracic extension, without any movement of the pelvis. This test should be

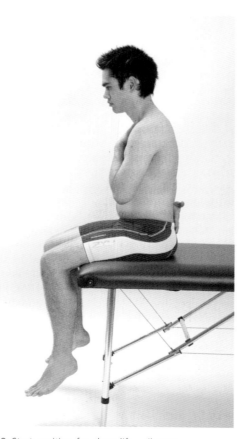

Figure 5.49 Start position for chest lift – tilt test

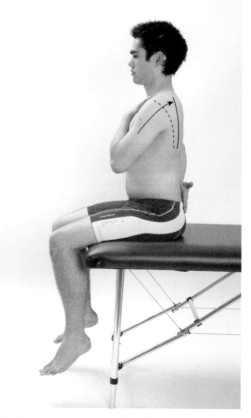

Figure 5.50 Benchmark for chest lift – tilt test

performed without any feedback (self-palpation, vision, tape, etc.) or cueing for correction.

Lumbar extension UCM

The person complains of extension-related symptoms in the lumbar spine. The lumbar spine has UCM into anterior pelvic tilt and lumbar multi-segmental hyperextension relative to the thoracic spine under extension load. During active thoracic extension, the pelvis starts to anteriorly tilt and the lumbar spine increases extension (increased lordosis) before achieving end-range thoracic extension. During the attempt to dissociate the pelvic tilt and lumbar extension from independent thoracic extension, the person either cannot control the UCM or has to concentrate and try hard.

When iliocostalis (global mobiliser) is the dominant trunk extensor, it produces concurrent thoracolumbar extension and lumbopelvic extension. If the lumbopelvic flexor stabiliser muscles can actively resist lumbopelvic extension (with internal oblique abdominal stabiliser activation) while the segmental thoracolumbar spinal stabiliser muscles actively extend the thorax, then iliocostalis must be inhibited to some extent. The internal oblique abdominals (global stabilisers) will probably contribute more to the control of lumbopelvic extension because they are less directly inhibited by the thoracic extension chest lift.

- If increased extension (increased lumbar lordosis) of the whole lumbar region and increased anterior pelvic tilt are observed, but no one particular vertebral level is dominant from the adjacent vertebrae, then the UCM is interpreted as a *multisegmental hyperextension*.

Clinical assessment note for direction-specific motor control testing

If some other movement (e.g. a small amount of flexion or rotation) is observed during a motor control (dissociation) test of extension control, *do not* score this as uncontrolled extension. The flexion and rotation motor control tests will identify if the observed movement is uncontrolled. A test for lumbar extension UCM is only positive if uncontrolled lumbar extension is demonstrated.

Rating and diagnosis of lumbar extension UCM

(T10.1 and T10.2)

Correction

The person sits tall with the feet on the floor and with the lumbar spine and pelvis positioned in the neutral. Monitor thoracolumbar motion by placing one hand on the sternum. Monitor lumbopelvic motion by placing the other hand on the sacrum. Without letting the lumbopelvic region move (pelvis and sacral hand does not move) lift the sternum up into independent thoracic extension.

In some cases it may be useful to tension a strip of adhesive strapping tape across the anterior abdomen (e.g. from the ASIS to the lower antero-lateral ribcage or along the rectus abdominis muscle). If the person cannot prevent spinal extension or anterior pelvic tilt across this multi-segmental group, the tape pulls the skin to provide sensory feedback about the UCM. Visual feedback (e.g. observation in a mirror) is also a useful retraining tool.

Ideally, the subject should have the ability to dissociate the lumbar spine from thoracic extension as evidenced by the ability to keep the lumbopelvic region neutral while independently extending the thoracic region from a position of flexion through extension. Lift the chest into the thoracic extension, but only as far as the neutral lumbopelvic position can be maintained (Figure 5.51). There must be no loss of neutral or UCM into lumbar extension or anterior pelvic tilt. There should be no provocation of any symptoms under flexion load, so long as the flexion give can be controlled.

The person should monitor the lumbar alignment and control with a variety of feedback options (T10.3). As the ability to independently control movement of the thoracic spine and lumbopelvic region gets easier and the pattern of dissociation feels less unnatural, the exercise can be progressed to performing concurrent thoracic flexion with lumbopelvic extension.

If control is poor, the upper body and trunk weight can be supported on hands and knees. Position the pelvis over the knees and the shoulders over the hands with the knees and hands comfortably apart. Rock the pelvis backwards and forwards from the sacrum (posterior and anterior

T10.1 Assessment and rating of low threshold recruitment efficiency of the Chest Lift – Tilt Test

CHEST LIFT – (TILT) TEST – SITTING

ASSESSMENT

Control point:
• prevent anterior pelvic tilt and lumbar extension
Movement challenge: thoracic extension (sitting)
Benchmark range: full available dissociated thoracic extension (sternum upwards and forwards) without compensation

RATING OF LOW THRESHOLD RECRUITMENT EFFICIENCY FOR CONTROL OF DIRECTION

	✓ or ✗		✓ or ✗
• Able to prevent 'UCM' into the test direction. Correct dissociation pattern of movement Prevent lumbar UCM into: hyperextension (multisegmental) and anterior pelvic tilt and move thoracic extension	☐	• Looks easy, and in the opinion of the assessor, is performed with confidence	☐
		• Feels easy, and the subject has sufficient awareness of the movement pattern that they confidently prevent 'UCM' into the test direction	☐
• Dissociate movement through the benchmark range of: full available thoracic extension *If there is more available range than the benchmark standard, only the benchmark range needs to be actively controlled*	☐	• The pattern of dissociation is smooth during concentric and eccentric movement	☐
		• Does not (consistently) use *end range movement into the opposite direction to prevent the UCM*	☐
• Without holding breath (though it is acceptable to use an alternate breathing strategy)	☐	• No extra feedback needed *(tactile, visual or verbal cueing)*	☐
		• Without external support or unloading	☐
• Control during eccentric phase	☐	• Relaxed natural breathing *(even if not ideal – so long as natural pattern does not change)*	☐
• Control during concentric phase	☐	• No fatigue	☐

CORRECT DISSOCIATION PATTERN   **RECRUITMENT EFFICIENCY**

T10.2 Diagnosis of the site and direction of UCM from the Chest Lift – Tilt Test

CHEST LIFT (TILT) TEST – SITTING

Site	Direction	Segmental/ multisegmental	✗✗ or ✓✗
Lumbar	Extension	Multisegmental hyperextension	☐

T10.3 Feedback tools to monitor retraining

FEEDBACK TOOL	PROCESS
Self-palpation	Palpation monitoring of joint position
Visual observation	Observe in a mirror or directly watch the movement
Adhesive tape	Skin tension for tactile feedback
Cueing and verbal correction	Listen to feedback from another observer
Flexicurve positional marker	Visual and sensory feedback of positional alignment

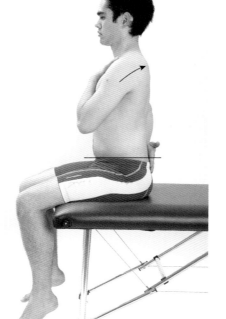

Figure 5.51 Ideal control of lumbopelvic extension

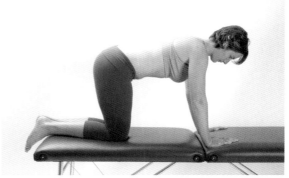

Figure 5.52 Correction (neutral start position)

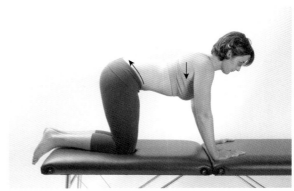

Figure 5.53 Correction (thoracic extension followed by lumbar flexion)

tilt) until the lumbar spine is in a long *shallow* lordosis. Then, push the body gently away from the hands without flexing the thoracic spine or lowering the head. Then lift the head (without chin poke) so that the back of the head touches an imaginary line connecting the sacrum and mid-thoracic spine. Use minimal effort to maintain this neutral spine position (Figure 5.52).

When control is poor, rather than specific dissociation, for some patients it is easier to use a recruitment reversal exercise to start with:

- Actively extend the thoracic spine and then flex the lumbar spine and posteriorly tilt the pelvis. (Figure 5.53).
- The reverse order of this same pattern may also be used. That is, actively flex the lumbar spine and posteriorly tilt the pelvis and then extend the thoracic spine (Figure 5.54).

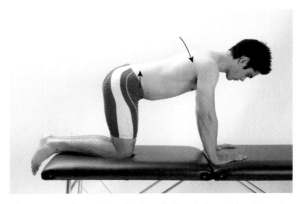

Figure 5.54 Correction (lumbar flexion followed by thoracic extension)

When the pattern of this recruitment reversal feels easy, then progress back to the sitting dissociation.

As the ability to independently control movement of the thoracic spine and lumbopelvic region gets easier and the pattern of dissociation feels less unnatural, the exercise can be progressed to standing. Stand upright with the knees and hips slightly flexed (unlocked) to prevent hip flexor tightness influencing the pelvis. Without letting the lumbopelvic region move (pelvis and sacrum do not move), lift the sternum and chest (thoracic extension). Once the pattern of dissociation is efficient and feels familiar it should be integrated into various functional postures and positions.

T11 SITTING: FORWARD LEAN TEST (tests for lumbar extension UCM)

This dissociation test assesses the ability to actively dissociate and control lumbar extension and anterior pelvic tilt then lean the trunk forwards (activates the back extensors to support the trunk load) while sitting.

Test procedure

The person should have the ability to actively lean forwards by flexing at the hips while controlling the lumbar spine and pelvis. The person sits tall with the feet on the floor and with the lumbar spine and pelvis positioned in the neutral (Figure 5.55). Lumbopelvic motion is monitored by the therapist. The therapist monitors the lumbosacral neutral position by palpating the spinous process of L2, L5 and S2 with their finger tips. During testing, if the palpating fingers do not move, the lumbosacral region is able to maintain neutral. If the palpating fingers move closer together, uncontrolled lumbar extension is identified.

The person is instructed to sit tall and to lean the trunk forwards from the hips, keeping the back straight (neutral spine). Ideally, the subject should have the ability to maintain a neutral lumbar spine and prevent uncontrolled lumbar extension when the back extensors activate to support the trunk through 30° of forward leaning (Hamilton et al 1998) (Figure 5.56). This test should be performed without any feedback (self-palpation, vision, tape, etc.) or cueing for correction.

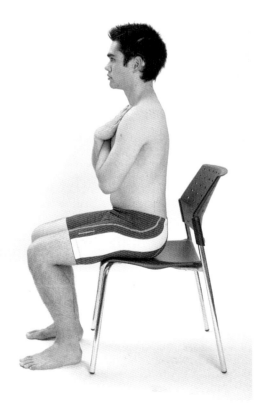

Figure 5.55 Start position for forward lean test

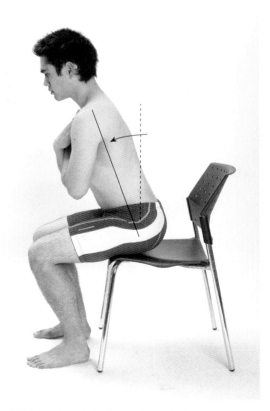

Figure 5.56 Benchmark for forward lean test

Lumbar extension UCM

The person complains of extension-related symptoms in the lumbar spine. The lumbar spine has UCM into extension relative to the hips under extension load. During active hip flexion and forward lean of the trunk in sitting, the lumbar spine starts to extend before achieving 30° forward lean. During the attempt to maintain a neutral lumbar spine and prevent uncontrolled lumbar extension when the back extensors activate to support the trunk, the person either cannot control the UCM or has to concentrate and try hard.

- If increased extension (increased lumbar lordosis) of the whole lumbar region and increased anterior pelvic tilt is observed, but no one particular vertebral level is dominant from the adjacent vertebrae, then the UCM is interpreted as a *multisegmental hyperextension*.

Clinical assessment note for direction-specific motor control testing

If some other movement (e.g. a small amount of flexion or rotation) is observed during a motor control (dissociation) test of extension control, *do not* score this as uncontrolled extension. The flexion and rotation motor control tests will identify if the observed movement is uncontrolled. A test for lumbar extension UCM is only positive if uncontrolled lumbar extension is demonstrated.

Rating and diagnosis of lumbar extension UCM

(T11.1 and T11.2)

Correction

The person sits tall with the feet on the floor and with the lumbar spine and pelvis positioned in the neutral. The person should monitor the lumbar alignment and control with a variety of feedback options (T11.3). They monitor the lumbosacral neutral position by palpating the spinous process of L2, L5 and S2 with their fingers. The person is instructed to sit tall and to lean the trunk forwards from the hips, keeping the back straight (neutral spine). If the palpating fingers do not move closer together, lumbar extension is being controlled.

Palpation feedback and visual feedback (e.g. observation in a mirror) are the most useful retraining tools. Ideally, the subject should have the ability to dissociate the lumbar spine from hip flexion, as evidenced by 30° forward lean while preventing lumbar extension. There should be no provocation of any symptoms under extension load, within the range that the flexion UCM can be controlled.

If control is poor, the pattern of forward leaning with a straight back and independent hip flexion should be performed *only* as far as lumbar extension can be actively controlled or prevented. Also, the upper body and trunk weight can be supported by weight bearing through the arms to decrease the load that must be controlled by the local and global stabiliser muscles. As the ability to control the UCM gets easier and the pattern of dissociation feels less unnatural, the exercise can be progressed to the unsupported position. Once the pattern of dissociation is efficient and feels familiar it should be integrated into various functional postures and positions.

T11.1 Assessment and rating of low threshold recruitment efficiency of the Forward Lean Test

FORWARD LEAN TEST – SITTING

ASSESSMENT

Control point:
• prevent lumbar extension
Movement challenge: forward lean of the trunk with back extensor activation (sitting)
Benchmark range: 30° forward lean of trunk without compensation

RATING OF LOW THRESHOLD RECRUITMENT EFFICIENCY FOR CONTROL OF DIRECTION

	✓ or ✗		✓ or ✗

• Able to prevent 'UCM' into the test direction. Correct dissociation pattern of movement
Prevent lumbar UCM into:
   hyperextension (multisegmental) and anterior
      pelvic tilt
and move forward lean of trunk (hip flexion)
	☐	• Looks easy, and in the opinion of the assessor, is performed with confidence	☐

		• Feels easy, and the subject has sufficient awareness of the movement pattern that they confidently prevent 'UCM' into the test direction	☐
• Dissociate movement through the benchmark range of: 30° of independent forward lean of trunk *If there is more available range than the benchmark standard, only the benchmark range needs to be actively controlled*	☐	• The pattern of dissociation is smooth during concentric and eccentric movement	☐
		• Does not (consistently) use *end range* movement into the opposite direction to prevent the UCM	☐
• Without holding breath (though it is acceptable to use an alternate breathing strategy)	☐	• No extra feedback needed *(tactile, visual or verbal cueing)*	☐
		• Without external support or unloading	☐
		• Relaxed natural breathing *(even if not ideal – so long as natural pattern does not change)*	☐
• Control during eccentric phase	☐	• No fatigue	☐
• Control during concentric phase	☐		

CORRECT DISSOCIATION PATTERN   **RECRUITMENT EFFICIENCY**

T11.2 Diagnosis of the site and direction of UCM from the Forward Lean Test

FORWARD LEAN TEST – SITTING

Site	Direction	Segmental/ multisegmental	✗✗ or ✓✗
Lumbar	Extension	Multisegmental hyperextension	☐

T11.3 Feedback tools to monitor retraining

FEEDBACK TOOL	PROCESS
Self-palpation	Palpation monitoring of joint position
Visual observation	Observe in a mirror or directly watch the movement
Adhesive tape	Skin tension for tactile feedback
Cueing and verbal correction	Listen to feedback from another observer

139

T12 4 POINT: FORWARD ROCKING TEST (tests for lumbar extension UCM)

This dissociation test assesses the ability to actively dissociate and control lumbar extension/anterior pelvic tilt and rock the body forwards, shifting weight onto the hands by moving the hips forwards into extension while in 4 point kneeling (hands and knees).

Test procedure

The person should have the ability to actively rock the body weight forwards over the hands by extending the hips and controlling the lumbar spine and pelvis. The person positions themselves in 4 point kneeling (hands and knees) with the lumbar spine and pelvis in neutral alignment (Figure 5.57). Lumbopelvic motion is monitored by the therapist. The therapist monitors the lumbosacral neutral position by palpating the spinous process of L2, L5 and S2 with their finger tips (Figure 5.58).

During testing, if the palpating fingers do not move, the lumbosacral region is able to maintain neutral. If the palpating fingers move closer together, uncontrolled segmental lumbar extension hinge is identified.

The person is instructed to rock forwards from the hips and shift their body weight forwards over their hands, keeping the back straight (neutral spine). Ideally, the neutral lumbar lordosis should be maintained until the trunk is in a straight line with the thighs (about 0° of hip extension) (Figure 5.59).

Ideally, the person should have the ability to dissociate the lumbar spine and pelvis from hip extension, as evidenced by 0° of hip flexion during forward rocking while preventing lumbar extension or anterior pelvic tilt. The lumbar spine and pelvis should return to a neutral position as the subject rocks backwards to the starting position. The pelvis should have good symmetry; that is, no lateral tilt or rotation. This test should be

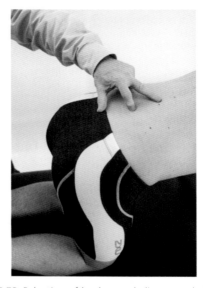

Figure 5.58 Palpation of lumbosacral alignment during test

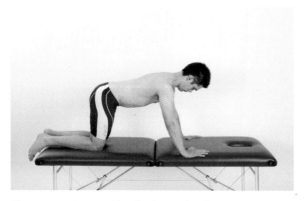

Figure 5.57 Start position for forward rocking test

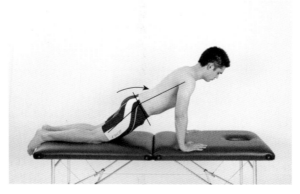

Figure 5.59 Benchmark for forward rocking test

performed without any feedback (self-palpation, vision, tape, etc.) or cueing for correction.

Lumbar extension UCM

The person complains of extension-related symptoms in the lumbar spine. The lumbar spine has UCM into extension relative to the hips under extension load. During rocking forwards over the hands, while the hips are extending, the lumbar spine starts to extend before achieving 0° of hip extension. During the attempt to dissociate the lumbar spine and pelvis from independent hip extension, the person either cannot control the UCM or has to concentrate and try hard.

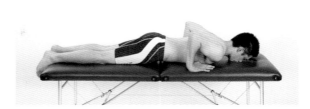

Figure 5.60 Correction with prone start position

- If only one spinous process is observed as prominent and protruding 'out of line' compared to the other vertebrae, then the UCM is interpreted as a *segmental extension hinge*. The specific hinging segment should be noted and recorded.
- If excessive lumbopelvic extension is observed, but no one particular spinous process is hinging from the adjacent vertebrae, then the UCM is interpreted as a *multisegmental hyperextension*.

Clinical assessment note for direction-specific motor control testing

If some other movement (e.g. a small amount of flexion or rotation) is observed during a motor control (dissociation) test of extension control, *do not* score this as uncontrolled extension. The flexion and rotation motor control tests will identify if the observed movement is uncontrolled. A test for lumbar extension UCM is only positive if uncontrolled lumbar extension is demonstrated.

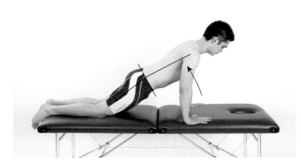

Figure 5.61 Correction with ideal control in rocking forward

Rating and diagnosis of lumbar extension UCM

(T12.1 and T12.2)

Correction

If control is poor, start with the person lying flat in a prone position, with the hands positioned as if to perform a 'push up' (Figure 5.60). Then,

keeping the trunk, pelvis and hips from moving, and with the knees staying on the floor, slowly push through the hands to lift the trunk away from the floor. This 'push up from the knees' action does not require any active hip extension. Instead, the hip starts in extension and just has to prevent any further extension (Figure 5.61) during the push up from the knees.

As control improves, the person positions themselves in 4 point kneeling (hands and knees) with the lumbar spine and pelvis in neutral alignment. The person then rocks forwards shifting partial weight towards their hands, but only as far as lumbar extension and anterior pelvic tilt can be actively controlled or prevented (Figure 5.62). There should be no provocation of any symptoms, so long as the extension UCM can be controlled. Progress until good control through

141

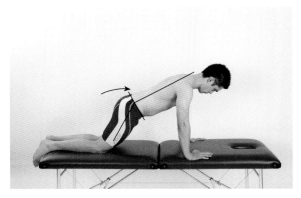

Figure 5.62 Correction with partial rocking forward from hands and knees position

0° hip extension is easy, but not beyond this range.

The person should self-monitor the lumbo-pelvic alignment and control with a variety of feedback options (T12.3). Visual feedback (e.g. observation in a mirror) is also a useful retraining tool.

Once the pattern of dissociation is efficient and feels familiar, it should be integrated into various functional postures and positions.

T12.1 Assessment and rating of low threshold recruitment efficiency of the Forward Rocking Test

FORWARD ROCKING TEST – 4 POINT KNEELING

ASSESSMENT

Control point:
- prevent multisegmental lumbar extension and anterior pelvic tilt
- prevent segmental extension hinge and anterior tilt

Movement challenge: hip extension (4 point kneeling)

Benchmark range: forward rocking of pelvis to shift weight onto hands with independent 0° hip extension

RATING OF LOW THRESHOLD RECRUITMENT EFFICIENCY FOR CONTROL OF DIRECTION

	✓ or ✗		✓ or ✗

• Able to prevent 'UCM' into the test direction. Correct dissociation pattern of movement
Prevent lumbar UCM into:
   hyperextension (multisegmental) and anterior pelvic tilt
   forward pelvic sway and extension hinge (single segment)
and move hip extension
	☐	• Looks easy, and in the opinion of the assessor, is performed with confidence	☐

		• Feels easy, and the subject has sufficient awareness of the movement pattern that they confidently prevent 'UCM' into the test direction	☐
• Dissociate movement through the benchmark range of: 0° forward rocking at pelvis with independent hip extension *If there is more available range than the benchmark standard, only the benchmark range needs to be actively controlled*	☐	• The pattern of dissociation is smooth during concentric and eccentric movement	☐
		• Does not (consistently) use *end range* movement into the opposite direction to prevent the UCM	☐
• Without holding breath (though it is acceptable to use an alternate breathing strategy)	☐	• No extra feedback needed *(tactile, visual or verbal cueing)*	☐
		• Without external support or unloading	☐
• Control during eccentric phase	☐	• Relaxed natural breathing *(even if not ideal – so long as natural pattern does not change)*	☐
• Control during concentric phase	☐	• No fatigue	☐
CORRECT DISSOCIATION PATTERN		**RECRUITMENT EFFICIENCY**	

T12.2 Diagnosis of the site and direction of UCM from the Forward Rocking Test

FORWARD ROCKING TEST – 4 POINT KNEELING

Site	Direction	Segmental/ multisegmental	✗✗ or ✓✗
Lumbar	Extension	Segmental extension hinge (indicate level)	☐
		Multisegmental hyperextension	☐

T12.3 Feedback tools to monitor retraining

FEEDBACK TOOL	PROCESS
Self-palpation	Palpation monitoring of joint position
Visual observation	Observe in a mirror or directly watch the movement
Adhesive tape	Skin tension for tactile feedback
Cueing and verbal correction	Listen to feedback from another observer

T13 CROOK: DOUBLE BENT LEG LOWER TEST
(tests for lumbar extension UCM)

This dissociation test assesses the ability to actively dissociate and control lumbar extension and anterior pelvic tilt then lower both feet to the floor by actively extending the hips (from flexion) in a crook lying position.

Test procedure

The person should have the ability to lower both feet to the floor (in crook lying) by extending the hips from 90° flexion to 45° flexion, while concurrently controlling the lumbar spine and pelvis. The person lies on the back in crook lying (hips and knees bent and feet resting on the floor), with the lumbar spine and pelvis relaxed in neutral alignment (Figure 5.63). Lumbopelvic motion is monitored by the placement of a Pressure Biofeedback Unit (PBU) (Stabilizer – Chattanooga) under the back, centred at L3 in the middle of the lumbar lordosis (Figures 5.14 and 5.15). During limb load tests and exercises the PBU can objectively monitor the functional stability of the trunk. In crook lying the PBU is inflated to a base pressure of 40 mmHg (Figure 5.16). This pressure is used to position and support the lumbar spine in neutral alignment. Under functional limb load or movement, no pressure change = no loss of neutral position = good control. If the lumbar spine extends beyond the neutral starting position a decrease in pressure is registered by the PBU.

The person is permitted to watch the PBU to monitor the accuracy of their ability to control the lumbar spine and prevent lumbar extension. The PBU is initially inflated to a base pressure of 40 mmHg while the lumbar spine is relaxed and supported in a neutral resting position. During the leg movement phase, some small movement of the pelvis is normal. This is accounted for in the test by allowing a small tolerance of pressure change during the leg movement phase. Therefore, a pressure *increase* or *decrease* of 10 mmHg either side of the base pressure of 40 mmHg is acceptable.

The therapist then passively lifts both feet off the floor until the hips are flexed to 90° (Figure 5.64). Normally a pressure increase is noted at this point as the back flexes slightly onto the PBU. Keeping the thighs vertical with the hips at 90° (supported passively by the therapist), the person is instructed to actively reposition the pelvic tilt to return the back to neutral and the base pressure to 40 mmHg keeping the hips at 90° (Figure 5.65). The person is then required to actively take the weight of their legs and hold this position and keep the PBU pressure at 40 mmHg for at least 5 seconds without therapist support. If the person cannot maintain the unsupported leg position at 90° of hip flexion and the pressure at 40 mmHg, the test is discontinued. So long as the person can maintain the pressure at 40 mmHg they are then instructed to slowly lower both heels (simultaneously) to the floor while keeping the back stable (no pressure change).

Ideally, the person should be able to slowly lower both feet towards the floor and maintain the pressure at 40 mmHg (±10 mmHg while the legs are moving). The person should hold the legs steady just a few millimetres off the floor (45° hip flexion) while keeping the pressure constant

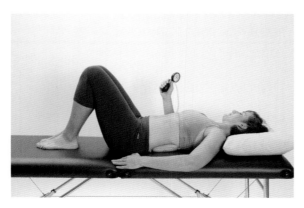

Figure 5.63 Start position for double bent leg lower test

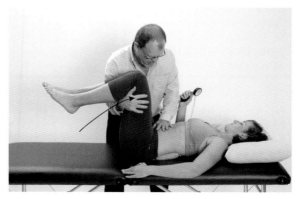

Figure 5.64 Passive support to 90° of hip flexion and reposition lumbar spine to achieve 40 mmHg

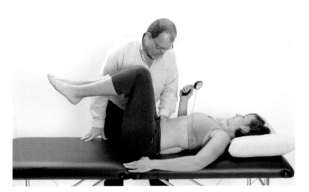

Figure 5.65 Unsupported leg load

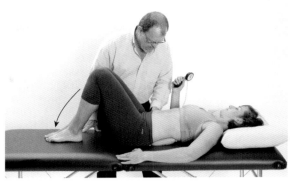

Figure 5.66 Benchmark for double bent leg lower test

at 40 mmHg (Figure 5.66). As soon as any pressure decrease (towards 30 mmHg) is registered the movement must stop and the feet be returned (one at a time) back to the start position.

If no PBU is available the therapist should place their hand under the lumbar lordosis instead of the PBU. It has been anecdotally claimed that the hand is sensitive to a pressure change roughly equivalent to 40 mmHg. So, if no pressure decrease is detected by the hand, the control would seem to be within the limits as determined by the PBU.

Lumbar extension UCM

The person complains of extension-related symptoms in the lumbar spine. The lumbar spine has UCM into extension relative to the hips under extension load. During a double leg lower in crook lying, the lumbar spine starts to extend before the feet reach the floor. During the attempt to control lumbar extension and anterior pelvic tilt from independent hip extension, the person either cannot control the UCM or has to concentrate and try hard.

In the process of trying to keep the back neutral, the pelvis must not tilt anteriorly and extend the lumbar spine. A pressure decrease of more than 10 mmHg (decrease to more than 30 mmHg) indicates excessive uncontrolled anterior tilt and a loss of stability into spinal extension. As soon as any pressure increase (beyond 50 mmHg) is registered the leg movement must stop and the feet lower back to the start position. If control is poor, a series of graduated progressions using

relatively less load and specific facilitation of the oblique abdominals can be used.

- If increased extension (increased lumbar lordosis) of the whole lumbar region and increased anterior pelvic tilt are observed, but no one particular vertebral level is dominant from the adjacent vertebrae, then the UCM is interpreted as a *multisegmental hyperextension*.

Clinical assessment note for direction-specific motor control testing

If some other movement (e.g. a small amount of flexion or rotation) is observed during a motor control (dissociation) test of extension control, *do not* score this as uncontrolled extension. The flexion and rotation motor control tests will identify if the observed movement is uncontrolled. A test for lumbar extension UCM is only positive if uncontrolled lumbar extension is demonstrated.

Rating and diagnosis of lumbar extension UCM

(T13.1 and T13.2)

Correction

The person lies in crook lying with the lumbar spine and pelvis relaxed in neutral alignment. Lumbopelvic position is monitored by the placement of a PBU under the back, centred at L3 in the middle of the lumbar lordosis. Inflate the PBU to a base pressure of 40 mmHg. The PBU maintains the neutral spine.

145

The person is permitted to watch the PBU to monitor the accuracy of their ability to control the lumbar spine and prevent lumbar extension. During all retraining of uncontrolled lumbar extension a pressure increase of 10 mmHg is acceptable during unsupported leg movements. That is, if the start pressure is 40 mmHg a pressure increase of 10 mmHg (up to 50 mmHg) is acceptable during leg movement. Likewise, if the start pressure is 45 mmHg (with oblique abdominal facilitation) a pressure increase of 10 mmHg (up to 55 mmHg) is acceptable during leg movement. However, when leg movement stops the pressure must be maintained at the original start pressure.

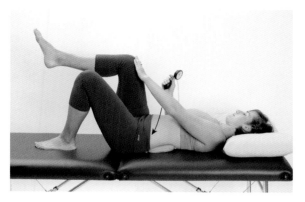

Figure 5.67 Facilitation with opposite knee to hand push

Oblique abdominal facilitation

If uncontrolled lumbar extension is identified, facilitation of the oblique abdominals is encouraged. Take a relaxed breath in and breathe out. Do not breathe as the low lateral abdominal wall is hollowed (drawn up and in) in an attempt to flatten the lumbar lordosis and increase pressure on the pad. Specific external oblique abdominal facilitation is achieved by cueing active lower ribcage depression. Ensure that no pelvic tilt occurs. The pad maintains the neutral spine. Hold this contraction and breathe gently.

Ideally, with efficient oblique abdominal recruitment, the pressure should increase by 8–10 mmHg (from 40 mmHg to approximately 48–50 mmHg). The pressure increase should be able to be consistently maintained.

A pressure increase of 15–20 mmHg (55–60 mmHg) indicates posterior tilt and reversal of the lumbar lordosis to the flat position. This pressure change is associated with bracing strategies. (A bracing strategy is acceptable under double leg load when strength training is the aim, rather than motor control training.)

Static diagonal: isometric opposite knee to hand push

First facilitate the oblique abdominals (PBU held at 48–50 mmHg or other hand to monitor that no pressure change = spinal control), slowly lift one knee towards the opposite hand and push them isometrically against each other on a diagonal line (Figure 5.67). Push for 10 seconds and repeat 10 times so long as stability is maintained (no pressure change). As soon as any pressure

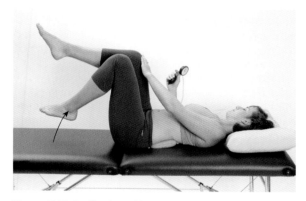

Figure 5.68 Facilitation with second leg lift

increase or decrease is registered the movement must stop and return to the start position. Do not stabilise with the opposite foot or allow substitution or fatigue.

Static diagonal heel lift: isometric knee to hand push + 2nd heel lift

First facilitate the oblique abdominals (PBU held at 48–50 mmHg or other hand to monitor that no pressure change = spinal control), slowly lift one knee towards the opposite hand and push them isometrically against each other on a diagonal line. While keeping this pressure, slowly lift the second heel off the floor and bring it up beside the first leg. (Figure 5.68) Hold this position for 10 seconds and repeat 10 times so long as stability is maintained (no pressure change).

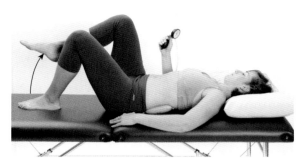

Figure 5.69 Progression: first leg lift

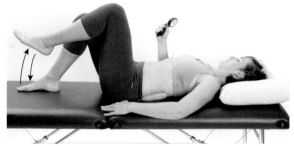

Figure 5.71 Progression: first leg lower

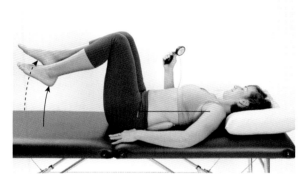

Figure 5.70 Progression: second leg lift

As soon as any pressure increase or decrease is registered the movement must stop and return to the start position. The point of greatest risk of losing stability is when the second heel leaves the floor. Do not allow substitution or fatigue.

Alternate single leg heel touch: (Sahrmann level 1)

First facilitate the oblique abdominals (PBU held at 48–50 mmHg or other hand to monitor that no pressure change = spinal stability), slowly lift one foot off the floor (Figure 5.69) and then lift the second foot off the floor and bring it up beside the first leg (Figure 5.70). Crook lying with hips flexed to 90° and *both* feet off the floor is the starting position.

Hold this position and, keeping the back stable (no pressure change), slowly lower one heel to the floor (Figure 5.71) and lift it back to the start position. Repeat this movement, slowly alternating legs, for 10 seconds so long as stability is maintained (no pressure change), and then return both feet to the floor. Repeat the whole process 10 times.

As soon as any pressure decrease (or increase) is registered the movement must stop and return to the start position. The point of greatest risk of losing stability is when the heel is lowering to the floor. Do not allow substitution or fatigue.

The person should self-monitor the lumbopelvic alignment and control with a variety of feedback options (T13.3). It is very useful to use a PBU for precise monitoring of lumbar position. Taping will also provide sensory feedback and some degree of mechanical support to the control of extension. Visual feedback (e.g. observation in a mirror) is also a useful retraining tool.

If control is poor, the leg lift with a controlled back and independent hip flexion should be performed *only* as far as lumbar extension and anterior pelvic tilt can be actively controlled or prevented. There should be no provocation of any symptoms, so long as the lumbar extension can be controlled. Once the pattern of dissociation is efficient and feels familiar, it should be integrated into various functional postures and positions.

T13.1 Assessment and rating of low threshold recruitment efficiency of the Double Bent Leg Lower Test

DOUBLE BENT LEG LOWER TEST – CROOK LYING

ASSESSMENT

Control point:
• prevent lumbar extension and anterior pelvic tilt
Movement challenge: hip extension (crook lying)
Benchmark range: 90° flexion to 45° bilateral hip extension

RATING OF LOW THRESHOLD RECRUITMENT EFFICIENCY FOR CONTROL OF DIRECTION

	✓ or ✗		✓ or ✗
• Able to prevent 'UCM' into the test direction. Correct dissociation pattern of movement Prevent lumbar UCM into: hyperextension (multisegmental) and anterior pelvic tilt and move hip extension	☐	• Looks easy, and in the opinion of the assessor, is performed with confidence	☐
		• Feels easy, and the subject has sufficient awareness of the movement pattern that they confidently prevent 'UCM' into the test direction	☐
• Dissociate movement through the benchmark range of: bilateral independent hip extension from 90° hip flexion to 45° and: Maintain the PBU at 40 mmHg ± 10 mmHg while the legs are moving Hold the PBU at 40 mmHg with hips flexed at 90° for 5 seconds and with the heels held just above the floor for 5 seconds *If there is more available range than the benchmark standard, only the benchmark range needs to be actively controlled*	☐	• The pattern of dissociation is smooth during concentric and eccentric movement	☐
		• Does not (consistently) use *end range* movement into the opposite direction to prevent the UCM	☐
		• No extra feedback needed *(tactile, visual or verbal cueing)*	☐
		• Without external support or unloading	☐
		• Relaxed natural breathing *(even if not ideal – so long as natural pattern does not change)*	☐
• Without holding breath (though it is acceptable to use an alternate breathing strategy)	☐	• No fatigue	☐
• Control during eccentric phase	☐		
• Control during concentric phase	☐		
CORRECT DISSOCIATION PATTERN		**RECRUITMENT EFFICIENCY**	

T13.2 Diagnosis of the site and direction of UCM from the Double Bent Leg Lower Test

DOUBLE BENT LEG LOWER TEST – CROOK LYING

Site	Direction	Segmental/ multisegmental	✗✗ or ✓✗
Lumbar	Extension	Multisegmental hyperextension	☐

T13.3 Feedback tools to monitor retraining

FEEDBACK TOOL	PROCESS
Self-palpation	Palpation monitoring of joint position
Visual observation	Observe in a mirror or directly watch the movement
Adhesive tape	Skin tension for tactile feedback
Pressure biofeedback	Visual confirmation of the control of position
Cueing and verbal correction	Listen to feedback from another observer

T14 PRONE: DOUBLE KNEE BEND TEST (tests for lumbar extension UCM)

This dissociation test assesses the ability to actively dissociate and control lumbar extension and anterior pelvic tilt, then actively flex both knees to engage the point where rectus femoris tension starts to pull the pelvis into anterior tilt while lying prone.

Test procedure

In prone lying the lumbar spine is positioned in neutral alignment (long shallow lordosis) by actively anteriorly or posteriorly tilting the pelvis from the sacrum (Figure 5.72). Monitor lumbopelvic motion by placing the one hand (opposite to the knee flexion) with fingers spread across the low lumbar vertebrae and across the sacrum (alternative lumbopelvic monitoring: place hands on lateral iliac crest). The person is instructed to bend both knees simultaneously. The lumbopelvic region should maintain a neutral position and not move into anterior tilt or increase in the depth of the lordosis (monitor lumbar spine and sacrum) as the knees actively flex to approximately 120° (Figure 5.73). As soon as any anterior tilt or increase of lumbar lordosis is observed (indicating a loss of neutral into extension), the knee flexion must stop and return back to the start position.

Ideally, the person should have the ability to dissociate the lumbar spine from the rectus femoris tension pulling the pelvis into anterior tilt and lumbar extension, as evidenced by maintenance of lumbar spine in a neutral position during active knee flexion to 120°. Normally, there will be paraspinal muscle activation but there should be no increase in multisegmental lumbar extension or segmental shear into an extension hinge (marked skin crease) in the low lumbar spine. This test should be performed without any feedback (self-palpation, vision, tape, etc.) or cueing for correction.

Lumbar extension UCM

The person complains of extension-related symptoms in the lumbar spine. The lumbar spine has UCM into extension relative to rectus femoris tension and anterior tilt loading under extension load. The pelvis anteriorly tilts or the lumbar spine starts to extend before the knees reach 120° flexion. During the attempt to maintain a neutral lumbar spine and prevent uncontrolled lumbar extension when rectus femoris tension pulls on the pelvis, the person either cannot control the UCM or has to concentrate and try hard.

- Note if one vertebral level appears to translate forwards excessively, producing a skin crease as it hinges backwards into extension. If this segment is observed as hinging into translation 'out of line' compared to the other vertebrae, then the UCM is interpreted as a *segmental extension hinge*. The specific hinging segment should be noted and recorded.
- If increased extension (increased lumbar lordosis) of the whole lumbar region and increased anterior pelvic tilt is observed, but no one particular vertebral level is dominant from the adjacent vertebrae, then the UCM is interpreted as a *multisegmental hyperextension*.

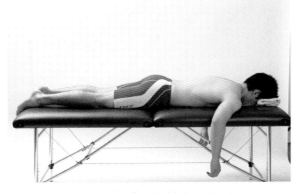

Figure 5.72 Start position for double knee bend test

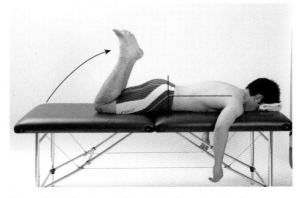

Figure 5.73 Benchmark for double knee bend test

Clinical assessment note for direction-specific motor control testing

If some other movement (e.g. a small amount of flexion or rotation) is observed during a motor control (dissociation) test of extension control, *do not* score this as uncontrolled extension. The flexion and rotation motor control tests will identify if the observed movement is uncontrolled. A test for lumbar extension UCM is only positive if uncontrolled lumbar extension is demonstrated.

Rating and diagnosis of lumbar extension UCM

(T14.1 and T14.2)

Correction

In prone lying position the lumbar spine is in neutral alignment (long shallow lordosis). Monitor the lumbar spine and sacrum position. The person is instructed to bend both knees simultaneously. The lumbopelvic region should maintain a neutral position and not move into anterior tilt or increase in the depth of the lordosis as the knees actively flex. As soon as any an-terior tilt or increase of lumbar lordosis is observed (indicating a loss of neutral into extension), the knee flexion must stop and return back to the start position.

Ideally, the person should have the ability to dissociate the lumbar spine from the rectus femoris tension pulling the pelvis into anterior tilt and lumbar extension, as evidenced by maintenance of lumbar spine in a neutral position during active knee flexion to 120°. Normally, there will be paraspinal muscle activation but there should be no increase in multisegmental lumbar extension or segmental shear into an extension hinge (marked skin crease) in the low lumbar spine. Only bend the knees as far as the neutral lumbopelvic position (monitored with feedback) can be maintained. The person should self-monitor the lumbopelvic alignment and control with a variety of feedback options (T14.3). Palpation feedback is the most useful retraining tool. There should be no provocation of any symptoms within the range that the extension UCM can be controlled. There must be no loss of neutral or UCM into extension or anterior tilt.

If control is poor, start retraining with unilateral knee flexion, but only as far as the neutral

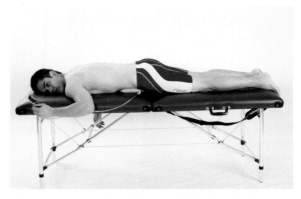

Figure 5.74 Correction with PBU positioned under the abdominal wall

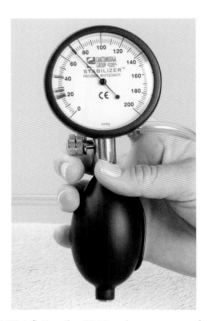

Figure 5.75 Inflating the PBU to a base pressure of 70 mmHg

lumbopelvic position can be maintained. There must be no loss of neutral or give into extension. As control of extension improves, the training can progress to bilateral knee flexion.

In some cases it may be useful to use a PBU to monitor control of the UCM. In prone lying the lumbar spine is positioned in neutral alignment. Place the PBU under the abdomen (centred about the umbilicus) (Figure 5.74). Inflate the pad to a base pressure of 70 mmHg (Figure 5.75). Take a

T14.1 Assessment and rating of low threshold recruitment efficiency of the Double Knee Bend Test

DOUBLE KNEE BEND TEST – PRONE

ASSESSMENT

Control point:
- prevent lumbar extension and anterior pelvic tilt
- prevent segmental hinging into extension/translation

Movement challenge: anterior tilt force from rectus femoris (prone)

Benchmark range: 120° bilateral knee flexion without compensation

RATING OF LOW THRESHOLD RECRUITMENT EFFICIENCY FOR CONTROL OF DIRECTION

	✓ or ✗		✓ or ✗
• Able to prevent 'UCM' into the test direction. Correct dissociation pattern of movement Prevent lumbar UCM into: extension hinge (single segment) hyperextension (multisegmental) and anterior pelvic tilt and move bilateral knee flexion	☐	• Looks easy, and in the opinion of the assessor, is performed with confidence	☐
		• Feels easy, and the subject has sufficient awareness of the movement pattern that they confidently prevent 'UCM' into the test direction	☐
• Dissociate movement through the benchmark range of: 120° of knee flexion *If there is more available range than the benchmark standard, only the benchmark range needs to be actively controlled*	☐	• The pattern of dissociation is smooth during concentric and eccentric movement	☐
		• Does not (consistently) use *end range* movement into the opposite direction to prevent the UCM	☐
• Without holding breath (though it is acceptable to use an alternate breathing strategy)	☐	• No extra feedback needed *(tactile, visual or verbal cueing)*	☐
		• Without external support or unloading	☐
• Control during eccentric phase	☐	• Relaxed natural breathing *(even if not ideal – so long as natural pattern does not change)*	☐
• Control during concentric phase	☐	• No fatigue	☐

CORRECT DISSOCIATION PATTERN | **RECRUITMENT EFFICIENCY**

T14.2 Diagnosis of the site and direction of UCM from the Double Knee Bend Test

DOUBLE KNEE BEND TEST – PRONE

Site	Direction	Segmental/ multisegmental	✗✗ or ✓✗
Lumbar	Extension	Segmental extension hinge (indicate level)	☐
		Multisegmental hyperextension	☐

T14.3 Feedback tools to monitor retraining

FEEDBACK TOOL	PROCESS
Self-palpation	Palpation monitoring of joint position
Visual observation	Observe in a mirror or directly watch the movement
Adhesive tape	Skin tension for tactile feedback
Cueing and verbal correction	Listen to feedback from another observer

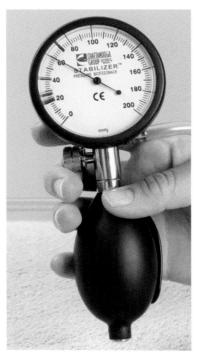

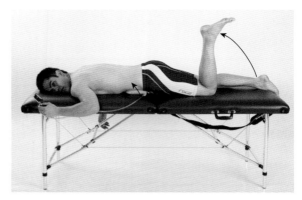

Figure 5.77 Correction with abdominal pre-activation and flexion of one knee

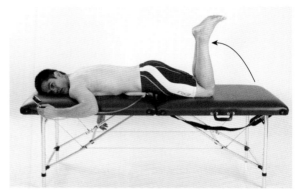

Figure 5.78 Progression: abdominal pre-activation and flexion of both knees

Figure 5.76 Correct abdominal pre-activation decreases PBU pressure to 60 mmHg

relaxed breath in and breathe out. Do not breathe as the low lateral abdominal wall is hollowed (drawn up and in) in an attempt to flatten the lumbar lordosis and decrease pressure on the pad. Ensure that no obvious pelvic tilt occurs. Hold this abdominal contraction. Ideally, the pressure should decrease by 8–10 mmHg (from 70 mmHg to approximately 60–62 mmHg) (Figure 5.76). The pressure decrease should be able to be consistently maintained. No pressure change indicates an efficient co-activation of the global and local stability muscles. A pressure increase indicates ineffective hollowing and substitution with a bracing action.

Keeping the pre-activation of the abdominal muscles (extension control), the person is instructed to fully bend one knee (Figure 5.77). Progress to bilateral knee flexion (Figure 5.78). The lumbopelvic region should maintain a neutral position (no pressure change) as the knee actively flexes (approximately 120°) As soon as any pressure increase is registered (from 60 mmHg towards 70 mmHg) indicating a loss of control into extension, the movement must stop and return back to the start position.

If no PBU is available, the subject may place their opposite hand across the lumbopelvic junction to monitor for any loss of neutral position. The knees may bend only as far as the neutral lumbopelvic position can be maintained without straining or trying too hard. At this point the feet are slowly eccentrically lowered back towards the floor while also maintaining lumbopelvic neutral.

T15 PRONE (TABLE): HIP EXTENSION LIFT TEST
(tests for lumbar extension UCM)

This dissociation test assesses the ability to actively dissociate and control lumbar extension and anterior pelvic tilt, then actively extend one hip while lying prone with hips over the edge of a table.

Test procedure

The person supports their trunk on a table, plinth or bed, with the pelvis at the edge of the table and both feet supported on the floor (the knees slightly flexed) (Figure 5.79). The lumbar spine is positioned in neutral alignment (long shallow lordosis) by actively anteriorly or posteriorly tilting the pelvis from the sacrum. Monitor lumbopelvic motion by placing the one hand (opposite to the leg extension) with fingers spread across the low lumbar vertebrae and across the sacrum (alternative lumbopelvic monitoring: place hands on lateral iliac crest). The person is instructed to slowly extend one knee and then to slowly lift the straight leg off the floor into hip extension to reach the horizontal position (0° hip 'neutral'). The lumbopelvic region should maintain a neutral position with no anterior pelvic tilt or increase in the depth of the lordosis (monitor lumbar spine and sacrum) as the hip actively extends to approximately thigh horizontal (Figure 5.80). As soon as any movement indicating a loss of neutral into extension is observed,

the movement must stop and return back to the start position.

Ideally, the lumbopelvic region should maintain a neutral position as the hip actively extends as far as neutral (i.e. approximately horizontal). Hip extension should be initiated and maintained by gluteus maximus. The hamstrings will participate in the movement but should not dominate. There will be paraspinal muscle activation (asymmetrically biased) but there should be no increase in multisegmental lumbar extension or segmental shear into an extension hinge (marked skin crease) in the low lumbar spine. The hip extension must be independent of any lumbopelvic motion. Assess both sides. Note any excessive lumbar extension under hip extension load. This test should be performed without any feedback (self-palpation, vision, tape, etc.) or cueing for correction.

Lumbar extension UCM

The person complains of extension-related symptoms in the lumbar spine. The lumbar spine has UCM into extension relative to the hips under extension load. The pelvis anteriorly tilts or the lumbar spine starts to extend before the hip reaches 0° extension. The hamstrings may appear to be relatively more active than gluteus maximus during hip extension or overactivation of the back extensor muscles and lumbar extension may even initiate hip extension. During the attempt to maintain a neutral lumbar spine and prevent uncontrolled lumbar extension during active hip extension, the person either cannot

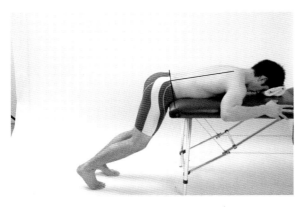

Figure 5.79 Start position for hip extension lift test

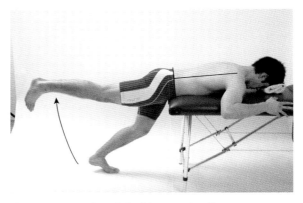

Figure 5.80 Benchmark for hip extension lift test

control the UCM or has to concentrate and try hard.

- Note if one vertebral level appears to translate forwards excessively, producing a skin crease as it hinges backwards into extension. If this segment is observed as hinging into translation 'out of line' compared to the other vertebrae, then the UCM is interpreted as a *segmental extension hinge*. The specific hinging segment should be noted and recorded.
- If increased extension (increased lumbar lordosis) of the whole lumbar region and increased anterior pelvic tilt is observed, but no one particular vertebral level is dominant from the adjacent vertebrae, then the UCM is interpreted as a *multisegmental hyperextension*.

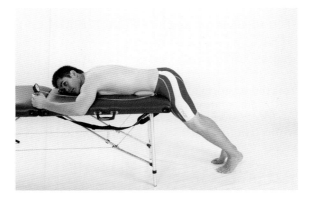

Figure 5.81 Correction with PBU positioned under the abdominal wall

Clinical assessment note for direction-specific motor control testing

If some other movement (e.g. a small amount of flexion or rotation) is observed during a motor control (dissociation) test of extension control, *do not* score this as uncontrolled extension. The flexion and rotation motor control tests will identify if the observed movement is uncontrolled. A test for lumbar extension UCM is only positive if uncontrolled lumbar extension is demonstrated.

Rating and diagnosis of lumbar extension UCM

(T15.1 and T15.2)

Correction

The person supports their trunk on a table, with both feet supported on the floor and the lumbar spine positioned in neutral alignment (long shallow lordosis). Monitor lumbopelvic motion. The person is instructed to slowly extend one knee and then to slowly lift the straight leg off the floor into hip extension.

Ideally, the person should have the ability to dissociate the lumbar spine and pelvis as evidenced by maintenance of the lumbar spine in a neutral position during active hip extension to 0° or thigh horizontal. The abdominal and gluteal muscles are co-activated to control the neutral spine and to prevent excessive lumbar extension. Only lift the hip into extension as far as the neutral lumbopelvic position (monitored with

feedback) can be maintained. The person should self-monitor the lumbopelvic alignment and control with a variety of feedback options (T15.3). Palpation feedback is the most useful retraining tool. There should be no provocation of any symptoms within the range that the extension UCM can be controlled. There must be no loss of neutral or UCM into extension or anterior tilt.

If control is poor it may be useful to use a PBU to monitor control of the UCM. In prone lying over the edge of the table, the lumbar spine is positioned in neutral alignment. Place the PBU unit under the abdomen (centred about the umbilicus) (Figure 5.81). Inflate the pad to a base pressure of 70 mmHg (Figure 5.82). Take a relaxed breath in and breathe out. Do not breathe as the low lateral abdominal wall is hollowed (drawn up and in) in an attempt to flatten the lumbar lordosis and decrease pressure on the pad. Ensure that no pelvic tilt occurs. Hold this abdominal contraction. Ideally, the pressure should decrease by 8–10 mmHg (from 70 mmHg to approximately 60–62 mmHg) (Figure 5.83). The pressure decrease should be able to be consistently maintained. No pressure change indicates inefficient co-activation of the global and local stability muscles. A pressure increase indicates ineffective hollowing and substitution with a bracing action.

Keeping the pre-activation of the abdominal muscles (extension control), the person is instructed to fully extend one knee and then lift the straight leg into hip extension (Figure 5.84). The lumbopelvic region should maintain a neutral position (no pressure change) as the hip

T15.1 Assessment and rating of low threshold recruitment efficiency of the Hip Extension Lift Test

HIP EXTENSION LIFT TEST – PRONE (TABLE)

ASSESSMENT

Control point:
- prevent lumbar extension and anterior pelvic tilt
- prevent segmental hinging into extension/translation

Movement challenge: extension of the hip (prone over a table)

Benchmark range: 0° unilateral hip extension without compensation

RATING OF LOW THRESHOLD RECRUITMENT EFFICIENCY FOR CONTROL OF DIRECTION

	✓ or ✗		✓ or ✗

• Able to prevent 'UCM' into the test direction. Correct dissociation pattern of movement
Prevent lumbar UCM into:
    extension hinge (single segment)
    hyperextension (multisegmental) and anterior
      pelvic tilt
and move single hip extension
	☐	• Looks easy, and in the opinion of the assessor, is performed with confidence	☐

		• Feels easy, and the subject has sufficient awareness of the movement pattern that they confidently prevent 'UCM' into the test direction	☐
• Dissociate movement through the benchmark range of: 0° hip extension (thigh horizontal) *If there is more available range than the benchmark standard, only the benchmark range needs to be actively controlled*	☐	• The pattern of dissociation is smooth during concentric and eccentric movement	☐
		• Does not (consistently) use *end range* movement into the opposite direction to prevent the UCM	☐
• Without holding breath (though it is acceptable to use an alternate breathing strategy)	☐	• No extra feedback needed *(tactile, visual or verbal cueing)*	☐
		• Without external support or unloading	☐
• Control during eccentric phase	☐	• Relaxed natural breathing *(even if not ideal – so long as natural pattern does not change)*	☐
• Control during concentric phase	☐	• No fatigue	☐

CORRECT DISSOCIATION PATTERN   RECRUITMENT EFFICIENCY

T15.2 Diagnosis of the site and direction of UCM from the Hip Extension Lift Test

HIP EXTENSION LIFT TEST – PRONE (TABLE)

Site	Direction	Segmental/ multisegmental	✗✗ or ✓✗
Lumbar	Extension	Segmental extension hinge (indicate level)	☐
		Multisegmental hyperextension	☐

T15.3 Feedback tools to monitor retraining

FEEDBACK TOOL	PROCESS
Self-palpation	Palpation monitoring of joint position
Visual observation	Observe in a mirror or directly watch the movement
Adhesive tape	Skin tension for tactile feedback
Cueing and verbal correction	Listen to feedback from another observer

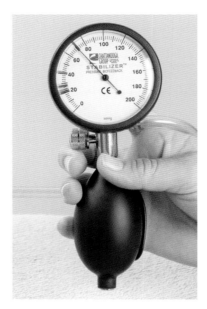

Figure 5.82 Inflating the PBU to a base pressure of 70 mmHg

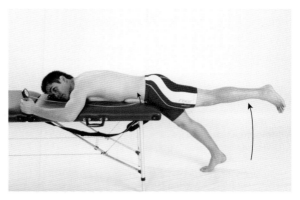

Figure 5.84 Correction with abdominal pre-activation and lifting one leg

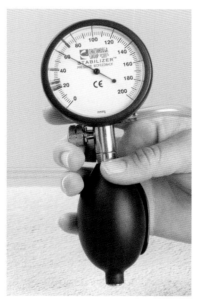

Figure 5.83 Correct abdominal pre-activation decreases PBU pressure to 60 mmHg

actively extends (thigh horizontal – approximately 0°).

If no PBU is available, the subject may place their opposite hand across the lumbopelvic junction to monitor for any loss of neutral position. Only lift the hip into extension as far as the neutral lumbopelvic position (monitored with the PBU) can be maintained without straining or trying too hard. As soon as any pressure increase is registered (from 60 mmHg towards 70 mmHg), indicating a loss of control into extension, the movement must stop and return back to the start position. At this point the leg is slowly eccentrically lowered back towards the floor while also maintaining lumbopelvic neutral.

If control is particularly poor, the person may only be able to dissociate the lumbar spine (neutral) from hip extension to within 40° from horizontal. As the ability to control lumbopelvic extension gets easier and the pattern of dissociation feels less unnatural, the exercise can be progressed to hip extension level with the horizontal (0°) and eventually into the full range of hip extension (10–15° of extension above the horizontal).

T16 STANDING: HIP EXTENSION TOE SLIDE TEST
(tests for lumbar extension UCM)

This dissociation test assesses the ability to actively dissociate and control pelvic forward sway and lumbar extension, then actively extend one hip while standing.

Test procedure

The person stands tall and unsupported with legs straight and the lumbar spine and pelvis positioned in the neutral. The head is positioned directly over the shoulders without chin poke (Figure 5.85). Without letting the lumbopelvic region move into forward sway, or the pelvis move into anterior tilt and increased lumbar extension, the person should have the ability to extend the hip 10–15° past the midline. The lumbar spine is positioned in neutral alignment (long shallow lordosis) by actively anteriorly or posteriorly tilting the pelvis from the sacrum. Monitor lumbopelvic motion by placing the one hand (opposite to the leg extension) with fingers spread across the low lumbar vertebrae and across the sacrum (alternat ive lumbopelvic monitoring: place hands on lateral iliac crest).

The person is instructed to slowly bend one knee, allowing the heel to lift, and keep the toes in contact with the floor. The hip should now be resting in 15–20° of flexion (Figure 5.86). From this starting position, slowly slide the toes backwards along the floor so that the hip extends. Slide the toes back far enough to ensure that the hip extends past the midline to approximately 10–15° of extension (Figure 5.87). The lumbopelvic region should maintain a neutral position with no anterior pelvic tilt or increase in the depth of the lordosis (monitor lumbar spine and

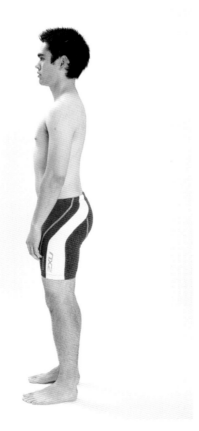

Figure 5.85 Neutral standing

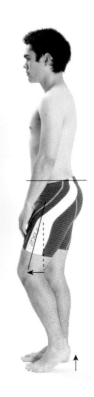

Figure 5.86 Start position for hip extension toe slide test

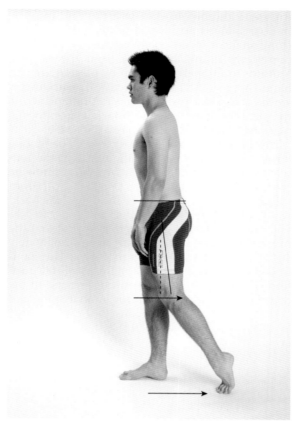

Figure 5.87 Benchmark for hip extension toe slide test

Lumbar extension UCM

The person complains of extension-related symptoms in the lumbar spine. The lumbar spine has UCM into extension relative to the hips under extension load. The pelvis anteriorly tilts or the lumbar spine starts to extend before the hip reaches 10–15° extension. During the attempt to maintain a neutral lumbar spine and prevent uncontrolled lumbar extension during active hip extension, the person either cannot control the UCM or has to concentrate and try hard.

- Note if one vertebral level appears to translate forwards, excessively, producing a skin crease as it hinges backwards into extension. If this segment is observed as hinging into translation 'out of line' compared to the other vertebrae, then the UCM is interpreted as a *segmental extension hinge*. The specific hinging segment should be noted and recorded.
- If increased extension (increased lumbar lordosis) of the whole lumbar region and increased anterior pelvic tilt is observed, but no one particular vertebral level is dominant from the adjacent vertebrae, then the UCM is interpreted as a *multisegmental hyperextension*.

Clinical assessment note for direction-specific motor control testing

If some other movement (e.g. a small amount of flexion or rotation) is observed during a motor control (dissociation) test of extension control, *do not* score this as uncontrolled extension. The flexion and rotation motor control tests will identify if the observed movement is uncontrolled. A test for lumbar extension UCM is only positive if uncontrolled lumbar extension is demonstrated.

Rating and diagnosis of lumbar extension UCM

(T16.1 and T16.2)

Correction

The person stands tall with their thighs right up against a bench or table to limit any pelvic sway or rotation (Figure 5.88). The abdominal and gluteal muscles are co-activated to control the neutral spine and to prevent excessive lumbar

sacrum) and no forward sway of the pelvis (monitor the pelvis) as the hip actively extends past the midline. As soon as any movement indicating a loss of neutral into extension is observed, the movement must stop and return back to the start position.

Ideally, the lumbopelvic region should maintain a neutral position as the hip actively extends 10–15° past neutral. There will be paraspinal muscle activation (asymmetrically biased) but there should be no increase in multisegmental lumbar extension (increased lordosis) or sway into a segmental extension hinge (marked skin crease) in the low lumbar spine. The hip extension must be independent of any lumbopelvic motion. Assess both sides. Note any uncontrolled lumbar extension under hip extension load. This test should be performed without any feedback (self-palpation, vision, tape, etc.) or cueing for correction.

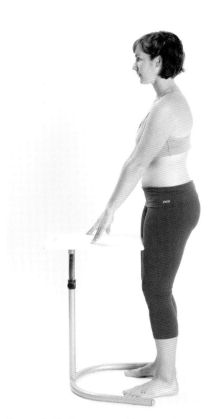

Figure 5.88 Correction with support

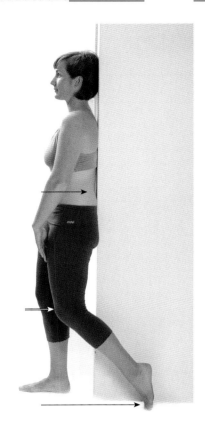

Figure 5.89 Correction using wall fixation

extension and anterior tilt. Monitor lumbopelvic motion with the hands if required. Bend one knee, allowing the heel to lift with the toes in contact with the floor. The hip should now be resting in 15–20° of flexion. From this starting position, the hip is independently extended, by sliding the unweighted foot backwards (toes slide), but only as far as the neutral lumbopelvic position (monitored with feedback) can be maintained and without swaying the upper body or shoulders backwards.

The person should self-monitor the lumbopelvic alignment and control with a variety of feedback options (T16.3). There should be no provocation of any symptoms within the range that the extension UCM can be controlled. There must be no loss of lumbar neutral or UCM into lumbar extension or pelvic sway. As the ability to control lumbar extension or pelvic sway gets easier and the pattern of dissociation feels less

unnatural, the exercise can be progressed to the unsupported position without a bench or table.

If control is very poor, start standing in a doorway or at a wall corner. Position the feet so that one foot can slide backwards (hip extension) behind the body while the back is supported by the doorway or wall. Activate the abdominals and gluteals to flatten the back towards the wall. Maintain pressure against the wall as the unweighted hip extends (toe slides backwards behind the body). The hip is independently extended (Figure 5.89) by sliding the unweighted foot backwards, but only as far as the neutral lumbopelvic position can be maintained and the back does increase extension or the pelvis sway off the wall.

Lumbar extension UCM summary

(Table 5.5)

T16.1 Assessment and rating of low threshold recruitment efficiency of the Hip Extension Toe Slide Test

HIP EXTENSION TOE SLIDE TEST – STANDING

ASSESSMENT

Control point:
- prevent lumbar extension and anterior pelvic tilt
- prevent forward pelvic sway into segmental hinging into extension translation

Movement challenge: extension of the hip (prone over a table)

Benchmark range: 0° unilateral hip extension without compensation

RATING OF LOW THRESHOLD RECRUITMENT EFFICIENCY FOR CONTROL OF DIRECTION

	✓ or ✗		✓ or ✗

• Able to prevent 'UCM' into the test direction. Correct dissociation pattern of movement
Prevent lumbar UCM into:
  forward pelvic sway and extension hinge (single segment)
  hyperextension (multisegmental) and anterior pelvic tilt
and move single hip extension
	☐	• Looks easy, and in the opinion of the assessor, is performed with confidence	☐

		• Feels easy, and the subject has sufficient awareness of the movement pattern that they confidently prevent 'UCM' into the test direction	☐
• Dissociate movement through the benchmark range of: 10–15° hip extension (thigh past the midline) *If there is more available range than the benchmark standard, only the benchmark range needs to be actively controlled*	☐	• The pattern of dissociation is smooth during concentric and eccentric movement	☐
		• Does not (consistently) use *end range* movement into the opposite direction to prevent the UCM	☐
		• No extra feedback needed *(tactile, visual or verbal cueing)*	☐
• Without holding breath (though it is acceptable to use an alternate breathing strategy)	☐	• Without external support or unloading	☐
		• Relaxed natural breathing *(even if not ideal – so long as natural pattern does not change)*	☐
• Control during eccentric phase	☐	• No fatigue	☐
• Control during concentric phase	☐		

CORRECT DISSOCIATION PATTERN   **RECRUITMENT EFFICIENCY**

T16.2 Diagnosis of the site and direction of UCM from the Hip Extension Toe Slide Test

HIP EXTENSION TOE SLIDE TEST – STANDING

Site	Direction	Segmental/ multisegmental	✗✗ or ✓✗
Lumbar	Extension	Segmental extension hinge (indicate level)	☐
		Multisegmental hyperextension	☐

T16.3 Feedback tools to monitor retraining

FEEDBACK TOOL	PROCESS
Self-palpation	Palpation monitoring of joint position
Visual observation	Observe in a mirror or directly watch the movement
Adhesive tape	Skin tension for tactile feedback
Cueing and verbal correction	Listen to feedback from another observer

Table 5.5 Summary and rating of lumbar extension tests

UCM DIAGNOSIS AND TESTING

SITE: LUMBAR	DIRECTION: EXTENSION	CLINICAL PRIORITY ☐
TEST	**RATING** (✓✓ or ✓✗ or ✗✗) and rationale	
Standing: thoracic extension (sway)		
Standing: thoracic extension (tilt)		
Sitting: chest lift (tilt)		
Sitting: forward lean		
4 point: forward rocking		
Crook: double bent leg lower		
Prone: double knee bend		
Prone (table): hip extension lift		
Standing: hip extension toe slide		

Tests of lumbopelvic rotation control

LUMBOPELVIC ROTATION (ASYMMETRICAL/UNILATERAL) CONTROL TESTS AND ROTATION CONTROL REHABILITATION

These asymmetrical and unilateral load tests assess the extent of rotation, side-bend or side-shift UCM in the lumbar spine and pelvic regions and assess the ability of the dynamic stability system to adequately control rotation or lateral load and strain. It is a priority to assess for rotation UCM if the person complains of or demonstrates unilaterally biased symptoms or disability or asymmetry of alignment.

Rotation or lateral stability dysfunctions are usually superimposed on top of a flexion or extension dysfunction. It is important to identify the direction of rotational or shift UCM. There are many tests that identify rotational stability dysfunction. There is no particular progression implied by the order that they are presented. They all use different co-activation synergies and different loads. It is a priority to assess for extension UCM if the patient complains of or demonstrates extension-related symptoms or disability. The tests that identify dysfunction can also be used to guide and direct rehabilitation strategies.

Unlike flexion and extension control problems, lumbopelvic rotation control does not have obvious direct links to functional movements. Rotation control faults are usually combined with lumbar flexion or extension UCMs which do have functional links. The uncontrolled rotation contributes to asymmetry of alignment and unilateral symptoms within lumbar flexion and extension UCM. It is very uncommon for a primary lumbar dysfunction to present solely with uncontrolled rotation while demonstrating good flexion and extension control. If a patient presents with lumbopelvic pain and demonstrates good flexion and extension control, while concurrently demonstrating poor control of rotation, this would suggest that the primary problem of UCM is related to the sacroiliac joints (SIJs), rather than the lumbar spine. UCM of the SIJ and pelvic girdle are consistently unilateral in nature and always demonstrate either open chain or closed chain uncontrolled rotation.

OBSERVATION AND ANALYSIS OF LUMBOPELVIC ROTATION ± SIDE-BEND

Description of ideal pattern

The subject is instructed to twist fully to the left and right as they normally would. Ideally, there should be even rotation throughout the spine as the patient actively rotates, with both the spine and legs concurrently contributing to the rotation. The upper body (monitored by the line across the acromions) should turn approximately 90°. The legs (monitored by the relative position of the pelvis) should contribute approximately 45°, while the spine should also contribute to the other 45° (position of upper body relative to the pelvis). Of the 45° of spinal rotation, approximately 10–15° should come from the lumbar spine while the thoracic spine should provide the majority of spinal rotation (30–35°). The pelvis should not sway forwards during rotation and there should be good symmetry of movement without any weight shift of the trunk or pelvis (Figures 5.90 and 5.91).

Movement faults associated with lumbopelvic rotation

Relative stiffness (restrictions)

- *Hip rotation restriction* – either hip may lack 35–40° of normal range of rotation in standing twisting or turning movements. The lumbar spine or pelvis frequently increases rotation to compensate for the lack of hip mobility. Hip rotation range can be tested passively and dynamically with manual examination.
- *Thoracic rotation restriction* – the middle and lower thoracic spine has a rotation restriction that may also contribute to compensatory increases in lumbopelvic range. This is confirmed with manual segmental assessment.

Relative flexibility (potential UCM)

- *Lumbopelvic rotation.* The lumbar spine and pelvis may initiate functional movements into rotation and contribute more during

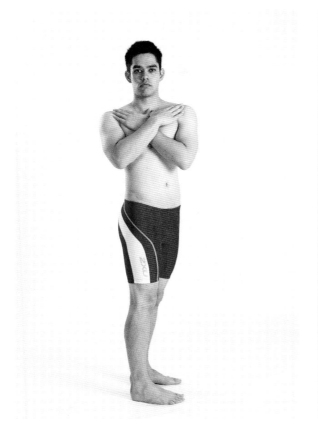

Figure 5.90 Ideal pattern of lumbopelvic rotation (side view)

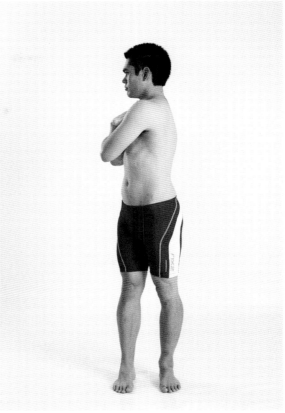

Figure 5.91 Ideal pattern of lumbopelvic rotation (front view)

turning or twisting while the hips and thoracic contributions start later and contribute less. At the limit of turning or twisting, excessive or hypermobile range of lumbopelvic rotation may be observed. During the return to neutral the lumbopelvic rotation persists and recovers later.

In the assessment of lumbopelvic rotation movement, the UCM can be identified as either open chain or closed chain.

Indications to test for lumbopelvic rotation UCM

Observe or palpate for:

1. hypermobile lumbopelvic rotation range
2. excessive initiation of rotation with lumbopelvic rotation

3. symptoms (pain, discomfort, strain) associated with lumbopelvic rotation
4. asymmetrical or unilateral symptoms associated with flexion or extension movements
5. asymmetrical posture or alignment, in the lumbopelvic region.

The person complains of asymmetrical or unilateral-related symptoms in the lumbar spine. Under rotation or unilateral load, the lumbar spine has UCM *into rotation* relative to the hips or relative to the thoracic spine. The dysfunction is confirmed with rotation dissociation tests.

Tests of open chain rotation control

T17 SUPINE: SINGLE HEEL SLIDE TEST (tests for lumbopelvic rotation UCM)

This dissociation test assesses the ability to actively dissociate and control lumbopelvic rotation and slide one heel along the floor (heel beside the straight knee) by moving one hip through flexion while in supine lying. During any unilateral or asymmetrical limb load or movement, a rotational force is transmitted to the lumbopelvic region.

Test procedure

In supine lying, place two PBUs, clipped together, under the lumbar lordosis (centred about L3 with the join along the spine) (Figure 5.92). Alternatively, place one PBU on one side of the spine and a folded towel on the other side (Figure 5.93). While lying relaxed with the legs straight, inflate the pad(s) to a base pressure of 40 mmHg. The PBU at this pressure maintains the neutral lordosis. A loss of control into rotation causes a pressure change on the pad(s). An increase in pressure on a pad indicates rotation of the lumbopelvic region towards that side. A decrease in pressure on a pad indicates rotation of the lumbopelvic region away from that side. No pressure change = no loss of neutral position = good control.

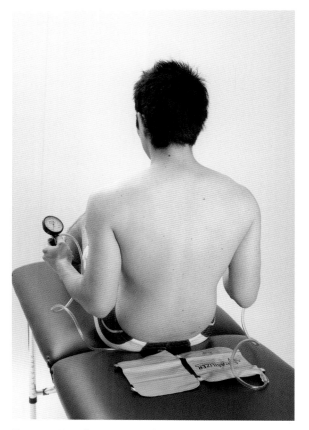

Figure 5.92 Self-positioning of two PBUs in the lumbar lordosis

When using two PBUs, if lumbopelvic rotation occurs, one pad will increase pressure while the other pad will decrease pressure. The change in pressure indicates the direction of lumbopelvic rotation (e.g. if the pressure in the right pad increases while the left decreases, then the pelvis is rotating to the right). Usually, one PBU demonstrates a greater pressure change than the other. For testing and retraining it is best that the person only has to monitor one PBU. They should monitor lumbopelvic rotation control only with the PBU that has the greatest change.

With the person lying supine and with legs extended and the feet together, both ASIS are checked for symmetry in the anteroposterior plane and both PBUs are set at 40 mmHg (Figure 5.94). If no PBUs are available the control of lumbopelvic position should be monitored with palpation and visual feedback. Using the PBU with the greatest pressure change to monitor the precision of lumbopelvic rotation control, the person is instructed to keep the pelvis as level as possible (no pressure change) and to slide one heel up along the floor to stop beside the other (straight) knee (Figure 5.95). The hip should be flexed to approximately 45°. Hold this position for about 5 seconds and then slowly straighten the leg and slide the leg out to the start position.

Ideally, the pelvis should not rotate and the ASIS positions should remain symmetrical as the hip flexes up and returns. There should be no significant pressure change in the pressure of both PBUs. A small change in pressure of less than 5 mmHg (2 graduations) is acceptable while the

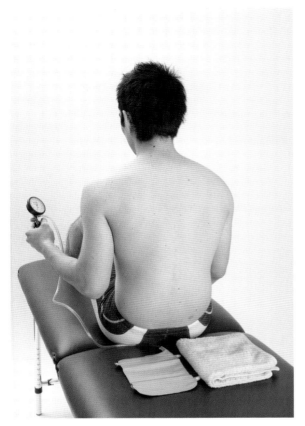

Figure 5.93 Self-positioning of one PBU and a towel

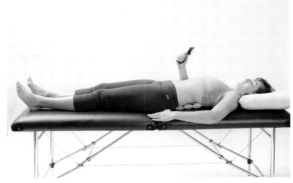

Figure 5.94 Start position for single heel slide test

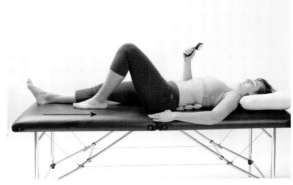

Figure 5.95 Benchmark for single heel slide test

leg is moving, so long as both pads can be stabilised at 40 mmHg when the leg is stationary.

The unilateral hip flexion must be independent of any lumbopelvic rotation. Assess both sides. Note any excessive lumbopelvic rotation under hip rotation load. The therapist should not rely solely on the PBU. They should also use palpation of the pelvis and visual observation to determine whether the control of rotation is adequate. This test should be performed without any feedback (self-palpation, vision, tape, etc.) or cueing for correction. The person is allowed to watch the PBU, however, because it is required for the precision of the testing range.

Lumbopelvic rotation UCM

The person complains of unilateral symptoms in the lumbar spine. During any unilateral or asymmetrical limb load a rotational force is transmitted to the lumbopelvic region. The trunk rotation stabilisers are not able to effectively control this rotation force. The lumbar spine has UCM into lumbopelvic rotation relative to the hips under unilateral hip flexion load. During a single leg heel slide in supine that produces unilateral hip flexion, the lumbopelvic region starts to rotate towards that side before the heel reaches the straight knee.

Uncontrolled rotation is identified by an excessive pressure increase in the PBU on that side as the low back and pelvis rotates onto the pad (ipsilateral ASIS moves posteriorly). Uncontrolled rotation can also be identified by an excessive pressure decrease in the PBU on the other side (straight leg side) as the low back and pelvis rotates away from the pad (contralateral ASIS moves anteriorly). A change in pressure of 5 mmHg (2 graduations) or more is not acceptable while the leg is moving. This indicates

165

uncontrolled lumbopelvic rotation. Uncontrolled lumbopelvic rotation is also identified if *both* pads cannot be symmetrically stabilised on 40 mmHg when the heel slide leg is stationary.

During the attempt to dissociate the lumbopelvic rotation from independent unilateral hip flexion, the person either cannot control the UCM or has to concentrate and try hard to dissociate the lumbopelvic rotation from independent hip movement. The movement must be assessed on both sides. Note the direction that the rotation cannot be controlled (i.e. is there uncontrolled lumbopelvic rotation to the left or the right). It may be unilateral or bilateral. If lumbopelvic rotation UCM presents bilaterally, one side may be better or worse than the other.

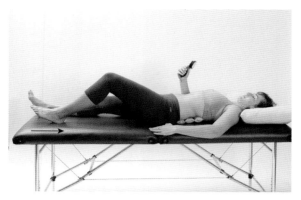

Figure 5.96 Correction: partial range heel slide

Clinical assessment note for direction-specific motor control testing

If some other movement (e.g. a small amount of flexion or extension) is observed during a motor control (dissociation) test of rotation control, *do not* score this as uncontrolled rotation. The flexion and extension motor control tests will identify if the observed movement is uncontrolled. A test for lumbopelvic rotation UCM is only positive if uncontrolled lumbopelvic rotation is demonstrated.

Rating and diagnosis of lumbopelvic rotation UCM

(T17.1 and T17.2)

Correction

With the person lying supine with legs extended and the feet together, both PBUs are set at 40 mmHg. If no PBUs are available the control of lumbopelvic position should be monitored with palpation and visual feedback. The person is instructed to keep the pelvis as level as possible (no pressure change) and to slide one heel up along the floor beside the other (straight) knee but only as far as neutral lumbopelvic rotation can be controlled (monitored with feedback) (Figure 5.96). At the point in range that the lumbopelvic region starts to lose control of rotation the movement should stop. The lumbopelvic position is restabilised; then hold this position for a few seconds and return to the start

position with control of the lumbopelvic rotation UCM.

Ideally, the pelvis should not rotate and the ASIS positions should remain symmetrical as the hip flexes and returns. A small change in pressure of less than 5 mmHg (2 graduations) is acceptable while the leg is moving, so long as both pads can be stabilised at 40 mmHg when the leg is stationary. The person should self-monitor the lumbopelvic alignment and control with a variety of feedback options (T17.3). There should be no provocation of any symptoms within the range that the rotation UCM can be controlled.

During any unilateral or asymmetrical limb load a rotational force is transmitted to the lumbopelvic region. The lumbopelvic rotation stability muscles control this rotational stress. The oblique abdominal muscles, anterior fascicles of psoas major and the superficial fibres of lumbar multifidus, which stabilise trunk rotation, must coordinate with the hip flexor/rotator muscles, which concentrically slide the leg up and eccentrically return the leg to the start position. The uncontrolled lumbopelvic rotation is often associated with inefficiency of the trunk stabilisers (especially the oblique abdominals) to coordinate with the limb muscles. (For example, the left external obliques and the right internal obliques control the lumbopelvic rotation stability as the right leg flexes and returns). If control is poor the person lies supine and actively contracts the lateral oblique abdominal muscles to improve control of lumbopelvic rotation. The contralateral external oblique abdominals and the ipsilateral internal oblique abdominals can be facilitated

T17.1 Assessment and rating of low threshold recruitment efficiency of the Single Heel Slide Test

SINGLE HEEL SLIDE TEST – SUPINE

ASSESSMENT

Control point:
• prevent lumbopelvic rotation
Movement challenge: unilateral hip flexion (supine)
Benchmark range: heel beside the straight knee (approx 45° hip flexion)

RATING OF LOW THRESHOLD RECRUITMENT EFFICIENCY FOR CONTROL OF DIRECTION

	✓ or ✗		✓ or ✗
• Able to prevent 'UCM' into the test direction. Correct dissociation pattern of movement Prevent lumbopelvic UCM into: rotation and move unilateral hip flexion	☐	• Looks easy, and in the opinion of the assessor, is performed with confidence	☐
		• Feels easy, and the subject has sufficient awareness of the movement pattern that they confidently prevent 'UCM' into the test direction	☐
• Dissociate movement through the benchmark range of: heel beside the straight knee (approx 45° hip flexion) *If there is more available range than the benchmark standard, only the benchmark range needs to be actively controlled*	☐	• The pattern of dissociation is smooth during concentric and eccentric movement	☐
		• Does not (consistently) use *end range* movement into the opposite direction to prevent the UCM	☐
• Without holding breath (though it is acceptable to use an alternate breathing strategy)	☐	• No extra feedback needed *(tactile, visual or verbal cueing)*	☐
• Control during eccentric phase	☐	• Without external support or unloading	☐
• Control during concentric phase	☐	• Relaxed natural breathing *(even if not ideal – so long as natural pattern does not change)*	☐
		• No fatigue	☐
CORRECT DISSOCIATION PATTERN		**RECRUITMENT EFFICIENCY**	

T17.2 Diagnosis of the site and direction of UCM from the Single Heel Slide Test

SINGLE HEEL SLIDE TEST – SUPINE

Site	Direction	Pelvis to the left (L)	Pelvis to the right (R)
		(check box)	(check box)
Lumbopelvic	Rotation (open chain)	☐	☐

T17.3 Feedback tools to monitor retraining

FEEDBACK TOOL	PROCESS
Self-palpation	Palpation monitoring of joint position
Visual observation	Observe in a mirror or directly watch the movement
Adhesive tape	Skin tension for tactile feedback
Pressure biofeedback	Visual confirmation of the control of position
Cueing and verbal correction	Listen to feedback from another observer

separately to identify which is more effective at controlling the rotation UCM.

External oblique abdominal recruitment

The instruction to actively pull the anterior lower ribcage down and posteriorly in towards the spine on the *contralateral* side is a good facilitation cue for the external oblique abdominals. This should be coordinated with the cue to 'pull in' the whole abdominal wall at the same time. (Do not use the transversus abdominis facilitation cue of only 'hollowing' the lower abdominal wall. Transversus abdominis does not adequately control trunk rotation.) Discourage bracing or bulging out of the abdominal wall.

Internal oblique abdominal recruitment

The instruction to actively push or lift the *ipsilateral* ASIS in an anterior or forward direction is a good facilitation cue for the internal oblique abdominals. Visualise 'pushing a button' with the ipsilateral ASIS. This should be coordinated with the cue to 'pull in' the whole abdominal wall at the same time. Discourage bracing or bulging out of the abdominal wall.

With an efficient 'preset' contraction of the appropriate oblique abdominals, the pressure should increase by 8–10 mmHg (from 40 mmHg to approximately 48–50 mmHg) on both PBU pads. This also provides a counter-rotation force for the uncontrolled lumbopelvic rotation under unilateral limb load. If a PBU is not available, the subject should palpate the ASIS on the contralateral side for feedback regarding loss of pelvic

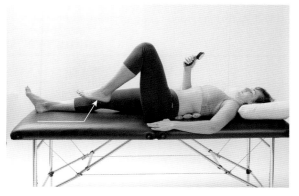

Figure 5.97 Progression: heel slide foot unsupported

neutral position into rotation. It is also useful to palpate the posterolateral iliac crest on the ipsilateral (leg movement) side for loss of pelvic neutral position. Some people will also need to have their head supported in flexion so that they can use visual feedback and watch for the loss of control.

Once effective oblique abdominal facilitation has been achieved, the person is then instructed to slowly slide one heel up towards the other knee. The heel slide can continue only as far as there is no rotation of the pelvis at all.

As the ability to control the lumbopelvic region during independent hip rotation gets easier and the pattern of dissociation feels less unnatural the exercise can be progressed. A basic progression would be to perform this movement then lift the heel beside the straight knee and hold it 5 cm off the floor (Figure 5.97).

T18 SUPINE: BENT KNEE FALL OUT TEST (tests for lumbopelvic rotation UCM)

This dissociation test assesses the ability to actively dissociate and control lumbopelvic rotation and lower the bent knee (heel beside the straight knee) by moving the hip through abduction/lateral rotation and back while in supine lying. During any unilateral or asymmetrical limb load or movement, a rotational force is transmitted to the lumbopelvic region.

Test procedure

In supine lying, place two PBUs, clipped together, under the lumbar lordosis (centred about L3 with the join along the spine). Alternatively, place one PBU on one side of the spine and a folded towel on the other side. While lying relaxed with the legs straight, inflate the pad(s) to a base pressure of 40 mmHg. The PBU at this pressure maintains the neutral lordosis. A loss of control into rotation causes a pressure change on the pad(s). An increase in pressure on a pad indicates rotation of the lumbopelvic region towards that side. A decrease in pressure on a pad indicates rotation of the lumbopelvic region away from that side. No pressure change = no loss of neutral position = good control.

> When using two PBUs, if lumbopelvic rotation occurs, one pad will increase pressure while the other pad will decrease pressure. The change in pressure indicates the direction of lumbopelvic rotation (e.g. if the pressure in the right pad increases while the left decreases, then the pelvis is rotating to the right). Usually, one PBU demonstrates a greater pressure change than the other. For testing and retraining it is best that the person only has to monitor one PBU. They should monitor lumbopelvic rotation control only with the PBU that has the greatest change.

With the person lying supine and with legs extended and the feet together, both ASIS are checked for symmetry in the anteroposterior plane and both PBUs are set at 40 mmHg (Figure 5.98). The person moves one heel up beside the other knee. Ideally, the pelvis should not be rotated here (no pressure change). If some rotation is present, correct the pelvic alignment to get the pelvis level (both PBUs back at 40 mmHg)

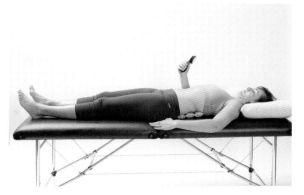

Figure 5.98 Preparation to set the PBU base pressure at 40 mmHg

(Figure 5.99). If no PBUs are available the control of lumbopelvic position should be monitored with palpation and visual feedback. Using the PBU with the greatest pressure change to monitor the precision of lumbopelvic rotation control, the person is instructed to keep the pelvis absolutely level (no pressure change) and to slowly lower the bent leg out to the side, keeping the foot supported beside the straight leg. Ideally, the bent leg should be able to be lowered out through at least 45° of the available range of hip abduction and lateral rotation (Figure 5.100) and returned, without associated pelvic rotation. A small change in pressure of less than 5 mmHg (2 graduations) is acceptable while the leg is moving, so long as both pads can be stabilised on 40 mmHg when the leg is stationary.

The unilateral hip rotation must be independent of any lumbopelvic rotation. Assess both sides. Note any excessive lumbopelvic rotation under hip rotation load. The therapist should not rely solely on the PBU. They should also use palpation of the pelvis and visual observation to determine whether the control of rotation is adequate. This test should be performed without any feedback (self-palpation, vision, tape, etc.) or cueing for correction. The person is allowed to watch the PBU, however, because it is required for the precision of the testing range.

Lumbopelvic rotation UCM

The person complains of unilateral symptoms in the lumbar spine. During any unilateral or asymmetrical limb load a rotational force is

169

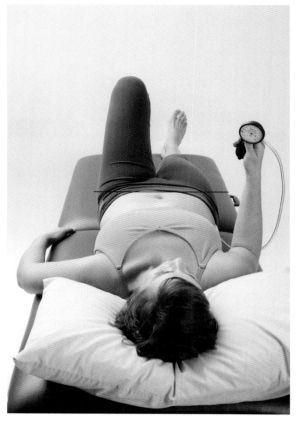

Figure 5.99 Start position of bent knee fall out test – reposition pelvis to achieve PBU pressure of 40 mmHg

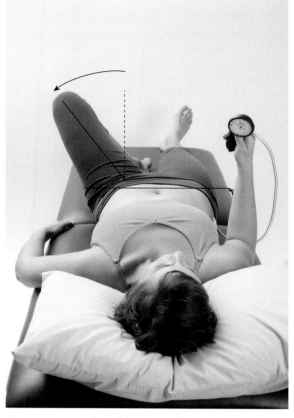

Figure 5.100 Benchmark bent knee fall out test

transmitted to the lumbopelvic region. The trunk rotation stabilisers are not able to effectively control this rotation force. The lumbar spine has UCM into rotation relative to the hips under unilateral hip rotation load. As the bent leg is lowered out to the side, the pelvis begins to rotate to follow the hip movement before 45° of rotation range is achieved. Uncontrolled lumbopelvic rotation is also identified if *both* pads cannot be symmetrically stabilised on 40 mmHg when the bent knee fall out leg is stationary. The rotation UCM is demonstrated by pressure increasing on the PBU on the side of leg movement as the low back and pelvis rotates onto the pad (ipsilateral ASIS moves posteriorly) or pressure decreasing on PBU on the contralateral side to the leg movement as the low back and pelvis rotates away from the pad (contralateral ASIS moves anteriorly).

The person is unable to dissociate movement in the hip from the lumbar spine and pelvis. A change in pressure of 5 mmHg (2 graduations) or more is not acceptable while the leg is moving. This indicates uncontrolled lumbopelvic rotation. Uncontrolled lumbopelvic rotation is also identified if *both* pads cannot be symmetrically stabilised on 40 mmHg when the leg is stationary.

During the attempt to dissociate the lumbopelvic rotation from independent unilateral hip flexion, the person either cannot control the UCM or has to concentrate and try hard to dissociate the lumbopelvic rotation from independent hip movement. The movement must be assessed on both sides. Note the direction that the rotation cannot be controlled (i.e. is there uncontrolled lumbopelvic rotation to the left or the right). It may be unilateral or bilateral. If lumbopelvic rotation UCM presents bilaterally, one side may be better or worse than the other.

Clinical assessment note for direction-specific motor control testing

If some other movement (e.g. a small amount of flexion or extension) is observed during a motor control (dissociation) test of rotation control, *do not* score this as uncontrolled rotation. The flexion and extension motor control tests will identify if the observed movement is uncontrolled. A test for lumbopelvic rotation UCM is only positive if uncontrolled lumbopelvic rotation is demonstrated.

Rating and diagnosis of lumbopelvic rotation UCM

(T18.1 and T18.2)

Correction

With the person lying supine and with legs extended and the feet together, both PBUs are set at 40 mmHg. If no PBUs are available, the control of lumbopelvic position should be monitored with palpation and visual feedback. The person is instructed to keep the pelvis as level as possible (no pressure change) and to place one heel up beside the other knee. If some rotation is present, correct the pelvic alignment to get the pelvis level (both PBUs back at 40 mmHg). Then, keeping the pelvis absolutely level (no pressure change), slowly lower the bent leg out to the side, but only as far as neutral lumbopelvic rotation can be controlled (monitored with feedback). Hold this position for a few seconds and then return the leg out to the start position. At the point in range that the lumbopelvic region starts to lose control of rotation the movement should stop. The lumbopelvic position is restabilised, then hold this position for a few seconds and return to the start position with control of the lumbopelvic rotation UCM.

Ideally, the pelvis should not rotate and the ASIS positions should remain symmetrical as the leg rotates and returns. A small change in pressure of less than 5 mmHg (2 graduations) is acceptable while the leg is moving, so long as both pads can be stabilised at 40 mmHg when the leg is stationary. The person should self-monitor the lumbopelvic alignment and control with a variety of feedback options (T18.3). There should be no provocation of any symptoms within the range that the rotation UCM can be controlled.

During any unilateral or asymmetrical limb load a rotational force is transmitted to the lumbopelvic region. The lumbopelvic rotation stability muscles control this rotational stress. The oblique abdominal muscles, anterior fascicles of psoas major and the superficial fibres of lumbar multifidus, which stabilise trunk rotation, must coordinate with the hip adductor/rotator muscles, which eccentrically lower the leg out to the side and concentrically return the leg to the start position. The uncontrolled lumbopelvic rotation is often associated with inefficiency of the trunk stabilisers (especially the oblique abdominals) to coordinate with the limb muscles. For example, the left external obliques and the right internal obliques control the lumbopelvic rotation stability as the right leg lowers out to the side. If control is poor, the person actively contracts the lateral oblique abdominal muscles to improve control of lumbopelvic rotation. The contralateral external oblique abdominals and the ipsilateral internal oblique abdominals can be facilitated separately to identify which is more effective at controlling the rotation UCM.

External oblique abdominal recruitment

The instruction to actively pull the anterior lower ribcage down and posteriorly in towards the spine on the *contralateral* side is a good facilitation cue for the external oblique abdominals. This should be coordinated with the cue to 'pull in' the whole abdominal wall at the same time. (Do not use the transversus abdominis facilitation cue of only 'hollowing' the lower abdominal wall. Transversus abdominis does not adequately control trunk rotation.) Discourage bracing or bulging out of the abdominal wall.

Internal oblique abdominal recruitment

The instruction to actively push or lift the *ipsilateral* ASIS in an anterior or forward direction is a good facilitation cue for the internal oblique abdominals. Visualise 'pushing a button' with the ipsilateral ASIS. This should be coordinated with the cue to 'pull in' the whole abdominal wall at the same time. Discourage bracing or bulging out of the abdominal wall.

T18.1 Assessment and rating of low threshold recruitment efficiency of the Bent Knee Fall Out Test

BENT KNEE FALL OUT TEST – SUPINE

ASSESSMENT

Control point:
• prevent lumbopelvic rotation
Movement challenge: unilateral lateral rotation and abduction (supine)
Benchmark range: 45° hip lateral rotation and abduction (heel beside the knee)

RATING OF LOW THRESHOLD RECRUITMENT EFFICIENCY FOR CONTROL OF DIRECTION

	✓ or ✗		✓ or ✗
• Able to prevent 'UCM' into the test direction. Correct dissociation pattern of movement Prevent lumbopelvic UCM into: rotation and move unilateral hip lateral rotation and abduction	☐	• Looks easy, and in the opinion of the assessor, is performed with confidence	☐
		• Feels easy, and the subject has sufficient awareness of the movement pattern that they confidently prevent 'UCM' into the test direction	☐
• Dissociate movement through the benchmark range of: 45° hip lateral rotation/abduction *If there is more available range than the benchmark standard, only the benchmark range needs to be actively controlled*	☐	• The pattern of dissociation is smooth during concentric and eccentric movement	☐
		• Does not (consistently) use *end range* movement into the opposite direction to prevent the UCM	☐
• Without holding breath (though it is acceptable to use an alternate breathing strategy)	☐	• No extra feedback needed (*tactile, visual or verbal cueing*)	☐
		• Without external support or unloading	☐
• Control during eccentric phase	☐	• Relaxed natural breathing (*even if not ideal – so long as natural pattern does not change*)	☐
• Control during concentric phase	☐	• No fatigue	☐
CORRECT DISSOCIATION PATTERN		**RECRUITMENT EFFICIENCY**	

T18.2 Diagnosis of the site and direction of UCM from the Bent Knee Fall Out Test

BENT KNEE FALL OUT TEST – SUPINE

Site	Direction	Pelvis to the left (L)	Pelvis to the right (R)
		(check box)	(check box)
Lumbopelvic	Rotation (open chain)	☐	☐

T18.3 Feedback tools to monitor retraining

FEEDBACK TOOL	PROCESS
Self-palpation	Palpation monitoring of joint position
Visual observation	Observe in a mirror or directly watch the movement
Adhesive tape	Skin tension for tactile feedback
Cueing and verbal correction	Listen to feedback from another observer
Pressure biofeedback	Visual confirmation of the control of position

With an efficient 'preset' contraction of the appropriate oblique abdominals, the pressure should increase by 8–10 mmHg (from 40 mmHg to approximately 48–50 mmHg) on both PBU pads. This also provides a counter-rotation force for the uncontrolled lumbopelvic rotation under unilateral limb load. If a PBU is not available, the subject should palpate the ASIS on the contralateral side for feedback regarding loss of pelvic neutral position into rotation. It is also useful to palpate the posterolateral iliac crest on the ipsilateral (leg movement) side for loss of pelvic neutral position. Some people will also need to have their head supported in flexion so that they can use visual feedback and watch for the loss of control.

Once effective oblique abdominal facilitation has been achieved, the person is then instructed to slowly slide and lower one knee out to the side. The bent knee fall out can continue only as far as there is no rotation of the pelvis at all.

As the ability to control the lumbopelvic region during independent hip rotation gets easier and the pattern of dissociation feels less unnatural, the exercise can be progressed. A basic progression would be to perform this movement with the leg unsupported. That is, lift the heel of the bent leg 5 cm off the supporting surface and control lumbopelvic rotation during an unsupported bent knee fall out.

T19 SIDE-LYING: TOP LEG TURN OUT TEST (tests for lumbopelvic rotation UCM)

This dissociation test assesses the ability to actively dissociate and control lumbopelvic rotation and lift the top knee (hip and knee flexion) by lifting the top hip through abduction/lateral rotation and back while in side-lying position During any unilateral or asymmetrical limb load or movement, a rotational force is transmitted to the lumbopelvic region.

Test procedure

The person lies on one side with hips flexed to 45° and the knees flexed to 90° and the feet together (Figure 5.101). The pelvis should be positioned in neutral rotation. For initial teaching of the test movement, a 'flexicurve' can be positioned so that one end of the 'flexicurve' contacts the ASIS of the pelvis to provide a reference marker for the control of lumbopelvic rotation. The person is instructed to keep the pelvis from rotating backwards (maintain ASIS contact with the flexicurve) and slowly lift the uppermost knee up and out to the side while keeping the heels together. Ideally, the top leg should be able to turn up and out to at least 15° (above horizontal) of hip abduction and lateral rotation (Figure 5.102) and return, without associated lumbopelvic rotation.

The unilateral hip rotation must be independent of any lumbopelvic rotation. Assess both sides. Note any excessive lumbopelvic rotation under hip rotation load. This test should be performed without any feedback (self-palpation, vision, flexicurve, etc.) or cueing for correction. The therapist should use visual observation of the pelvis to determine whether the control of lumbopelvic rotation is adequate when feedback is removed for testing.

Lumbopelvic rotation UCM

The person complains of unilateral symptoms in the lumbar spine. The lumbar spine has UCM into rotation relative to the hips under unilateral hip rotation load. As the top leg turns up and out to the side, the pelvis begins to rotate to follow the hip movement before 15° of rotation range above horizontal is achieved. Uncontrolled lumbopelvic rotation is also identified if the ASIS rotates away from contact with the flexicurve before 15° of lateral rotation range above horizontal is achieved (Figure 5.103).

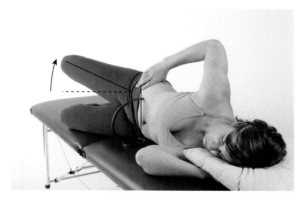

Figure 5.102 Benchmark top leg turn out test

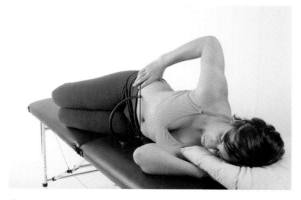

Figure 5.101 Start position top leg tun out test

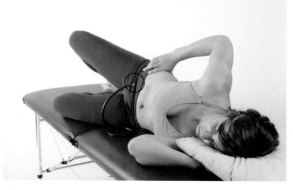

Figure 5.103 Monitoring uncontrolled movement with a flexicurve

During the attempt to dissociate the lumbopelvic rotation from independent unilateral hip lateral rotation and abduction, the person either cannot control the UCM or has to concentrate and try hard to dissociate the lumbopelvic rotation from independent hip movement. The movement must be assessed on both sides. Note the direction that the rotation cannot be controlled (i.e. is there uncontrolled lumbopelvic rotation to the left or the right). It may be unilateral or bilateral. If lumbopelvic rotation UCM presents bilaterally, one side may be better or worse than the other.

Clinical assessment note for direction-specific motor control testing

If some other movement (e.g. a small amount of flexion or extension) is observed during a motor control (dissociation) test of rotation control, *do not* score this as uncontrolled rotation. The flexion and extension motor control tests will identify if the observed movement is uncontrolled. A test for lumbopelvic rotation UCM is only positive if uncontrolled lumbopelvic rotation is demonstrated.

Rating and diagnosis of lumbopelvic rotation UCM

(T19.1 and T19.2)

Correction

With the person side-lying and the hips flexed to 45°, the knees flexed to 90° and the feet together, the pelvis should be positioned in neutral rotation. The person is instructed to keep the pelvis vertical and prevent the pelvis from rotating backwards as they lift the top leg up and out to the side. The heels stay together, and the 'turn out' is produced from independent hip lateral rotation and abduction. The top leg lifts into the turn out only as far as neutral lumbopelvic rotation can be controlled (monitored with feedback). Hold this position for a few seconds and then lower the leg out to the start position. At the point in range that the lumbopelvic region starts to lose control of rotation the movement should stop. The lumbopelvic position is restabilised, then hold this position for a few seconds and return to the start position with control of the lumbopelvic rotation UCM.

Ideally, the pelvis should not rotate as the leg turns out and returns. The person should self-monitor the lumbopelvic alignment and control with a variety of feedback options (T19.3). There should be no provocation of any symptoms within the range that the rotation UCM can be controlled.

During any unilateral or asymmetrical limb load a rotational force is transmitted to the lumbopelvic region. The lumbopelvic rotation stability muscles control this rotational stress. The oblique abdominal muscles, anterior fascicles of psoas major and the superficial fibres of lumbar multifidus, which stabilise trunk rotation, must coordinate with the hip abductor/rotator muscles, which concentrically lift the leg out to the side and eccentrically lower the leg to the start position. The uncontrolled lumbopelvic rotation is often associated with inefficiency of the trunk stabilisers (especially the oblique abdominals) to coordinate with the limb muscles. (For example, the left external obliques and the right internal obliques control the lumbopelvic rotation stability as the right leg lifts out to the side.) If control is poor, the person actively contracts the lateral oblique abdominal muscles to improve control of lumbopelvic rotation. The contralateral external oblique abdominals and the ipsilateral internal oblique abdominals can be facilitated separately to identify which is more effective at controlling the rotation UCM.

External oblique abdominal recruitment

The instruction to actively pull the anterior lower ribcage down and posteriorly in towards the spine on the *contralateral* side is a good facilitation cue for the external oblique abdominals. This should be coordinated with the cue to 'pull in' the whole abdominal wall at the same time. (Do not use the transversus abdominis facilitation cue of only 'hollowing' the lower abdominal wall. Transversus abdominis does not adequately control trunk rotation.) Discourage bracing or bulging out of the abdominal wall.

Internal oblique abdominal recruitment

The instruction to actively push or lift the *ipsilateral* ASIS in an anterior or forward direction is a good facilitation cue for the internal oblique abdominals. Visualise 'pushing a button' with the ipsilateral ASIS. This should be coordinated with

T19.1 Assessment and rating of low threshold recruitment efficiency of the Top Leg Turn Out Test

TOP LEG TURN OUT TEST – SIDE LYING

ASSESSMENT

Control point:
• prevent lumbopelvic rotation
Movement challenge: unilateral hip lateral rotation and abduction (side lying)
Benchmark range: 15° hip lateral rotation and abduction above horizontal (heels together)

RATING OF LOW THRESHOLD RECRUITMENT EFFICIENCY FOR CONTROL OF DIRECTION

	✓ or ✗		✓ or ✗
• Able to prevent 'UCM' into the test direction. Correct dissociation pattern of movement Prevent lumbopelvic UCM into: rotation and move unilateral hip lateral rotation and abduction	☐	• Looks easy, and in the opinion of the assessor, is performed with confidence	☐
		• Feels easy, and the subject has sufficient awareness of the movement pattern that they confidently prevent 'UCM' into the test direction	☐
• Dissociate movement through the benchmark range of: 15° hip lateral rotation/abduction *If there is more available range than the benchmark standard, only the benchmark range needs to be actively controlled*	☐	• The pattern of dissociation is smooth during concentric and eccentric movement	☐
		• Does not (consistently) use *end range* movement into the opposite direction to prevent the UCM	☐
• Without holding breath (though it is acceptable to use an alternate breathing strategy)	☐	• No extra feedback needed *(tactile, visual or verbal cueing)*	☐
		• Without external support or unloading	☐
• Control during eccentric phase	☐	• Relaxed natural breathing *(even if not ideal – so long as natural pattern does not change)*	☐
• Control during concentric phase	☐	• No fatigue	☐

CORRECT DISSOCIATION PATTERN   **RECRUITMENT EFFICIENCY**

T19.2 Diagnosis of the site and direction of UCM from the Top Leg Turn Out Test

TOP LEG TURN OUT TEST – SIDE-LYING

Site	Direction	Pelvis to the left (L)	Pelvis to the right (R)
		(check box)	(check box)
Lumbopelvic	Rotation (open chain)	☐	☐

T19.3 Feedback tools to monitor retraining

FEEDBACK TOOL	PROCESS
Self-palpation	Palpation monitoring of joint position
Visual observation	Observe in a mirror or directly watch the movement
Adhesive tape	Skin tension for tactile feedback
Flexicurve positional marker	Visual and sensory feedback of positional alignment
Cueing and verbal correction	Listen to feedback from another observer

the cue to 'pull in' the whole abdominal wall at the same time. Discourage bracing or bulging out of the abdominal wall.

Once effective oblique abdominal facilitation has been achieved, the person is instructed to slowly lift the top knee up and out to the side. The top leg turn out can continue only as far as there is no rotation of the pelvis at all.

If lumbopelvic rotation control is very poor, the use of the 'flexicurve' positioned at the ASIS, or using hand palpation on the iliac crest to self-monitor the lumbopelvic rotation control, is essential. It may even be useful to perform the retraining exercise on the floor with the pelvis, thoracic spine and heels supported back against a wall for additional support and feedback.

As the ability to control the lumbopelvic region during independent hip rotation gets easier and the pattern of dissociation feels less unnatural the exercise can be progressed. A basic progression would be to perform this movement with the leg unsupported. That is, lift the heel of the top leg 5 cm from the other heel and control lumbopelvic rotation during an unsupported top leg turn out.

T20 PRONE: SINGLE HIP ROTATION TEST (tests for lumbopelvic rotation UCM)

This dissociation test assesses the ability to actively dissociate and control lumbopelvic rotation and rotate hip through medial and lateral rotation while lying prone. During any unilateral or asymmetrical limb load or movement, a rotational force is transmitted to the lumbopelvic region.

Test procedure

The person lies in prone with the legs extended and the lumbopelvic region supported in neutral. The hip is positioned in neutral rotation and one knee is flexed to 90° with the lower leg vertical (Figure 5.104). The person is instructed to prevent lumbopelvic rotation and rotate the hip by moving the foot from one side to the other. Moving the foot out to the side medially rotates the hip (Figure 5.105) while moving the foot in across the body laterally rotates the hip (Figure 5.106). Ideally, the neutral lumbopelvic position should be controlled through at least 30° hip medial and lateral rotation each side of neutral (vertical lower leg) and returned, without associated pelvic rotation.

The unilateral hip rotation must be independent of any lumbopelvic rotation. Assess both sides. Note any excessive lumbopelvic rotation under hip rotation load. This test should be performed without any feedback (self-palpation, vision, etc.) or cueing for correction. When feedback is removed for testing the therapist should use visual observation of the pelvis to determine whether the control of lumbopelvic rotation is adequate.

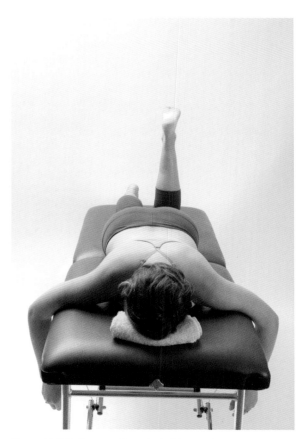

Figure 5.104 Start position single hip rotation test

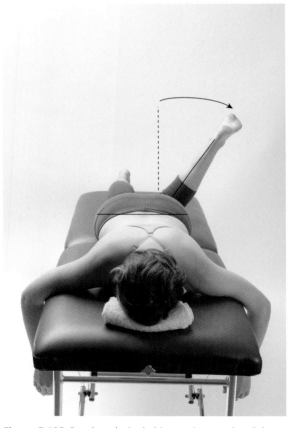

Figure 5.105 Benchmark single hip rotation test (medial rotation)

bilaterally, one side may be better or worse than the other.

Rating and diagnosis of lumbopelvic rotation UCM

(T20.1 and T20.2)

Correction

The person lies prone with the legs extended and together with the lumbopelvic region supported in neutral. One knee is flexed to 90° and the hip is positioned in neutral rotation with the lower leg vertical. They are instructed to maintain a neutral pelvic position and prevent the pelvis from rotating to either side as the hip rotates to each side. The hip should rotate only as far as neutral lumbopelvic rotation can be controlled (monitored with feedback). At the point in range that the lumbopelvic region starts to lose control of rotation the movement should stop. The lumbopelvic position is restabilised, then hold this position for a few seconds and return to the start position with control of the lumbopelvic rotation UCM.

Ideally, the pelvis should not rotate as the hip rotates and returns. The person should self-monitor the lumbopelvic alignment and control with a variety of feedback options (T20.3). Self-palpation of the pelvis is especially useful (Figures 5.107 and 5.108). There should be no provocation of any symptoms within the range that the rotation UCM can be controlled.

During any unilateral or asymmetrical limb load a rotational force is transmitted to the lumbopelvic region. The lumbopelvic rotation stability muscles control this rotational stress. The oblique abdominal muscles, anterior fascicles of psoas major and the superficial fibres of lumbar

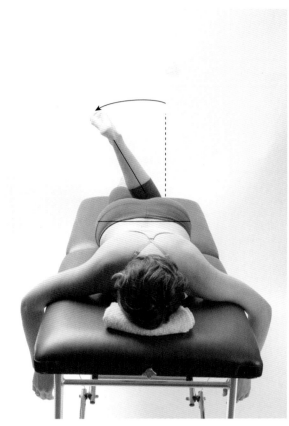

Figure 5.106 Benchmark single hip rotation test (lateral rotation)

Lumbopelvic rotation UCM

The person complains of unilateral symptoms in the lumbar spine. The lumbar spine has UCM into rotation relative to the hips under unilateral hip rotation load. As the hip rotates medially or laterally, the pelvis begins to rotate to follow the hip movement before 30° of rotation range is achieved.

During the attempt to dissociate the lumbopelvic rotation from independent unilateral hip lateral rotation and abduction, the person either cannot control the UCM or has to concentrate and try hard to dissociate the lumbopelvic rotation from independent hip movement. The movement must be assessed on both sides. Note the direction that the rotation cannot be controlled (i.e. is there uncontrolled lumbopelvic rotation to the left or the right). It may be unilateral or bilateral. If lumbopelvic rotation UCM presents

T20.1 Assessment and rating of low threshold recruitment efficiency of the Single Hip Rotation Test

SINGLE HIP ROTATION TEST – PRONE

ASSESSMENT

Control point:
- prevent lumbopelvic rotation

Movement challenge: unilateral hip medial rotation and lateral rotation (prone)

Benchmark range: 30° hip medial rotation and lateral rotation either side of the vertical lower leg (knees together)

RATING OF LOW THRESHOLD RECRUITMENT EFFICIENCY FOR CONTROL OF DIRECTION

	✓ or ✗		✓ or ✗

• Able to prevent 'UCM' into the test direction. Correct dissociation pattern of movement
Prevent lumbopelvic UCM into:
  rotation
and move unilateral hip rotation
  hip medial rotation
  hip lateral rotation
	☐	• Looks easy, and in the opinion of the assessor, is performed with confidence	☐

		• Feels easy, and the subject has sufficient awareness of the movement pattern that they confidently prevent 'UCM' into the test direction	☐
• Dissociate movement through the benchmark range of: 30° hip rotation each side of neutral (lower leg vertical) *If there is more available range than the benchmark standard, only the benchmark range needs to be actively controlled*	☐	• The pattern of dissociation is smooth during concentric and eccentric movement	☐
		• Does not (consistently) use *end range* movement into the opposite direction to prevent the UCM	☐
		• No extra feedback needed *(tactile, visual or verbal cueing)*	☐
• Without holding breath (though it is acceptable to use an alternate breathing strategy)	☐	• Without external support or unloading	☐
		• Relaxed natural breathing *(even if not ideal – so long as natural pattern does not change)*	☐
• Control during eccentric phase	☐	• No fatigue	☐
• Control during concentric phase	☐		

CORRECT DISSOCIATION PATTERN   **RECRUITMENT EFFICIENCY**

T20.2 Diagnosis of the site and direction of UCM from the Single Hip Rotation Test

SINGLE HIP ROTATION TEST – PRONE

Site	Direction	Pelvis to the left (L)	Pelvis to the right (R)
		(check box)	(check box)
Lumbopelvic	Rotation (open chain)	☐ (L) hip lateral rotation (R) hip medial rotation	☐ (R) hip lateral rotation (L) hip medial rotation

T20.3 Feedback tools to monitor retraining

FEEDBACK TOOL	PROCESS
Self-palpation	Palpation monitoring of joint position
Visual observation	Observe in a mirror or directly watch the movement
Adhesive tape	Skin tension for tactile feedback
Cueing and verbal correction	Listen to feedback from another observer

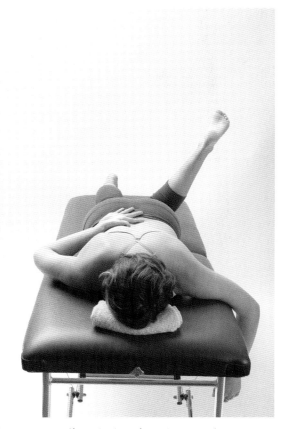

Figure 5.107 Self-monitoring of rotation control

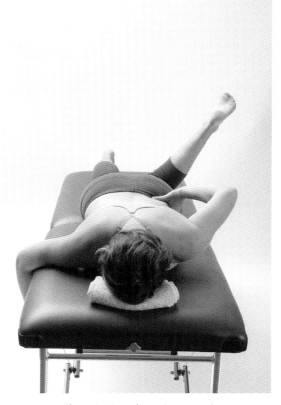

Figure 5.108 Self-monitoring of rotation control

multifidus, which stabilise trunk rotation, must coordinate with the hip extensor/rotator muscles, which eccentrically lower the leg to the side and concentrically return the leg to the start position. The uncontrolled lumbopelvic rotation is often associated with inefficiency of the trunk stabilisers (especially the oblique abdominals) to coordinate with the limb muscles. For example, the left external obliques and the right internal obliques control the lumbopelvic rotation stability as the right leg moves out to the side. If control is poor, the person actively contracts the lateral oblique abdominal muscles to improve control of lumbopelvic rotation. The contralateral external oblique abdominals and the ipsilateral internal oblique abdominals can be facilitated separately to identify which is more effective at controlling the rotation UCM.

External oblique abdominal recruitment

The instruction to actively pull the anterior lower ribcage down and posteriorly in towards the spine on the *contralateral* side is a good facilitation cue for the external oblique abdominals. This should be coordinated with the cue to 'pull in' the whole abdominal wall at the same time. (Do not use the transversus abdominis facilitation cue of only 'hollowing' the lower abdominal wall. Transversus abdominis does not adequately control trunk rotation.) Discourage bracing or bulging out of the abdominal wall.

Internal oblique abdominal recruitment

The instruction to actively push or lift the *ipsilateral* ASIS in an anterior or forward direction is a good facilitation cue for the internal oblique

181

abdominals. Visualise 'pushing a button' with the ipsilateral ASIS. This should be coordinated with the cue to 'pull in' the whole abdominal wall at the same time. Discourage bracing or bulging out of the abdominal wall.

Once effective oblique abdominal facilitation has been achieved, the person is then instructed to slowly rotate the leg out to the side. The leg can rotate only as far as there is no rotation of the pelvis at all.

As the ability to control the lumbopelvic region during independent hip rotation gets easier, and the pattern of dissociation feels less unnatural, the exercise can be progressed. A basic progression would be to perform this movement with a boot or light weight attached to the foot.

T21 PRONE: SINGLE KNEE FLEXION TEST (tests for lumbopelvic rotation UCM)

This dissociation test assesses the ability to actively dissociate and control lumbopelvic rotation and then actively flex one knee to engage the point where rectus femoris tension starts to pull the pelvis into rotation while lying prone.

Test procedure

In prone lying, the lumbar spine is positioned in neutral alignment (long shallow lordosis) by actively anteriorly or posteriorly tilting the pelvis from the sacrum (Figure 5.109). The person is instructed to bend one knee. The lumbopelvic region should maintain a neutral position and not move into lumbopelvic rotation (monitor lumbar spine and sacrum) as the knee actively flexes to approximately 120° (Figure 5.110). As

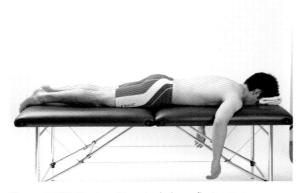

Figure 5.109 Start position single knee flexion test

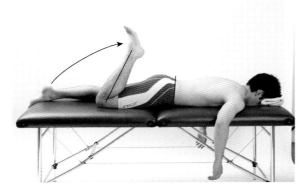

Figure 5.110 Benchmark single knee flexion test

soon as any lumbopelvic rotation occurs (indicating a loss of neutral), the knee flexion must stop and return back to the start position. This test should be performed without any feedback (self-palpation, vision, flexicurve, etc.) or cueing for correction. When feedback is removed for testing the therapist should use visual observation of the pelvis to determine whether the control of lumbopelvic rotation is adequate.

Ideally, the person should have the ability to dissociate the lumbar spine from the rectus femoris tension pulling the pelvis into rotation as evidenced by maintenance of the lumbar spine in a neutral position during active knee flexion to 120°. Normally, there will be paraspinal muscle activation but there should be no increase in lumbopelvic rotation. This test should be performed without any feedback (self-palpation, vision, tape, etc.) or cueing for correction.

Lumbopelvic rotation UCM

The person complains of unilateral symptoms in the lumbar spine. The lumbar spine has uncontrolled movement into rotation relative to the hips under unilateral knee flexion load. As the knee flexes, the pelvis begins to rotate before 120° of knee flexion range.

During the attempt to dissociate the lumbopelvic rotation from independent unilateral knee flexion and rectus femoris tension, the person either cannot control the UCM or has to concentrate and try hard to dissociate the lumbopelvic rotation from independent leg movement. The movement must be assessed on both sides. Note the direction that the rotation cannot be controlled (i.e. is there uncontrolled lumbopelvic rotation to the left or the right). It may be unilateral or bilateral. If lumbopelvic rotation UCM presents bilaterally, one side may be better or worse than the other.

Clinical assessment note for direction-specific motor control testing

If some other movement (e.g. a small amount of flexion or extension) is observed during a motor control (dissociation) test of rotation control, *do not* score this as uncontrolled rotation. The flexion and extension motor control tests will identify if the observed movement is uncontrolled. A test for lumbopelvic rotation UCM is only positive if uncontrolled lumbopelvic rotation is demonstrated.

Rating and diagnosis of lumbopelvic rotation UCM

(T21.1 and T21.2)

Correction

In prone lying, position the lumbar spine in neutral alignment (long shallow lordosis). Monitor lumbopelvic motion by placing the one hand (opposite to the knee flexion) with fingers spread across the low lumbar vertebrae and across the sacrum (alternative lumbopelvic monitoring: place hands on lateral iliac crest). The person is instructed to bend one knee.

The knee flexes only as far as neutral lumbopelvic rotation can be controlled (monitored with feedback). Hold this position for a few seconds and then lower the leg out to the start position. At the point in range that the lumbopelvic region starts to lose control of rotation the movement should stop. The lumbopelvic position is restabilised and the leg is returned to the start position with control of the lumbopelvic rotation UCM.

Ideally, the pelvis should not rotate as the knee flexes. The person should self-monitor the lumbopelvic alignment and control with a variety of feedback options (T21.3). There should be no provocation of any symptoms within the range that the rotation UCM can be controlled.

T21.1 Assessment and rating of low threshold recruitment efficiency of the Single Knee Flexion Test

SINGLE KNEE FLEXION TEST – PRONE

ASSESSMENT

Control point:
• prevent lumbopelvic rotation
Movement challenge: anterior tilt force from rectus femoris (prone)
Benchmark range: 120° unilateral knee flexion without compensation

RATING OF LOW THRESHOLD RECRUITMENT EFFICIENCY FOR CONTROL OF DIRECTION

	✓ or ✗		✓ or ✗
• Able to prevent 'UCM' into the test direction. Correct dissociation pattern of movement Prevent lumbopelvic UCM into: rotation and move unilateral knee flexion	☐	• Looks easy, and in the opinion of the assessor, is performed with confidence	☐
		• Feels easy, and the subject has sufficient awareness of the movement pattern that they confidently prevent 'UCM' into the test direction	☐
• Dissociate movement through the benchmark range of: 120° of knee flexion *If there is more available range than the benchmark standard, only the benchmark range needs to be actively controlled*	☐	• The pattern of dissociation is smooth during concentric and eccentric movement	☐
		• Does not (consistently) use *end range* movement into the opposite direction to prevent the UCM	☐
• Without holding breath (though it is acceptable to use an alternate breathing strategy)	☐	• No extra feedback needed *(tactile, visual or verbal cueing)*	☐
• Control during eccentric phase	☐	• Without external support or unloading	☐
• Control during concentric phase	☐	• Relaxed natural breathing *(even if not ideal – so long as natural pattern does not change)*	☐
		• No fatigue	☐

CORRECT DISSOCIATION PATTERN **RECRUITMENT EFFICIENCY**

T21.2 Diagnosis of the site and direction of UCM from the top Single Knee Flexion Test

SINGLE KNEE FLEXION TEST – PRONE

Site	Direction	To the left (L)	To the right (R)
		(check box)	(check box)
Lumbopelvic	Rotation (open chain)	☐	☐

T21.3 Feedback tools to monitor retraining

FEEDBACK TOOL	PROCESS
Self-palpation	Palpation monitoring of joint position
Visual observation	Observe in a mirror or directly watch the movement
Adhesive tape	Skin tension for tactile feedback
Cueing and verbal correction	Listen to feedback from another observer

185

T22 PRONE (TABLE): HIP EXTENSION LIFT TEST
(tests for lumbopelvic rotation UCM)

This dissociation test assesses the ability to actively dissociate and control lumbopelvic rotation, when actively extending one hip while lying prone with hips over the edge of a table. During any unilateral or asymmetrical limb load or movement, a rotational force is transmitted to the lumbopelvic region.

Test procedure

The person supports their trunk on a table, plinth or bed with the pelvis at the edge of the table and both feet supported on the floor (the knees slightly flexed) (Figure 5.111). The lumbar spine is positioned in neutral alignment (long shallow lordosis) by actively anteriorly or posteriorly tilting the pelvis from the sacrum. The person is instructed to slowly extend one knee and then to slowly lift the straight leg off the floor into hip extension to reach the horizontal position (0° hip 'neutral'). The lumbopelvic region should maintain a neutral position with no lumbopelvic rotation (monitor lumbar spine and sacrum) as the hip actively extends to where the thigh is approximately horizontal (Figure 5.112). As soon as any movement indicating a loss of neutral into lumbopelvic rotation is observed, the movement must stop and return back to the start position.

Ideally, the lumbopelvic region should maintain a neutral position as the hip actively extends as far as neutral (i.e. approximately horizontal). The hip extension must be independent of any lumbopelvic motion. Assess both sides. Note any excessive lumbopelvic rotation under unilateral hip extension load. This test should be performed without any feedback (self-palpation, vision, tape, etc.) or cueing for correction.

Lumbopelvic rotation UCM

The person complains of unilateral symptoms in the lumbar spine. The lumbar spine has UCM into rotation relative to the hips under unilateral hip extension load. The pelvis rotates before the hip reaches horizontal (0° extension).

During the attempt to dissociate the lumbopelvic rotation from independent unilateral hip extension, the person either cannot control the UCM or has to concentrate and try hard to dissociate the lumbopelvic rotation from independent hip movement. The movement must be assessed on both sides. Note the direction that the rotation cannot be controlled (i.e. is there uncontrolled lumbopelvic rotation to the left or the right). It may be unilateral or bilateral. If lumbopelvic rotation UCM presents bilaterally, one side may be better or worse than the other.

Clinical assessment note for direction-specific motor control testing

If some other movement (e.g. a small amount of flexion or extension) is observed during a motor control (dissociation) test of rotation control, *do not* score this as uncontrolled rotation. The flexion and extension motor control tests will identify if the observed movement is uncontrolled. A test for lumbopelvic rotation UCM is only positive if uncontrolled lumbopelvic rotation is demonstrated.

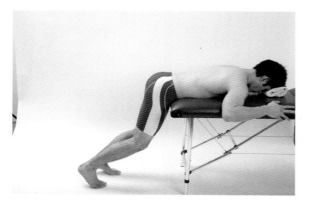
Figure 5.111 Start position hip extension lift test

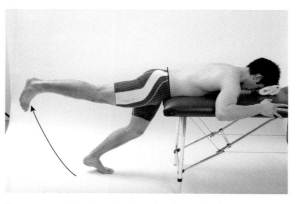
Figure 5.112 Benchmark hip extension lift test

Rating and diagnosis of lumbopelvic rotation UCM

(T22.1 and T22.2)

Correction

The person supports their trunk on a table, with both feet supported on the floor and the lumbar spine positioned in neutral alignment (long shallow lordosis). Monitor lumbopelvic motion by placing the one hand (opposite to the leg extension) with fingers spread across the low lumbar vertebrae and across the sacrum (alternative lumbopelvic monitoring: place hands on lateral iliac crest). The person is instructed to slowly extend one knee and then to slowly lift the straight leg off the floor into hip extension.

Hip extension should be initiated and maintained by gluteus maximus. The hamstrings will participate in the movement but should not dominate. There will be good contralateral paraspinal muscle activation (asymmetrically biased) but there should be no increase in lumbopelvic rotation.

Ideally, the person should have the ability to dissociate the lumbar spine and pelvis as evidenced by maintenance of lumbar spine in a neutral position during active hip extension to 0° or thigh horizontal. The abdominal and gluteal muscles are co-activated to control the neutral spine and to prevent excessive lumbar extension. Only lift the hip into extension as far as the neutral lumbopelvic position (monitored with feedback) can be maintained. The person should self-monitor the lumbopelvic alignment and control with a variety of feedback options (T22.3). Palpation feedback is the most useful retraining tool. There should be no provocation of any symptoms within the range that the extension UCM can be controlled. There must be no loss of neutral or UCM into lumbopelvic rotation.

If control is poor, the person may only be able to dissociate the lumbar spine (neutral) from unilateral hip extension to within 40° from horizontal. As the ability to control lumbopelvic rotation gets easier and the pattern of dissociation feels less unnatural, the exercise can be progressed to hip extension level with the horizontal (0°) and eventually into the full range of hip extension (10–15° of extension above the horizontal).

T22.1 Assessment and rating of low threshold recruitment efficiency of the Hip Extension Lift Test

HIP EXTENSION LIFT TEST – PRONE (TABLE)

ASSESSMENT

Control point:
- prevent lumbopelvic rotation

Movement challenge: extension of the hip (prone over a table)

Benchmark range: 0° unilateral hip extension without compensation

RATING OF LOW THRESHOLD RECRUITMENT EFFICIENCY FOR CONTROL OF DIRECTION

	✓ or ✗		✓ or ✗
• Able to prevent 'UCM' into the test direction. Correct dissociation pattern of movement Prevent lumbopelvic UCM into: rotation and move single hip extension	☐	• Looks easy, and in the opinion of the assessor, is performed with confidence	☐
		• Feels easy, and the subject has sufficient awareness of the movement pattern that they confidently prevent 'UCM' into the test direction	☐
• Dissociate movement through the benchmark range of: 0° hip extension (thigh horizontal) *If there is more available range than the benchmark standard, only the benchmark range needs to be actively controlled*	☐	• The pattern of dissociation is smooth during concentric and eccentric movement	☐
		• Does not (consistently) use *end range* movement into the opposite direction to prevent the UCM	☐
• Without holding breath (though it is acceptable to use an alternate breathing strategy)	☐	• No extra feedback needed *(tactile, visual or verbal cueing)*	☐
• Control during eccentric phase	☐	• Without external support or unloading	☐
• Control during concentric phase	☐	• Relaxed natural breathing *(even if not ideal – so long as natural pattern does not change)*	☐
		• No fatigue	☐

CORRECT DISSOCIATION PATTERN | | **RECRUITMENT EFFICIENCY**

T22.2 Diagnosis of the site and direction of UCM from the Hip Extension Lift Test

HIP EXTENSION LIFT TEST – PRONE (TABLE)

Site	Direction	To the left (L)	To the right (R)
		(check box)	(check box)
Lumbopelvic	Rotation (open chain)	☐	☐

T22.3 Feedback tools to monitor retraining

FEEDBACK TOOL	PROCESS
Self-palpation	Palpation monitoring of joint position
Visual observation	Observe in a mirror or directly watch the movement
Adhesive tape	Skin tension for tactile feedback
Cueing and verbal correction	Listen to feedback from another observer

T23 SITTING: SINGLE KNEE EXTENSION TEST
(tests for lumbopelvic rotation UCM)

This dissociation test assesses the ability to actively dissociate and control lumbopelvic rotation while sitting, then actively extend one knee to engage the point where hamstring tension starts to unilaterally pull the pelvis into rotation. During any unilateral or asymmetrical limb load or movement, a rotational force is transmitted to the lumbopelvic region.

Test procedure

The person sits tall with the feet off the floor and with the lumbar spine and pelvis positioned in neutral and with both feet off the floor. Make the spine as tall or as long as possible to position the normal curves in an elongated 'S' with the acromions vertical over the ischiums (do not lean backwards) (Figure 5.113.). Without letting the lumbopelvic region move they should then straighten one knee to within 10–15° of full extension, keeping the back straight (neutral spine) and without leaning back or allowing lumbopelvic rotation (Figure 5.114). Ideally, the person should have the ability to maintain the lumbopelvic region neutral and prevent the hamstrings pulling the pelvis into lumbopelvic rotation. This test should be performed without any feedback (self-palpation, vision, tape, etc.) or cueing for correction.

Lumbopelvic rotation UCM

The person complains of unilateral symptoms in the lumbar spine. The lumbar spine has UCM into rotation under unilateral hamstring tension and lumbopelvic rotation occurs before the knee reaches 10–15° from full extension.

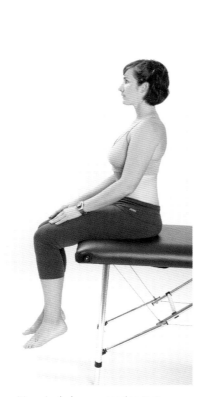

Figure 5.113 Start position single knee extension test

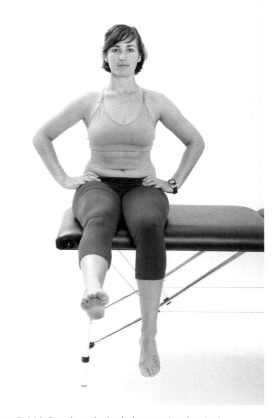

Figure 5.114 Benchmark single knee extension test

During the attempt to dissociate the lumbopelvic rotation from unilateral hamstring tension, the person either cannot control the UCM or has to concentrate and try hard to dissociate the lumbopelvic rotation. The movement must be assessed on both sides. Note the direction that the rotation cannot be controlled (i.e. is there uncontrolled lumbopelvic rotation to the left or the right). It may be unilateral or bilateral. If lumbopelvic rotation UCM presents bilaterally, one side may be better or worse than the other.

Clinical assessment note for direction-specific motor control testing

If some other movement (e.g. a small amount of flexion or extension) is observed during a motor control (dissociation) test of rotation control, *do not* score this as uncontrolled rotation. The flexion and extension motor control tests will identify if the observed movement is uncontrolled. A test for lumbopelvic rotation UCM is only positive if uncontrolled lumbopelvic rotation is demonstrated.

Rating and diagnosis of lumbopelvic rotation UCM

(T23.1 and T23.2)

Correction

The person sits tall with the feet off the floor and with the lumbar spine and pelvis positioned in the neutral. They should monitor the lumbopelvic rotation control by palpating the iliac crest or sacrum. The person is instructed to keep the back straight (neutral spine) and without leaning back, slowly straighten one knee and prevent the pelvis from rotating backwards as tension is produced in the hamstrings. Only move as far as neutral lumbopelvic rotation can be controlled (monitored with feedback). Hold this position for a few seconds and then lower the leg to the start position. At the point in range that the lumbopelvic region starts to lose control of rotation the movement should stop. The lumbopelvic position is restabilised and the leg is returned to the start position with control of the lumbopelvic rotation UCM.

Ideally, the pelvis should not rotate as the knee extends. The person should self-monitor the lumbopelvic alignment and control with a variety of feedback options (T23.3). Visual feedback (e.g. observation in a mirror) is also a useful retraining tool. There should be no provocation of any symptoms within the range that the rotation UCM can be controlled.

If control is poor, it is acceptable to start with unilateral (then progress to bilateral) knee extension with a straight back, but only as far as the neutral lumbopelvic position can be maintained. Beware neurodynamic symptoms associated with positive slump responses. Unload the neural system with ankle plantarflexion or partial cervical extension. Once the pattern of dissociation is efficient and feels familiar it should be integrated into various functional postures and positions.

T23.1 Assessment and rating of low threshold recruitment efficiency of the Single Knee Extension Test

SINGLE KNEE EXTENSION TEST – SITTING

ASSESSMENT

Control point:
• prevent lumbopelvic rotation
Movement challenge: rotation force from unilateral hamstring tension (sitting)
Benchmark range: 10–15° from full knee extension (unilateral)

RATING OF LOW THRESHOLD RECRUITMENT EFFICIENCY FOR CONTROL OF DIRECTION

✓ or ✗		✓ or ✗	
• Able to prevent 'UCM' into the test direction. Correct dissociation pattern of movement Prevent lumbopelvic UCM into: rotation and move unilateral knee extension	☐	• Looks easy, and in the opinion of the assessor, is performed with confidence	☐
		• Feels easy, and the subject has sufficient awareness of the movement pattern that they confidently prevent 'UCM' into the test direction	☐
• Dissociate movement through the benchmark range of: 10–15° from full knee extension *If there is more available range than the benchmark standard, only the benchmark range needs to be actively controlled*	☐	• The pattern of dissociation is smooth during concentric and eccentric movement	☐
		• Does not (consistently) use *end range* movement into the opposite direction to prevent the UCM	☐
• Without holding breath (though it is acceptable to use an alternate breathing strategy)	☐	• No extra feedback needed *(tactile, visual or verbal cueing)*	☐
• Control during eccentric phase	☐	• Without external support or unloading	☐
• Control during concentric phase	☐	• Relaxed natural breathing *(even if not ideal – so long as natural pattern does not change)*	☐
		• No fatigue	☐

CORRECT DISSOCIATION PATTERN | **RECRUITMENT EFFICIENCY**

T23.2 Diagnosis of the site and direction of UCM from the Single Knee Extension Test

SINGLE KNEE EXTENSION – SITTING

Site	Direction	Pelvis to the left (L)	Pelvis to the right (R)
		(check box)	(check box)
Lumbopelvic	Rotation (open chain)	☐	☐

T23.3 Feedback tools to monitor retraining

FEEDBACK TOOL	PROCESS
Self-palpation	Palpation monitoring of joint position
Visual observation	Observe in a mirror or directly watch the movement
Adhesive tape	Skin tension for tactile feedback
Cueing and verbal correction	Listen to feedback from another observer

Tests of closed chain rotation control

T24 CROOK LYING: SINGLE LEG BRIDGE EXTENSION TEST
(tests for lumbopelvic rotation UCM)

This dissociation test assesses the ability to actively dissociate and control lumbopelvic rotation and lift the pelvis into a bridge and straighten one leg while in supine lying. During any unilateral or asymmetrical limb load or movement, a rotational force is transmitted to the lumbopelvic region.

Test procedure

The person lies in crook lying with the heels and knees together (Figure 5.115). Keeping the spine in neutral, lift the pelvis just clear (5 cm) of the floor and hold this position. Slowly shift weight onto one foot and extend the other knee, keeping the knees and thighs side by side. Ideally, there should be no change to hip position (no flexion or extension). Maintain the neutral lumbopelvic position and do not allow the pelvis to rotate or to shift laterally during the weight transfer and the unilateral leg extension (Figure 5.116). Return the foot to the floor and repeat the movement with the opposite leg. As soon as any lumbopelvic rotation (indicating a loss of neutral) or cramping of the weight bearing hamstrings occurs, the movement must stop and return back to the start position. Do not allow the arms to brace the trunk by pushing down onto the floor. This test should be performed without any feedback (self-palpation, vision, etc.) or cueing for correction. When feedback is removed for testing the therapist should use visual observation of the pelvis to determine whether the control of lumbopelvic rotation is adequate.

Lumbopelvic rotation UCM

The person complains of unilateral symptoms in the lumbar spine. During any unilateral or asymmetrical limb load a rotational force is transmitted to the lumbopelvic region. The trunk rotation stabilisers are not able to effectively control this rotation force. The lumbar spine has UCM into rotation under unilateral long lever leg load. As the weight is transferred to one foot and the other leg extends, the pelvis begins to rotate and drop down on the unweighted extended leg side. The person is unable to control lumbopelvic rotation. Cramping of the weight bearing hamstrings (substitution) indicates an inefficient pattern of gluteal recruitment.

During the attempt to dissociate the lumbopelvic rotation from unilateral leg loading, the person either cannot control the UCM or has to concentrate and try hard to control the lumbopelvic rotation. The movement must be assessed on both sides. Note the direction that the rotation cannot be controlled (i.e. is there uncontrolled lumbopelvic rotation to the left or the right). It may be unilateral or bilateral. If lumbopelvic rotation UCM presents bilaterally, one side may be better or worse than the other.

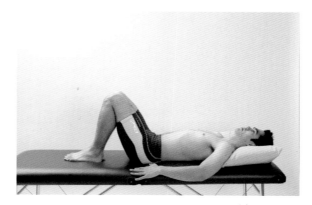

Figure 5.115 Start position single leg bridge extension

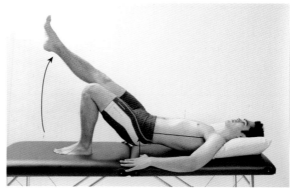

Figure 5.116 Benchmark single leg bridge extension

Clinical assessment note for direction-specific motor control testing

If some other movement (e.g. a small amount of flexion or extension) is observed during a motor control (dissociation) test of rotation control, *do not* score this as uncontrolled rotation. The flexion and extension motor control tests will identify if the observed movement is uncontrolled. A test for lumbopelvic rotation UCM is only positive if uncontrolled lumbopelvic rotation is demonstrated.

Rating and diagnosis of lumbopelvic rotation UCM

(T24.1 and T24.2)

Correction

Starting in crook lying with the feet and knees together, the person lifts the pelvis 5 cm off the floor while maintaining neutral alignment. Initially, transfer weight to one foot and only lift the other heel a few centimetres from the floor (Figure 5.117). A further progression is to transfer weight to one foot and only lift the other foot a few centimetres from the floor while partially extending the unweighted leg. The unweighted leg is progressively extended until full extension is achieved. The person should only lift and extend the unweighted leg as far as neutral lumbopelvic rotation can be controlled (monitored with feedback). At the point in range that the lumbopelvic region starts to lose control of rotation the movement should stop. The lumbopelvic position is restabilised, then hold this position for a few seconds and return to the start position (crook lying with pelvis resting) with control of the lumbopelvic rotation UCM. Make sure that good control of lumbopelvic rotation and side-shift is maintained. Make sure that the gluteal muscles on the weight bearing leg are active and do not allow the hamstrings to cramp.

A final progression would be to maintain lumbopelvic neutral and extend the knee as above (no rotation or pelvic tilt), and then slowly flex the hip and knee. Hip and knee flexion continues until there is 90° of both hip and knee flexion (Figure 5.118). Then the hip and knee are extended to reach the starting position but the hip continues to extend until the heel is lowered to the horizontal position (Figure 5.119). The hip then

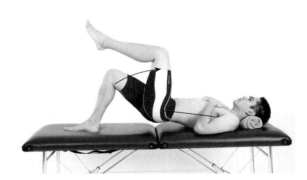

Figure 5.118 Progression: bridge with hip and knee flexion to 90°

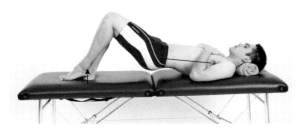

Figure 5.117 Correction: bridge with weight transfer and single heel lift

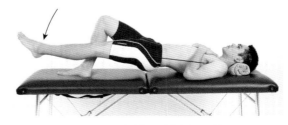

Figure 5.119 Progression: bridge with hip and knee extension to horizontal

returns to the starting position. At all times the pelvis stays unsupported and hip and knee movement occurs only as far as the rotation is controlled and as far as any restriction allows.

The person should self-monitor the lumbopelvic alignment and control with a variety of feedback options (T24.3). There should be no provocation of any symptoms within the range that the rotation UCM can be controlled.

During any unilateral or asymmetrical limb load a rotational force is transmitted to the lumbopelvic region. The lumbopelvic rotation stability muscles control this rotational stress. In closed chain rotation control training, the trunk rotator stabiliser muscles (the oblique abdominal muscles, anterior fascicles of psoas major and the superficial fibres of lumbar multifidus) must coordinate with the hip rotator stabiliser muscles (the deep gluteals, adductor brevis, pectineus and iliacus) to control lumbopelvic rotation from above and below the pelvis. The uncontrolled lumbopelvic rotation is often associated with inefficiency of the trunk stabilisers (especially the oblique abdominals) to coordinate with the limb muscles (especially the gluteals). The person is encouraged and trained to actively contract the lateral oblique abdominal muscles and the deep gluteals to improve control of lumbopelvic rotation.

If control is very poor, starting in crook lying with the feet and knees together, the person lifts the pelvis 5 cm off the floor while maintaining neutral alignment. Initially, transfer weight to one foot and only take partial weight off the other foot (e.g. heel marching – heel lift but continue to take weight on the ball of the foot).

The person can actively recruit the lateral oblique abdominal muscles to control pelvic rotation. The contralateral external oblique abdominals are facilitated with contralateral ribcage depression and the ipsilateral internal oblique abdominals can be facilitated by holding the ASIS forward. This should be coordinated with the cue to 'hollow' or 'pull the whole abdominal wall in' at the same time. Discourage bracing or bulging out of the abdominal wall. Also, preset a deep gluteal contraction. Palpate for definite contraction near the superior ischium without a maximal lateral gluteal contraction posterior to the trochanter. Discourage the maximal 'butt squeeze' or the 'butt gripping' action.

Once oblique abdominal and deep gluteal facilitation has been achieved in crook lying with the heels and knees together, the person is then instructed to keep the spine and pelvis in neutral, then lift the pelvis just clear of the floor and hold this position. In this neutral bridge position, the person is then instructed to slowly shift weight onto one foot and, keeping the knees together, extend the other knee. One knee is extended and returned to the floor, but only as far as the neutral lumbopelvic position can be maintained. There must be no loss of neutral or give into rotation. There should be no provocation of any symptoms under unilateral load, so long as the lumbopelvic rotation UCM can be controlled.

T24.1 Assessment and rating of low threshold recruitment efficiency of the Single Leg Bridge Extension Test

SINGLE LEG BRIDGE EXTENSION TEST – CROOK LYING

ASSESSMENT

Control point:
• prevent lumbopelvic rotation
Movement challenge: unilateral leg load from an unsupported pelvis (bridge)
Benchmark range: fully extended leg (knees side by side)

RATING OF LOW THRESHOLD RECRUITMENT EFFICIENCY FOR CONTROL OF DIRECTION

	✓ or ✗		✓ or ✗
• Able to prevent 'UCM' into the test direction. Correct dissociation pattern of movement Prevent lumbopelvic UCM into: rotation and move weight transfer to one leg and unilateral leg extension	☐	• Looks easy, and in the opinion of the assessor, is performed with confidence	☐
		• Feels easy, and the subject has sufficient awareness of the movement pattern that they confidently prevent 'UCM' into the test direction	☐
• Dissociate movement through the benchmark range of: full leg extension (knees side by side) *If there is more available range than the benchmark standard, only the benchmark range needs to be actively controlled*	☐	• The pattern of dissociation is smooth during concentric and eccentric movement	☐
		• Does not (consistently) use *end range* movement into the opposite direction to prevent the UCM	☐
		• No extra feedback needed *(tactile, visual or verbal cueing)*	☐
• Without holding breath (though it is acceptable to use an alternate breathing strategy)	☐	• Without external support or unloading	☐
		• Relaxed natural breathing *(even if not ideal – so long as natural pattern does not change)*	☐
• Control during eccentric phase	☐	• No fatigue	☐
• Control during concentric phase	☐		
CORRECT DISSOCIATION PATTERN		**RECRUITMENT EFFICIENCY**	

T24.2 Diagnosis of the site and direction of UCM from the Single Leg Bridge Extension Test

SINGLE LEG BRIDGE EXTENSION TEST – CROOK LYING

Site	Direction	Pelvis to the left (L)	Pelvis to the right (R)
		(check box)	(check box)
Lumbopelvic	Rotation (closed chain)	☐	☐

T24.3 Feedback tools to monitor retraining

FEEDBACK TOOL	PROCESS
Self-palpation	Palpation monitoring of joint position
Visual observation	Observe in a mirror or directly watch the movement
Adhesive tape	Skin tension for tactile feedback
Pressure biofeedback	Visual confirmation of the control of position
Cueing and verbal correction	Listen to feedback from another observer

T25 STANDING: THORACIC ROTATION TEST
(tests for lumbopelvic rotation UCM)

This dissociation test assesses the ability to actively dissociate and control lumbopelvic rotation and rotate the thoracic spine while standing. During any asymmetrical or non-sagittal trunk movement a rotational force is transmitted to the lumbopelvic region.

Test procedure

The person stands with the feet hip-width apart (heels approximately 10–15 cm apart) with the inside borders of the feet parallel (not turned out). Stand upright with the upper body vertical and the weight balanced over the midfoot. Perform a 'small knee bend' (SKB) by flexing at the knees and dorsiflexing the ankles while keeping both heels on the floor, as if sliding the back down a wall. Keep the trunk vertical and do not lean the trunk forwards (Figure 5.120). Keep the knees a little further apart than the heels to orientate the long axis of the femur (the line of the thigh) out over the middle toes.

Then, while standing with feet under hips, with arms crossed and hands touching opposite shoulders, the person is instructed to rotate the shoulders and upper trunk around to each side (to approximately 40°) but keep the low lumbar spine and pelvis from moving. They should have the ability to actively rotate the upper trunk and thoracic spine independently of the lumbopelvic region. Ideally, there should be symmetrical rotation of the thoracic spine to both sides without lumbopelvic rotation. Ultimately, there should be approximately 40° of independent thoracic rotation, without any pelvic rotation or lateral shift/ weight transfer (Figure 5.121). As soon as any

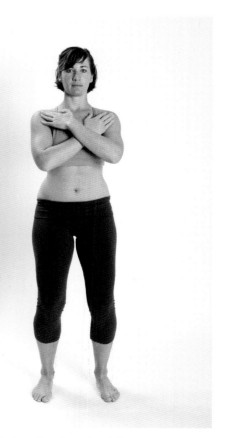

Figure 5.120 Start position thoracic rotation

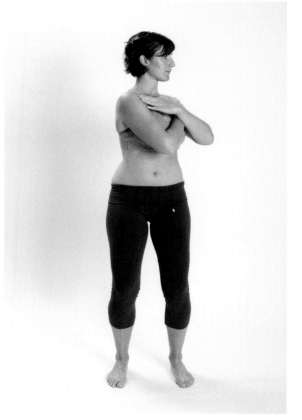

Figure 5.121 Benchmark thoracic rotation

lumbopelvic rotation occurs, the movement must stop and return back to the start position. This test should be performed without any feedback (self-palpation, vision, etc.) or cueing for correction. The therapist should use visual observation of the pelvis to determine whether the control of lumbopelvic rotation is adequate when feedback is removed for testing. Assess both sides.

Lumbopelvic rotation UCM

The person complains of unilateral symptoms in the lumbopelvic region. Lumbopelvic rotation begins to follow the upper trunk before the thorax reaches 40° of independent rotation range. The lumbar spine has UCM into rotation relative to the thoracic spine under rotation load. In some cases the lumbopelvic region may even initiate the upper trunk rotation.

If the lumbopelvic rotation stabilisers are not able to effectively control this rotation force many maladaptive substitution strategies may be observed during rotation of the upper trunk:

- Rotation of the pelvis (hip rotation) to follow the upper trunk rotation. There is no dissociation of rotation between the lumbar and thoracic regions. Instead they appear rigid and the rotation occurs primarily at the hips.
- Rotation of the pelvis initiates the movement and the upper trunk appears to 'tag along' after the pelvis.
- Counter rotation of the pelvis occurs in the opposite direction to upper trunk rotation. Occasionally, the pelvic counter-rotation may initiate the movement.
- During rotation, the trunk flexes (this is often related to a restriction of thoracic rotation).
- During rotation, the pelvis sways forwards into uncontrolled extension.
- During rotation, the thoracolumbar region extends (sternal lift) along with scapular retraction (rhomboids substituting for thoracis paraspinal stabilisers to rotate the thorax).
- During rotation, there is lateral shift of body weight and the lumbopelvic region moves into side-shift of the pelvis away from the side of rotation (most common). Occasionally, it side-shifts towards the side of rotation. Side-bending of the trunk accompanies lateral movement of the pelvis.

The uncontrolled lumbopelvic rotation is often associated with inefficiency of the stability function of the oblique abdominals or the hip rotation stabilisers. (For example, the left external obliques and the right internal obliques control the lumbopelvic rotation UCM to the right, while the right posterior gluteus medius and maximus control pelvic rotation to the right when weight bearing.) During any asymmetrical or non-sagittal trunk movement, a rotational force is transmitted to the lumbopelvic region. The lumbopelvic rotation stability muscles control this rotational load. The oblique abdominal muscles, anterior fascicles of psoas major and superficial fibres of lumbar multifidus, which stabilise trunk rotation, must coordinate with the weight bearing deep hip muscles, which concentrically and eccentrically control rotation of the pelvis from below.

During the attempt to dissociate the lumbopelvic rotation from thoracic rotation, the person either cannot control the UCM or has to concentrate and try hard to control the lumbopelvic rotation. The movement must be assessed on both sides. Note the direction that the rotation cannot be controlled (i.e. is there uncontrolled lumbopelvic rotation to the left or the right). It may be unilateral or bilateral. If lumbopelvic rotation UCM presents bilaterally, then one side may be better or worse than the other.

Clinical assessment note for direction-specific motor control testing

If some other movement (e.g. a small amount of flexion or extension) is observed during a motor control (dissociation) test of rotation control, *do not* score this as uncontrolled rotation. The flexion and extension motor control tests will identify if the observed movement is uncontrolled. A test for lumbopelvic rotation UCM is only positive if uncontrolled lumbopelvic rotation is demonstrated.

Rating and diagnosis of lumbopelvic rotation UCM

(T25.1 and T25.2)

Correction

The person stands in a 'small knee bend' with the feet hip width apart (heels approx 10–15 cm apart) with the inside borders of the feet parallel (not turned out), flexing at the knees and dorsi-flexing the ankles while keeping both heels on the floor, as if sliding the back down a wall. Then, with the arms crossed, the person is instructed to actively rotate the upper trunk and thoracic spine independently of the lumbopelvic region to each side. Only rotate the thorax as far as lumbopelvic rotation can be controlled (monitored with self-feedback). At the point in range that the lumbopelvic region starts to lose control of rotation the movement should stop. The lumbopelvic position is restabilised, then hold this position for a few seconds and return to the start position with control of the lumbopelvic rotation UCM.

The person should self-monitor the lumbopelvic alignment and control with a variety of feedback options (T25.3). There should be no provocation of any symptoms within the range that the rotation UCM can be controlled.

If control is particularly poor, the pattern of correct movement may be taught with the person sitting in neutral trunk alignment on a fixed chair with the feet on the floor. The lumbopelvic region should be either manually supported or supported by a low lumbar back support during the active thoracic rotation. Once the pattern of dissociation is established, progress to standing where the person positions the ischiums (touching but not weight bearing) against the edge of a table or bench for feedback about lumbopelvic rotation control (Figure 5.122).

Additional facilitation can come from active setting of the scapula in neutral and by active pre-setting of the oblique abdominals.

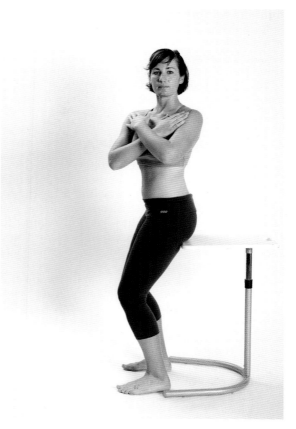

Figure 5.122 Correction with ischial support

T25.1 Assessment and rating of low threshold recruitment efficiency of the Thoracic Rotation Test

THORACIC ROTATION TEST – STANDING

ASSESSMENT

Control point:
- prevent lumbopelvic rotation

Movement challenge: thoracic rotation (standing: small knee bend)

Benchmark range: 40° independent thoracic rotation

RATING OF LOW THRESHOLD RECRUITMENT EFFICIENCY FOR CONTROL OF DIRECTION

	✓ or ✗		✓ or ✗
• Able to prevent 'UCM' into the test direction. Correct dissociation pattern of movement Prevent lumbopelvic UCM into: rotation and move thoracic rotation	☐	• Looks easy, and in the opinion of the assessor, is performed with confidence	☐
		• Feels easy, and the subject has sufficient awareness of the movement pattern that they confidently prevent 'UCM' into the test direction	☐
• Dissociate movement through the benchmark range of: 40° thoracic rotation *If there is more available range than the benchmark standard, only the benchmark range needs to be actively controlled*	☐	• The pattern of dissociation is smooth during concentric and eccentric movement	☐
		• Does not (consistently) use *end range* movement into the opposite direction to prevent the UCM	☐
• Without holding breath (though it is acceptable to use an alternate breathing strategy)	☐	• No extra feedback needed *(tactile, visual or verbal cueing)*	☐
• Control during eccentric phase	☐	• Without external support or unloading	☐
• Control during concentric phase	☐	• Relaxed natural breathing *(even if not ideal – so long as natural pattern does not change)*	☐
		• No fatigue	☐

CORRECT DISSOCIATION PATTERN   **RECRUITMENT EFFICIENCY**

T25.2 Diagnosis of the site and direction of UCM from the Thoracic Rotation Test

THORACIC ROTATION TEST – STANDING: SMALL KNEE BEND

Site	Direction	Pelvis to the left (L)	Pelvis to the right (R)
		(check box)	(check box)
Lumbopelvic	Rotation (closed chain)	☐	☐

T25.3 Feedback tools to monitor retraining

FEEDBACK TOOL	PROCESS
Self-palpation	Palpation monitoring of joint position
Visual observation	Observe in a mirror or directly watch the movement
Adhesive tape	Skin tension for tactile feedback
Cueing and verbal correction	Listen to feedback from another observer

T26 STANDING: DOUBLE KNEE SWING TEST
(tests for lumbopelvic rotation UCM)

This dissociation test assesses the ability to actively dissociate and control lumbopelvic rotation and asymmetrically rotate legs while standing. During any unilateral or asymmetrical limb load or movement, a rotational force is transmitted to the lumbopelvic region.

Test procedure

The person stands with the feet hip width apart (heels approx 10–15 cm apart) with the inside borders of the feet parallel (not turned out). Stand upright with the upper body vertical and the weight balanced over the midfoot. Perform a 'small knee bend' (SKB) by flexing at the knees and dorsiflexing the ankles while keeping both heels on the floor, as if sliding the back down a wall. Keep the trunk vertical and do not lean the trunk forwards (Figure 5.123). Keep the knees a little further apart than the heels to orientate the long axis of the femur (the line of the thigh) out over the middle.

Then, while standing with the feet under hips in the SKB, with arms relaxed, the person is instructed to keep the trunk and pelvis from moving and swing both knees at least 20–30° (hip rotation) to the same side (Figure 5.124). This requires simultaneous but asymmetrical hip rotation to be coordinated with lumbopelvic rotation control. When the knees swing to the right, the right hip laterally rotates while the left hip simultaneously medially rotates and vice versa to the other side. It is essential the foot pronation and supination coordinates with the hip movement. So, when the knees swing to the right, the right foot should supinate as the knee

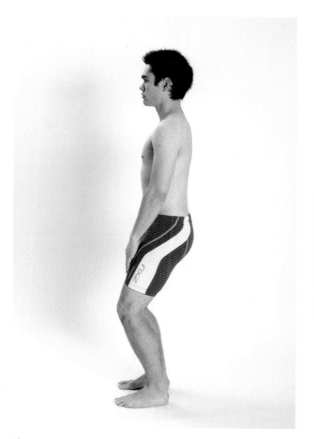

Figure 5.123 Start position double knee swing

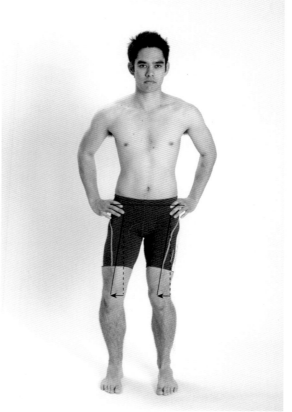

Figure 5.124 Benchmark double knee swing

moves lateral to the 2nd metatarsal; and the left foot should pronate when the knee moves medial to the 2nd metatarsal.

Many people will experience a sensation of a lack of the required hip rotation range. This is rarely a real loss of hip rotation as evidenced by assessment of hip rotation when moving each hip independently, one at a time. This test requires that, during testing for UCM, the knees swing at least 20–30° each side so that the compensation and UCM can be identified.

Ideally, there should be approximately 20–30° of independent double knee swing (asymmetrical hip rotation), without any lumbopelvic rotation, lateral pelvic shift or weight transfer at the feet. Body weight should stay equally distributed on each foot and there should be no lateral shift of the pelvis. The feet should supinate and pronate following the knee movement. The 1st metatarsal head (at the base of the big toe) should stay in contact with the floor as the foot supinates on the laterally rotating side. The metatarsal head should not lift off into foot inversion. This test should be performed without any feedback (self-palpation, vision, etc.) or cueing for correction. When feedback is removed for testing the therapist should use visual observation of the pelvis to determine whether the control of lumbopelvic rotation is adequate. Assess both directions.

Lumbopelvic rotation UCM

The person complains of unilateral symptoms in the lumbopelvic region. Lumbopelvic rotation begins to rotate to follow the hips before the double knee swing reaches 20–30° of independent range. The lumbar spine has UCM into rotation relative to the hips under rotation load.

The uncontrolled lumbopelvic rotation is often associated with inefficiency of the stability function of the oblique abdominals or the hip rotation stabilisers. (For example, the left external obliques and the right internal obliques control the lumbopelvic rotation UCM to the right, while the right posterior gluteus medius and maximus control pelvic rotation to the right when weight bearing.) During any asymmetrical or non-sagittal trunk movement, a rotational force is transmitted to the lumbopelvic region. The lumbopelvic rotation stability muscles control this rotational load. The oblique abdominal muscles, anterior fascicles of psoas major and superficial fibres of lumbar multifidus, which stabilise trunk rotation,

must coordinate with the weight bearing deep hip muscles, which concentrically and eccentrically control rotation of the pelvis from below.

During the attempt to dissociate the lumbopelvic rotation from thoracic rotation, the person either cannot control the UCM or has to concentrate and try hard to control the lumbopelvic rotation. The movement must be assessed on both sides. Note the direction that the rotation cannot be controlled (i.e. is there uncontrolled lumbopelvic rotation to the left or the right). It may be unilateral or bilateral. If lumbopelvic rotation UCM presents bilaterally, then one side may be better or worse than the other.

Clinical assessment note for direction-specific motor control testing

If some other movement (e.g. a small amount of flexion or extension) is observed during a motor control (dissociation) test of rotation control, *do not* score this as uncontrolled rotation. The flexion and extension motor control tests will identify if the observed movement is uncontrolled. A test for lumbopelvic rotation UCM is only positive if uncontrolled lumbopelvic rotation is demonstrated.

Rating and diagnosis of lumbopelvic rotation UCM

(T26.1 and T26.2)

Correction

The person stands in a SKB position with the trunk supported, leaning against a wall. They should monitor lumbopelvic rotation control by palpating both iliac crests for feedback regarding loss of position. Some people will also need to use a mirror so that they can watch for the loss of control. The person should actively contract the lateral abdominal muscles (especially the external obliques with ribcage depression) to flatten the lumbar spine, especially on the contralateral side to knee swing. This also provides a counter-rotation force for the uncontrolled lumbopelvic rotation. The lumbar spine may be supported in a neutral position with a folded towel if desired.

While maintaining a neutral lumbopelvic position and using the wall for support, the person is instructed to actively swing the knees to the side, only as far as there is no rotation of the pelvis at all. At the point in range that the lumbopelvic region starts to lose control of rotation, the knee movement should stop, the lumbopelvic position is restabilised and the knees return to the start position with control of the lumbopelvic rotation UCM. Allow the feet to roll into supination and pronation to follow the knees. As the ability to control the lumbopelvic region during independent hip rotation gets easier and the pattern of dissociation feels less unnatural the exercise can be progressed. A basic progression would be to perform this movement without the support of the wall.

The person should self-monitor the lumbopelvic alignment and control with a variety of feedback options (T26.3). There should be no provocation of any symptoms within the range that the rotation UCM can be controlled.

If control is poor, the pattern of correct movement may be taught with the person in the small knee bend position with the trunk supported, leaning against a wall. Maintaining a neutral lumbopelvic position and using the wall for support,

the person is then instructed to swing *one knee at a time* to the left then to the right (photo sequence A (R) leg only: Figures 5.125, 5.126, 5.127; photo sequence B one leg at a time swing to (R): Figures 5.128, 5.129). Allow the feet to roll into supination and pronation but keep all metatarsal heads on the floor. Next, practise the same movement with both knees moving to the same side but one after the other (not simultaneously). Then repeat the pattern to the other side. Finally, progress to swinging both knees to the same side, at the same time, with the trunk still supported against the wall.

An alternative option is to use a walk stance or lunge position with the trunk upright and the lumbopelvic region in neutral and facing forwards (Figure 5.130). Take approximately $\frac{2}{3}$ of the weight on the front foot and $\frac{1}{3}$ of the weight on the rear foot. Maintain control of lumbopelvic rotation and swing the front knee independently from side to side to rotate the hip (Figures 5.131 and 5.132). Maintain control of lumbopelvic rotation and swing the rear knee independently from side to side to rotate the hip (Figures 5.133 and 5.134). Practise with the right foot forward and left foot forward.

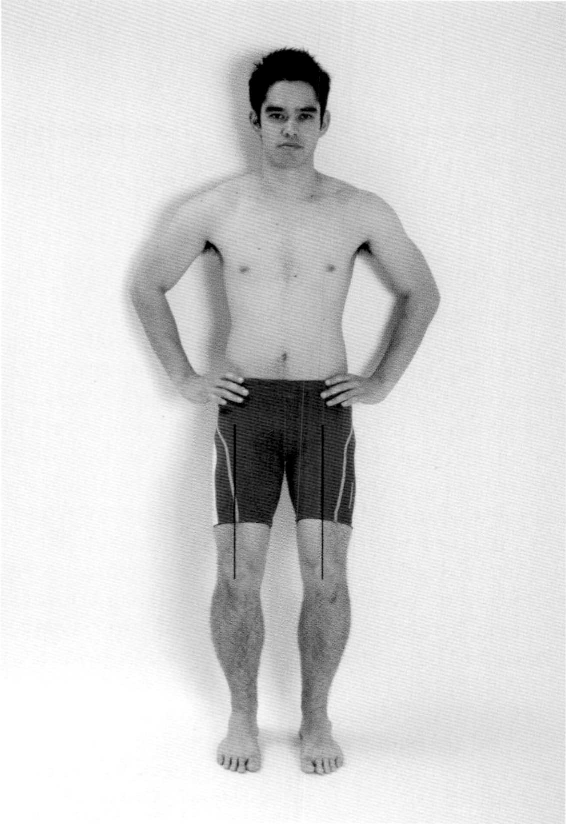

Figure 5.125 Correction sequence A(i): start position

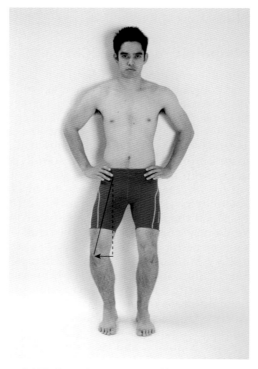

Figure 5.126 Correction sequence A(ii): one leg swings out

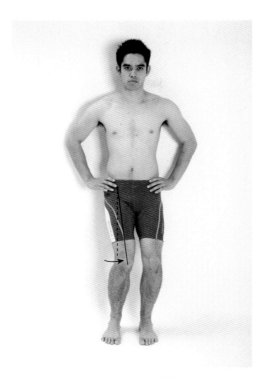

Figure 5.127 Correction sequence A(iii): same leg swings in

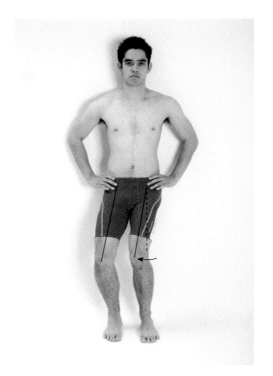

Figure 5.129 Correction sequence B(ii): other leg swings in

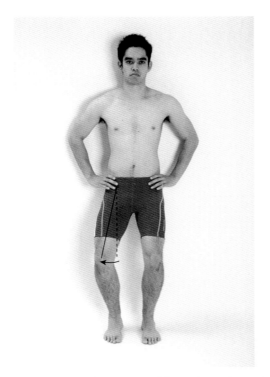

Figure 5.128 Correction sequence B(i): one leg swings out

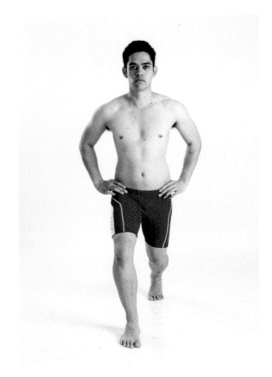

Figure 5.130 Correction sequence C(i) ½ lunge: start position

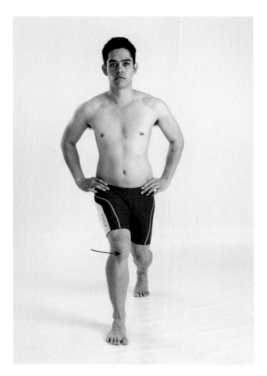

Figure 5.131 Correction sequence C(ii) ½ lunge: front leg swings in

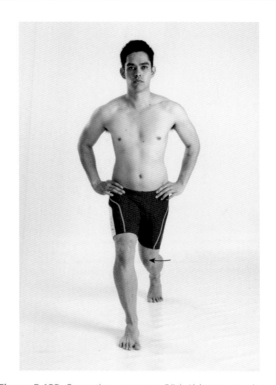

Figure 5.133 Correction sequence C(iv) ½ lunge: rear leg swings in

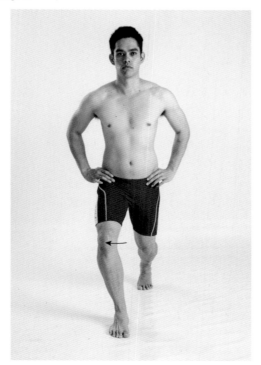

Figure 5.132 Correction sequence C(iii) ½ lunge: front leg swings out

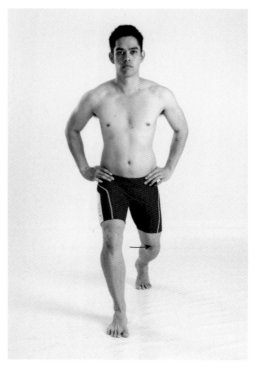

Figure 5.134 Correction sequence C(v) ½ lunge: rear leg swings out

T26.1 Assessment and rating of low threshold recruitment efficiency of the Double Knee Swing Test

DOUBLE KNEE SWING TEST – STANDING

ASSESSMENT

Control point:
- prevent lumbopelvic rotation

Movement challenge: simultaneous asymmetrical hip rotation (standing: small knee bend)

Benchmark range: 20–30° independent double knee swing (hip rotation)

RATING OF LOW THRESHOLD RECRUITMENT EFFICIENCY FOR CONTROL OF DIRECTION

	✓ or ✗		✓ or ✗
• Able to prevent 'UCM' into the test direction. Correct dissociation pattern of movement Prevent lumbopelvic UCM into: rotation and move simultaneous asymmetrical hip rotation	☐	• Looks easy, and in the opinion of the assessor, is performed with confidence	☐
		• Feels easy, and the subject has sufficient awareness of the movement pattern that they confidently prevent 'UCM' into the test direction	☐
• Dissociate movement through the benchmark range of: 20–30° double knee swing (hip rotation) *If there is more available range than the benchmark standard, only the benchmark range needs to be actively controlled*	☐	• The pattern of dissociation is smooth during concentric and eccentric movement	☐
		• Does not (consistently) use *end range* movement into the opposite direction to prevent the UCM	☐
• Without holding breath (though it is acceptable to use an alternate breathing strategy)	☐	• No extra feedback needed *(tactile, visual or verbal cueing)*	☐
		• Without external support or unloading	☐
• Control during eccentric phase	☐	• Relaxed natural breathing *(even if not ideal – so long as natural pattern does not change)*	☐
• Control during concentric phase	☐	• No fatigue	☐
CORRECT DISSOCIATION PATTERN		**RECRUITMENT EFFICIENCY**	

T26.2 Diagnosis of the site and direction of UCM from the Double Knee Swing Test

DOUBLE KNEE SWING TEST – STANDING: SMALL KNEE BEND

Site	Direction	Pelvis to the left (L)	Pelvis to the right (R)
		(check box)	(check box)
Lumbopelvic	Rotation (closed chain)	☐	☐

T26.3 Feedback tools to monitor retraining

FEEDBACK TOOL	PROCESS
Self-palpation	Palpation monitoring of joint position
Visual observation	Observe in a mirror or directly watch the movement
Adhesive tape	Skin tension for tactile feedback
Cueing and verbal correction	Listen to feedback from another observer

T27 STANDING: TRUNK SIDE-BEND TEST (tests for lumbopelvic rotation UCM)

This dissociation test assesses the ability to actively dissociate and control lumbopelvic rotation and side-bend the trunk while standing. During any asymmetrical or non-sagittal trunk movement, a rotational force is transmitted to the lumbopelvic region.

Test procedure

The person stands with the back resting on a wall, the feet at least shoulder width apart, and with the knees slightly flexed (hip flexors unloaded and wide base of support). The arms are crossed with hands touching opposite shoulders and the pelvis rolled back to flatten the back onto the wall (Figure 5.135). Then, keeping the pelvis level and stationary against the wall, they are instructed to side-bend against the wall, first to one side, then the other. Ideally, there should be at least 30° lateral flexion range (measured from the mid-sternal line) throughout the spine, without any lumbopelvic rotation, lateral tilt or side-shift of the pelvis (Figure 5.136). There should be no increase in spinal flexion or extension in the attempt to reach 30° side-bend. There should also be good symmetry of range to each side. This procedure requires that during testing for UCM, the spine side-bends to at least 30° each side so that any compensation and UCM can be identified.

This test should be performed without any extra feedback (self-palpation, vision, etc.) or cueing for correction. When feedback is removed for testing the therapist should use visual observation of the pelvis relative to the wall to determine whether the control of lumbopelvic rotation is adequate. Assess both directions.

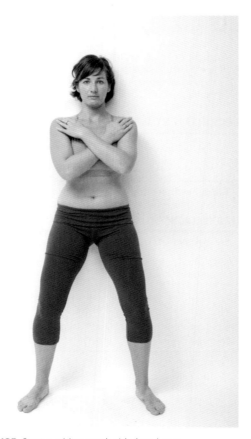

Figure 5.135 Start position trunk side-bend test

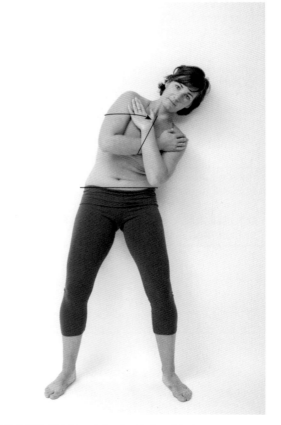

Figure 5.136 Benchmark trunk side-bend test

Lumbopelvic rotation UCM

The person complains of unilateral symptoms in the lumbopelvic region. Lumbopelvic rotation or lateral shift or lateral tilt occurs before the spinal side-bend on the wall reaches 30° of independent range. The lumbopelvic region has UCM into rotation relative to the trunk under side-bending load. Look for the presence of a segmental hinge as well as multi-segmental rotation and extension UCM. (Beware – acute discal pathology may produce protective responses that may be misinterpreted.)

The uncontrolled lumbopelvic rotation or lateral shift is often associated with inefficiency of the stability function of the oblique abdominals or the hip rotation stabilisers. (For example, the left external obliques and the right internal obliques control the lumbopelvic rotation UCM to the right, while the right posterior gluteus medius and maximus control pelvic rotation to the right when weight bearing.) During any asymmetrical or non-sagittal trunk movement, a rotational force is transmitted to the lumbopelvic region. The lumbopelvic rotation stability muscles control this rotational load. The oblique abdominal muscles, anterior fascicles of psoas major and superficial fibres of lumbar multifidus, which stabilise trunk rotation, must coordinate with the weight bearing deep hip muscles, which concentrically and eccentrically control rotation of the pelvis from below.

There may be significant compensation within side-bending motion as a means of adapting to either asymmetry of length or a myofascial restriction of quadratus lumborum or iliocostalis, or due to asymmetry of stabiliser control. If the lumbopelvic rotation stabilisers are not able to effectively control rotation force, many maladaptive substitution strategies can be observed during spinal side-bending:

- A marked pelvic tilt down (dropping) on the side-bending side, associated with unlocking the ipsilateral knee and allowing the pelvis to drop into lateral tilt to follow the spinal side-bend.
- A marked pelvic tilt up (hitching) on the contralateral side to the side-bending movement is associated with shifting body weight onto the ipsilateral leg and lifting the contralateral heel. This allows the pelvis to lift into lateral tilt to follow the spinal side-bend.

- Side-bending movement of the trunk can be initiated with lateral shift of the pelvis (i.e. the pelvis moving under the trunk instead of the trunk moving of the pelvis).
- One of the most common compensations is to rotate the pelvis and extend the trunk or to rotate the pelvis and flex the trunk into side-bending function. Lumbar side-bending or lateral flexion movement can be associated with excessive or asymmetrical pelvic rotation. Rotation forward of the ipsilateral pelvis is frequently combined with spinal extension or pelvic forward sway, while rotation backward of the ipsilateral pelvis is frequently combined with spinal flexion.

During side-bending of the trunk with the back flattened on the wall (or neutral), the person lacks the ability to keep the back flat on the wall during this movement. There are a variety of compensatory patterns of substitution dysfunction: i) the pelvis may rotate and twist off the wall; ii) the pelvis may laterally shift or tilt excessively on the wall; iii) the lumbar spine may extend off the wall; iv) the pelvis may sway forwards off the wall; and v) the upper back may flex and roll off the wall. All of these compensations, when present with side-bending away from the midline, are biomechanically linked to uncontrolled lumbopelvic rotation.

During the attempt to dissociate the lumbopelvic rotation from spinal side-bending, the person either cannot control the UCM or has to concentrate and try hard to control the lumbopelvic rotation. The movement must be assessed on both sides. Note the direction that the rotation cannot be controlled (i.e. is there uncontrolled lumbopelvic rotation to the left or the right). It may be unilateral or bilateral. If lumbopelvic rotation UCM presents bilaterally, one side may be better or worse than the other.

Clinical assessment note for direction-specific motor control testing

If some other movement (e.g. a small amount of flexion or extension) is observed during a motor control (dissociation) test of rotation control, *do not* score this as uncontrolled rotation. The flexion and extension motor control tests will identify if the observed movement is uncontrolled. A test for lumbopelvic rotation UCM is only positive if uncontrolled lumbopelvic rotation is demonstrated.

Rating and diagnosis of lumbopelvic rotation UCM

(T27.1 and T27.2)

Correction

The person stands in a wide stance SKB position with the trunk supported, leaning against a wall. They should monitor lumbopelvic rotation control by palpating both iliac crests for feedback regarding loss of position. Some people will also need to use a mirror so that they can watch for the loss of control. The person should actively contract the lateral abdominal muscles (especially the external obliques with ribcage depression) to flatten the lumbar spine, and to resist lumbopelvic rotation. (The lumbar spine may be supported in a neutral position with a folded towel if desired.)

Then, keeping the pelvis level and stationary against the wall, they are instructed to side-bend to the side, only moving as far as the back can be maintained on the wall without compensation or substitution. At the point in range that the lumbopelvic region starts to lose control of rotation, the spinal side-bending movement must stop, the lumbopelvic position is restabilised and the trunk returned to the start position with control of the lumbopelvic rotation UCM. There must be *no pelvic or trunk rotation*. Likewise, there should be no lumbar extension or anterior pelvic tilt, no trunk flexion or forward sway of the pelvis and no lateral tilt or shift of the pelvis.

Side-bending is performed only through the range that the UCM can be actively controlled and as far as any restriction allows. Easy control through symmetry of range is the goal. As the ability to control the UCM gets easier and the pattern of dissociation feels less unnatural, the exercise can be progressed to an unsupported position away from the wall in free standing. The person should self-monitor the lumbopelvic alignment and control with a variety of feedback options (T27.3). There should be no provocation of any symptoms within the range that the rotation UCM can be controlled.

T27.1 Assessment and rating of low threshold recruitment efficiency of the Trunk Side-Bend Test

TRUNK SIDEBEND TEST – STANDING WALL

ASSESSMENT

Control point:
- prevent lumbopelvic rotation

Movement challenge: spinal sidebend (standing: wall)

Benchmark range: 30° independent sidebend (mid-sternal line)

RATING OF LOW THRESHOLD RECRUITMENT EFFICIENCY FOR CONTROL OF DIRECTION

	✓ or ✗		✓ or ✗
• Able to prevent 'UCM' into the test direction. Correct dissociation pattern of movement Prevent lumbopelvic UCM into: rotation and move spinal sidebend	☐	• Looks easy, and in the opinion of the assessor, is performed with confidence • Feels easy, and the subject has sufficient awareness of the movement pattern that they confidently prevent 'UCM' into the test direction	☐ ☐
• Dissociate movement through the benchmark range of: 30° sidebend (mid-sternal line) *If there is more available range than the benchmark standard, only the benchmark range needs to be actively controlled*	☐	• The pattern of dissociation is smooth during concentric and eccentric movement • Does not (consistently) use *end range* movement into the opposite direction to prevent the UCM	☐ ☐
• Without holding breath (though it is acceptable to use an alternate breathing strategy)	☐	• No extra feedback needed *(tactile, visual or verbal cueing)*	☐
• Control during eccentric phase	☐	• Without external support or unloading	☐
• Control during concentric phase	☐	• Relaxed natural breathing *(even if not ideal – so long as natural pattern does not change)* • No fatigue	☐ ☐

CORRECT DISSOCIATION PATTERN **RECRUITMENT EFFICIENCY**

T27.2 Diagnosis of the site and direction of UCM from the Trunk Side-Bend Test

TRUNK SIDE-BEND TEST – STANDING: WALL

Site	Direction	Pelvis to the left (L)	Pelvis to the right (R)
		(check box)	(check box)
Lumbopelvic	Rotation (closed chain)	☐	☐

T27.3 Feedback tools to monitor retraining

FEEDBACK TOOL	PROCESS
Self-palpation	Palpation monitoring of joint position
Visual observation	Observe in a mirror or directly watch the movement
Adhesive tape	Skin tension for tactile feedback
Cueing and verbal correction	Listen to feedback from another observer

T28 STANDING: PELVIC SIDE-SHIFT TEST (tests for lumbopelvic rotation UCM)

This dissociation test assesses the ability to actively dissociate and control lumbopelvic rotation and side-shift the pelvis while standing. During any asymmetrical or non-sagittal trunk movement, a rotational force is transmitted to the lumbopelvic region.

Test procedure

The person stands with the back resting on a wall, the feet at least shoulder width apart and with the knees slightly flexed (hip flexors unloaded and wide base of support). The arms are crossed with hands touching opposite shoulders and the pelvis rolled back to flatten the back onto the wall

(Figure 5.137). Then, keeping the shoulders level and stationary against the wall, they are instructed to side-shift the pelvis laterally against the wall, first to one side, then the other. Ideally, there should be at least 5 cm lateral pelvis movement without any lumbopelvic rotation, lateral tilt of the shoulders or side-shift of the chest (Figure 5.138). There should be no increase in spinal flexion or extension in the attempt to reach 5 cm lateral pelvic shift. There should also be good symmetry of range to each side. This procedure requires that during testing for UCM, the pelvis side-shifts to at least 5 cm each side so that any compensation and UCM can be identified.

This test should be performed without any extra feedback (self-palpation, vision, etc.) or cueing for correction. When feedback is removed for testing the therapist should use visual observation of the pelvis relative to the wall to determine

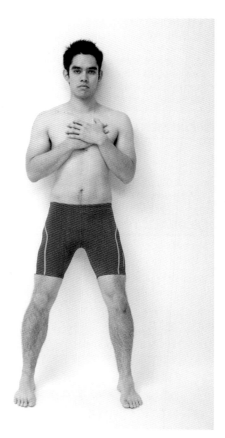

Figure 5.137 Start position pelvic side-shift test

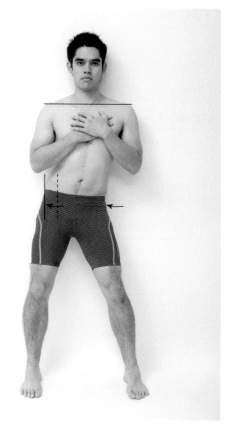

Figure 5.138 Benchmark pelvic side-shift test

whether the control of lumbopelvic rotation is adequate. Assess both directions.

Lumbopelvic rotation UCM

The person complains of unilateral symptoms in the lumbopelvic region. Lumbopelvic rotation or lateral tilt of the chest occurs before the lateral pelvic shift on the wall reaches 5 cm of independent range. The lumbopelvic region has UCM into rotation relative to the trunk under a side-shift load. (Beware – acute discal pathology may produce protective responses that may be misinterpreted.)

The uncontrolled lumbopelvic rotation is often associated with inefficiency of the stability function of the oblique abdominals or the hip rotation stabilisers. During any asymmetrical or non-sagittal trunk movement, a rotational force is transmitted to the lumbopelvic region. The lumbopelvic rotation stability muscles control this rotational load. The oblique abdominal muscles, anterior fascicles of psoas major and superficial fibres of lumbar multifidus, which stabilise trunk rotation, must coordinate with the weight bearing deep hip muscles, which concentrically and eccentrically control rotation of the pelvis from below.

There may be significant compensation within side-bending motion as a means of adapting to either asymmetry of length or a myofascial restriction of quadratus lumborum or iliocostalis, or due to asymmetry of stabiliser control. If the lumbopelvic rotation stabilisers are not able to effectively control rotation force, many maladaptive substitution strategies can be observed during spinal side-bending:

- A marked shift of the head and shoulders along with the shift of the pelvis to follow the pelvic shift. This transfers body weight onto one leg.
- A marked lateral tilt (drop) of the shoulders and lateral flexion of the upper trunk away from the pelvic shift to adapt to the pelvic shift.
- A marked pelvic tilt up (hitching) on the side of the pelvis side-shift movement is associated with excessive substitution of quadratus lumborum and iliocostalis mobiliser muscles instead of the trunk rotation stabiliser muscles.
- One of the most common compensations is to rotate the pelvis and extend the trunk or

to rotate the pelvis and flex the trunk into lateral side-shift function.

During side-shift of the pelvis with the back flattened on the wall (or neutral), the person lacks the ability to keep the back flat on the wall during this movement. There are a variety of compensatory patterns of substitution dysfunction. The pelvis may rotate and twist off the wall. The shoulders may laterally tilt excessively on the wall. The lumbar spine may extend off the wall. The pelvis may sway forward off the wall. The upper back may flex and roll off the wall. All of these compensations, when present with pelvic side-shift away from the midline, are biomechanically linked to uncontrolled lumbopelvic rotation.

During the attempt to dissociate the lumbopelvic rotation from pelvic side-shift, the person either cannot control the UCM or has to concentrate and try hard to control the lumbopelvic rotation. The movement must be assessed on both sides. Note the direction that the rotation cannot be controlled (i.e. is there uncontrolled lumbopelvic rotation to the left or the right). It may be unilateral or bilateral. If lumbopelvic rotation UCM presents bilaterally, one side may be better or worse than the other.

Clinical assessment note for direction-specific motor control testing:

If some other movement (e.g. a small amount of flexion or extension) is observed during a motor control (dissociation) test of rotation control, *do not* score this as uncontrolled rotation. The flexion and extension motor control tests will identify if the observed movement is uncontrolled. A test for lumbopelvic rotation UCM is only positive if uncontrolled lumbopelvic rotation is demonstrated.

Rating and diagnosis of lumbopelvic rotation UCM

(T28.1 and T28.2)

Correction

The person stands in a wide stance SKB position with the trunk supported, leaning against a wall. They should monitor lumbopelvic rotation

T28.1 Assessment and rating of low threshold recruitment efficiency of the Pelvic Side-Shift Test

PELVIC SIDE SHIFT TEST – STANDING WALL

ASSESSMENT

Control point:
• prevent lumbopelvic rotation
Movement challenge: pelvic side shift (standing: wall)
Benchmark range: 5 cm independent lateral pelvic side shift

RATING OF LOW THRESHOLD RECRUITMENT EFFICIENCY FOR CONTROL OF DIRECTION

	✓ or ✗		✓ or ✗
• Able to prevent 'UCM' into the test direction. Correct dissociation pattern of movement Prevent lumbopelvic UCM into: rotation and move lateral pelvic side shift	☐	• Looks easy, and in the opinion of the assessor, is performed with confidence	☐
		• Feels easy, and the subject has sufficient awareness of the movement pattern that they confidently prevent 'UCM' into the test direction	☐
• Dissociate movement through the benchmark range of: 5 cm lateral side shift *If there is more available range than the benchmark standard, only the benchmark range needs to be actively controlled*	☐	• The pattern of dissociation is smooth during concentric and eccentric movement	☐
		• Does not (consistently) use *end range* movement into the opposite direction to prevent the UCM	☐
• Without holding breath (though it is acceptable to use an alternate breathing strategy)	☐	• No extra feedback needed *(tactile, visual or verbal cueing)*	☐
• Control during eccentric phase	☐	• Without external support or unloading	☐
• Control during concentric phase	☐	• Relaxed natural breathing *(even if not ideal – so long as natural pattern does not change)*	☐
		• No fatigue	☐
CORRECT DISSOCIATION PATTERN		**RECRUITMENT EFFICIENCY**	

T28.2 Diagnosis of the site and direction of UCM from the Pelvic Side-Shift Test

PELVIC SIDE-SHIFT TEST – STANDING: WALL

Site	Direction	Pelvis to the left (L)	Pelvis to the right (R)
		(check box)	(check box)
Lumbopelvic	Rotation (closed chain)	☐	☐

T28.3 Feedback tools to monitor retraining

FEEDBACK TOOL	PROCESS
Self-palpation	Palpation monitoring of joint position
Visual observation	Observe in a mirror or directly watch the movement
Adhesive tape	Skin tension for tactile feedback
Cueing and verbal correction	Listen to feedback from another observer

control by palpating both iliac crests for feedback regarding loss of position. Some people will also need to use a mirror so that they can watch for the loss of control. The person should actively contract the lateral abdominal muscles (especially the external obliques with ribcage depression) to flatten the lumbar spine, and to resist lumbopelvic rotation. (The lumbar spine may be supported in a neutral position with a folded towel if desired.)

Then, keeping the shoulders level and the head and chest stationary against the wall, they are instructed to side-shift the pelvis laterally, only moving as far as the back can be maintained on the wall without compensation or substitution. At the point in range that the lumbopelvic region starts to lose control of rotation, the pelvic side-shift movement must stop, the lumbopelvic position is restabilised and the trunk returned to the start position with control of the lumbopelvic rotation UCM. There must be *no pelvic or trunk rotation*. Likewise, there should be no lumbar extension or anterior pelvic tilt, no trunk flexion or forward sway of the pelvis and no lateral tilt of the shoulders and head.

Pelvic side-shift is performed only through the range that the UCM can be actively controlled and as far as any restriction allows. Easy control through symmetry of range is the goal. As the ability to control the UCM gets easier and the pattern of dissociation feels less unnatural, the exercise can be progressed to an unsupported position away from the wall in free-standing. The person should self-monitor the lumbopelvic alignment and control with a variety of feedback options (T28.3). There should be no provocation of any symptoms within the range that the rotation UCM can be controlled.

Rotation (unilateral) UCM summary

(Tables 5.6 and 5.7).

Table 5.6 Summary and rating of lumbopelvic open chain rotation tests		
UCM DIAGNOSIS AND TESTING		
SITE: LUMBAR	DIRECTION: ROTATION (OPEN)	**CLINICAL PRIORITY** ☐
TEST	**RATING** (✓✓ or ✓✗ or ✗✗) and rationale	
	(L)	(R)
Supine: single heel slide		
Supine: bent knee fall out		
Side-lying: top leg turn out		
Prone: single hip rotation		
Prone: single knee flexion		
Prone: hip extension lift		
Sitting: single knee extension		

Table 5.7 Summary and rating of lumbopelvic closed chain rotation tests

UCM DIAGNOSIS AND TESTING		
SITE: **LUMBAR**	**DIRECTION:** **ROTATION (CLOSED)**	**CLINICAL PRIORITY** ☐
TEST	**RATING** (✓✓ or ✓✗ or ✗✗) and rationale	
	(L)	(R)
Crook lying: single leg bridge extension		
Standing: thoracic rotation		
Standing: double knee swing		
Standing: trunk side-bend		
Standing: pelvic side-shift		

REFERENCES

Airaksinen, O., Brox, J.I., Cedraschi, C., Hildebrandt, J., Klaber-Moffett, J., Kovacs, F., et al., 2006. COST B13 Working Group on Guidelines for Chronic Low Back Pain. Chapter 4. European guidelines for the management of chronic nonspecific low back pain. European Spine Journal 15 (Suppl. 2), S192–S300.

Bogduk, N., 1997. Clinical anatomy of the lumbar spine and sacrum, ed 3. Churchill Livingstone, Edinburgh.

Cibulka, M.T., 2002. Understanding sacroiliac joint movement as a guide to the management of a patient with unilateral low back pain. Manual Therapy 7 (4), 215–221.

Dankaerts, W., O'Sullivan, P., Burnett, A., Straker, L., 2006. Altered patterns of superficial trunk muscle activation during sitting in nonspecific chronic low back pain patients: importance of subclassification. Spine 31 (17), 2017–2023.

Dankaerts, W., O'Sullivan, P.B., Burnett, A.F., Straker, L.M., 2007. The use of a mechanism-based classification system to evaluate and direct management of a patient with non-specific chronic low back pain and motor control impairment – a case report. Manual Therapy 12 (2), 181–191.

Fritz, J.M., Cleland, J.A., Childs, J.D., 2007. Subgrouping patients with low back pain: evolution of a classification approach to physical therapy. Journal of Orthopaedic and Sports Physical Therapy 37 (6), 290–302.

Gombatto, S.P., Collins, D.R., Sahrmann, S.A., Engsberg, J.R., Van Dillen, L.R., 2007. Patterns of lumbar region movement during trunk lateral bending in 2 subgroups of people with low back pain. Physical Therapy 87 (4), 441–454.

Greenman, P.E., 2003. Principles of manual medicine, 3rd ed. Lippincott Williams & Wilkins.

Hall, L., Tsao, H., Macdonald, D., Coppieters, M., Hodges, P.W., 2007. Immediate effects of co-contraction training on motor control of the trunk muscles in people with recurrent low back pain. Journal of Electromyography and Kinesiology 19 (5), 763–773.

Hamilton, C., Richardson, C., 1998. Active control of the neutral lumbopelvic posture: a comparison between back pain and non back pain subjects. In: Vleeming, A., Mooney, V., Tilsher, H., Dorman, T., Snijders, C. (Eds.), 3rd Interdisciplinary World Congress on low back pain and pelvic pain, Vienna, Austria.

Hides, J.A., Jull, G.A., Richardson, C.A., 2001. Long-term effects of specific stabilizing exercises for first-episode low back pain. Spine 26 (11), E243–E248.

Hodges, P.W., 2003. Core stability exercise in chronic low back pain. Orthopedic Clinics of North America 34 (2), 245–254.

Hungerford, B., Gilleard, W., Hodges, P., 2003. Evidence of altered lumbopelvic muscle recruitment in the presence of sacroiliac joint pain. Spine 28 (14), 1593–1600.

Hungerford, B., Gilleard, W., Lee, D., 2004. Altered patterns of pelvic bone motion determined in subjects with posterior pelvic pain using skin markers. Clinical Biomechanics (Bristol, Avon) 19 (5), 456–464.

Hungerford, B.A., Gilleard, W., Moran, M., Emmerson, C., 2007. Evaluation of the ability of physical therapists to palpate intrapelvic motion with the Stork test on the support side. Physical Therapy 87 (7), 879–887.

Jull, G., Richardson, C.A., Toppenberg, R., Comerford, M., Bui, B., 1993. Towards a measurement of active muscle control for lumbar stabilisation. Australian Journal of Physiotherapy 39, 187–193.

Laslett, M., Aprill, C.N., McDonald, B., Young, S.B., 2005. Diagnosis of sacroiliac joint pain: validity of individual provocation tests and composites of tests. Manual Therapy 10 (3), 207–218.

Lee, D., 2004. The pelvic girdle. Elsevier, Edinburgh.

Luomajoki, H., Kool, J., de Bruin, E.D., Airaksinen, O., 2007. Reliability of movement control tests in the lumbar spine. BMC Musculoskeletal Disorders 8, 90.

Luomajoki, H., Kool, J., de Bruin, E.D., Airaksinen, O., 2008. Movement control tests of the low back: evaluation of the difference between patients with low back pain and healthy controls. BMC Musculoskeletal Disorders 9, 170.

Luomajoki, H., Kool, J., de Bruin, E.D., Airaksinen, O., 2010. Improvement in low back movement control, decreased pain and disability, resulting from specific exercise intervention. Sports Medicine, Arthroscopy, Rehabilitation, Therapy and Technology 23 (2), 11.

Macedo, L.G., Maher, C.G., Latimer, J., McAuley, J.H., 2009. Motor control exercise for persistent, nonspecific low back pain: a systematic review. Physical Therapy 89 (1), 9–25. Epub 2008.

Maitland, G., Hengeveld, E., Banks, K., English, K., 2005. Maitland's vertebral manipulation. Butterworth Heinemann, Oxford.

Maluf, K.S., Sahrmann, S.A., Van Dillen, L.R., 2000. Use of a classification system to guide nonsurgical management of a patient with chronic low back pain. Physical Therapy 80 (11), 1097–1111.

Mens, J.M., Vleeming, A., Snijders, C.J., Koes, B.W., Stam, H.J., 2002. Validity of the active straight leg raise test for measuring disease severity in patients with posterior pelvic pain after pregnancy. Spine (Phila Pa 1976) 27 (2), 196–200.

Mitchell, F., Moran, P., Pruzzo, N., 1979. An evaluation and treatment manual of osteopathic muscle energy procedures. Mitchell Moran and Pruzzo Associates, Missouri.

Morrissey, D., Morrissey, M.C., Driver, W., King, J.B., Woledge, R.C., 2008. Manual landmark identification and tracking during the medial rotation test of the shoulder: an accuracy study using three dimensional ultrasound and motion analysis measures. Manual Therapy 13 (6), 529–535.

Moseley, L., 2002. Combined physiotherapy and education is efficacious for chronic low back pain. Australian Journal of Physiotherapy 48 (4), 297–302.

O'Sullivan, P., 2005. Diagnosis and classification of chronic low back pain disorders: maladaptive movement and motor control impairments as underlying mechanism. Manual Therapy 10 (4), 242–255.

O'Sullivan, P.B., Beales, D.J., 2007a. Changes in pelvic floor and diaphragm kinematics and respiratory patterns in subjects with sacroiliac joint pain following a motor learning intervention: a case series. Manual Therapy 12 (3), 209–218.

O'Sullivan, P.B., Beales, D.J., 2007b. Diagnosis and classification of pelvic girdle pain disorders. Part 2: illustration of the utility of a classification system via case studies. Manual Therapy 12 (2), e1–e12.

O'Sullivan, P.B., Grahamslaw, K.M., Kendell, M., Lapenskie, S.C., Möller, N.E., Richards, K.V., 2002a. The effect of different standing and sitting postures on trunk muscle activity in a pain-free population. Spine 27 (11), 1238–1244.

O'Sullivan, P.B., Beales, D.J., Beetham, J.A., Cripps, J., 2002b. Altered motor control strategies in subjects with sacroiliac joint pain during the active straight leg raise test. Spine 27 (1), E1–E8.

O'Sullivan, P.B., Burnett, A., Floyd, A.N., Gadsdon, K., Logiudice, J., Miller, D., et al., 2003. Lumbar repositioning in a specific low back pain population. Spine 28 (10), 1074–1079.

O'Sullivan, P.B., Grahamslaw, K.M., Kendell, M., Lapenskie, S.C., Moller, N.E., Richards, K.V., 2002. The effect of different standing and sitting postures on trunk muscle activity in a pain-free population. Spine 27 (11), 1238–1244.

O'Sullivan, P.B., Mitchell, T., Bulich, P., Waller, R., Holte, J., 2006. The relationship between posture and back muscle endurance in industrial workers with flexion-related low back pain. Manual Therapy 11 (4), 264–271.

O'Sullivan, P.B., Twomey, L., Allison, G., 1997. Evaluation of specific

stabilising exercises in the treatment of chronic low back pain with radiological diagnosis of spondylosis or spondylolisthesis. Spine 22 (24), 2959–2967.

Oh, J.S., Cynn, H.S., Won, J.H., Kwon, O.Y., Yi, C.H., 2007. Effects of performing an abdominal drawing-in maneuver during prone hip extension exercises on hip and back extensor muscle activity and amount of anterior pelvic tilt. Journal of Orthopaedic and Sports Physical Therapy 37 (6), 320–324.

Panjabi, M.M., 1992. The stabilising system of the spine. Part II. Neutral zone and instability hypothesis. Journal of Spinal Disorders 5 (4), 390–397.

Pool-Goudzwaard, A.L., Vleeming, A., Stoeckart, R., Snijders, C.J., Mens, J.M., 1998. Insufficient lumbopelvic stability: a clinical, anatomical and biomechanical approach to 'a-specific' low back pain. Manual Therapy 3 (1), 12–20.

Richardson, C.A., Jull, G.A., Toppenberg, R., Comerford, M.J., 1992. Techniques for active lumbar stabilisation for spinal protection: a pilot study. Australian Journal of Physiotherapy 38, 105–112.

Richardson, C.A., Snijders, C.J., Hides, J.A., 2002. The relationship between the transversus abdominis muscles sacroiliac joint mechanics and low back pain. Spine 27 (4), 399–405.

Riddle, D.L., Freburger, J.K., 2002. Evaluation of the presence of sacroiliac joint region dysfunction using a combination of tests: a multicenter intertester reliability study. Physical Therapy 82 (8), 772–781.

Roussel, N.A., Nijs, J., Mottram, S., van Moorsel, A., Truijen, S., Stassijns, G., 2009. Altered lumbopelvic movement control but not generalised joint hypermobility is associated with increased injury in dancers. A prospective study. Manual Therapy 14 (6), 630–635.

Sahrmann, S.A., 2002. Diagnosis and treatment of movement impairment syndromes. Mosby, St Louis.

Stuge, B., Veierod, M.B., Laerum, E., Vollestad, N., 2004. The efficacy of a treatment program focusing on specific stabilizing exercises for pelvic girdle pain after pregnancy: a two-year follow-up of a randomized clinical trial. Spine 29 (10), E197–E203.

Sturesson, B., Selvic, G., Uden, A., 1989. Movements of the sacroiliac joints: a roentgen stereophotogrammetric analysis. Spine 14 (2), 162–165.

Teyhen, D.S., Flynn, T.W., Childs, J.D., Abraham, L.D., 2007. Arthrokinematics in a subgroup of patients likely to benefit from a lumbar stabilization exercise program. Physical Therapy 87 (3), 313–325.

Trudelle-Jackson, E., Sarvaiya-Shah, S.A., Wang, S.S., 2008. Interrater reliability of a movement impairment-based classification system for lumbar spine syndromes in patients with chronic low back pain. Journal of Orthopaedic and Sports Physical Therapy 38 (6), 371–376.

Tsao, H., Hodges, P.W., 2008. Persistence of improvements in postural strategies following motor control training in people with recurrent low back pain. Journal of Electromyography and Kinesiology 18 (4), 559–567.

Van Dillen, L.R., Maluf, K.S., Sahrmann, S.A., 2009. Further examination of modifying patient-preferred movement and alignment strategies in patients with low back pain during symptomatic tests. Manual Therapy 14 (1), 52–60.

Vibe Fersum, K., O'Sullivan, P.B., Kvåle, A., Skouen, J.S., 2009. Inter-examiner reliability of a classification system for patients with non-specific low back pain. Manual Therapy 4 (5), 555–561.

CHAPTER 6
THE CERVICAL SPINE

Chapter | 6 |

The cervical spine

INTRODUCTION

In the past two decades there has been an increase in research into cervical musculoskeletal disorders with many movement impairments and pathophysiological disorders subsequently identified. These include changes in the sensory and motor systems, in sensorimotor function and psychological features associated with whiplash, headache and neck pain (Jull et al 2008). Although the management of neck pain does include the assessment and retraining of muscle function, assessment of dynamic movement faults, known to be a significant factor in musculoskeletal disorders, are still poorly described, utilised and researched in the cervical spine (Jull et al 2008). Fritz & Brennan (2007) have highlighted the importance of developing a classification system for subgroups of patients with neck pain. This chapter sets out to explore the assessment and retraining of uncontrolled movement (UCM) in the cervical spine. Before details of the assessment and retraining of UCM in the cervical region are explained, a brief review of cervical spine structure and function, changes in muscle function and movement and postural control in the region are presented.

Cervical spine muscle function

The cervical spine supports and orients the head in space relative to the thorax (Jull et al 2008). To do this effectively and efficiently the cervical muscle system, comprising both deep and superficial muscles, must work in synergy and provide the movement and stability. The 'stability system', characterised by deep segmentally attaching muscles, should be able to maintain control of the cervical spine segments during low load postural control tasks, functional movements and high load fatiguing activities. The co-activation of the stability muscles should control abnormal intersegmental translation at the motion segments, give segmental support to the spinal neutral curves, maintain the head balance on the upper cervical spine and dynamically balance the head and neck on the trunk. The anatomical connections between the cervical spine, temporomandibular joint (TMJ), thorax and shoulder girdle, with the musculoskeletal and neurovascular structures, make movement control function complex. Further influences come from respiratory function.

There is evidence to demonstrate changes in cervical and scapulothoracic muscle function in people with neck pain. Falla & Farina (2007) describe in detail the altered control strategies and peripheral changes in cervical muscles in people with pain which lead to limited endurance, greater fatiguability, less strength, altered proprioception and reorganisation of muscle coordination. Figure 6.1 illustrates the interrelationships between pain, altered control strategies and peripheral changes in the cervical muscles (Falla & Farina 2007). Similarly, recruitment of

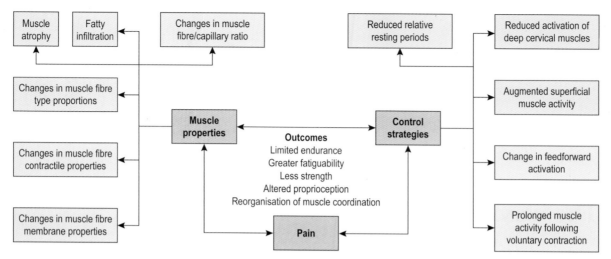

Figure 6.1 Inter-relationships between pain, altered control strategies and peripheral changes in the cervical muscles (Falla & Farina 2007)

the scapulothoracic muscles has been identified in people with neck pain (Nederhand et al 2000; Falla et al 2004b; Szeto et al 2005a; Johnston et al 2008b; Szeto et al 2008) along with histological changes in upper trapezius (Lindman 1991a, b).

UCM in the cervical spine

The current literature suggests people with cervical pain have altered movement control strategies and that these changes are associated with pain and disability (Falla et al 2004b; Johnston et al 2008a, b). Altered movement strategies have been associated with the clinical presentations of whiplash (Nederhand et al 2002; Jull et al 2004; Sterling et al 2003, 2005), cervicogenic headaches (Jull et al 2002; Fernández-de-las-Peñas et al 2008), neck pain (Jull et al 2004; O'Leary et al 2007; Falla et al 2004a, b) and work-related musculoskeletal disorders (Johnston 2008a, b; Szeto et al 2008). The pathophysiological and psychosocial mechanisms identified in people with neck pain are proposed to be a cause of respiratory disorders (Kapreli et al 2008).

These altered strategies will influence the control of movement which can present as both uncontrolled translatatory movement and uncontrolled range or physiological motion. Either movement dysfunction will present clinically as areas of relative flexibility. Increases in translational movements have been highlighted at C4–5

and C5–6 in people with disc degeneration (Miyazaki et al 2008). With disc degeneration the intersegmental motion changes from the normal state to an unstable phase and subsequently to an ankylosed stage with increased stability and loss of function in late stage degeneration. Further literature indicates how alteration in the cervical motion is seen at segmental levels in subjects with neck pain (White et al 1975; Amevo et al 1992; Panjabi 1992; Singer et al 1993; Dvorak et al 1998; Cheng et al 2007; Grip et al 2008).

Changes in alignment in the cervical spine may result in a forward head posture position demonstrating an increase in low cervical flexion (Szeto et al 2005b; Falla et al 2007; Fernández-de-las-Peñas et al 2007; Straker et al 2008). Yip and colleagues (2008) noted the greater the forward head posture, the greater the disability. Regions and segments of less mobility have been noted in the cervical spine which will present clinically as regions of relative stiffness (Dall'Alba et al 2001, Dvorak et al 1988).

Introduction to rehabilitation for cervical spine dysfunction

Systematic reviews indicate that different treatment modalities have an effect on neck disorders with exercise being a key element in the management of pain disability and dysfunction (Kjellman et al 1999; Gross et al 2004; Verhagen et al 2004). In addition, there is a growing body of evidence that supports the efficacy of exercise in the management of cervical pain (Jull et al 2002; Falla et al 2006, 2007). Along with the identification and correction of movement control dysfunction, it is important to address the altered control strategies and peripheral changes in the cervical muscles (Jull et al 2008, ch. 4 p. 50). Psychosocial and physiological factors also have a role in the development and maintenance of cervical pain (Jull et al 2008 , ch. 7 p. 97) and influence how it is managed appropriately.

It is important to consider other postural influences when retraining the control of neck movements as it has been demonstrated that there is better recruitment of postural neck muscles with facilitation of a good lumbar position (Falla et al 2007). Researchers have further demonstrated that improving postural alignment of the thoracic spine and the head and neck also has benefits for recruitment of the deep neck stability muscles. Changes in muscle function have been identified in functional activities, highlighting the importance of linking the rehabilitation of movement control with functional activities (Falla et al 2004b; Szeto et al 2008).

Identifying UCM in the cervical spine

This body of evidence indicates it is important to be able to identify control impairments in people with neck pain and relate these to their symptom presentation and disability. The classification in terms of site and direction of UCM has been proposed (Mottram 2003; Comerford & Mottram 2011), and a diagnosis based on movement impairment (Sahrmann 2002; McDonnell et al 2005; Caldwell et al 2007). The influence of the scapula on neck symptoms and range of movement needs to be considered in treating UCM in the cervical spine. Passive scapula elevation has been shown to decrease neck symptoms and increase range of movement (Van Dillen et al 2007). This chapter details the assessment of

UCM at the cervical spine region and describes retraining strategies.

DIAGNOSIS OF THE SITE AND DIRECTION OF UCM IN THE CERVICAL SPINE

The diagnosis of site and direction of UCM at the cervical spine can be identified in terms of site: upper cervical spine, mid-cervical spine and lower cervical spine, and direction of flexion, extension and asymmetry (Table 6.1). As with all UCMs, they can present as uncontrolled translational movements (e.g. at C4/5 (Cheng et al 2007)) or uncontrolled range movements (e.g. low cervical flexion (Straker et al 2008)).

A diagnosis of UCM requires evaluation of its clinical priority. This is based on the relationship between the UCM and the presenting symptoms. The therapist should look for a link between the direction of UCM and the direction of symptom provocation: a) does the site of uncontrolled movement relate to the site or joint that the patient complains of as the source of symptoms? b) does the direction of movement or load testing relate to the direction or position of provocation of symptoms? *This identifies the clinical priorities.*

The site and direction of UCM at the cervical spine can be linked with different clinical presentations, postures and activities aggravating symptoms. The typical assessment findings in the cervical spine are identified in Table 6.2.

IDENTIFYING THE SITE AND DIRECTION OF UCM AT THE CERVICAL SPINE

The key principles for assessment and classification of UCM have previously been described in Chapter 3. All dissociation tests are performed

Table 6.1 Site and direction of UCM in the cervical spine			
	UPPER CERVICAL SPINE	**MID-CERVICAL SPINE**	**LOW CERVICAL SPINE**
Direction	• Extension • Flexion • Rotation/side-bend	• Extension • Rotation/side-bend	• Flexion • Rotation/side-bend

Table 6.2 The link between site and direction of UCM at the cervical spine and different clinical presentations

SITE AND DIRECTION OF UCM	CLINICAL EXAMPLES OF SYMPTOM/PRESENTATIONS	PROVOCATIVE MOVEMENTS, POSTURES AND ACTIVITIES
LOWER CERVICAL FLEXION Can present as: • uncontrolled translation at one segment or uncontrolled range of the cervicothoracic region into flexion (± hypermobile flexion range)	• Symptoms in low cervical spine, cervicothoracic region and posterior shoulder • ± Referral from myofascial, articular and neural structures • May present with segmental pain pattern	Symptoms provoked by flexion movements and postures (especially sustained); for example, reading, driving, office work, sustained sitting, bending forwards
UPPER CERVICAL EXTENSION Can present as: • uncontrolled translation at one segment or uncontrolled range of the cervicothoracic region into extension (± hypermobile extension range)	• Localised upper cervical pain • Headaches – referral to head and face • ± TMJ signs and symptoms • Often associated with thoracic outlet symptoms	Symptoms provoked with extension stress to upper cervical spine; for example, reading, driving, office work, sustained sitting, looking up, sustained extension
UPPER CERVICAL FLEXION Uncommon: • usually presents following a flexion based mechanism of injury; for example, fall from horse, dive into shallow water, whiplash into flexion or pathological instability (e.g. rheumatoid arthritis)	• Localised upper cervical pain • ± Signs and symptoms of upper cervical spine instability; for example, unilateral tongue anaesthesia, persistent/worsening non-radicular deep neck pain, dizziness	Symptoms often provoked by both flexion and extension activities and posture; for example, lifting the head up from supine lying, sustained rotation, sustained arm loading, looking down
MID-CERVICAL TRANSLATION (into EXTENSION) Can present as: • uncontrolled translation (shear) especially at C3–4–5, and uncontrolled range into extension (± hypermobile extension range)	• Localised mid-cervical pain • ± Referral (articular, myofascial, neural)	Symptoms provoked with extension stress to upper cervical spine; for example, reading, driving, office work, sustained sitting, looking up, sustained extension
ROTATION/SIDE-BEND ASYMMETRY (superimposed on any UCM above) Can present as: • uncontrolled rotation or uncontrolled side-bend in either the upper cervical spine or the mid/lower cervical spine. The rotation or side-bend UCM is usually more pronounced to either the right or left side	• Unilateral symptoms ± unilateral radiation • Symptom can be localised to the upper, the middle or the lower cervical regions • Coupled with any of the above (upper, mid- or low cervical spine) UCM	Unilateral symptoms provoked by movements or sustained postures away from the midline; for example, rotation or side-bend with symptoms usually worse in one direction more than another Unilateral symptoms provoked by either flexion or extension activities or sustained postures linked to the above UCM

with the cervical spine in the neutral training region.

Cervical spine neutral: positioning cervical, scapula and temporomandibular neutral

• Guideline to assess and reposition low cervical neutral

Position the mid–low cervical neutral line in neutral alignment by placing an appropriate thickness of folded towel behind the occiput so that the low cervical line is vertical in standing or sitting and horizontal in lying. It is acceptable for the low cervical neutral line to be positioned within 10° of vertical in standing/sitting or horizontal in lying (neutral ± 10° is within acceptable variability for a normal population distribution).

Generally, the occiput should be positioned about 1–2 cm forward of a line connecting the sacrum and thoracic kyphosis. That is, 1–2 cm forward of a wall in standing/sitting or 1–2 cm forward of the plinth in lying supine. The low cervical spine should not feel like it is at end-range extension. *If the thoracic kyphosis is flattened the occiput may rest on the wall in standing or sitting or on the plinth in lying. If the thoracic spine has an exaggerated kyphosis the occiput may be 3–5 cm away from the wall or the plinth.*

See Figure 6.2. Visualise a line across the upper neck (A), which follows the line of the jaw towards C2. Bisect this line (i). Visualise a second line across the lower neck (B), which follows the line of the clavicle towards the cervicothoracic junction. Bisect this line (ii). A line (C) that joins the bisectors (i) and (ii) ideally should be vertical in standing and sitting or horizontal in lying or within 10° of forward inclination.

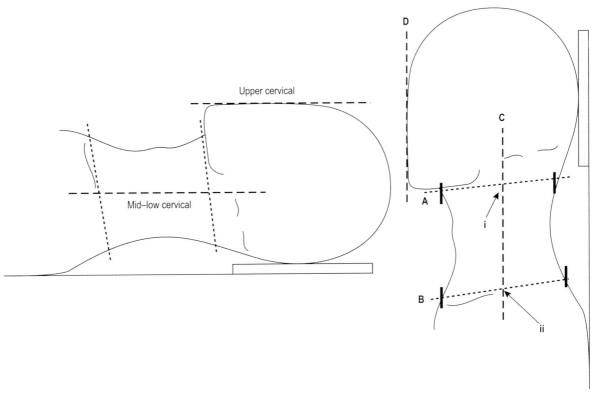

Figure 6.2 Guidelines for determining the upper and lower cervical neutral alignment (reproduced with permission of Comera Movement Science)

223

- **Guideline to assess and reposition upper cervical neutral**

Position the upper cervical neutral line parallel to the mid–low cervical neutral line. The upper cervical spine should not be in end-range flexion or 'chin tuck'.

See Figure 6.2. Visualise a line in the plane of the face (D). This line ideally should be parallel to or within 10° of the low cervical neutral line (C).

- **Guideline to assess and reposition scapula neutral**

Position the scapula midway between elevation and depression and let the scapula *relax* on the wall in standing or back towards the plinth in lying.

- **Guideline to assess and reposition temporomandibular joint (TMJ) neutral**

Place the tip of the tongue on the roof of the mouth behind the teeth and rest the tongue on the roof of the hard palate. Then allow the jaw to *relax* open. Ideally, the teeth should separate about 1 cm. Do not force the jaw open. Once the jaw is relaxed open, allow the tongue to rest naturally. Do not maintain the tongue held against the roof of the mouth as this provides increased distal fixation for the hyoids and encourages substitution from these cervical mobilisers.

The cervical spine neutral position needs to be observed with consideration of thoracic and lumbar postures in sitting, standing and functional positions as one region may influence another (Straker et al 2008). Cervical postural dysfunction is frequently most evident in sitting, but both sitting and standing will often demonstrate significant lumbopelvic alignment abnormalities, which may influence cervicothoracic alignment. Facilitation of lumbopelvic and thoracolumbar neutral alignment may well change cervical posture. It is important to consider the positions of symptom provocation in function.

Resting posture is individual, and people with restrictions may not present with an 'ideal' resting position. Instead, they present with a resting or 'natural' alignment that reflects how they have adapted to their restrictions. For example, if someone has a marked restriction of low cervical extension, they may develop a head forward posture as they adaptively find a mid-point within the available neutral region (somewhere midway between the ends of range). If the attempt to position the low cervical line in an 'ideal' neutral results in the low cervical joints being sustained at end range of the restricted extension, it then becomes necessary to reposition the low cervical spine within mid-range; preferably close to the neutral line. Box 6.1 illustrates some clinical pointers which may help the clinician achieve the neutral training position.

Box 6.1 Clinical pointers which may help the clinician achieve the neutral training position

- A plumb line from the ear lobe should drop just posterior to the clavicle (with the scapula in neutral). The plumb line falling on or forward of the clavicle indicates a forward head posture.
- Viewed from the side, the plane of the anterior neck and the line of the lower jaw should be distinctly different (i.e. not a continuous curve).
- Retracted chin posture (loss of normal lordosis) is often indicative of guarding or protective spasm.
- A mid-cervical crease, at rest, may be indicative of a mid-cervical translational pivot.
- A line from the mid-thoracic region to the sacrum should be slightly posterior to the back of the head (1–2 cm).
- When assessing asymmetry (rotation/lateral flexion) ask the person how a corrected neutral feels – if it feels 'odd' then an asymmetrical alignment is indicated.
- A flat multisegmental region between T2 and T6 may reflect a neural response, overactive or short rhomboids or serratus posterior superior indicative of poor scapular control, or stiff cervicothoracic segments, which are compensated for by increased thoracic extension.
- Check what influence correction of lumbopelvic alignment has on cervical posture.
- Neural sensitivity issues may influence postural alignment. There is usually an elevated shoulder girdle at rest.
- Alignment assessment should differentiate between upper cervical extension (chin poke) and mid-cervical extension (head back posture).
- Alignment assessment should differentiate between upper cervical extension (chin poke) or mid-cervical extension (head back posture) and head forward posture, although both often occur together.
- The mastoid, acromion and ischium should be in vertical alignment.

CERVICAL SPINE TESTS FOR UCM

Cervical flexion control

OBSERVATION AND ANALYSIS OF NECK FLEXION

Description of ideal pattern

While sitting tall with feet unsupported and the pelvis in neutral, the low and upper cervical spine is positioned in the neutral training region. The scapula and TMJ are also positioned in neutral. When instructed to flex the head forwards and look down towards the feet, a pattern of smooth and even cervicothoracic flexion should be observed with flattening (or slight flexion) at the upper and mid-cervical lordosis. There should be concurrent upper and lower cervical movement. The range should be such that the chin moves to within two finger-breadths of the sternum without compensation.

Movement faults associated with cervical flexion

In the assessment of flexion the UCM can be identified as either segmental or multisegmental. If only one spinous process is observed as prominent and protruding 'out of line' compared to the other vertebrae, then the UCM is interpreted as a *segmental flexion hinge*. The specific hinging segment should be noted and recorded. If, on the other hand, excessive cervicothoracic flexion is observed, but no one particular spinous process is prominent from the adjacent vertebrae, then the UCM is interpreted as a *multisegmental hyperflexion*.

Relative stiffness (restrictions)

- *Restriction of upper or mid-cervical flexion* – the upper/mid-cervical spine maintains the lordosis during flexion. At the end of neck flexion range the cervical lordosis does not flatten or reverse. The restriction may be due to a loss of articular motion or due to a loss of extensibility of myofascial structures. Cervical flexion joint mobility can be tested passively, and passive manual examination will identify any significant articular restriction of segmental flexion range of motion. Posterior myofascial restrictions of flexion can be tested with passive extensibility of the suboccipital extensors, sternocleidomastoid, splenius capitis, levator scapula and the ligamentum nuchae.
- *Restriction of thoracic flexion* – mid- and upper thoracic flexion restriction are not so common, but if present they are easily tested.

Relative flexibility (potential UCM)

- *Cervicothoracic flexion* – the low cervical spine may initiate the movement into flexion; or, during the return to neutral, the head may stay in a head forward position. The posture resulting from this is often described as a cervicothoracic bump or dowager's hump and may be observed as excessive protuberance or 'step' of C6–T1 spinous processes.
- *Upper cervical flexion* – this is uncommon but is usually associated with a traumatic forced flexion incident (requires assessment of upper cervical instability).

Asymmetry

- Asymmetry may be a feature with UCM into rotation and side-bending. If deviation into rotation or side-bending is noted on sagittal plane tests of flexion or extension control, detailed evaluation of rotation or side-bending control tests should be independently assessed.

Tests of low cervical flexion control

T29 OCCIPUT LIFT TEST – NODDING (tests for low cervical flexion UCM)

This dissociation test assesses the ability to actively dissociate and control low cervical flexion and move the upper cervical spine into flexion.

Test procedure

The person sits tall with their feet unsupported and the pelvis in neutral. The low and upper cervical spine is positioned in the neutral training region. The scapula and TMJ are also positioned in neutral (Figure 6.3). Without letting the head move forwards, the person is instructed to lift the chin into partial upper cervical extension and then to independently flex the upper cervical spine by visualising sliding the occiput vertically up an imaginary wall placed at the back of the head. This should be a nodding action (through a transverse axis of the upper cervical spine, not a chin tuck or retraction action). There should be no low cervical flexion (head moving forwards) or loss of scapula position (observe for scapula elevation, forward tilt or downward rotation). The jaw should stay relaxed (Figure 6.4). Ideally, the person should be able to easily maintain the low cervical spine neutral alignment and prevent the head moving forwards while actively moving the upper cervical spine through range from extension to flexion (chin lift to chin drop) by using a 'nodding' action of the head.

While teaching, allow the person to initially learn and practise the test movement using feedback from a wall or the therapist's hand. Keep the occiput in contact with a supporting surface to monitor and control the low cervical neutral

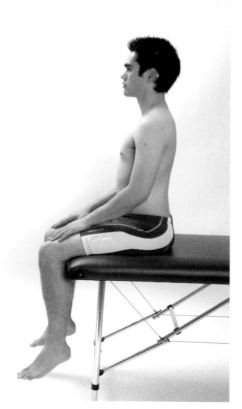

Figure 6.3 Start position occiput lift test

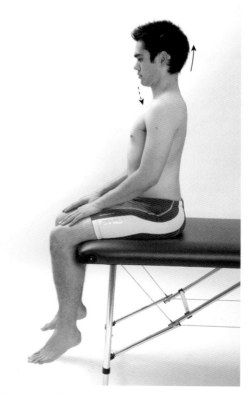

Figure 6.4 Benchmark occiput lift test

position until awareness of the correct movement is achieved. The therapist should monitor the control of the low cervical neutral position. Scapula control is important. It may be necessary to unload the neural and myofascial structures by supporting the scapula in upward rotation. If the upper cervical spine has concurrent UCM, only move the upper cervical spine from neutral to flexion (no extension) to avoid provoking upper cervical symptoms.

Low cervical flexion UCM

The person complains of flexion-related symptoms at the cervicothoracic region. The low cervical spine has greater movement into flexion than the upper cervical segments under flexion load. During active upper cervical flexion, the cervicothoracic region demonstrates uncontrolled low cervical flexion. During the attempt to dissociate the low cervical spine from independent upper cervical flexion, the person either cannot control the movement or has to concentrate and try too hard.

- If only one spinous process is observed as prominent and protruding 'out of line' compared to the other vertebrae, then the UCM is interpreted as a *segmental flexion hinge*. The specific hinging segment should be noted and recorded.
- If excessive cervicothoracic flexion is observed, but no one particular spinous process is prominent from the adjacent vertebrae, then the UCM is interpreted as a *multisegmental hyperflexion*.

Clinical assessment note for direction-specific motor control testing:

If some other movement (e.g. a small amount of cervical rotation) is observed during a motor control (dissociation) test of low cervical flexion, *do not* score this as uncontrolled low cervical flexion. The cervical rotation motor control tests will identify if the observed unrelated movement is uncontrolled. *A test for low cervical flexion UCM is only positive if uncontrolled low cervical **flexion** is demonstrated.*

Rating and diagnosis of cervical flexion UCM

(T29.1 and T29.2)

Correction

Initially, position the lower and upper cervical spine in neutral with the head supported. This can be done in sitting or standing with the thoracic spine and the back of the head against a wall (Figure 6.5). Using the feedback and support of the supporting surface, the person is trained to perform independent upper cervical flexion (nodding). The upper cervical spine can flex only so far as there is no low cervical flexion and the scapulae and TMJ do not lose their neutral position. If control is poor, start in supine lying with the occiput supported on a small folded towel (Figure 6.6). Initially the scapula may need to be supported. As the ability to control upper cervical extension gets easier and the pattern of dissociation feels less unnatural the exercise can be progressed from head and shoulder girdle supported to head and shoulder girdle unsupported postures.

A useful progression is performed standing with the forearms vertical on a wall. Keep the scapula in mid-position and push the body and head away from the wall (Figure 6.7). Keeping the head back over the shoulders slowly perform independent upper cervical flexion (nodding) (Figure 6.8). The upper cervical spine can flex only so far as there is no low cervical flexion and the scapulae do not lose their neutral position.

The person should self-monitor the control of low cervical flexion UCM with a variety of feedback options (T29.3). There should be no provocation of any symptoms within the range that the flexion UCM can be controlled.

Once the pattern of dissociation feels familiar it should be integrated into various functional postures and positions. T29.4 illustrates some retraining options.

227

T29.1 Assessment and rating of low threshold recruitment efficiency of the Occiput Lift Test

RATING AND DIAGNOSIS OF CERVICAL FLEXION UCM OCCIPUT LIFT TEST – NODDING

ASSESSMENT

Control point:
- prevent low cervical flexion

Movement challenge: upper cervical flexion (nodding) (sitting)

Benchmark range: plane of the face inclines past vertical

RATING OF LOW THRESHOLD RECRUITMENT EFFICIENCY FOR CONTROL OF DIRECTION

	✓ or ✗		✓ or ✗
• Able to prevent UCM into the test direction Correct dissociation pattern of movement Prevent low cervical (cervicothoracic) UCM into: • flexion (multisegmental) • flexion (single segment) and move upper cervical flexion	☐	• Looks easy, and in the opinion of the assessor, is performed with confidence	☐
		• Feels easy, and the subject has sufficient awareness of the movement pattern that they confidently prevent UCM into the test direction	☐
• Dissociate movement through the benchmark range of: plane of face inclines forwards past vertical *If there is more available range than the benchmark standard, only the benchmark range needs to be actively controlled*	☐	• The pattern of dissociation is smooth during concentric and eccentric movement	☐
		• Does not (consistently) use *end-range* movement into the opposite direction to prevent the UCM	☐
• Without holding breath (though it is acceptable to use an alternate breathing strategy)	☐	• No extra feedback needed *(tactile, visual or verbal cueing)*	☐
		• Without external support or unloading	☐
• Control during eccentric phase	☐	• Relaxed natural breathing *(even if not ideal – so long as natural pattern does not change)*	☐
• Control during concentric phase	☐	• No fatigue	☐

CORRECT DISSOCIATION PATTERN **RECRUITMENT EFFICIENCY**

T29.2 Diagnosis of the site and direction of UCM from the Occiput lift test

OCCIPUT LIFT TEST – NODDING

Site	Direction	Segmental/multisegmental	
Low cervical	Flexion	Segmental flexion hinge (indicate level)	☐
		Multisegmental hyperflexion	☐

T29.3 Feedback tools to monitor retraining

FEEDBACK TOOL	PROCESS
Self-palpation	Palpation monitoring of joint position
Visual observation	Observe in a mirror or directly watch the movement
Adhesive tape	Skin tension for tactile feedback
Cueing and verbal correction	Listen to feedback from another observer

---

T29.4 Functional positions for retraining low cervical flexion control

- Sitting
- Standing
- Supine (bias anterior muscles)
- Recline sitting backwards (bias anterior muscles)
- Side-lying
- Prone (bias posterior muscles)
- 4 point kneeling (bias posterior muscles)
- Incline sitting forwards (bias posterior muscles)
- Standing forward lean (bias posterior muscles)
- Functional activities

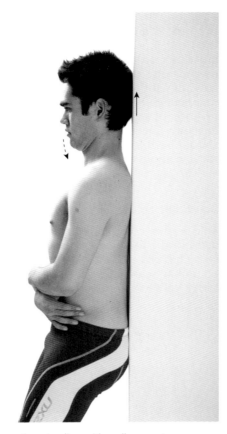

Figure 6.5 Correction standing with wall support

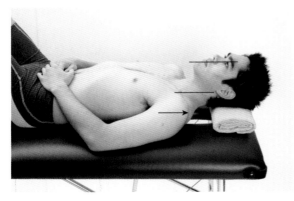

Figure 6.6 Correction supine with folded towel

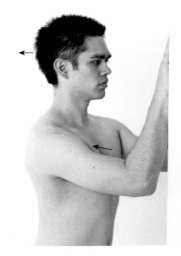

Figure 6.7 Progression: hands on wall, head unsupported low cervical control – start position

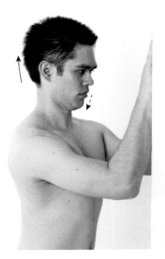

Figure 6.8 Progression: hands on wall, head unsupported – correction

T30 THORACIC FLEXION TEST (tests for low cervical flexion UCM)

This dissociation test assesses the ability to actively dissociate and control low cervical flexion and move the thoracic spine into flexion.

Test procedure

The person should have the ability to actively flex the thoracic spine while controlling low cervical and head neutral. The person sits tall with feet unsupported and pelvis neutral. The low and upper cervical spine is positioned in the neutral training region. The scapula and TMJ are also positioned in neutral. The plane of the face should be vertical (Figure 6.9). Thoracolumbar motion is monitored by placing one hand on the sternum and head and cervical motion

monitored by placing the thumb on the jaw and the middle finger on the forehead. Without letting the head move forwards or down (monitor jaw and forehead) allow the sternum to lower (drop) towards the pelvis. Ideally, the person should have the ability to keep the head neutral while independently flexing the thoracic region from a position of extension through to flexion, without any movement of the head. Ideally, the person should be able to perform this dissociated movement without feedback from their hands (Figure 6.10).

Low cervical flexion UCM

The person complains of flexion-related symptoms in the low cervical region. The low cervical spine has greater give into flexion than the thoracolumbar segments under flexion load. During active thoracic flexion, the low cervical region

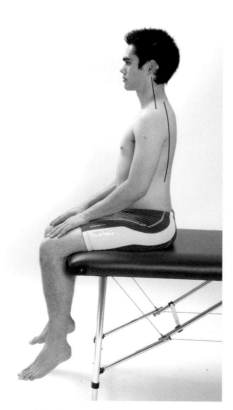

Figure 6.9 Start position thoracic flexion test

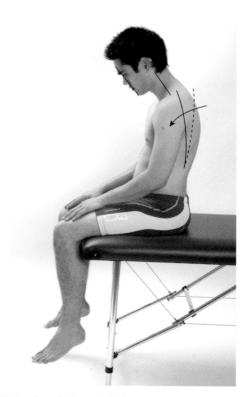

Figure 6.10 Benchmark thoracic flexion test

gives excessively into flexion. During the attempt to dissociate the low cervical spine from independent thoracic flexion, the person either cannot control the UCM or has to concentrate and try too hard.

- If only one spinous process is observed as prominent and protruding 'out of line' compared to the other vertebrae, then the UCM is interpreted as a *segmental flexion hinge*. The specific hinging segment should be noted and recorded.
- If excessive cervicothoracic flexion is observed, but no one particular spinous process is prominent from the adjacent vertebrae, then the UCM is interpreted as a *multisegmental hyperflexion*.

Clinical assessment note for direction-specific motor control testing

If some other movement (e.g. a small amount of cervical rotation) is observed during a motor control (dissociation) test of low cervical flexion, *do not* score this as uncontrolled low cervical flexion. The cervical rotation motor control tests will identify if the observed unrelated movement is uncontrolled. *A test for low cervical flexion UCM is only positive if uncontrolled low cervical* **flexion** *is demonstrated.*

Rating and diagnosis of cervical flexion UCM

(T30.1 and T30.2)

Correction

The person sits tall with feet unsupported and pelvis neutral. The low and upper cervical spine is positioned in the neutral training region. The scapula and TMJ are also positioned in neutral. The plane of the face should be vertical. Monitor thoracolumbar motion by placing one hand on the sternum. Monitor head and cervical motion by placing the thumb on the jaw and the middle finger on the forehead. Without letting the head move forwards or down (monitor jaw and forehead) allow the sternum to lower (drop) towards the pelvis. Ideally, the person should have the ability to keep the head neutral while independently flexing the thoracic region from a position of extension through to flexion, without any movement of the head. As the ability to independently control movement of the low cervical spine gets easier and the pattern of dissociation feels less unnatural, the exercise can be progressed to performing the exercise without palpation feedback.

The person should self-monitor the control of low cervical flexion UCM with a variety of feedback options (T30.3). There should be no provocation of any symptoms within the range that the flexion UCM can be controlled.

Once the pattern of dissociation feels familiar it should be integrated into various functional postures and positions. T30.4 illustrates some retraining options.

T30.1 Assessment and rating of low threshold recruitment efficiency of the Thoracic Flexion Test

THORACIC FLEXION TEST

ASSESSMENT

Control point:
- prevent low cervical flexion

Movement challenge: thoracic flexion (sitting)

Benchmark range: full end range of independent thoracic flexion

RATING OF LOW THRESHOLD RECRUITMENT EFFICIENCY FOR CONTROL OF DIRECTION

	✓ or ✗		✓ or ✗
• Able to prevent UCM into the test direction Correct dissociation pattern of movement Prevent low cervical (cervicothoracic) UCM into: • flexion (multisegmental) • flexion (single segment) and move thoracic flexion	☐	• Looks easy, and in the opinion of the assessor, is performed with confidence	☐
		• Feels easy, and the subject has sufficient awareness of the movement pattern that they confidently prevent UCM into the test direction	☐
• Dissociate movement through the benchmark range of: full end range of independent thoracic flexion *If there is more available range than the benchmark standard, only the benchmark range needs to be actively controlled*	☐	• The pattern of dissociation is smooth during concentric and eccentric movement	☐
		• Does not (consistently) use *end-range* movement into the opposite direction to prevent the UCM	☐
• Without holding breath (though it is acceptable to use an alternate breathing strategy)	☐	• No extra feedback needed *(tactile, visual or verbal cueing)*	☐
		• Without external support or unloading	☐
• Control during eccentric phase	☐	• Relaxed natural breathing *(even if not ideal – so long as natural pattern does not change)*	☐
• Control during concentric phase	☐	• No fatigue	☐

CORRECT DISSOCIATION PATTERN   **RECRUITMENT EFFICIENCY**

T30.2 Diagnosis of the site and direction of UCM from the Thoracic Flexion Test

THORACIC FLEXION TEST

Site	Direction	Segmental/multisegmental	
Low cervical	Flexion	Segmental flexion hinge (indicate level)	☐
		Multisegmental hyperflexion	☐

T30.3 Feedback tools to monitor retraining

FEEDBACK TOOL	PROCESS
Self-palpation	Palpation monitoring of joint position
Visual observation	Observe in a mirror or directly watch the movement
Adhesive tape	Skin tension for tactile feedback
Cueing and verbal correction	Listen to feedback from another observer

---

T30.4 Functional positions for retraining low cervical flexion control

- Sitting
- Supine (bias anterior muscles)
- Recline sitting backwards (bias anterior muscles)
- Side-lying
- Prone (bias posterior muscles)
- 4 point kneeling (bias posterior muscles)
- Incline sitting forwards (bias posterior muscles)
- Functional activities

T31 OVERHEAD ARM LIFT TEST
(tests for low cervical flexion UCM)

This dissociation test assesses the ability to actively dissociate and control low cervical flexion and move the shoulders through overhead flexion.

Test procedure

The person should have the ability to actively perform shoulder flexion through full range to the overhead position while concurrently controlling low cervical spine and head neutral. The person stands with the arms resting by the side in neutral rotation (palm in) and with the scapula in a neutral position. The low and upper cervical spine is positioned in the neutral training region. The scapula and TMJ are also positioned in neutral. The plane of the face should be vertical (Figure 6.11).

Without letting the head move forwards or look down, the person is instructed to keep the low cervical spine and the head in the neutral position and lift both arms overhead, through full 180° of shoulder flexion, and lower the arms back to the side. The neutral arm rotation (palm in) should be maintained. Ideally, the person should have the ability to keep the head neutral while independently flexing the shoulders and lifting the arms to a vertical overhead position (180° flexion) and lowering them back to the side (Figure 6.12).

Low cervical flexion UCM

The person complains of flexion-related symptoms in the low cervical region. The low cervical spine has greater give into flexion than the shoulder girdle under arm flexion load. During active shoulder flexion, the low cervical region gives excessively into flexion. During the attempt to dissociate the low cervical spine from independent shoulder flexion, the person either cannot control the UCM or has to concentrate and try too hard.

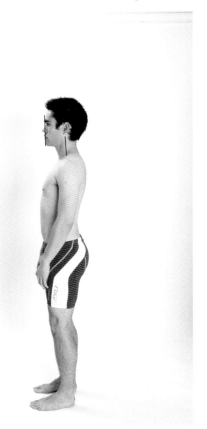

Figure 6.11 Start position overhead arm lift test

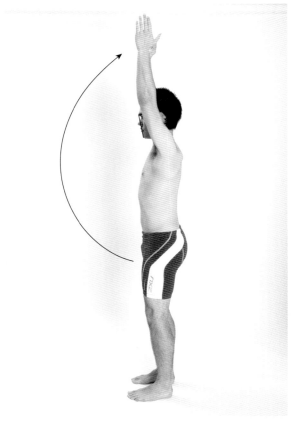

Figure 6.12 Benchmark overhead arm lift test

- If only one spinous process is observed as prominent and protruding 'out of line' compared to the other vertebrae, then the UCM is interpreted as a *segmental flexion hinge*. The specific hinging segment should be noted and recorded.
- If excessive cervicothoracic flexion is observed, but no one particular spinous process is prominent from the adjacent vertebrae, then the UCM is interpreted as a *multisegmental hyperflexion*.

Clinical assessment note for direction-specific motor control testing

If some other movement (e.g. a small amount of cervical rotation) is observed during a motor control (dissociation) test of low cervical flexion, *do not* score this as uncontrolled low cervical flexion. The cervical rotation motor control tests will identify if the observed unrelated movement is uncontrolled. *A test for low cervical flexion UCM is only positive if uncontrolled low cervical **flexion** is demonstrated.*

Rating and diagnosis of cervical flexion UCM

(T31.1 and T31.2)

Correction

The person stands with the arms resting by the side in neutral rotation (palm in) and with the scapula in a neutral position. The low and upper cervical spine is positioned in the neutral training region. The scapula and TMJ are also positioned in neutral. The plane of the face should be vertical.

Without letting the head move forwards or look down, lift both arms to a vertical overhead position (180° shoulder flexion). The person should keep the head neutral while independently flexing the shoulder. If control is poor, stand with the head and thoracic spine supported against a wall for feedback and support. Start doing unilateral arm lifts (Figure 6.13) and progress to bilateral

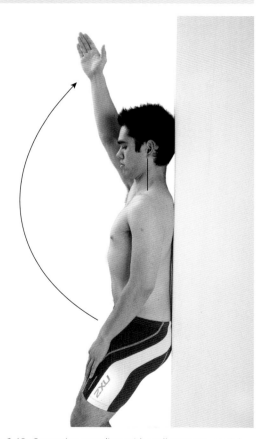

Figure 6.13 Correction standing with wall support, partial range

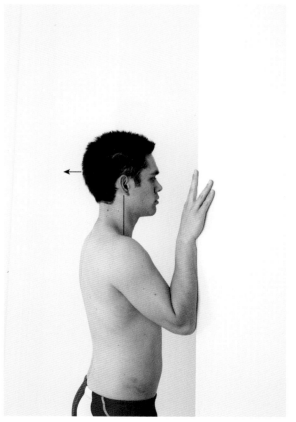

Figure 6.14 Progression: forearms on wall – low cervical control start position

arm lifts as control improves. Initially reduce the arm load by lifting a short lever (elbow bent) and only through reduced range (e.g. 90° then 120°, etc.). As the ability to independently control movement of the low cervical spine gets easier and the pattern of dissociation feels less unnatural, the exercise can be progressed to performing the exercise to long lever full overhead range against light resistance.

An alternative progression is to face the wall with the forearms vertical on the wall. Keep the scapula in mid-position and push the body and head away from the wall (Figure 6.14). Keeping the head back over the shoulders, slowly slide one forearm vertically up the wall (Figures 6.15 and 6.16) only so far as there is no low cervical flexion.

The person should self-monitor the control of low cervical flexion UCM with a variety of feedback options (T31.3). There should be no provocation of any symptoms within the range that the flexion UCM can be controlled.

Once the pattern of dissociation feels familiar it should be integrated into various functional postures and positions. T31.4 illustrates some retraining options.

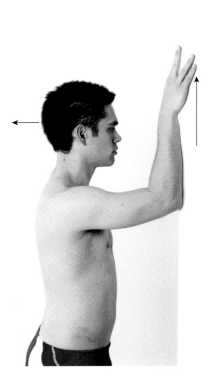

Figure 6.15 Progression: forearm wall slide – 90°

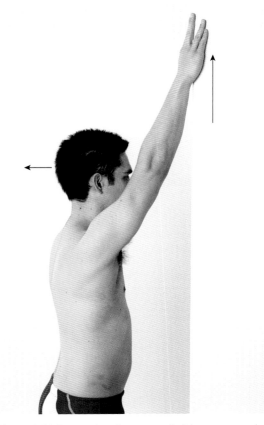

Figure 6.16 Progression: forearm wall slide – arms overhead

T31.1 Assessment and rating of low threshold recruitment efficiency of the Overhead Arm Lift Test

OVERHEAD ARM LIFT TEST

ASSESSMENT

Control point:
• prevent low cervical flexion
Movement challenge: shoulder flexion (standing)
Benchmark range: 180° bilateral shoulder flexion (vertical overhead)

RATING OF LOW THRESHOLD RECRUITMENT EFFICIENCY FOR CONTROL OF DIRECTION

	✓ or ✗		✓ or ✗
• Able to prevent UCM into the test direction Correct dissociation pattern of movement Prevent low cervical (cervicothoracic) UCM into: • flexion (multisegmental) • flexion (single segment) and move shoulder flexion	☐	• Looks easy, and in the opinion of the assessor, is performed with confidence	☐
		• Feels easy, and the subject has sufficient awareness of the movement pattern that they confidently prevent UCM into the test direction	☐
• Dissociate movement through the benchmark range of: 180° bilateral shoulder flexion (arms vertical overhead) *If there is more available range than the benchmark standard, only the benchmark range needs to be actively controlled*	☐	• The pattern of dissociation is smooth during concentric and eccentric movement	☐
		• Does not (consistently) use *end-range* movement into the opposite direction to prevent the UCM	☐
• Without holding breath (though it is acceptable to use an alternate breathing strategy)	☐	• No extra feedback needed *(tactile, visual or verbal cueing)*	☐
		• Without external support or unloading	☐
• Control during eccentric phase	☐	• Relaxed natural breathing *(even if not ideal – so long as natural pattern does not change)*	☐
• Control during concentric phase	☐	• No fatigue	☐

CORRECT DISSOCIATION PATTERN   **RECRUITMENT EFFICIENCY**

T31.2 Diagnosis of the site and direction of UCM from the Overhead Arm Lift Test

OVERHEAD ARM LIFT TEST

Site	Direction	Segmental/multisegmental	
Low cervical	Flexion	Segmental flexion hinge (indicate level)	☐
		Multisegmental hyperflexion	☐

T31.3 Feedback tools to monitor retraining

FEEDBACK TOOL	PROCESS
Self-palpation	Palpation monitoring of joint position
Visual observation	Observe in a mirror or directly watch the movement
Adhesive tape	Skin tension for tactile feedback
Cueing and verbal correction	Listen to feedback from another observer

---

T31.4 Functional positions for retraining low cervical flexion control

• Sitting
• Standing
• Supine (bias anterior muscles)
• Recline sitting backwards (bias anterior muscles)

• Prone (bias posterior muscles)
• 4 point kneeling (bias posterior muscles)
• Incline sitting forwards (bias posterior muscles)
• Functional activities

Test of upper cervical flexion control

T32 FORWARD HEAD LEAN TEST (tests for upper cervical flexion UCM)

This dissociation test assesses the ability to actively dissociate and control upper cervical flexion and move the low cervical spine into flexion.

Test procedure

The person sits tall with feet unsupported and pelvis neutral. The low and upper cervical spine is positioned in the neutral training region. The scapula and TMJ are also positioned in neutral (Figure 6.17). The therapist monitors the upper cervical neutral position by palpating the occiput with one finger and palpating the C2 spinous process with another finger (Figure 6.19). During testing, if the palpating fingers do not move, the upper cervical segments are able to maintain neutral. If the palpating fingers move apart, uncontrolled upper cervical flexion is identified.

Without letting chin drop or tuck in, the person is instructed to move the low cervical spine through flexion by tilting the head to lean forwards from the base of the neck. The person is to only move through the range where the ability to control the upper cervical spine is effective (Figure 6.18). There should be no upper cervical flexion (palpating fingers move apart or chin drop or tuck is observed) or loss of scapula

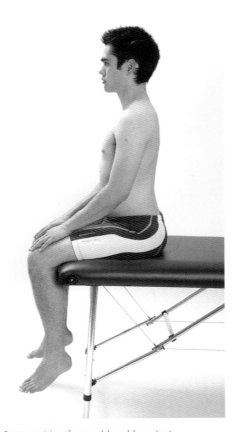

Figure 6.17 Start position forward head lean test

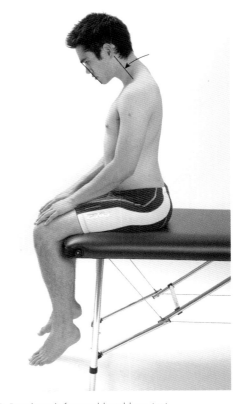

Figure 6.18 Benchmark forward head lean test

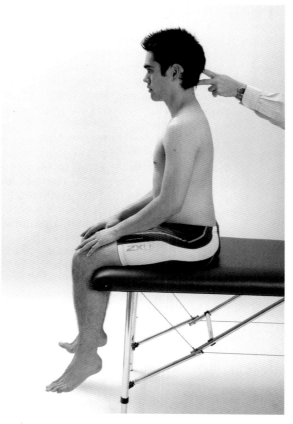

Figure 6.19 Therapist palpating for upper cervical movement

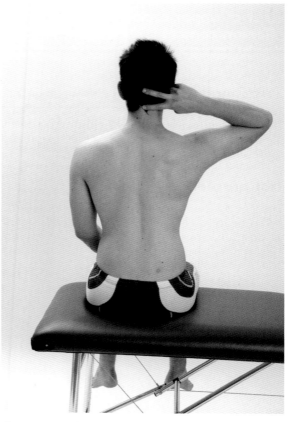

Figure 6.20 Self-palpation for teaching and training

position (especially observe for scapula elevation, retraction or forward tilt). The jaw should stay relaxed.

Ideally, the person should be able to easily prevent the chin from tucking or dropping and maintain the upper cervical spine neutral (palpating fingers do not move apart) while independently moving the lower cervical spine through range from extension to flexion (head starts upright and leans forwards).

While teaching, allow the person to initially learn and practise the test movement using feedback from palpation with their own fingers to monitor and control the upper cervical neutral position until awareness of the correct movement is achieved (Figure 6.20).

Upper cervical flexion UCM

The person complains of flexion-related symptoms in the upper cervical spine region. The upper cervical spine has greater give *into flexion* than the lower cervical spine under flexion load. During active lower cervical flexion, the upper cervical gives excessively into *segmental flexion and translational shear*. This uncontrolled flexion can occur at the C0–1, the C1–2, or the C2–3 segmental levels. Segmental laxity can be confirmed with manual articular assessment or upper cervical ligamentous stability tests. During the attempt to dissociate the upper cervical spine from independent lower cervical flexion, the person either cannot control the UCM or has to concentrate and try too hard.

- If only one spinous process is observed as prominent and protruding 'out of line' compared to the other vertebrae, then the UCM is interpreted as a *segmental flexion hinge*. The specific hinging segment should be noted and recorded.
- If excessive cervicothoracic flexion is observed, but no one particular spinous process is prominent from the adjacent vertebrae, then the UCM is interpreted as a *multisegmental hyperflexion*.

Clinical assessment note for direction-specific motor control testing

If some other movement (e.g. a small amount of cervical rotation) is observed during a motor control (dissociation) test of upper cervical flexion, *do not* score this as uncontrolled upper cervical flexion. The cervical rotation motor control tests will identify if the observed unrelated movement is uncontrolled. *A test for upper cervical flexion UCM is only positive if uncontrolled upper cervical* **flexion** *is demonstrated*.

Rating and diagnosis of cervical flexion UCM

(T32.1 and T32.2)

Correction

Initially, in sitting or standing, the thoracic spine and the back of the head should be supported upright against a wall. The low cervical spine is in slight extension. The upper cervical spine is positioned in neutral by actively lifting and dropping the chin through the full range of upper cervical movement, then positioning in the middle of this range. Ideally, the plane of the face should incline forwards about 45° (Figure 6.21). Using feedback from palpating the occiput with one finger and C2 with another finger, the person is trained to perform independent lower cervical flexion.

The person should prevent the chin from tucking or dropping and maintain the upper cervical spine neutral (palpating fingers do not move apart) while independently moving the lower cervical spine through range from extension to flexion (head starts upright and leans forwards). The lower cervical spine can flex and the head leans forwards from the base of the neck only so far as there is no upper cervical flexion and the scapula and TMJ do not lose their neutral position. As the ability to control upper cervical extension gets easier and the pattern of dissociation feels less unnatural, the exercise can be progressed from head and shoulder girdle supported to head and shoulder girdle unsupported postures (Figure 6.22).

The person should self-monitor the control of low cervical flexion UCM with a variety of feedback options (T32.3). There should be no provocation of any symptoms within the range that the flexion UCM can be controlled.

Once the pattern of dissociation feels familiar it should be integrated into various functional postures and positions. T32.4 illustrates some retraining options.

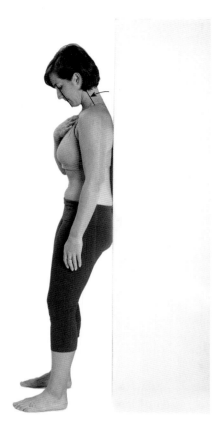

Figure 6.21 Correction standing with wall support

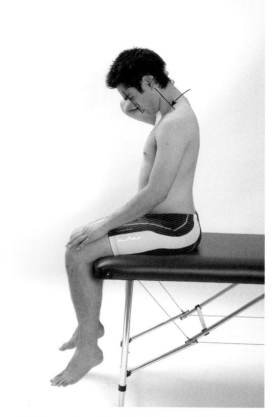

Figure 6.22 Correction with self-palpation and head unsupported

T32.1 Assessment and rating of low threshold recruitment efficiency of the Forward Head Lean Test

FORWARD HEAD LEAN TEST

ASSESSMENT

Control point:
- prevent upper cervical flexion

Movement challenge: low cervical flexion (sitting)

Benchmark range: plane of the face inclines past 45°

RATING OF LOW THRESHOLD RECRUITMENT EFFICIENCY FOR CONTROL OF DIRECTION

	✓ or ✗		✓ or ✗
• Able to prevent UCM into the test direction Correct dissociation pattern of movement Prevent upper cervical UCM into: • flexion (multisegmental) • flexion (single segment) and move low cervical flexion	☐	• Looks easy, and in the opinion of the assessor, is performed with confidence	☐
		• Feels easy, and the subject has sufficient awareness of the movement pattern that they confidently prevent UCM into the test direction	☐
• Dissociate movement through the benchmark range of: plane of face inclines forwards past 45° *If there is more available range than the benchmark standard, only the benchmark range needs to be actively controlled*	☐	• The pattern of dissociation is smooth during concentric and eccentric movement	☐
		• Does not (consistently) use *end-range* movement into the opposite direction to prevent the UCM	☐
• Without holding breath (though it is acceptable to use an alternate breathing strategy)	☐	• No extra feedback needed *(tactile, visual or verbal cueing)*	☐
		• Without external support or unloading	☐
• Control during eccentric phase	☐	• Relaxed natural breathing *(even if not ideal – so long as natural pattern does not change)*	☐
• Control during concentric phase	☐	• No fatigue	☐

CORRECT DISSOCIATION PATTERN   **RECRUITMENT EFFICIENCY**

T32.2 Diagnosis of the site and direction of UCM from the Forward Head Lean Test

FORWARD HEAD LEAN TEST

Site	Direction	Segmental/multisegmental	
Upper cervical	Flexion	Segmental flexion hinge (indicate level)	☐
		Multisegmental hyperflexion	☐

T32.3 Feedback tools to monitor retraining

FEEDBACK TOOL	PROCESS
Self-palpation	Palpation monitoring of joint position
Visual observation	Observe in a mirror or directly watch the movement
Cueing and verbal correction	Listen to feedback from another observer

---

T32.4 Functional positions for retraining upper cervical flexion control

- Sitting
- Standing
- Recline sitting backwards (bias anterior muscles)

- 4 point kneeling (bias posterior muscles)
- Incline sitting forwards (bias posterior muscles)
- Standing forward lean (bias posterior muscles)
- Functional activities

T33 ARM EXTENSION TEST
(tests for upper cervical flexion UCM)

This dissociation test assesses the ability to actively dissociate and control upper cervical flexion/head retraction and move the shoulders through extension.

Test procedure

The person should have the ability to actively perform shoulder extension through full range while concurrently controlling cervical spine and head neutral. The person stands with the arms resting by the side in neutral rotation (palm in) and with the scapula in a neutral position. The low and upper cervical spine is positioned in the neutral training region. The scapula and TMJ are also positioned in neutral. The plane of the face should be vertical (Figure 6.23).

Without letting the chin tuck in towards the neck, or the scapula tilting forwards or retracting, the person is instructed to keep the cervical spine and the head in the neutral position and reach back with both arms, through 15–20° of shoulder extension. The neutral arm rotation (palm in) should be maintained. Ideally, the person should have the ability to keep the head and scapulae neutral while independently extending the shoulders and reaching back with the arms to end range (Figure 6.24).

Upper cervical flexion UCM

The person complains of flexion-related symptoms in the upper cervical region. The upper cervical spine has greater give into flexion than the shoulder girdle under arm extension load. During active shoulder extension, the upper cervical region gives excessively into flexion or head retraction. During the attempt to dissociate

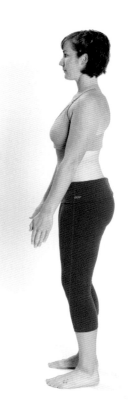

Figure 6.23 Start position arm extension test

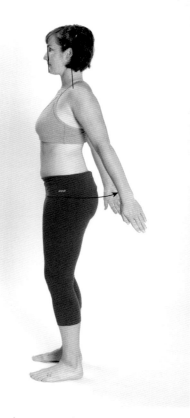

Figure 6.24 Benchmark arm extension test

the upper cervical spine from independent shoulder extension, the person either cannot control the UCM or has to concentrate and try too hard.

- If only one spinous process is observed as prominent and protruding 'out of line' compared to the other vertebrae, then the UCM is interpreted as a *segmental flexion hinge*. The specific hinging segment should be noted and recorded.
- If excessive cervicothoracic flexion is observed, but no one particular spinous process is prominent from the adjacent vertebrae, then the UCM is interpreted as a *multisegmental hyperflexion*.

Clinical assessment note for direction-specific motor control testing

If some other movement (e.g. a small amount of cervical rotation) is observed during a motor control (dissociation) test of upper cervical flexion, *do not* score this as uncontrolled upper cervical flexion. The cervical rotation motor control tests will identify if the observed unrelated movement is uncontrolled. *A test for upper cervical flexion UCM is only positive if uncontrolled upper cervical* **flexion** *is demonstrated.*

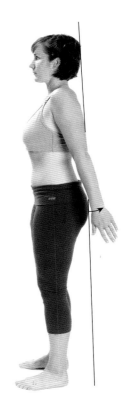

Figure 6.25 Correction unilateral arm extension

Rating and diagnosis of cervical flexion UCM

(T33.1 and T33.2)

Correction

The person stands with the arm resting by the side in neutral rotation (palm in) and with the scapula in a neutral position. The low and upper cervical spine is positioned in the neutral training region. The scapula and TMJ are also positioned in neutral. The plane of the face should be vertical.

Without letting the chin tuck in towards the neck, or the scapula tilting forwards or retracting, the person is instructed to keep the cervical spine and the head in the neutral position and reach back with both arms, through 15–20° of shoulder extension. The person should keep the head neutral while independently extending the shoulder. If control is poor, stand with the head and thoracic spine supported against a wall for feedback and support. Start doing unilateral arm extension (Figure 6.25) and progress to bilateral arm extension as control improves. Initially, reduce the arm load by lifting a short lever (elbow bent) and only through reduced range (e.g. 5° then 10°, etc.). As the ability to independently control movement of the upper and low cervical spine gets easier and the pattern of dissociation feels less unnatural, the exercise can be progressed to performing the exercise to long lever full range against light resistance.

The person should self-monitor the control of low cervical flexion UCM with a variety of feedback options (T33.3). There should be no provocation of any symptoms within the range that the flexion UCM can be controlled.

Once the pattern of dissociation feels familiar it should be integrated into various functional postures and positions. T33.4 illustrates some retraining options.

T33.1 Assessment and rating of low threshold recruitment efficiency of the Arm Extension Test

ARM EXTENSION TEST

ASSESSMENT

Control point:
- prevent upper cervical flexion and head retraction

Movement challenge: shoulder extension (standing)

Benchmark range: 15–20° bilateral shoulder extension

RATING OF LOW THRESHOLD RECRUITMENT EFFICIENCY FOR CONTROL OF DIRECTION

	✓ or ✗		✓ or ✗
• Able to prevent UCM into the test direction Correct dissociation pattern of movement Prevent upper cervical UCM into: • flexion (multisegmental) • flexion (single segment) and move shoulder extension	☐	• Looks easy, and in the opinion of the assessor, is performed with confidence	☐
		• Feels easy, and the subject has sufficient awareness of the movement pattern that they confidently prevent UCM into the test direction	☐
• Dissociate movement through the benchmark range of: 15–20° bilateral shoulder extension *If there is more available range than the benchmark standard, only the benchmark range needs to be actively controlled*	☐	• The pattern of dissociation is smooth during concentric and eccentric movement	☐
		• Does not (consistently) use *end-range* movement into the opposite direction to prevent the UCM	☐
• Without holding breath (though it is acceptable to use an alternate breathing strategy)	☐	• No extra feedback needed *(tactile, visual or verbal cueing)*	☐
		• Without external support or unloading	☐
• Control during eccentric phase	☐	• Relaxed natural breathing *(even if not ideal – so long as natural pattern does not change)*	☐
• Control during concentric phase	☐	• No fatigue	☐

CORRECT DISSOCIATION PATTERN | **RECRUITMENT EFFICIENCY**

T33.2 Diagnosis of the site and direction of UCM from the Arm Extension Test

ARM EXTENSION TEST

Site	Direction	Segmental/ multisegmental	
Upper cervical	Flexion	Segmental flexion hinge (indicate level)	☐
		Multisegmental hyperflexion	☐

T33.3 Feedback tools to monitor retraining

FEEDBACK TOOL	PROCESS
Self-palpation	Palpation monitoring of joint position
Visual observation	Observe in a mirror or directly watch the movement
Cueing and verbal correction	Listen to feedback from another observer

---

T33.4 Functional positions for retraining upper and low cervical flexion control

- Sitting
- Standing
- Recline sitting backwards (bias anterior muscles)

- Prone (bias posterior muscles)
- 4 point kneeling (bias posterior muscles)
- Incline sitting forwards (bias posterior muscles)
- Functional activities

Cervical extension control

OBSERVATION AND ANALYSIS OF NECK EXTENSION

Description of ideal pattern

While sitting tall with their feet unsupported and the pelvis in neutral, the low and upper cervical spine is positioned in the neutral training region. The scapula and TMJ are also positioned in neutral. When instructed to extend the neck backwards and look up towards the ceiling, a pattern of smooth and even neck extension should be observed. There should be concurrent upper and lower cervical movement. The range should be such that the plane of the face gets to within 15–20° from horizontal without compensation.

During active neck extension there is a normal palpation finding if translation is not excessive. The therapist palpates the tip of the spinous process. As extension is initiated some normal anterior translation is felt, but this stops early and as the neck continues to extend the therapist should feel that the vertebra then moves backwards as the head moves backwards over the shoulders.

Movement faults associated with cervical extension

If translation is excessive, the therapist feels the initial anterior translation does not appear to stop but instead seems to continue forwards. The palpating finger tip may appear to be caught between the spinous processes either side. When anterior translation has been habitually excessive, a skin crease develops transversely across the posterior neck at the level of the UCM. This skin crease is present even when the neck is in its resting or neutral posture. (Note: there is always a normal posterior skin crease at end-range extension.)

In the assessment of extension, the UCM can be identified as either segmental or multisegmental. If excessive upper or mid-cervical extension is observed but no one particular spinous process is excessively displacing anteriorly from the adjacent vertebrae, then the UCM is interpreted as a *multisegmental hyperextension*. If, on the other hand, only one spinous process is observed as

excessively displacing anteriorly and translating forwards 'out of line' compared to the other vertebrae, then the UCM is interpreted as a *segmental extension hinge*. The specific hinging segment should be noted and recorded.

Relative stiffness (restrictions)

- *Upper cervicothoracic restriction of extension* – this can be assessed by passive low cervical extension. Stabilise the upper back below T2 and position the upper cervical in flexion (Figure 6.26). Passively move the head backwards over the shoulders to extend the cervicothoracic junction. Ideally the mid–low cervical neutral line should be 10–15° past vertical (Figure 6.27).
- *Articular restriction* – passive manual examination will identify any significant segmental articular restriction of extension range of motion.
- *Myofascial restriction* – scalene muscle relative stiffness and tightness can limit lower cervical extension. If the anterior scalene muscle lacks extensibility, lower cervical extension is limited. Passive examination of low cervical extension should be reassessed with the cervicothoracic neuromuscular structures unloaded along with relative stiffness and length changes in the scalenes.

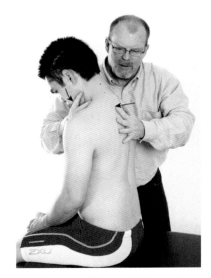

Figure 6.26 Passive test of low cervical extension range – hand position

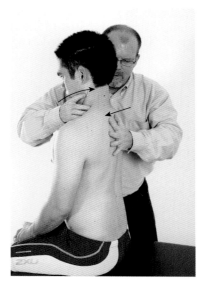

Figure 6.27 Passive test of low cervical extension range – ideal range

If the hyoid muscles lack extensibility, end-range extension is only achieved if the jaw is open. When the jaw is closed, a lack of full end-range neck extension is noted.

- *Fascial restriction of extension* – if the posterior neck fascias (from a region of the occiput to the posterior acromions to T4) are posturally short, they may compress the cervicothoracic segments in flexion and limit normal extension.

Relative flexibility (potential UCM)

- *Upper cervical extension*. The upper cervical spine may initiate the movement into extension. Cervicothoracic extension is often limited or late. During the return to neutral from extension the head may stay in upper cervical extension with chin protrusion. Excessive upper and mid-cervical extension observed, but no one particular vertebral level dominates. The UCM is interpreted as a *multisegmental hyperextension*. The posture resulting from this is often described as a chin poke posture.
- *Mid-cervical shear*. This is more difficult to observe but palpation is useful to identify increased anterior translation and pain provocation at C3–4–5 during active extension. One spinous process is palpated as excessively displacing anteriorly during active neck extension 'out of line' compared to the other extending vertebrae then the UCM is interpreted as a *segmental extension hinge*. The specific hinging segment should be noted and recorded.

Asymmetry

- Asymmetry may be a feature and UCM into rotation and side-bending. If deviation into rotation or side-bending is noted on sagittal plane tests of extension or flexion control, detailed evaluation of rotation or side-bending control tests should be independently assessed.

Tests of upper cervical extension control

T34 BACKWARD HEAD LIFT TEST (tests for upper cervical extension UCM)

This dissociation test assesses the ability to actively dissociate and control upper cervical extension and move the low cervical spine into extension.

Test procedure

The person sits tall with feet unsupported and the pelvis, scapula and TMJ are positioned in their neutral training region. The low cervical spine is positioned in flexion by allowing the head to hang forwards fully. The upper cervical spine is then positioned in neutral by actively lifting and dropping the chin through the full range of upper cervical movement, then positioning in the middle of this range (Figure 6.28).

The therapist monitors the upper cervical neutral position by palpating the occiput with one finger and C2 with another finger. During testing, if the palpating fingers do not move the upper cervical segments are able to maintain neutral. If the palpating fingers move closer together, uncontrolled upper cervical extension is identified.

Without letting the chin lift or retract, the person is instructed to move the low cervical spine through extension by lifting the head upright. The head should move backwards from the base of the neck, only through range of good upper cervical control. There should be no upper cervical extension (palpating fingers move closer together or chin lift or retraction is observed) or loss of scapula position (especially observe for scapula elevation, retraction or forward tilt). The jaw should stay relaxed (Figure 6.29).

Ideally, the person should be able to easily prevent the chin from lifting or retracting and maintain the upper cervical spine neutral (palpating fingers do not move together) while independently moving the lower cervical spine through range from flexion to extension (head starts forwards and lifts to upright) and return.

While teaching, allow the person to initially learn and practise the test movement using

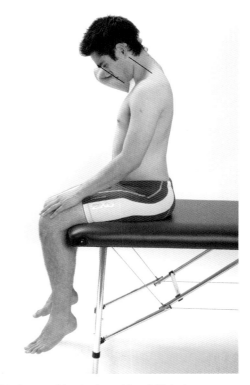

Figure 6.28 Start position backward head lift test

feedback from palpation with their own fingers to monitor and control the upper cervical neutral position until awareness of the correct movement is achieved (Figure 6.30).

Upper cervical extension UCM

The person complains of extension-related symptoms in the upper cervical spine region. The upper cervical spine has greater give into extension than the lower cervical spine under extension load. During active lower cervical extension, the upper cervical gives excessively into segmental extension and translational shear (primarily at C0–1–2, but potentially also at C2–3) or it gives excessively into upper cervical hyperextension. During the attempt to dissociate the upper cervical spine from independent lower cervical extension, the person either cannot control the UCM or has to concentrate and try too hard.

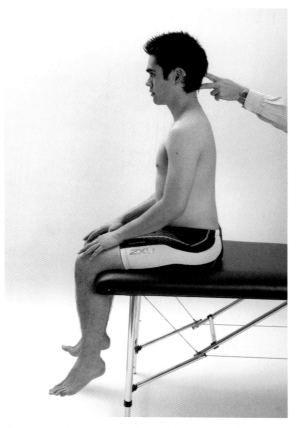

Figure 6.29 Benchmark backward head lift test with therapist palpation

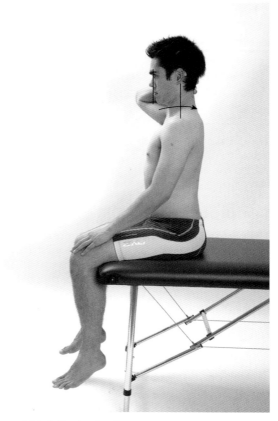

Figure 6.30 Self-palpation for teaching and training

- If only one spinous process is observed as prominent and protruding 'out of line' compared to the other vertebrae, then the UCM is interpreted as a *segmental extension hinge*. The specific hinging segment should be noted and recorded.
- If excessive cervicothoracic flexion is observed, but no one particular spinous process is prominent from the adjacent vertebrae, then the UCM is interpreted as a *multisegmental hyperextension*.

Clinical assessment note for direction-specific motor control testing

If some other movement (e.g. a small amount of cervical rotation) is observed during a motor control (dissociation) test of upper cervical extension, *do not* score this as uncontrolled upper cervical extension. The cervical rotation motor control tests will identify if the observed unrelated movement is uncontrolled. *A test for upper cervical extension UCM is only positive if uncontrolled upper cervical* **extension** *is demonstrated.*

Rating and diagnosis of cervical extension UCM

(T34.1 and T34.2)

Correction

Initially, in sitting or standing with the thoracic spine supported upright against a wall, the head is allowed to hang forwards so that the low cervical spine is in flexion. The upper cervical spine is then positioned in neutral by actively lifting and dropping the chin through the full range of upper cervical movement, then positioning in the middle of this range. Using feedback from palpating the occiput with one finger and C2 with another finger, the person is trained to perform independent lower cervical extension.

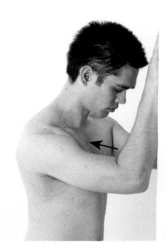

Figure 6.31 Progression: hands on wall, head unsupported upper cervical control – start position

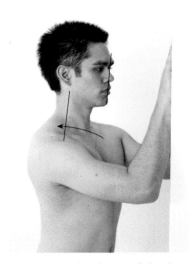

Figure 6.32 Progression: hands on wall, head unsupported – correction

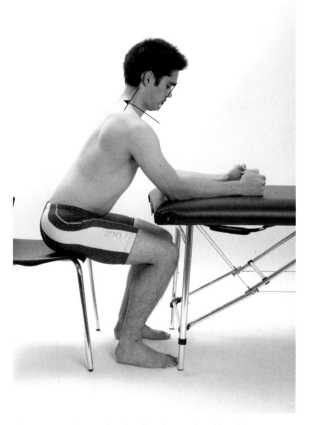

Figure 6.33 Correction leaning forwards with table support

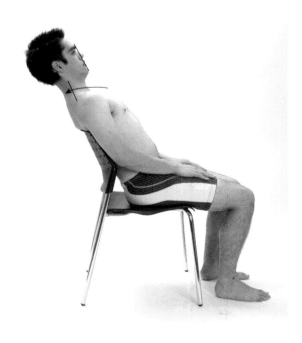

Figure 6.34 Correction leaning backwards with chair support

T34.1 Assessment and rating of low threshold recruitment efficiency of the Backward Head Lift Test

BACKWARD HEAD LIFT TEST

ASSESSMENT

Control point:
- prevent upper cervical extension

Movement challenge: low cervical extension (sitting)

Benchmark range: lower cervical neutral line inclines 10° backwards past vertical

RATING OF LOW THRESHOLD RECRUITMENT EFFICIENCY FOR CONTROL OF DIRECTION

	✓ or ✗		✓ or ✗
• Able to prevent UCM into the test direction Correct dissociation pattern of movement Prevent upper cervical UCM into: • extension (multisegmental) • extension (single segment) and move low cervical extension	☐	• Looks easy, and in the opinion of the assessor, is performed with confidence	☐
		• Feels easy, and the subject has sufficient awareness of the movement pattern that they confidently prevent UCM into the test direction	☐
• Dissociate movement through the benchmark range of: low cervical neutral line inclines 10° backwards past vertical *If there is more available range than the benchmark standard, only the benchmark range needs to be actively controlled*	☐	• The pattern of dissociation is smooth during concentric and eccentric movement	☐
		• Does not (consistently) use *end-range* movement into the opposite direction to prevent the UCM	☐
• Without holding breath (though it is acceptable to use an alternate breathing strategy)	☐	• No extra feedback needed *(tactile, visual or verbal cueing)*	☐
		• Without external support or unloading	☐
• Control during eccentric phase	☐	• Relaxed natural breathing *(even if not ideal – so long as natural pattern does not change)*	☐
• Control during concentric phase	☐	• No fatigue	☐

CORRECT DISSOCIATION PATTERN　　　　　**RECRUITMENT EFFICIENCY**

T34.2 Diagnosis of the site and direction of UCM from the Backward Head Lift Test

BACKWARD HEAD LIFT TEST

Site	Direction	Segmental/ multisegmental	
Upper cervical	Extension	Segmental extension hinge (indicate level)	☐
		Multisegmental hyperextension	☐

T34.3 Feedback tools to monitor retraining

FEEDBACK TOOL	PROCESS
Self-palpation	Palpation monitoring of joint position
Visual observation	Observe in a mirror or directly watch the movement
Cueing and verbal correction	Listen to feedback from another observer

---

T34.4 Functional positions for retraining upper cervical extension control

- Sitting
- Standing
- Supine (bias anterior muscles)

- 4 point kneeling (bias posterior muscles)
- Incline sitting forwards (bias posterior muscles)
- Standing forward lean (bias posterior muscles)
- Functional activities

The person should prevent the chin from lifting or retracting and maintain the upper cervical spine neutral (palpating fingers do not move together) while independently moving the lower cervical spine through range from flexion to extension (head starts forwards and lifts to upright). The lower cervical spine can extend and the head lifts backwards from the base of the neck only so far as there is no upper cervical extension and the scapula and TMJ do not lose their neutral position. As the ability to control upper cervical extension gets easier and the pattern of dissociation feels less unnatural, the exercise can be progressed from head and shoulder girdle supported to head and shoulder girdle unsupported postures.

An alternative progression is to face the wall with the forearms vertical on the wall. Keep the scapula in mid-position and push the body and allow the head to hang forwards. Position the upper cervical spine in neutral mid-position (Figure 6.31). Keeping the upper cervical spine neutral slowly lift the head back over the shoulders only so far as there is no upper cervical extension or chin poke (Figure 6.32).

The person should self-monitor the control of upper cervical extension UCM with a variety of feedback options (T34.3). There should be no provocation of any symptoms within the range that the extension UCM can be controlled.

Once the pattern of dissociation feels familiar it should be integrated into various functional postures and positions (Figures 6.33 and 6.34). T34.4 illustrates some retraining options.

T35 HORIZONTAL RETRACTION TEST (tests for upper cervical extension UCM)

This dissociation test assesses the ability to actively dissociate and control upper cervical extension and move the shoulders through horizontal extension and retraction.

Test procedure

The person should have the ability to actively perform shoulder extension through full range while concurrently controlling cervical spine and head neutral. The person stands with the arms reaching forwards (at 90° flexion) and with the scapula in a neutral position. The low and upper cervical spine is positioned in the neutral training region. The scapula and TMJ are also positioned in neutral. The plane of the face should be vertical (Figure 6.35).

Without letting the chin poke forwards (upper cervical extension) or the head move forwards (low cervical flexion), the person is instructed to keep the cervical spine and the head in the neutral position and pull both arms backwards. The elbows should bend and the forearms stay horizontal and the scapulae should retract to reach 15–20° of shoulder horizontal extension. Ideally, the person should have the ability to keep the head neutral while independently extending the shoulders and reaching back with the arms to end range and bringing them back to the side (Figure 6.36).

Upper cervical extension UCM

The person complains of extension-related symptoms in the upper cervical region. The upper cervical spine has greater give into extension than the

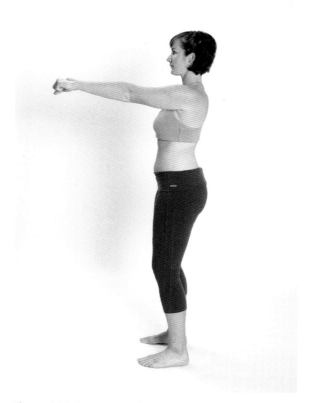

Figure 6.35 Start position horizontal retraction test

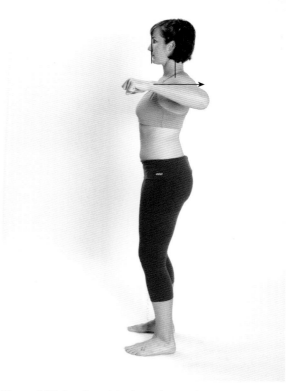

Figure 6.36 Benchmark horizontal retraction test

shoulder girdle under arm extension load. During active shoulder horizontal retraction, the upper cervical region gives excessively into extension. During the attempt to dissociate the upper cervical spine from independent shoulder horizontal retraction, the person either cannot control the UCM or has to concentrate and try too hard.

- If only one spinous process is observed as prominent and protruding 'out of line' compared to the other vertebrae, then the UCM is interpreted as a *segmental extension hinge*. The specific hinging segment should be noted and recorded.
- If excessive cervicothoracic flexion is observed, but no one particular spinous process is prominent from the adjacent vertebrae then the UCM is interpreted as a *multisegmental hyperextension*.

Clinical assessment note for direction-specific motor control testing

If some other movement (e.g. a small amount of cervical rotation) is observed during a motor control (dissociation) test of upper cervical extension, *do not* score this as uncontrolled upper cervical extension. The cervical rotation motor control tests will identify if the observed unrelated movement is uncontrolled. *A test for upper cervical extension UCM is only positive if uncontrolled upper cervical **extension** demonstrated.*

Rating and diagnosis of cervical extension UCM

(T35.1 and T35.2)

Correction

The person stands with the arms reaching forwards (at 90° flexion) with the scapula in a neutral position. The low and upper cervical spine is positioned in the neutral training region. The scapula and TMJ are also positioned in neutral. The plane of the face should be vertical.

Without letting the chin poke forwards (upper cervical extension) or the head move forwards (low cervical flexion), the person is instructed to pull both arms backwards. The elbows should bend and the forearms stay horizontal and the scapulae should retract to reach 15–20° of shoulder horizontal extension. If control is poor, stand with the head and thoracic spine supported against a wall (at a corner) for feedback and

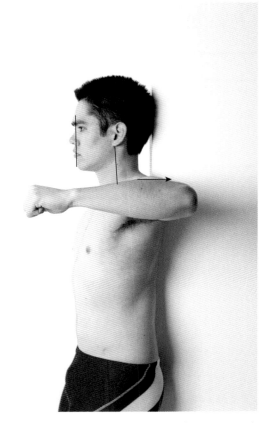

Figure 6.37 Correction – unilateral horizontal retraction with trunk support on wall

support (Figure 6.37). Start doing unilateral horizontal retraction and progress to bilateral arm movement as control improves. Initially move only through reduced range (e.g. 5° then 10°, etc.). As the ability to independently control movement of the upper and low cervical spine gets easier and the pattern of dissociation feels less unnatural, the exercise can be progressed to performing the exercise to long lever full range against light resistance.

The person should self-monitor the control of upper cervical extension UCM with a variety of feedback options (T35.3). There should be no provocation of any symptoms within the range that the extension UCM can be controlled.

Once the pattern of dissociation feels familiar it should be integrated into various functional postures and positions. T35.4 illustrates some retraining options.

T35.1 Assessment and rating of low threshold recruitment efficiency of the Horizontal Retraction Test

HORIZONTAL RETRACTION TEST

ASSESSMENT

Control point:
- prevent upper cervical extension

Movement challenge: shoulder horizontal retraction/extension (standing)

Benchmark range: 15–20° bilateral shoulder horizontal retraction/extension

RATING OF LOW THRESHOLD RECRUITMENT EFFICIENCY FOR CONTROL OF DIRECTION

	✓ or ✗		✓ or ✗
• Able to prevent UCM into the test direction Correct dissociation pattern of movement Prevent upper cervical UCM into: • extension (multisegmental) • extension (single segment) and move shoulder horizontal retraction/ extension	☐	• Looks easy, and in the opinion of the assessor, is performed with confidence	☐
		• Feels easy, and the subject has sufficient awareness of the movement pattern that they confidently prevent UCM into the test direction	☐
• Dissociate movement through the benchmark range of: 15–20° bilateral shoulder horizontal retraction *If there is more available range than the benchmark standard, only the benchmark range needs to be actively controlled*	☐	• The pattern of dissociation is smooth during concentric and eccentric movement	☐
		• Does not (consistently) use *end-range* movement into the opposite direction to prevent the UCM	☐
		• No extra feedback needed *(tactile, visual or verbal cueing)*	☐
• Without holding breath (though it is acceptable to use an alternate breathing strategy)	☐	• Without external support or unloading	☐
		• Relaxed natural breathing *(even if not ideal – so long as natural pattern does not change)*	☐
• Control during eccentric phase	☐	• No fatigue	☐
• Control during concentric phase	☐		

CORRECT DISSOCIATION PATTERN   **RECRUITMENT EFFICIENCY**

T35.2 Diagnosis of the site and direction of UCM from the Horizontal Retraction Test

HORIZONTAL RETRACTION TEST

Site	Direction	Segmental/ multisegmental	
Upper cervical	Extension	Segmental extension hinge (indicate level)	☐
		Multisegmental hyperextension	☐

T35.3 Feedback tools to monitor retraining

FEEDBACK TOOL	PROCESS
Self-palpation	Palpation monitoring of joint position
Visual observation	Observe in a mirror or directly watch the movement
Adhesive tape	Skin tension for tactile feedback
Cueing and verbal correction	Listen to feedback from another observer

---

T35.4 Functional positions for retraining upper and low cervical flexion control

- Sitting
- Standing
- Recline sitting backwards (bias anterior muscles)
- Prone (bias posterior muscles)
- 4 point kneeling (bias posterior muscles)
- Incline sitting forwards (bias posterior muscles)
- Functional activities

Tests of mid-cervical extension (translation) control

T36 HEAD BACK HINGE TEST (tests for mid-cervical translation/ extension UCM)

This dissociation test assesses the ability to actively dissociate and control mid-cervical translation during extension and move the low cervical spine into extension.

Test procedure

The person sits tall with feet unsupported and pelvis, scapula and TMJ are positioned in their neutral training region. The low cervical spine is positioned in flexion by allowing the head to hang forwards fully. The upper and mid-cervical spine is then positioned in neutral by actively lifting and dropping the chin through the full range of upper cervical movement, then positioning in the middle of this range. The therapist monitors the mid-cervical neutral position by palpating (with one finger tip) the spinous process of the hinge point: C3 or C4 (Figure 6.38).

Without letting the chin lift or retract, the person is instructed to lift the head upright by moving backwards from the base of the neck, only through the range of mid-cervical control. There should be no uncontrolled mid-cervical hinge or palpable forward translation of the spinous process during active low cervical extension. The person is instructed to lift the head back to the upright position by pushing back into the palpating finger on the spinous process (Figure 6.39). The palpating finger should feel the spinous process of C3 or C4 moving backwards and inferiorly as the head lifts and the articular surface of the upper segment glides backwards on the lower segment (Box 6.2). There should be no chin lift or retraction, or loss of scapula position (especially observe for scapula elevation, retraction or forward tilt). The jaw should stay relaxed.

Mid-cervical uncontrolled forward translation during extension

The person complains of extension-related symptoms in the mid-cervical spine region. The mid-cervical spine has greater give *into forward*

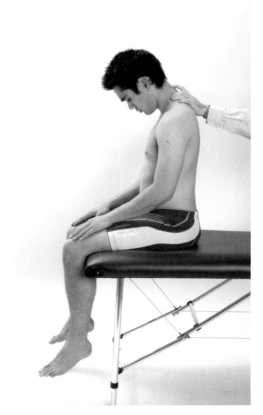

Figure 6.38 Start position head back hinge test

translation/extension than the lower cervical spine under extension load. During active lower cervical extension, the mid-cervical segments give excessively into *segmental extension hinge and translational shear* (primarily at C3–4 and C4–5, and occasionally at C5–6). During the attempt to dissociate the mid-cervical hinge from independent low cervical extension, the person either cannot control the UCM or has to concentrate and try too hard.

If uncontrolled mid-cervical hinge or forward translation occurs during extension, the palpating finger of the spinous process of C3 or C4 suddenly starts to sink into the neck, instead of moving backwards with the head and the adjacent vertebrae. Occasionally, chin lift or retraction is observed, or loss of scapula position (especially observe for scapula elevation, retraction or forward tilt). The jaw should stay relaxed.

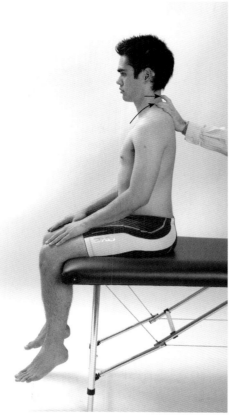

Figure 6.39 Benchmark head back hinge test with therapist palpation

---

Clinical assessment note for direction-specific motor control testing

If some other movement (e.g. a small amount of cervical rotation) is observed during a motor control (dissociation) test of mid-cervical extension hinge, *do not* score this as uncontrolled mid-cervical extension hinge. The cervical rotation motor control tests will identify if the observed unrelated movement is uncontrolled. *A test for mid-cervical extension hinge UCM is only positive if uncontrolled mid-cervical **extension hinge** is demonstrated.*

Rating and diagnosis of cervical extension UCM

(T36.1 and T36.2)

Box 6.2   Palpation of the mid-cervical spine on extension

Normal translation during active extension

At the initiation of active extension the palpating finger should feel the spinous process of C3 or C4 displace slightly forwards (as the articular surfaces close and compress). This forward displacement should then appear to stop early in extension range. As the head lifts and moves backwards over the shoulders, the spinous process should then start to move posteriorly and inferiorly as the articular surface of the upper segment glides backwards on the lower segment.

Abnormal translation during active extension

An abnormal mid-cervical translational shear or 'hinge' is identified by palpation of one spinous process that during active extension demonstrates excessive anterior displacement of the spinous process (spinous process moving forwards too far). The spinous process seems to 'sink in' to the neck excessively while the adjacent levels above and below do not. As active neck extension continues through range there is a lack of resistance to the anterior displacement and a failure to feel the normal posterior displacement as extension continues.

This is most commonly observed at C3 or C4. When excessive anterior translation has been habitually excessive, a postural skin crease develops transversely across the posterior neck at the level of the uncontrolled translation. This skin crease is present even when the neck is in its resting or neutral posture. (Note: there is always a normal posterior skin crease at end-range extension.)

Ideally, the person should be able to easily prevent excessive forward translation of mid-cervical vertebrae (palpating finger does not sink in to the neck) and prevent the chin from lifting or retracting while independently moving the lower cervical spine through range from flexion to extension (head starts forwards and lift to upright) and return.

While teaching, allow the person to initially learn and practise the test movement using feedback from palpation with their own fingers to monitor and control the mid-cervical translation (hinge) until awareness of the correct movement is achieved.

Correction

Initially, in sitting or standing with the thoracic spine supported upright against a wall. The head is allowed to hang forwards so that the low cervical spine is in flexion. The upper and mid-cervical spine is then positioned in neutral by actively lifting and dropping the chin through the full range of upper cervical movement, then

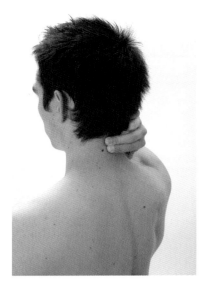

Figure 6.40 Self-palpation for teaching and training

positioning in the middle of this range. Using feedback from palpating the spinous process of C3 or C4, the person is trained to perform independent lower cervical extension (Figure 6.40).

The person should prevent the chin from lifting or retracting and maintain control of the mid-cervical hinge. Maintain a backward pressure at the spinous process during backward movement (push back into the palpating finger tip) while independently moving the lower cervical spine through range from flexion to extension (head starts forwards and lifts to upright). The lower cervical spine can extend and the head lifts backwards from the base of the neck only so far as there is no mid-cervical hinge and the scapula and TMJ do not lose their neutral position.

As the ability to control upper cervical extension gets easier and the pattern of dissociation feels less unnatural, the exercise can be progressed from head and shoulder girdle supported to head and shoulder girdle unsupported postures.

The person should self-monitor the control of mid-cervical translation during extension UCM with a variety of feedback options (T36.3). There should be no provocation of any symptoms within the range that the extension UCM can be controlled.

Once the pattern of dissociation feels familiar it should be integrated into various functional postures and positions. T36.4 illustrates some retraining options.

T36.1 Assessment and rating of low threshold recruitment efficiency of the Head Back Hinge Test

HEAD BACK HINGE TEST

ASSESSMENT

Control point:
- prevent mid-cervical anterior translation during extension

Movement challenge: low cervical extension (sitting)

Benchmark range: lower cervical neutral line inclines 10° backwards past vertical

RATING OF LOW THRESHOLD RECRUITMENT EFFICIENCY FOR CONTROL OF DIRECTION

	✓ or ✗		✓ or ✗
• Able to prevent UCM into the test direction Correct dissociation pattern of movement Prevent mid-cervical UCM into: • hinge or forward translation during extension (single segment) and move low cervical extension	☐	• Looks easy, and in the opinion of the assessor, is performed with confidence	☐
		• Feels easy, and the subject has sufficient awareness of the movement pattern that they confidently prevent UCM into the test direction	☐
• Dissociate movement through the benchmark range of: low cervical neutral line inclines 10° backwards past vertical *If there is more available range than the benchmark standard, only the benchmark range needs to be actively controlled*	☐	• The pattern of dissociation is smooth during concentric and eccentric movement	☐
		• Does not (consistently) use *end-range* movement into the opposite direction to prevent the UCM	☐
• Without holding breath (though it is acceptable to use an alternate breathing strategy)	☐	• No extra feedback needed *(tactile, visual or verbal cueing)*	☐
		• Without external support or unloading	☐
• Control during eccentric phase	☐	• Relaxed natural breathing *(even if not ideal – so long as natural pattern does not change)*	☐
• Control during concentric phase	☐	• No fatigue	☐

CORRECT DISSOCIATION PATTERN   **RECRUITMENT EFFICIENCY**

T36.2 Diagnosis of the site and direction of UCM from the Head Back Hinge Test

HEAD BACK HINGE TEST

Site	Direction	Segmental/multisegmental	
Mid-cervical	Translation Extension	Segmental extension hinge (indicate level)	☐

T36.3 Feedback tools to monitor retraining

FEEDBACK TOOL	PROCESS
Self-palpation	Palpation monitoring of joint position
Visual observation	Observe in a mirror or directly watch the movement
Adhesive tape	Skin tension for tactile feedback
Cueing and verbal correction	Listen to feedback from another observer

---

T36.4 Functional positions for retraining mid-cervical translation (in extension) control

- Sitting
- Standing
- Supine (bias anterior muscles)
- Recline sitting backwards (bias anterior muscles)
- Side-lying

- Incline sitting forwards (bias posterior muscles)
- Standing forward lean (bias posterior muscles)
- Functional activities

T37 CHIN LIFT HINGE TEST (tests for mid-cervical translation/ extension UCM)

This dissociation test assesses the ability to actively dissociate and control mid-cervical translation during extension and move the upper cervical spine into extension.

Test procedure

The person sits tall with feet unsupported and pelvis neutral. The low and upper cervical spine is positioned in the neutral training region. The scapula and TMJ are also positioned in neutral.

The therapist monitors the mid-cervical neutral position by palpating (with one finger tip) the spinous process of the hinge point: C3 or C4 (Figure 6.41).

Without letting the head move forwards or the chin poke forwards, the person is instructed to independently lift the chin (vertically) through upper cervical extension, visualising flattening the lordosis against an imaginary wall placed at the back of the head. There should be no uncontrolled mid-cervical hinge or palpable forward translation during active upper cervical extension. The person is instructed to lift the chin up and back (not up and forwards) and elongate the back of the neck by pushing back into the palpating finger on the spinous process (Figure 6.42). The

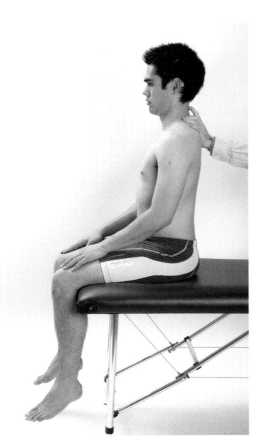

Figure 6.41 Start position chin lift hinge test

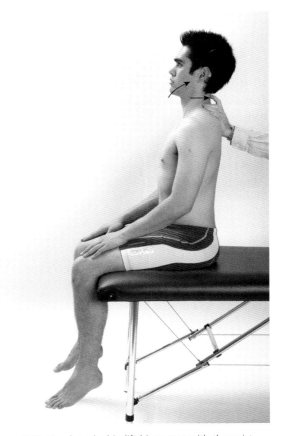

Figure 6.42 Benchmark chin lift hinge test with therapist palpation

palpating finger should feel that the spinous process of C3 or C4 does not move forwards ('sink' into the neck) as the chin lifts (see T36.1 in the previous section). There should be no low cervical flexion (head moving forwards), chin poke forwards or loss of scapula position (especially observe for scapula elevation or forward tilt). The jaw should stay relaxed.

Ideally, the person should be able to easily prevent excessive forward translation of mid-cervical vertebrae (palpating finger does not sink in to the neck) while independently moving the upper cervical spine through range from flexion to extension and return.

While teaching, allow the person to initially learn and practise the test movement using feedback from palpation with their own fingers to monitor and control the mid-cervical translation (hinge) until awareness of the correct movement is achieved.

Mid-cervical uncontrolled forward translation during extension

The person complains of extension-related symptoms in the mid-cervical spine region. The mid-cervical spine has greater give *into forward translation/extension* than the upper cervical spine under extension load. During active upper cervical extension, the mid-cervical segments give excessively into *segmental extension hinge and translational shear* (primarily at C3–4 and C4–5, and occasionally at C5–6). During the attempt to dissociate the mid-cervical hinge from independent upper cervical extension, the person either cannot control the UCM or has to concentrate and try too hard.

If uncontrolled mid-cervical hinge or forward translation occurs during extension, the palpating finger of the spinous process of C3 or C4 suddenly starts to 'sink' forwards into the neck, instead of moving backwards with the head and the adjacent vertebrae. Occasionally, chin poke and forward movement of the head is observed; or loss of scapula position (especially observe for scapula elevation, retraction or forward tilt). The jaw should stay relaxed.

Clinical assessment note for direction-specific motor control testing

If some other movement (e.g. a small amount of cervical rotation) is observed during a motor control (dissociation) test of mid-cervical extension hinge, *do not* score this as uncontrolled mid-cervical extension hinge. The cervical rotation motor control tests will identify if the observed unrelated movement is uncontrolled. *A test for mid-cervical extension hinge UCM is only positive if uncontrolled mid-cervical **extension hinge** is demonstrated.*

Rating and diagnosis of cervical extension UCM

(T37.1 and T37.2)

Correction

Initially, position the lower cervical spine in neutral with the head supported and the upper cervical spine slightly flexed by allowing the chin to drop towards the throat. This can be done in sitting or standing with the thoracic spine and the back of the head against a wall. Using the feedback and support of the supporting surface, the person is trained to perform independent upper cervical extension (vertical chin lift). The person is instructed to lift the chin up and back (not up and forwards) and elongate the back of the neck by pushing back into the palpating finger on the spinous process. The palpating finger should feel that the spinous process of C3 or C4 does not move forwards ('sink' into the neck) as the chin lifts.

The upper cervical spine can extend only so far as there is no forward movement of the head, no forward chin poke and the scapula and TMJ do not lose their neutral position. Using feedback from palpating the spinous process of C3 or C4 the person is trained to perform independent upper cervical extension while controlling mid-cervical translation. If control is poor, start in supine lying with the occiput supported on a small folded towel. The person should prevent the chin from poking forwards or the head from moving forwards and maintain control of the mid-cervical hinge. Maintain a backward pressure at the spinous process (push back into the palpating finger tip) while independently moving the upper cervical spine through range from flexion to extension (vertical chin lift). Only move so far as there is no mid-cervical hinge and the scapula and TMJ do not lose their neutral position.

As the ability to control upper cervical extension gets easier and the pattern of dissociation feels less unnatural, the exercise can be progressed from head and shoulder girdle supported to head and shoulder girdle unsupported postures (Figure 6.43).

The person should self-monitor the control of mid-cervical translation during extension UCM with a variety of feedback options (T37.3). There should be no provocation of any symptoms within the range that the extension UCM can be controlled.

Once the pattern of dissociation feels familiar it should be integrated into various functional postures and positions. T37.4 illustrates some retraining options.

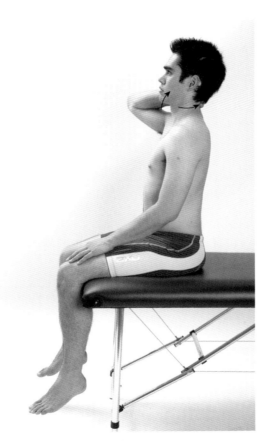

Figure 6.43 Correction with self-palpation

T37.1 Assessment and rating of low threshold recruitment efficiency of the Chin Lift Hinge Test

CHIN LIFT HINGE TEST

ASSESSMENT

Control point:
- prevent mid-cervical anterior translation during extension

Movement challenge: upper cervical extension (sitting)

Benchmark range: plane or face (upper cervical neutral line) extends backwards 10–15° past vertical

RATING OF LOW THRESHOLD RECRUITMENT EFFICIENCY FOR CONTROL OF DIRECTION

	✓ or ✗		✓ or ✗
• Able to prevent UCM into the test direction Correct dissociation pattern of movement Prevent mid-cervical UCM into: • hinge or forward translation during extension (single segment) and move upper cervical extension	☐	• Looks easy, and in the opinion of the assessor, is performed with confidence • Feels easy, and the subject has sufficient awareness of the movement pattern that they confidently prevent UCM into the test direction	☐ ☐
• Dissociate movement through the benchmark range of: plane of face (low cervical neutral line) extends backwards 10–15° past vertical *If there is more available range than the benchmark standard, only the benchmark range needs to be actively controlled*	☐	• The pattern of dissociation is smooth during concentric and eccentric movement • Does not (consistently) use *end-range* movement into the opposite direction to prevent the UCM • No extra feedback needed *(tactile, visual or verbal cueing)*	☐ ☐ ☐
• Without holding breath (though it is acceptable to use an alternate breathing strategy) • Control during eccentric phase • Control during concentric phase	☐ ☐ ☐	• Without external support or unloading • Relaxed natural breathing *(even if not ideal – so long as natural pattern does not change)* • No fatigue	☐ ☐ ☐

CORRECT DISSOCIATION PATTERN   **RECRUITMENT EFFICIENCY**

T37.2 Diagnosis of the site and direction of UCM from the Chin Lift Hinge Test

CHIN LIFT HINGE TEST

Site	Direction	Segmental/multisegmental	
Mid-cervical	Translation	Segmental extension hinge (indicate level)	☐
	Extension	Multisegmental hyperextension	☐

T37.3 Feedback tools to monitor retraining

FEEDBACK TOOL	PROCESS
Self-palpation	Palpation monitoring of joint position
Visual observation	Observe in a mirror or directly watch the movement
Cueing and verbal correction	Listen to feedback from another observer

---

T37.4 Functional positions for retraining mid-cervical translation (in extension) control

- Sitting
- Standing
- Supine (bias anterior muscles)
- Recline sitting backwards (bias anterior muscles)
- Side-lying
- Incline sitting forwards (bias posterior muscles)
- Standing forward lean (bias posterior muscles)
- Functional activities

Control of unilateral movements – rotation (± side-bend)

OBSERVATION AND ANALYSIS OF NATURAL NECK ROTATION

Description of ideal pattern

While sitting tall with their feet unsupported and the pelvis in neutral, the person's low and upper cervical spine is positioned in the neutral training region. The scapula and TMJ are also positioned in neutral. When instructed to turn the head to the side to look behind over the shoulders, a pattern of smooth and even head rotation should be observed. There should be concurrent upper and lower cervical movement. The plane of the face should stay vertical with the eyes horizontal and not tilt into side-bending compensation or compensate with chin poke and upper cervical extension (Figure 6.44).

The range should be such that the head can turn to 70–80° from the midline without compensation. There should be symmetrical range of rotation (Kapandji 1982) (Figure 6.45).

Movement faults associated with cervical rotation

Relative stiffness (restrictions)

*   This is noted by a significant asymmetry of rotation range or an obvious decrease in standard normal range of motion when compensations and uncontrolled motion are actively or passively controlled (Figure 6.46). If natural head rotation demonstrates reasonable range of motion but there is

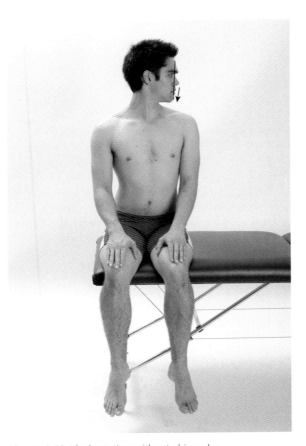

Figure 6.44 Ideal rotation without chin poke

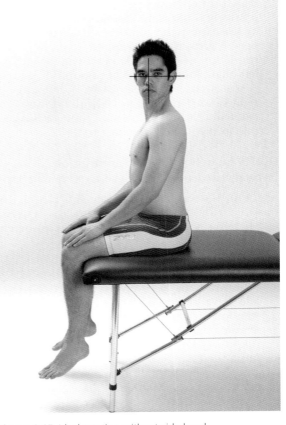

Figure 6.45 Ideal rotation without side-bend

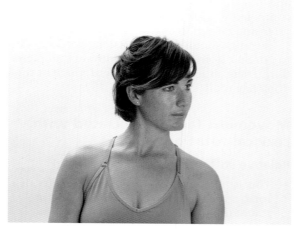

Figure 6.46 Significant restriction of neck rotation

observable compensation such as head lateral tilt or chin poke, the therapist should passively support and correct the movement by preventing the compensation while the person actively tries to rotate again. A restriction of rotation is identified if there is less than 70–80° range of rotation or if there is significant asymmetry between left and right sides. This does not identify if the restriction is due to articular influences or due to myofascial influences.

Useful guidelines for differentiation between articular and myofascial restrictions

Absolute differentiation between structures is not possible. However, this clinical analysis is useful for helping to differentiate between different tissues affecting functional movement.

- *Articular restriction.* If the cervical myofascial tissues and neural structures are unloaded ipsilaterally by passively upwardly rotating and elevating the scapula, and full range of rotation (70–80°) cannot be achieved (there is no or only slight increased range of rotation), the articular structures are implicated as a source of restriction. This is confirmed with rotation manual segmental assessment (e.g. Maitland PPIVMs or PAIVMs) and treatment is directed towards manual mobilisation or manipulation of the segmental articular restriction.

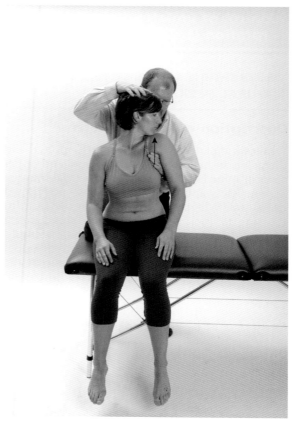

Figure 6.47 Unloading of ipsilateral scapula demonstrates increased neck rotation range

- *Myofascial/neural restriction.* If the cervical myofascial tissues and neural structures are unloaded ipsilaterally by passively lifting the scapula off the dropped shoulder position and upwardly rotating/elevating the scapula, and full range of rotation returns or a significant increase in rotation range is achieved, then the myofascial or neural tissues are implicated as a source of functional restriction (Figure 6.47). This is confirmed by re-loading these structures with ipsilateral scapula depression and a significant decrease in rotation range is noted (Figure 6.48).

Excessive tension in either the levator scapula (upper cervical attachments) or the scalenes (lower cervical attachments) on the ipsilateral side is implicated with altered side-bend rotation coupling mechanics,

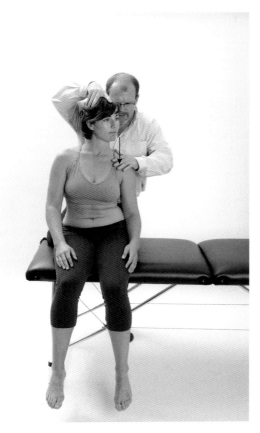

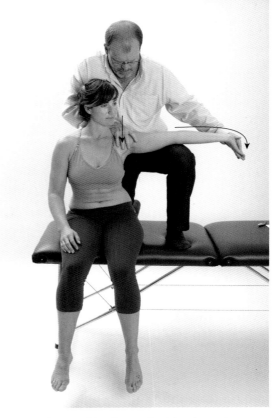

Figure 6.48 Ipsilateral scapular depression demonstrates decreased neck rotation range

Figure 6.49 Start position for myofascial and neural differentiation

producing a functional loss of head rotation. Excessive tension can arise from abnormally shortened muscles pulling on the cervical attachments or from an abnormally dropped (downwardly rotated or depressed) scapula adding excessive tension on the lateral neck via normal muscles. Treatment is directed towards stability rehabilitation of the scapula ± addressing neural sensitivity. Passive elevation of the scapulae has been shown to decrease symptoms with rotation in neck pain patients (Van Dillen et al 2007).

• *Differentiating between primary myofascial and primary neural mechanisms in function (non-articular) restriction.* If myofascial or neural involvement contributes to a functional restriction, a useful clinical test can help to differentiate whether the primary mechanism

is a neural sensitisation/protection problem or if the primary mechanism is a myofascial extensibility or scapular control problem.

Load the ipsilateral myofascial and neural structures together with scapula depression plus shoulder abduction to 90° and external rotation with relaxed elbow extension, forearm supination and slight wrist and finger extension. This incorporates the basic elements of the upper limb tension test 1 (ULTT1) (Butler 2000). Then rotate the head towards the ipsilateral shoulder to engage the point of restriction (Figure 6.49). Maintain the myofascial loading component with scapula depression while unloading the neural component by releasing the distal components of ULTT 1 (that is, flex the

265

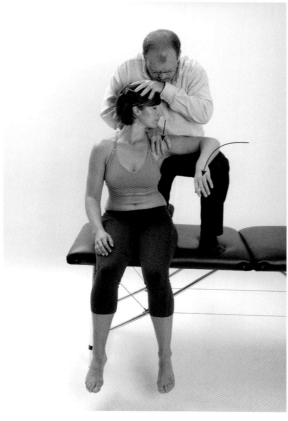

Figure 6.50 Maintaining myofascial loading while unloading neural tissues

elbow, internally rotate the shoulder and allow the wrist and fingers to relax into flexion) (Figure 6.50). It is normal for symptoms to decrease when the neural system is unloaded, but if the range of rotation significantly increases when the neural system only is unloaded, neural mobility or sensitivity is implicated as the primary dysfunction and further assessment should be considered (Butler 2000; Shacklock 2005).

If range of rotation stays restricted when the neural system is unloaded then the myofascial system is implicated as the primary dysfunction. If myofascial tissue changes are identified as the primary mechanism implicated in the restriction, this may be related to increased tension and lack of extensibility of the levator scapula or scalene muscles. This can be confirmed with muscle length tests. The increased tension in the levator scapulae and the scalene muscles and resultant functional restriction may also be due to muscles of normal length being placed under tension by a dropped shoulder position. Increased tension can result from a poor scapular control and a dropped scapula position placing passive tension on these muscles as the shoulder girdle 'hangs' off the neck. Analysis of scapula control will differentiate this (see Chapter 8).

Clinical note: restriction of movement can sometimes be observed when there is an articular hypermobile uncontrolled segment. This hypermobile motion contributes to a relative impingement process which in turn generates pain and subsequent protective guarding responses. When this hypermobility is actively stabilised with the deep neck flexors, or passively stabilised, provocation is controlled and range increases.

Relative flexibility (potential UCM)

- *Upper cervical extension.* The upper cervical spine may compensate for a restriction of rotation. Rotation may be limited due to articular or myofascial influences. Compensation with excessive upper cervical extension or a chin poke posture is observed in the attempt to increase rotation functional range (Figure 6.51).
- *Cervical side-bend.* Restrictions of rotation may be compensated for by tilting the head in to side-bending in an attempt to gain more functional range (Figure 6.52).
- *Segmental uncontrolled articular rotation.* This is identified as hypermobile articular rotation on passive manual assessment of intersegmental articular mobility (e.g. increased motion on testing with Maitland PPIVMs or PAIVMs).
- *Scapula compensation.* The scapula may also demonstrate a variety of compensation strategies associated with head rotation. Ideally, the scapula should be able to maintain a relatively neutral or mid-range position and allow full unrestricted

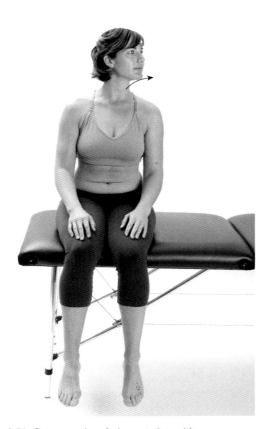

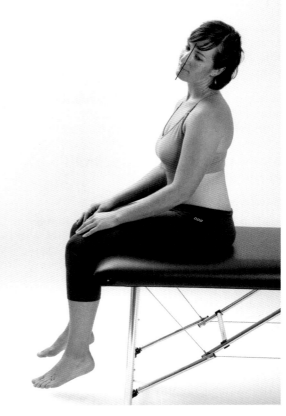

Figure 6.51 Compensation during rotation with upper cervical extension/chin poke

Figure 6.52 Compensation during rotation with side-bending

functional range of head rotation. If the scapula is depressed or downwardly rotated, increased passive tensile loading in shoulder girdle to neck muscles can contribute to a myofascial restriction and the chain of secondary compensation in the neck. Some people actively use excessive scapula retraction to initiate or assist neck rotation; in particular the rhomboids and levator scapula muscles are dominant in this strategy. Some people actively hitch the shoulder girdle into scapular elevation to unload any relative myofascial restriction to allow more functional range. With UCM associated with head rotation, the uncontrolled scapula is ipsilateral to (i.e. on the same side as) the direction of head rotation.

Control of unilateral movements – side-bend

OBSERVATION AND ANALYSIS OF NATURAL NECK SIDE-BENDING

Description of ideal pattern

While sitting tall with the feet unsupported and the pelvis in neutral, the low and upper cervical spine is positioned in the neutral training region. The scapula and TMJ are also positioned in neutral. When instructed to tilt the head laterally to the side as if moving the top tip of the ear towards the shoulder, a pattern of smooth and even head side-bending should be observed. There should be concurrent upper and lower cervical movement. The plane of the face should stay facing ahead (in the frontal plane) and not turn into rotation compensation or compensate with chin poke and upper cervical extension.

The range should be such that the head can side-bend to 40–45° from the mid-line without compensation. There should be symmetrical range of side-bending (Kapandji 1982).

Movement faults associated with cervical side-bend

Relative stiffness (restrictions)

- This is noted by a significant asymmetry of side-bend range or an obvious decrease in standard normal range of motion when compensations and uncontrolled motion are actively or passively controlled. If natural head side-bending demonstrates reasonable range of motion but there is observable compensation, such as head rotation or chin poke, the therapist should passively support and correct the movement by preventing the compensation while the person actively tries to side-bend again. A restriction of side-bending is identified if there is less than 40–45° range of lateral side-bend or if there is significant asymmetry between left and right sides. This does not identify if the restriction is due to articular influences or due to myofascial influences.

Guidelines for differentiation between articular and myofascial restrictions

Absolute differentiation between structures is not possible. However, this clinical analysis is useful for helping to differentiate between different components of the movement system.

- *Articular restriction.* If the cervical myofascial tissues and neural structures are unloaded contralaterally by passively upwardly rotating and elevating the scapula, and full range of side-bending (40–45°) cannot be achieved (there is no or only slight increase in the range of side-bend), the articular structures are implicated as a source of restriction. This is confirmed with lateral flexion manual segmental assessment (e.g. Maitland PPIVMs or PAIVMs) and treatment is directed towards

manual mobilisation or manipulation of the segmental articular restriction.

- *Myofascial/neural restriction.* If the cervical myofascial tissues and neural structures are unloaded contralaterally by passively lifting the scapula off the dropped shoulder position and upwardly rotating/elevating the scapula, and full range of side-bending returns or a significant increase in rotation range is achieved, then the myofascial or neural tissues are implicated as a source of functional restriction. This is confirmed by reloading these structures with contralateral scapula depression and a significant decrease in side-bending range is noted.

  Excessive tension in either the levator scapula (upper cervical attachments) or the scalenes (lower cervical attachments) on the contralateral side is implicated with altered side-bend rotation coupling mechanics producing a functional loss of head side-bending. Excessive tension can arise from abnormally shortened muscles pulling on the cervical attachments or from an abnormally dropped (downwardly rotated or depressed) scapula adding excessive tension on the lateral neck via normal muscles. Treatment is directed towards stability rehabilitation of the scapula ± addressing neural sensitivity. Passive elevation of the scapulae has been shown to decrease symptoms with side-bending in neck pain patients (Van Dillen et al 2007).

- *Differentiating between primary myofascial and primary neural mechanisms in function (non-articular) restriction.* If myofascial or neural involvement contributes to a functional restriction, a useful clinical test can help to differentiate whether the primary mechanism is a neural sensitisation/protection problem or if the primary mechanism is a myofascial extensibility or scapular control problem.

  Load the contralateral myofascial and neural structures together with scapula depression plus shoulder abduction to 90° and external rotation with relaxed elbow extension, forearm supination and slight wrist and finger extension. This incorporates the basic elements of the upper limb tension test 1 (ULTT1) (Butler 2000). Then, tilt the head laterally (towards the contralateral shoulder) to the point of restricted side-bend.

Maintain the myofascial loading component with scapula depression while unloading the neural component by releasing the distal components of ULTT 1. (That is, flex the elbow, internally rotate the shoulder and allow the wrist and fingers to relax into flexion.) It is normal for symptoms to decrease when the neural system is unloaded, but if the range of side-bending significantly increases when the neural system only is unloaded, neural mobility or sensitivity is implicated as the primary dysfunction and further assessment should be considered (Butler 2000; Shacklock 2005).

If range of side-bending stays restricted when the neural system is unloaded, then the myofascial system is implicated as the primary dysfunction. If myofascial tissue changes are identified as the primary mechanism implicated in the restriction, this may be related to increased tension and lack of extensibility of the levator scapula or scalene muscles. This can be confirmed with muscle length tests. The increased tension in the levator scapulae and the scalene muscles and resultant functional restriction may also be due to muscles of normal length being placed under tension by a dropped shoulder position. Increased tension can result from a poor scapular control and a dropped scapula position placing passive tension on these muscles as the shoulder girdle 'hangs' off the neck. Analysis of scapula control will differentiate this (see Chapter 8).

Clinical note: restriction of movement can sometimes be observed when there is an articular hypermobile uncontrolled segment. This hypermobile motion contributes to a relative impingement process which in turn generates pain and subsequent protective guarding responses. When this hypermobility is actively stabilised with the deep neck flexors, or passively stabilised, provocation is controlled and range increases.

Relative flexibility (potential UCM)

- *Upper cervical extension.* The upper cervical spine may compensate for a restriction of side-bending range. Side-bending may be limited due to articular or myofascial influences. Compensation with excessive upper cervical extension or a chin poke posture is observed in the attempt to increase side-bending functional range.
- *Cervical rotation.* Restrictions of side-bending may be compensated for by turning the head in to rotation in an attempt to gain more functional range.
- *Segmental uncontrolled articular side-bending.* This is identified as hypermobile articular side-bending on passive manual assessment of intersegmental articular mobility (e.g. increased motion on testing with Maitland PPIVMs or PAIVMs).
- *Segmental upper cervical.* Increased upper cervical side-bending may be observed as compensation for either an articular or myofascial restriction of low cervical side-bending.
- *Segmental lower cervical.* Increased lower cervical side-bending may be observed as compensation for either an articular or myofascial restriction of upper cervical side-bending.
- *Scapula compensation.* The scapula may also demonstrate a variety of compensation strategies associated with head side-bending. Ideally, the scapula should be able to maintain a relatively neutral or mid-range position and allow full unrestricted functional range of head side-bending. If the scapula is depressed or downwardly rotated, increased passive tensile loading in shoulder girdle to neck muscles can contribute to a myofascial restriction and the chain of secondary compensation in the neck. Some people actively hitch the shoulder girdle into scapular elevation to unload any relative myofascial restriction to allow more functional range. With UCM associated with head rotation, the uncontrolled scapula is contralateral to (i.e. on the opposite side to) the direction of head side-bending.

Tests of rotation/side-bend control

T38 HEAD TURN TEST
(tests for rotation/side-bend UCM)

This dissociation test assesses the ability to actively dissociate and control cervical side-bend and move the cervical spine into rotation.

Test procedure

The person sits tall with feet unsupported and pelvis neutral. The low and upper cervical spine is positioned in the neutral training region. The scapula is actively positioned in its neutral training region. Controlling the scapula neutral position is especially important if a myofascial restriction of functional head rotation is identified. The TMJ is also positioned in neutral and the jaw should stay relaxed (Figure 6.53).

The person is instructed to fully rotate the head by turning to look over one shoulder then the other. This should be a pure axial rotation and the person should be able to turn the head through approximately 70–80° of rotation, keeping the eyes horizontal (Figure 6.54). There should be no side-bending (lateral flexion compensating for poor rotation control) and there should be no chin poke (upper extension compensating for poor rotation control) or mid-cervical hinging into extension (translation). There should be no forward movement of the head (low cervical flexion) compensating for poor rotation control. The scapula should actively maintain a neutral position with scapula-trunk muscles dominant to the scapula-neck muscles. Ideally, the person should be able to easily prevent

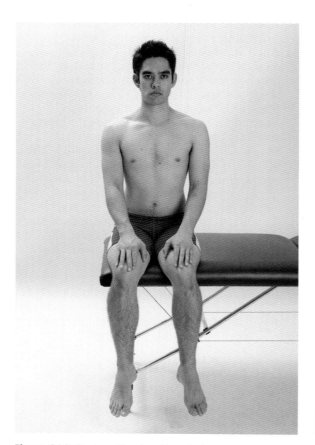

Figure 6.53 Start position head turn test

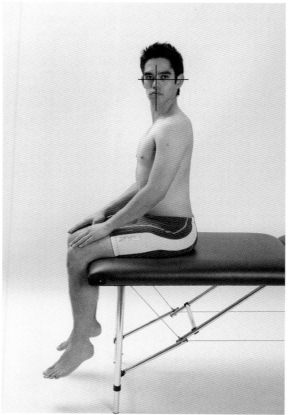

Figure 6.54 Benchmark head turn test

compensation and UCM and rotate the head through the 70–80° range.

While teaching, allow the person to initially learn and practise the test movement using feedback from head contact on a wall or observation using mirrors. Keep the occiput in contact with a supporting surface to monitor that the head turns into rotation (axial movement) and does not roll (side-bend) into rotation. Using a wall also provides support and feedback about scapula position and control during head rotation.

UCM during rotation

The person complains of unilateral symptoms in the neck. The cervical spine demonstrates UCM resulting from a variety of compensation strategies associated with head rotation (Table 6.3). The inability to prevent these compensation strategies during active rotation identifies UCM.

During the attempt to dissociate these compensations from independent cervical axial rotation, the person either cannot control the UCM or has to concentrate and try too hard.

The identification of UCM during head rotation needs to be assessed on both sides. Note the direction that the rotation cannot be controlled (i.e. does the chin poke or side-bend during rotation occur to the left or the right). It may be unilateral or bilateral.

The assessment of restricted motion is reliable only if any compensations/UCM are either actively or passively controlled. When compensations are eliminated, a lack of 70–80° range of head rotation identifies 'real' restriction which may be due to either a myofascial or articular restriction, or both combined. The uncontrolled rotation of the head may also be associated with a myofascial restriction holding the scapula in depression, or downward rotation caused by inefficiency of the stability function of the scapula-trunk muscles (serratus anterior and middle and lower trapezius).

Table 6.3 Compensation strategies associated with uncontrolled head rotation

• Cervical side-bend	• Scapular depression
• Upper cervical extension	• Scapular downward rotation
• Low cervical flexion	• Scapular retraction
• Mid-cervical hinge	• Scapular elevation

Clinical assessment note for direction-specific motor control testing

If some other movement (e.g. a small amount of thoracic flexion) is observed during a motor control (dissociation) test of cervical side-bend, *do not* score this as uncontrolled cervical side-bend. The thoracic flexion motor control tests will identify if the observed unrelated movement is uncontrolled. *A test for cervical side-bend UCM is only positive if uncontrolled cervical **side-bend** is demonstrated.*

Rating and diagnosis of cervical rotation/side-bend UCM

(T38.1 and T38.2)

Correction

The person sits or stands with the thoracic spine and head supported against a wall. Using a wall also provides support and feedback about scapula position and control during head rotation. Some people may find that initial retraining in supported supine positions is the preferred starting level (Figure 6.55). The low and upper cervical spine is positioned in the neutral training region. The TMJ is also positioned in neutral and the jaw should stay relaxed.

The ipsilateral scapula is initially passively positioned in upward rotation ± elevation to unload any myofascial restriction. The scapula is actively held against the wall for support and feedback. Controlling the scapula neutral position is especially important if a myofascial restriction of functional head rotation is identified. Some people

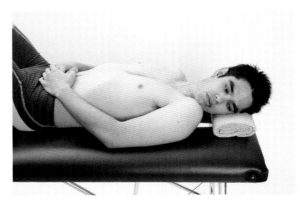

Figure 6.55 Correction in supine with head support

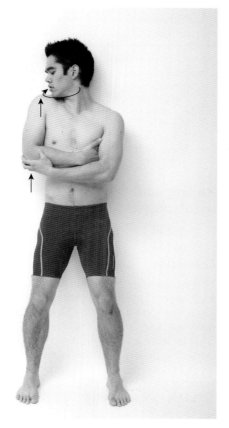

Figure 6.56 Correction standing with wall support and shoulder girdle unloaded

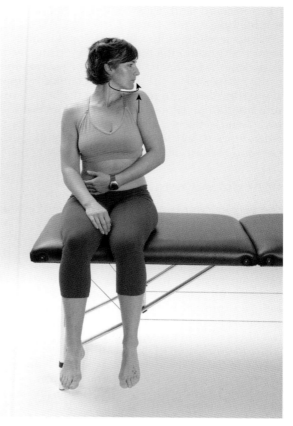

Figure 6.57 Correction sitting unsupported with active shoulder control

may need to passively support their ipsilateral shoulder girdle with their other hand at the elbow (like a sling), or use the armrest of a chair to maintain the unloaded shoulder girdle, or use taping in order to prevent the ipsilateral scalenes and levator scapula from generating increased tension and adding to the myofascial restriction.

The person is instructed to fully rotate the head by turning to look over one shoulder then the other (Figure 6.56). This should be a pure axial rotation and the person should be able to turn the head through approximately 70–80° of rotation, keeping the eyes horizontal. There should be no side-bending (lateral flexion compensating for poor rotation control) and there should be no chin poke (upper and mid-cervical extension compensating for poor rotation control). There should be no forward movement of the head (low cervical flexion compensating for poor rotation control). Keep the occiput in

contact with the wall to monitor that the head turns into rotation (axial movement) and does not roll (side-bend) into rotation. The scapula should actively maintain a neutral position without depression, downward rotation, retraction or elevation.

As control improves and symptoms decrease, the person should begin to actively control the scapula position supported on the wall during the neck rotation dissociation. The person should eventually progress to active control of the unsupported shoulder girdle off the wall while training neck rotation dissociation exercises through 70–80° range of rotation.

As the ability to control cervical rotation gets easier and the pattern of dissociation feels less unnatural, the exercise can be progressed from head and shoulder girdle supported to head and shoulder girdle unsupported postures (Figure 6.57).

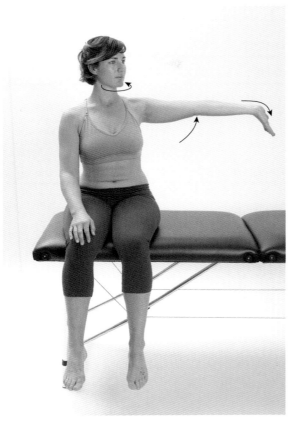

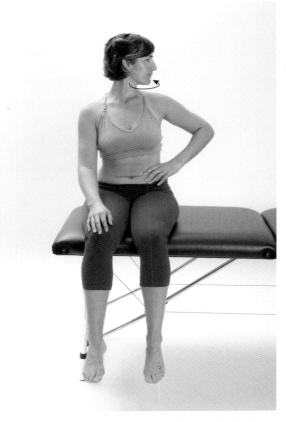

Figure 6.58 Correction unsupported with neural loading

Figure 6.59 Correction unsupported with neural unloading

The person should self-monitor the control of cervical side-bend UCM with a variety of feedback options (T38.3). There should be no provocation of any symptoms within the range that the side-bend UCM can be controlled.

Once the pattern of dissociation feels familiar it should be integrated into various functional postures and positions. T38.4 and Figures 6.58 and 6.59 illustrate some retraining positions (Figure 6.58 + neural load) (Figure 6.59 + neural unload).

T38.1 Assessment and rating of low threshold recruitment efficiency of the Head Turn Test

HEAD TURN TEST

ASSESSMENT

Control point:
- prevent cervical: side-bend, upper cervical extension, low cervical flexion, mid-cervical hinge
- prevent scapula: depression, downward rotation, retraction, elevation

Movement challenge: head rotation (sitting)

Benchmark range: head rotation to 70–80° from the midline with eyes horizontal

RATING OF LOW THRESHOLD RECRUITMENT EFFICIENCY FOR CONTROL OF DIRECTION

	✓ or ✗		✓ or ✗
• Able to prevent UCM into the test direction Correct dissociation pattern of movement Prevent cervical UCM into: • cervical side-bend • upper cervical extension • low cervical flexion • mid-cervical hinge Prevent scapula UCM into: • depression • downward rotation • retraction • elevation and move head rotation	☐	• Looks easy, and in the opinion of the assessor, is performed with confidence	☐
		• Feels easy, and the subject has sufficient awareness of the movement pattern that they confidently prevent UCM into the test direction	☐
		• The pattern of dissociation is smooth during concentric and eccentric movement	☐
		• Does not (consistently) use *end-range* movement into the opposite direction to prevent the UCM	☐
• Dissociate movement through the benchmark range of: 70–80° head rotation past midline (eyes horizontal) *If there is more available range than the benchmark standard, only the benchmark range needs to be actively controlled*	☐	• No extra feedback needed *(tactile, visual or verbal cueing)*	☐
• Without holding breath (though it is acceptable to use an alternate breathing strategy)	☐	• Without external support or unloading	☐
		• Relaxed natural breathing *(even if not ideal – so long as natural pattern does not change)*	☐
• Control during eccentric phase	☐	• No fatigue	☐
• Control during concentric phase	☐		

CORRECT DISSOCIATION PATTERN   **RECRUITMENT EFFICIENCY**

T38.2 Diagnosis of the site and direction of UCM from the Head Turn Test

HEAD TURN TEST

Site	Direction	To the (L)	To the (R)
Cervical	• Side-bend	☐	☐
Upper cervical	• Extension	☐	☐
Mid-cervical	• Hinge (into extension)	☐	☐
Low cervical	• Flexion	☐	☐
Scapula	• Depression	☐	☐
	• Downward rotation	☐	☐
	• Retraction	☐	☐
	• Elevation	☐	☐

T38.3 Feedback tools to monitor retraining	
FEEDBACK TOOL	**PROCESS**
Self-palpation	Palpation monitoring of joint position
Visual observation	Observe in a mirror or directly watch the movement
Cueing and verbal correction	Listen to feedback from another observer

T38.4 Functional positions for retraining cervical rotation control

- Sitting
- Standing
- Supine (bias anterior muscles)
- Recline sitting backwards (bias anterior muscles)
- Side-lying
- 4 point kneeling (bias posterior muscles)
- Incline sitting forwards (bias posterior muscles)
- Standing forward lean (bias posterior muscles)
- Functional activities

T39 HEAD TILT TEST (tests for rotation and/or side-bend UCM)

This dissociation test assesses the ability to actively dissociate and control cervical and scapula compensations and move the cervical spine into side-bend.

Test procedure

The person sits tall with feet unsupported and pelvis neutral. The low and upper cervical spine is positioned in the neutral training region. The scapula is actively positioned in its neutral training region. Controlling the scapula neutral position is especially important if a myofascial restriction of functional head rotation is identified. The TMJ is also positioned in neutral and the jaw should stay relaxed (Figure 6.60).

The person is instructed to fully side-bend the head by tilting the head towards one shoulder then the other. This should be a pure coronal side-bending and the person should be able to tilt the head through approximately 40° of side-bending keeping the plane of the face facing forwards in the frontal plane (Figure 6.61). There should be no turning (rotation compensating for poor side-bend control) and there should be no chin poke (upper cervical extension compensating for poor side-bend control) or mid-cervical translation. There should be no forward movement of the head (low cervical flexion) compensating for poor side-bend control. The scapula should actively maintain a neutral position with scapula-trunk muscles dominant to scapula-neck muscles.

Ideally, the person should be able to easily prevent chin poke, rotation or head forward compensation with a neutral scapular position and side-bend the cervical spine through 40° range of motion.

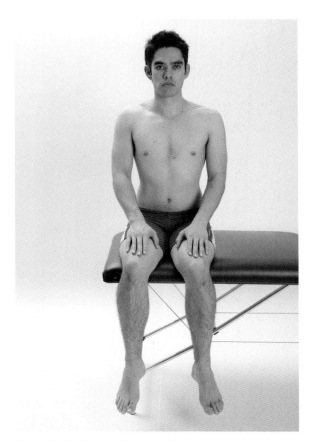

Figure 6.60 Start position head tilt test

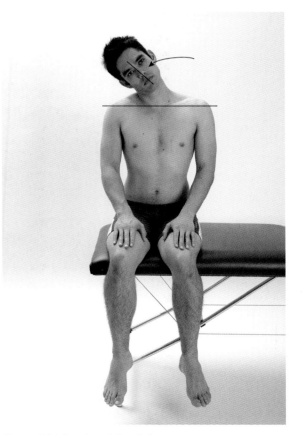

Figure 6.61 Benchmark head tilt test

Table 6.4 Compensation strategies associated with uncontrolled head side-bend	
• Cervical rotation	• Scapular depression
• Upper cervical extension	• Scapular downward
• Low cervical flexion	rotation
• Mid-cervical hinge	• Scapular elevation

Clinical assessment note for direction-specific motor control testing

If some other movement (e.g. a small amount of thoracic flexion) is observed during a motor control (dissociation) test of cervical rotation, *do not* score this as uncontrolled cervical rotation. The thoracic flexion motor control tests will identify if the observed unrelated movement is uncontrolled. *A test for cervical rotation UCM is only positive if uncontrolled cervical **rotation** is demonstrated.*

While teaching, allow the person to initially learn and practise the test movement using feedback from a wall or mirror. Keep the occiput in contact with a supporting surface to monitor that the head tilts into side-bend (coronal movement) and does not turn into rotation. Using a wall also provides support and feedback about scapula position and control during head rotation.

UCMs during side-bend

The person complains of unilateral symptoms in the neck. The cervical spine demonstrates UCM resulting from a variety of compensation strategies associated with head side-bending (Table 6.4). The inability to prevent these compensation strategies during active side-bending identifies UCM.

During the attempt to dissociate these compensations from independent cervical coronal side-bending, the person either cannot control the UCM or has to concentrate and try too hard.

The identification of UCM during cervical side-bending and head lateral tilt needs to be assessed on both sides. Note the direction that the side-bending cannot be controlled (i.e. does the chin poke or rotation during side-bending occur to the left or the right). It may be unilateral or bilateral.

The assessment of restricted motion is reliable only if any compensations/UCM are either actively or passively controlled. When compensations are eliminated, a lack of 40° range of head side-bending identifies 'real' restriction which may be due to either a myofascial or articular restriction or both combined. The uncontrolled side-bending of the head may also be associated with a myofascial restriction holding the scapula in depression or downward rotation caused by inefficiency of the stability function of the scapula-trunk muscles (serratus anterior and middle and lower trapezius).

Rating and diagnosis of cervical rotation/side-bend UCM

(T39.1 and T39.2)

Correction

The person sits or stands with the thoracic spine and head supported against a wall. Using a wall also provides support and feedback about scapula position and control during head side-bending. The low and upper cervical spine is positioned in the neutral training region. The TMJ is also positioned in neutral and the jaw should stay relaxed.

The contralateral scapula is initially passively positioned in upward rotation ± elevation to unload any myofascial restriction. The scapula is actively held against the wall for support and feedback (Figure 6.62). Controlling the scapula neutral position is especially important if a myofascial restriction of functional head side-bending is identified. Some people may need to passively support their contralateral shoulder girdle with their other hand at the elbow (like a sling), or use the armrest of a chair to maintain the unloaded shoulder girdle, or use taping in order to prevent the contralateral scalenes and levator scapula from generating increased tension and adding to the myofascial restriction.

The person is instructed to fully side-bend the head by tilting the ear towards one shoulder then the other. This should be a pure coronal side-bending and the person should be able to tilt the head through approximately 40° of side-bending keeping the plane of the face facing forwards in the frontal plane. There should be no turning (rotation compensating for poor side-bend control) and there should be no chin poke (upper and mid-cervical extension compensating for poor side-bend control). There should be no forward movement of the head (low cervical flexion) compensating for poor side-bend control. Keep the occiput in contact with the wall to monitor that the head tilts into side-bending (coronal movement) and does not turn into rotation. The scapula should actively maintain a neutral position without depression, downward rotation, retraction or elevation.

As control improves and symptoms decrease, the person should begin to actively control the scapula position supported on the wall during the neck side-bending dissociation. The person should eventually progress to active control of the unsupported shoulder girdle off the wall while training neck side-bending dissociation exercises through 40° range of side-bending.

As the ability to control cervical side-bending gets easier and the pattern of dissociation feels less unnatural, the exercise can be progressed from head and shoulder girdle supported to head and shoulder girdle unsupported postures (Figure 6.63).

The person should self-monitor the control of cervical rotation UCM with a variety of feedback options (T39.3). There should be no provocation of any symptoms within the range that the rotation UCM can be controlled.

Once the pattern of dissociation feels familiar it should be integrated into various functional postures and positions: (Figure 6.64 + neural load) (Figure 6.65 + neural unload). T39.4 illustrates some retraining options.

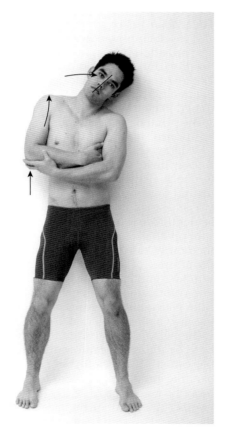

Figure 6.62 Correction standing with wall support and shoulder girdle unloaded

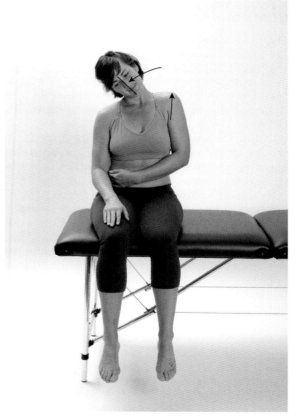

Figure 6.63 Correction sitting unsupported with active shoulder control

T39.1 Assessment and rating of low threshold recruitment efficiency of the Head Tilt Test

HEAD TILT TEST

ASSESSMENT

Control point:
- prevent cervical: rotation, upper cervical extension, low cervical flexion, mid-cervical hinge
- prevent scapula: depression, downward rotation, elevation

Movement challenge: head lateral tilt (sitting)

Benchmark range: head side-bend to 40° from the midline with plane of the face in the frontal plane

RATING OF LOW THRESHOLD RECRUITMENT EFFICIENCY FOR CONTROL OF DIRECTION

	✓ or ✗		✓ or ✗
• Able to prevent UCM into the test direction Correct dissociation pattern of movement	☐	• Looks easy, and in the opinion of the assessor, is performed with confidence	☐
Prevent cervical UCM into:		• Feels easy, and the subject has sufficient awareness of the movement pattern that they confidently prevent UCM into the test direction	☐
• cervical rotation			
• upper cervical extension			
• low cervical flexion		• The pattern of dissociation is smooth during concentric and eccentric movement	☐
• mid-cervical hinge			
Prevent scapula UCM into:		• Does not (consistently) use *end-range* movement into the opposite direction to prevent the UCM	☐
• depression			
• downward rotation			
• elevation		• No extra feedback needed *(tactile, visual or verbal cueing)*	☐
and move head side-bend			
• Dissociate movement through the benchmark range of: 40° head lateral tilt past midline (face in frontal plane) *If there is more available range than the benchmark standard, only the benchmark range needs to be actively controlled*	☐	• Without external support or unloading	☐
		• Relaxed natural breathing *(even if not ideal – so long as natural pattern does not change)*	☐
		• No fatigue	☐
• Without holding breath (though it is acceptable to use an alternate breathing strategy)	☐		
• Control during eccentric phase	☐		
• Control during concentric phase	☐		

CORRECT DISSOCIATION PATTERN   **RECRUITMENT EFFICIENCY**

T39.2 Diagnosis of the site and direction of UCM from the Head Tilt Test

HEAD TILT TEST

Site	Direction	To the (L)	To the (R)
Cervical	• Rotation	☐	☐
Upper cervical	• Extension	☐	☐
Mid-cervical	• Hinge (into extension)	☐	☐
Low cervical	• Flexion	☐	☐
Scapula	• Depression	☐	☐
	• Downward rotation	☐	☐
	• Elevation	☐	☐

T39.3 Feedback tools to monitor retraining	
FEEDBACK TOOL	**PROCESS**
Self-palpation	Palpation monitoring of joint position
Visual observation	Observe in a mirror or directly watch the movement
Cueing and verbal correction	Listen to feedback from another observer

T39.4 Functional positions for retraining cervical side-bend control

- Sitting
- Standing
- Recline sitting backwards (bias anterior muscles)
- Side-lying

- 4 point kneeling (bias posterior muscles)
- Incline sitting forwards (bias posterior muscles)
- Standing forward lean (bias posterior muscles)
- Functional activities

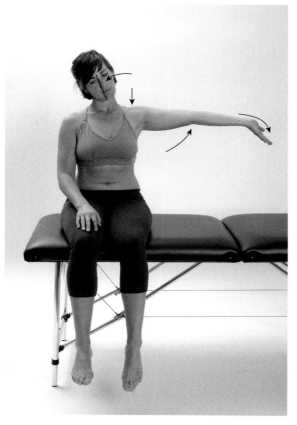

Figure 6.64 Correction unsupported with neural loading

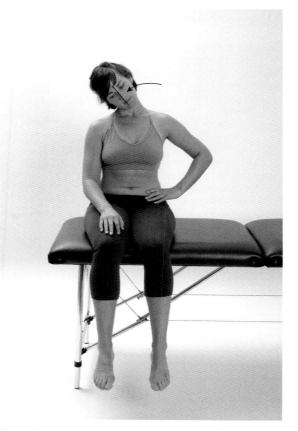

Figure 6.65 Correction unsupported with neural unloading

280

T40 UPPER NECK TILT TEST
(tests for rotation/side-bend UCM)

This dissociation test assesses the ability to actively dissociate and control low cervical side-bend and move the upper cervical spine into side-bend.

Test procedure

The person sits tall with feet unsupported and pelvis neutral. The low and upper cervical spine is positioned in the neutral training region. The scapula is actively positioned in its neutral training region. Controlling the scapula neutral position is especially important if a myofascial restriction of functional head rotation is identified. The TMJ is also positioned in neutral and the jaw should stay relaxed (Figure 6.66). The therapist monitors low cervical side-bend control by palpating the C4–7 spinous processes.

The person is instructed to prevent side-bending in the low cervical spine (do not move at the base of the neck) and then actively tilt the head through the available range of upper cervical side-bend by tilting the head at the base of the skull. As the ear drops towards the shoulder, the chin should move towards the opposite side (Figure 6.67). There should be no low cervical side-bend (monitor the C4–7 transverse or spinous processes) or uncontrolled compensation (e.g. head rotation or chin poke). This should be a pure coronal side-bending keeping the plane of the face facing forwards in the frontal plane. The scapula should actively maintain a neutral position.

Low cervical side-bend UCM

The person complains of unilateral symptoms at the base of the neck and low cervical spine. The low cervical spine and upper trunk has greater give *into side-bend* relative to the upper cervical

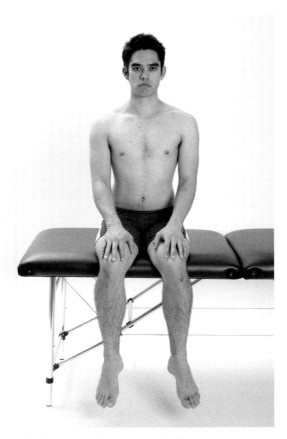

Figure 6.66 Start position upper neck tilt test

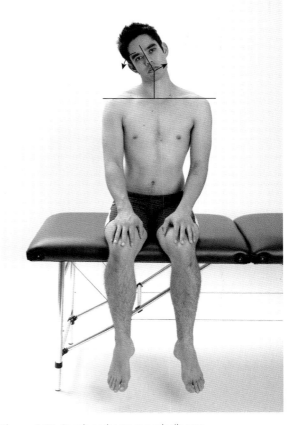

Figure 6.67 Benchmark upper neck tilt test

Table 6.5 Compensation strategies associated with uncontrolled side-bend

- Low cervical side-bend
- Upper cervical extension
- Upper cervical rotation
- Scapular elevation

spine and head under head side-bending or unilateral arm loading.

The person complains of unilateral symptoms in the lower neck and across the top of the shoulders. The cervical spine demonstrates UCM resulting from a variety of compensation strategies associated with head side-bending (Table 6.5). The inability to prevent these compensation strategies during active side-bending identifies UCM.

During the attempt to dissociate these compensations from independent upper cervical side-bending (face in the frontal plane), the person either cannot control the UCM or has to concentrate and try too hard.

The identification of UCM during upper cervical side-bending and head lateral tilt needs to be assessed on both sides. Note the direction that the side-bending cannot be controlled (i.e. does the chin poke or rotation during side-bending occur to the left or the right). It may be unilateral or bilateral.

The assessment of restricted motion is reliable only if any compensations/UCM are either actively or passively controlled. When compensations are eliminated, a lack of end range of upper cervical side-bending identifies 'real' restriction which may be due to either a myofascial or articular restriction or both combined. The uncontrolled upper cervical side-bending of the head may also be associated with a myofascial restriction holding the scapula in depression or downward rotation caused by inefficiency of the stability function of the scapula-trunk muscles (serratus anterior and middle and lower trapezius).

Clinical assessment note for direction-specific motor control testing

If some other movement (e.g. a small amount of thoracic flexion) is observed during a motor control (dissociation) test of low cervical side-bend, *do not* score this as uncontrolled low cervical side-bend. The thoracic flexion motor control tests will identify if the observed unrelated movement is uncontrolled. *A test for low cervical side-bend UCM is only positive if uncontrolled low cervical* **side-bend** *is demonstrated.*

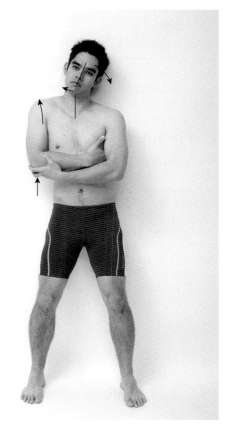

Figure 6.68 Correction standing with wall support and shoulder girdle unloaded

Rating and diagnosis of cervical rotation/side-bend UCM

(T40.1 and T40.2)

Correction

The person sits or stands with the thoracic spine and head supported against a wall. Using a wall also provides support and feedback about scapula position and control during head side-bending. The low and upper cervical spine is positioned in the neutral training region. The TMJ is also positioned in neutral and the jaw should stay relaxed.

The contralateral scapula is initially passively positioned in upward rotation ± elevation to unload any myofascial restriction. The scapula is actively held against the wall for support and feedback (Figure 6.68). Some people may need to

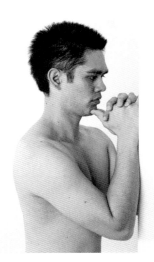

Figure 6.69 Correction – hand position for feedback

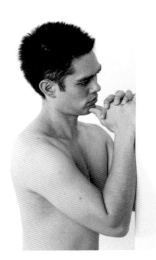

Figure 6.70 Correction with feedback

passively support their contralateral shoulder girdle with their other hand at the elbow (like a sling), or use the armrest of a chair to maintain the unloaded shoulder girdle, or use taping in order to prevent the contralateral scalenes and levator scapula from generating increased tension and adding to the myofascial restriction.

The person monitors low cervical side-bend control by palpating the C4–7 transverse and spinous processes. The person can also use their hand to provide manual fixation and support for the low cervical spine if necessary. The person is then instructed to actively tilt the head through the available range of upper cervical side-bend by tilting the head at the base of the skull while preventing side-bending in the low cervical spine. As the ear drops towards the shoulder the chin should move towards the opposite side.

As control improves and symptoms decrease the person should begin to actively control the scapula position supported on the wall during the neck side-bending dissociation. The person should eventually progress to active control of the unsupported shoulder girdle off the wall while training neck side-bending dissociation exercises.

An alternative progression is to face the wall with the forearms vertical on the wall. Keep the scapula in mid-position and push the body and head away from the wall, then clasp hands with the thumbs abducted and position the thumbs on the chin for feedback and support (Figure 6.69). Keeping the elbows on the wall, the head back over the shoulders and the chin in contact with the thumbs, slowly tilt the head side to side only so far as there is no low cervical side-bend (Figure 6.70). Pivot the chin off the thumbs to ensure that the movement is localised to the upper cervical spine.

The person should self-monitor the control of low cervical side-bend UCM with a variety of feedback options (T40.3). There should be no provocation of any symptoms within the range that the side-bend UCM can be controlled.

Once the pattern of dissociation feels familiar it should be integrated into various functional postures and positions. T40.4 illustrates some retraining options.

T40.1 Assessment and rating of low threshold recruitment efficiency of the Upper Neck Tilt Test

UPPER NECK TILT TEST

ASSESSMENT

Control point:
- prevent low cervical: side-bend
- prevent upper cervical rotation and extension
- prevent scapular elevation

Movement challenge: upper cervical side-bend (sitting)

Benchmark range: head side-bend through full available from the midline with plane of the face in the frontal plane

RATING OF LOW THRESHOLD RECRUITMENT EFFICIENCY FOR CONTROL OF DIRECTION

	✓ or ✗		✓ or ✗
• Able to prevent UCM into the test direction Correct dissociation pattern of movement	☐	• Looks easy, and in the opinion of the assessor, is performed with confidence	☐
Prevent low cervical UCM into:		• Feels easy, and the subject has sufficient awareness of the movement pattern that they confidently prevent UCM into the test direction	☐
• low cervical side-bend			
• upper cervical extension			
• low cervical rotation		• The pattern of dissociation is smooth during concentric and eccentric movement	☐
Prevent scapula UCM into:			
• depression		• Does not (consistently) use *end-range* movement into the opposite direction to prevent the UCM	☐
• downward rotation			
• elevation			
and move upper cervical side-bend		• No extra feedback needed *(tactile, visual or verbal cueing)*	☐
• Dissociate movement through the benchmark range of: full end-range upper cervical side-bend past midline (face in frontal plane) *If there is more available range than the benchmark standard, only the benchmark range needs to be actively controlled*	☐	• Without external support or unloading	☐
		• Relaxed natural breathing *(even if not ideal – so long as natural pattern does not change)*	☐
		• No fatigue	☐
• Without holding breath (though it is acceptable to use an alternate breathing strategy)	☐		
• Control during eccentric phase	☐		
• Control during concentric phase	☐		

CORRECT DISSOCIATION PATTERN   **RECRUITMENT EFFICIENCY**

T40.2 Diagnosis of the site and direction of UCM from the Upper Neck Tilt Test

UPPER NECK TILT TEST

Site	Direction	To the (L)	To the (R)
Low cervical	• Side-bend	☐	☐
Upper cervical	• Rotation • Extension	☐	☐
Scapula	• Elevation	☐	☐

T40.3 Feedback tools to monitor retraining

FEEDBACK TOOL	PROCESS
Self-palpation	Palpation monitoring of joint position
Visual observation	Observe in a mirror or directly watch the movement
Cueing and verbal correction	Listen to feedback from another observer

---

T40.4 Functional positions for retraining low cervical side-bend control

- Sitting
- Standing
- Recline sitting backwards (bias anterior muscles)
- Side-lying
- 4 point kneeling (bias posterior muscles)
- Incline sitting forwards (bias posterior muscles)
- Standing forward lean (bias posterior muscles)
- Functional activities

T41 LOWER NECK LEAN TEST (tests for rotation/side-bend UCM)

This dissociation test assesses the ability to actively dissociate and control upper cervical side-bend and move the low cervical spine into side-bend.

Test procedure

The person sits tall with feet unsupported and pelvis neutral. The low and upper cervical spine is positioned in the neutral training region. The scapula is actively positioned in its neutral training region. Controlling the scapula neutral position is especially important if a myofascial restriction of functional head rotation is identified. The TMJ is also positioned in neutral and the jaw should stay relaxed (Figure 6.71). The therapist monitors upper cervical side-bend control by palpating the C1–3 transverse and spinous processes.

The person is instructed to prevent side-bending in the upper cervical spine (do not move at the base of the skull) and then actively lean the head through the available range of low cervical side-bend by tilting the head at the base of the neck. As the head leans towards the shoulder, the chin should move towards the same side (Figure 6.72). There should be no upper cervical side-bend (monitor the C1–3 spinous processes) or uncontrolled compensation (upper cervical rotation or extension and low cervical flexion). This should be a pure coronal side-bending keeping the plane of the face facing forwards in the frontal plane. The scapula should actively maintain a neutral position with scapula-trunk muscles dominant to scapula-neck muscles.

Upper cervical side-bend UCM

The person complains of unilateral symptoms in the upper cervical spine or at the base of the skull. The upper cervical spine has greater give

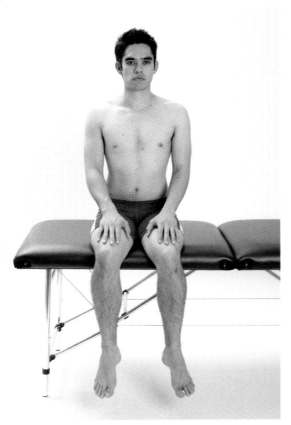

Figure 6.71 Start position lower neck lean test

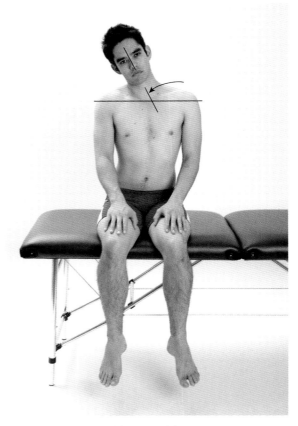

Figure 6.72 Benchmark lower neck lean test

Table 6.6 Compensation strategies associated with uncontrolled side-bend

- Upper cervical side-bend
- Upper cervical rotation
- Low cervical flexion
- Scapular elevation

into side-bend relative to the low cervical spine and head under head side-bending or unilateral arm loading.

The person complains of unilateral symptoms in the lower neck and across the top of the shoulders. The cervical spine demonstrates UCM resulting from a variety of compensation strategies associated with head side-bending (Table 6.6). The inability to prevent these compensation strategies during active side-bending identifies UCM.

During the attempt to dissociate these compensations from independent low cervical side-bending (face in the frontal plane), the person either cannot control the UCM or has to concentrate and try too hard.

The identification of UCM during low cervical side-bending and lateral tilt needs to be assessed on both sides. Note the direction that the side-bending cannot be controlled (i.e. does the rotation or chin poke during side-bending occur to the left or the right). It may be unilateral or bilateral.

The assessment of restricted motion is reliable only if any compensations/UCM are either actively or passively controlled. When compensations are eliminated, a lack of end range of low cervical side-bending identifies 'real' restriction, which may be due to either a myofascial or articular restriction or both combined. The uncontrolled cervical side-bending of the head may also be associated with a myofascial restriction holding the scapula in depression or downward rotation caused by inefficiency of the stability function of the scapula-trunk muscles (serratus anterior and middle and lower trapezius).

Clinical assessment note for direction-specific motor control testing

If some other movement (e.g. a small amount of thoracic flexion) is observed during a motor control (dissociation) test of upper cervical side-bend, *do not* score this as uncontrolled upper cervical side-bend. The thoracic flexion motor control tests will identify if the observed unrelated movement is uncontrolled. *A test for upper cervical side-bend UCM is only positive if uncontrolled upper cervical **side-bend** is demonstrated.*

Rating and diagnosis of cervical rotation/side-bend UCM

(T41.1 and T41.2)

Correction

The person sits or stands with the thoracic spine and head supported against a wall. Using a wall also provides support and feedback about scapula position and control during head side-bending. The low and upper cervical spine is positioned in the neutral training region. The TMJ is also positioned in neutral and the jaw should stay relaxed.

The contralateral scapula is initially passively positioned in upward rotation ± elevation to unload any myofascial restriction. The scapula is actively held against the wall for support and feedback (Figure 6.73). Some persons may need to passively support their contralateral shoulder

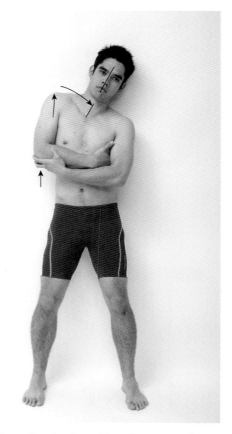

Figure 6.73 Correction standing with wall support and shoulder girdle unloaded

girdle with their other hand at the elbow (like a sling), or use the armrest of a chair to maintain the unloaded shoulder girdle, or use taping in order to prevent the contralateral scalenes and levator scapula from generating increased tension and adding to the myofascial restriction.

The person monitors upper cervical side-bend control by palpating the C0–3 transverse and spinous processes. The person can also use their hand to provide manual fixation and support for the upper cervical spine if necessary. The person is then instructed to actively tilt the head through the available range of lower cervical side-bend by tilting the head at the base of the neck while preventing side-bending in the upper cervical spine. As the ear drops towards the shoulder the chin should move towards the same side.

As control improves and symptoms decrease, the person should begin to actively control the scapula position supported on the wall during the neck side-bending dissociation. The person should eventually progress to active control of the unsupported shoulder girdle off the wall while training neck side-bending dissociation exercises.

The person should self-monitor the control of upper cervical side-bend UCM with a variety of feedback options (T41.3). There should be no provocation of any symptoms within the range that the side-bend UCM can be controlled.

Once the pattern of dissociation feels familiar it should be integrated into various functional postures and positions. T41.4 illustrates some retraining options.

T41.1 Assessment and rating of low threshold recruitment efficiency of the Lower Neck Lean Test

LOWER NECK LEAN TEST

ASSESSMENT

Control point:
- prevent upper cervical: side-bend, rotation
- prevent lower cervical flexion
- prevent scapular elevation

Movement challenge: low cervical side-bend (sitting)

Benchmark range: low cervical side-bend through full available from the midline with plane of the face in the frontal plane

RATING OF LOW THRESHOLD RECRUITMENT EFFICIENCY FOR CONTROL OF DIRECTION

	✓ or ✗		✓ or ✗
• Able to prevent UCM into the test direction Correct dissociation pattern of movement	☐	• Looks easy, and in the opinion of the assessor, is performed with confidence	☐
Prevent low cervical UCM into: • upper cervical side-bend • upper cervical extension • low cervical rotation		• Feels easy, and the subject has sufficient awareness of the movement pattern that they confidently prevent UCM into the test direction	☐
Prevent scapula UCM into: • elevation and move low cervical side-bend		• The pattern of dissociation is smooth during concentric and eccentric movement	☐
• Dissociate movement through the benchmark range of: full end-range 15° low cervical side-bend past midline (face in frontal plane) *If there is more available range than the benchmark standard, only the benchmark range needs to be actively controlled*	☐	• Does not (consistently) use *end-range* movement into the opposite direction to prevent the UCM	☐
		• No extra feedback needed *(tactile, visual or verbal cueing)*	☐
• Without holding breath (though it is acceptable to use an alternate breathing strategy)	☐	• Without external support or unloading	☐
		• Relaxed natural breathing *(even if not ideal – so long as natural pattern does not change)*	☐
• Control during eccentric phase	☐	• No fatigue	☐
• Control during concentric phase	☐		

CORRECT DISSOCIATION PATTERN   **RECRUITMENT EFFICIENCY**

T41.2 Diagnosis of the site and direction of UCM from the Lower Neck Lean Test

LOWER NECK LEAN TEST

Site	Direction	To the (L)	To the (R)
Upper cervical	• Rotation • Extension	☐ ☐	☐ ☐
Low cervical	• Flexion	☐	☐
Scapula	• Elevation	☐	☐

T41.3 Feedback tools to monitor retraining

FEEDBACK TOOL	PROCESS
Self-palpation	Palpation monitoring of joint position
Visual observation	Observe in a mirror or directly watch the movement
Cueing and verbal correction	Listen to feedback from another observer

---

T41.4 Functional positions for retraining upper cervical side-bend control

- Sitting
- Standing
- Recline sitting backwards (bias anterior muscles)
- Side-lying
- 4 point kneeling (bias posterior muscles)
- Incline sitting forwards (bias posterior muscles)
- Standing forward lean (bias posterior muscles)
- Functional activities

Cervical stability dysfunction summary

(Table 6.7)

Table 6.7 Summary and rating of cervical tests		
UCM DIAGNOSIS AND TESTING		
Test of stability control (site and direction)	Rating (✓✓ or ✓✗ or ✗✗) and rationale	
SITE: LOW CERVICAL	**DIRECTION: FLEXION**	**CLINICAL PRIORITY** ☐
Occiput lift test		
Thoracic flexion test		
Overhead arm lift test		
SITE: UPPER CERVICAL	**DIRECTION: FLEXION**	**CLINICAL PRIORITY** ☐
Forward head lean test		
Arm extension test		
SITE: UPPER CERVICAL	**DIRECTION: EXTENSION**	**CLINICAL PRIORITY** ☐
Backward head lift test		
Horizontal retraction test		
SITE: MID-CERVICAL	**DIRECTION: TRANSLATION (DURING EXTENSION)**	**CLINICAL PRIORITY** ☐
Head back hinge test		
Chin lift hinge test		
SITE: CERVICAL	**DIRECTION: SIDE-BEND**	**CLINICAL PRIORITY** ☐
Head turn test	(L)	(R)
SITE: CERVICAL	**DIRECTION: ROTATION**	**CLINICAL PRIORITY** ☐
Head tilt test	(L)	(R)
SITE: LOW CERVICAL	**DIRECTION: SIDE-BEND**	**CLINICAL PRIORITY** ☐
Upper neck tilt test	(L)	(R)
SITE: UPPER CERVICAL	**DIRECTION: SIDE-BEND**	**CLINICAL PRIORITY** ☐
Lower neck lean test	(L)	(R)

REFERENCES

Amevo, B., Aprill, C., Bogduk, N., 1992. Abnormal instantaneous axes of rotation in patients with neck pain. Spine 54 (2), 213–217.

Butler, D., 2000. The sensitive nervous system. NOI Publications, Adelaide, Australia.

Caldwell, C., Sahrmann, S., Van, D., 2007. Use of a movement system impairment diagnosis for physical therapy in the management of a patient with shoulder pain. Journal of Orthopaedic and Sports Physical Therpay 37 (9), 551–563.

Cheng, J.S., Liu, F., Komistek, R.D., Mahfouz, M.R., Sharma, A., Glaser, D., 2007. Comparison of cervical spine kinematics using a fluoroscopic model for adjacent segment degeneration. Invited submission from the Joint Section on Disorders of the Spine and Peripheral Nerves, March 2007. Journal of Neurosurgery, Spine 7 (5), 509–513.

Comerford, M.J., Mottram, S.L., 2011. Diagnosis of uncontrolled movement, subgroup classification and motor control retraining of the neck. Kinetic Control, UK.

Dall'Alba, P.T., Sterling, M.M., Treleaven, J.M., Edwards, S.L., Jull, G.A., 2001. Cervical range of motion discriminates between asymptomatic persons and those with whiplash. Spine 26 (19), 2090–2094.

Dvorak, J., Froehlich, D., Penning, L., Baumgartner, H., Panjabi, M.M., 1998. Functional radiographic diagnosis of the cervical spine: flexion/extension. Spine 13, 748–755.

Falla, D., Farina, D., 2007. Neural and muscular factors associated with motor impairment in neck pain. Current Rheumatology Reports 9 (6), 497–502.

Falla, D., Bilenkij, G., Jull, G., 2004b. Patients with chronic neck pain demonstrate altered patterns of muscle activation during performance of a functional upper limb task. Spine 29, 1436–1440.

Falla, D., Jull, G., Hodges, P., 2004a. Patients with neck pain demonstrate

reduced electromyographic activity of the deep cervical flexor muscles during performance of the craniocervical flexion test. Spine 29, 2108–2114.

Falla, D., Jull, G., Hodges, P., Vicenzino, B., 2006. An endurance-strength training regime is effective in reducing myoelectric manifestations of cervical flexor muscle fatigue in females with chronic neck pain. Clinical Neurophysiology 117, 828–837.

Falla, D., Jull, G., Russell, T., Vicenzino, B., Hodges, P., 2007. Effect of neck exercise on sitting posture in patients with chronic neck pain. Physical Therapy 87, 408–417.

Fernández-de-las-Peñas, C., Falla, D., Arendt-Nielsen, L., Farina, D., 2008. Cervical muscle co-activation in isometric contractions is enhanced in chronic tension-type headache patients. Cephalalgia 28 (7), 744–751.

Fernández-de-las-Peñas, C., Pérez-de-Heredia, M., Molero-Sánchez, A., Miangolarra-Page, J.C., 2007. Performance of the craniocervical flexion test, forward head posture, and headache clinical parameters in patients with chronic tension-type headache: a pilot study. Journal of Orthopaedic and Sports Physical Therapy 37 (2), 33–39.

Fritz, J.M., Brennan, G.P., 2007. Preliminary examination of a proposed treatment-based classification system for patients receiving physical therapy interventions for neck pain. Physical Therapy 87 (5), 513–524.

Grip, H., Sundelin, G., Gerdle, B., Karlsson, J.S., 2008. Cervical helical axis characteristics and its center of rotation during active head and upper arm movements – comparisons of whiplash-associated disorders, non-specific neck pain and asymptomatic individuals. Journal of Biomechanics doi:10.1016/j.jbiomech.2008.07.005.

Gross, A.R., Hoving, J.L., Haines, T.A., Goldsmith, C.H., Kay, T., Aker, P., et al., 2004. Cervical, Overview Group. A Cochrane review of manipulation and mobilization for

mechanical neck disorders. Spine 29, 1541–1548.

Johnston, V., Jull, G., Darnell, R., Jimmieson, N.L., Souvlis, T., Jull, G., et al., 2008b. Alterations in cervical muscle activity in functional and stressful tasks in female office workers with neck pain. European Journal of Applied Physiology 103 (3), 253–264.

Johnston, V., Jull, G., Souvlis T., Jimmieson, N.L., 2008a. Neck movements and muscle activity characteristics in office workers with neck pain. Spine 33 (5), 555–563.

Jull, G., Kristjansson, E., Dall'Alba, P., 2004. Impairment in the cervical flexors: a comparison of whiplash and insidious onset neck pain patients. Manual Therapy 9, 89–94.

Jull, G., Sterling, M., Falla, D., Treleaven, J., O'Leary, S., 2008. Whiplash, headache and neck pain. Elsevier, Edinburgh.

Jull, G., Trott, P., Potter, H., Zito, G., Niere, K., Shirley, D., et al., 2002. A randomized controlled trial of exercise and manipulative therapy for cervicogenic headache. Spine 27, 1835–1843.

Kapandji, I.A., 1982. The physiology of the joints, 5th edn. Vol 3. The trunk and vertebral column. Churchill Livingstone, Edinburgh.

Kapreli, E., Vourazanis, E., Strimpakos, N., 2008. Neck pain causes respiratory dysfunction. Medical Hypotheses 70 (5), 1009–1013.

Kjellman, G.V., Skargren, E.I., Oberg, B.E., 1999. A critical analysis of randomised clinical trials on neck pain and treatment efficiency. A review of the literature. Scandinavian Journal of Rehabilitation Medicine 31, 139–152.

Lindman, R., Eriksson, A., Thornell, L.E., 1991a. Fiber type composition of the human female trapezius muscle: enzyme – histochemical characteristics. American Journal of Anatomy 190 (4), 385–392.

Lindman, R., Hagberg, M., Karl-Axis, A., Soderlund, K., Hultman, E., Thornell, L.E., 1991b. Changes in muscle morphology in chronic trapezius myalgia. Scandinavian

Journal of Work, Environment and Health 17 (5), 347–355.

McDonnell, M.K., Sahrmann, S.A., Van Dillen, L., 2005. A specific exercise program and modification of postural alignment for treatment of cervicogenic headache: a case report. Journal of Orthopaedic and Sports Physical Therapy 35, 3–15.

Miyazaki, M., Hong, S.W., Yoon, S.H., Zou, J., Tow, B., Alanay, A., et al., 2008. Kinematic analysis of the relationship between the grade of disc degeneration and motion unit of the cervical spine. Spine 33 (2), 187–193.

Mottram, S.L., 2003. Dynamic stability of the scapula. In: Beeton, K.S. (Eds), Manual therapy masterclasses – the peripheral joints. Churchill Livingstone, Edinburgh.

Nederhand, M.J., Hermens, H.J., IJzerman, M.J., Turk, D.C., Zilvold, G., 2002. Cervical muscle dysfunction in chronic whiplash-associated disorder grade 2: the relevance of the trauma. Spine 27 (10), 1056–1061.

Nederhand, M.J., Ijzerman, M.J., Hermens, H., Baten, C.T., Zilvold, G., 2000. Cervical muscle dysfunction in the chronic whiplash associated disorder grade II (WAD-II). Spine 25 (15), 1938–1943.

O'Leary, S., Jull, G., Kim, M., Vicenzino, B., 2007. Cranio-cervical flexor muscle impairment at maximal, moderate, and low loads is a feature of neck pain. Manual Therapy 12, 34–39.

Panjabi, M.M., 1992. The stabilising system of the spine. Part II. Neutral zone and instability hypothesis. Journal of Spinal Disorders 5 (4), 390–397.

Sahrmann, S.A., 2002. Diagnosis and treatment of movement impairment syndromes. Mosby, St Louis, MO.

Shacklock, M., 2005. Clinical neurodynamics: a new system of neuromusculoskeletal treatment. Butterworth Heinmann, Edinburgh.

Singer, K.P., Fitzgerald, D., Milne, N., 1993. Neck retraction exercises and cervical disk disease. MPAA Conference proceedings, Australia.

Sterling, M., Jull, G., Vicenzino, B., Kenardy, J., Darnell, R., 2003. Development of motor system dysfunction following whiplash injury. Pain 103 (1–2), 65–73.

Sterling, M., Jull, G., Vicenzino, B., Kenardy, J., Darnell, R., 2005. Physical and psychological factors predict outcome following whiplash injury. Pain 114 (1–2), 141–148.

Straker, L.M., O'Sullivan, P.B., Smith, A.J., Perry, M.C., 2008. Relationships between prolonged neck/shoulder pain and sitting spinal posture in male and female adolescents. Manual Therapy, doi:10.1016/j.math.2008.04.004.

Szeto, G.P.Y., Straker, L., O'Sullivan, P., 2005a. A comparison of symptomatic and asymptomatic office workers performing monotonous keyboard work. 1: Neck and shoulder muscle recruitment patterns. Manual Therapy 10, 270–280.

Szeto, G.P.Y., Straker, L., O'Sullivan, P., 2005b. A comparison of symptomatic and asymptomatic office workers performing monotonous keyboard work. 2: Neck and shoulder kinematics. Manual Therapy 10, 281–291.

Szeto, G.P., Straker, L.M., O'Sullivan, P.B., 2008. Neck-shoulder muscle activity in general and task-specific resting postures of symptomatic computer users with chronic neck pain. Doi:10.1016/j.math.2008.05.001.

Van Dillen, L.R., McDonnell, M.K., Susco, T.M., Sahrmann, S.A., 2007. The immediate effect of passive scapular elevation on symptoms with active neck rotation in patients with neck pain. Clinical Journal of Pain 23 (8), 641–647.

Verhagen, A.P., Scholten-Peeters, G.G., de Bie, R.A., Bierma-Zeinstra, S.M., 2004. Conservative treatments for whiplash. Cochrane Database Syst. Rev. 1, CD003338.

White, 3rd., A.A., Johnson, R.M., Panjabi, M.M., Southwick, W.O., 1975. Biomechanical analysis of clinical stability in the cervical spine. Clinical Orthopaedics and Related Research (109), 85–96.

Yip, C.H., Chiu, T.T., Poon, A.T., 2008. The relationship between head posture and severity and disability of patients with neck pain. Manual Therapy 13 (2), 148–154.

CHAPTER 7
THE THORACIC SPINE

Chapter | **7** |

The thoracic spine

INTRODUCTION

The thoracic spine has been the focus of little research or review attention compared to the lumbar and cervical spine. This may partly be due to the lower frequency of thoracic spinal pain syndrome and partly because the thoracic region is well stabilised by the rib cage and rib articulations to the thoracic vertebrae (Watkins et al 2005). Almost all of the research and review literature available that is related to the thoracic spine is based on anatomical and biomechanical analysis of osteoligamentous and myofascial influences on articular function (Edmondston & Singer 1997; Maitland et al 2005). There is a lack of research and analysis of neurophysiological motor control changes associated with pain and dysfunction in the thorax.

Changes in movement and postural control in the thoracic spine

Most of the clinical interventions to address motor control dysfunction of the thoracic spine are extrapolated from the current research derived from the lumbar spine and cervical spine (Carrière 1996; Lee 1996, 2003; Lee et al 2005).

There are currently no significant studies published measuring uncontrolled movement (UCM) in the thoracic spine. Observations of thoracic UCM are largely anecdotal, and management guidelines are based on principles and strategies that have been developed from the extensive research conducted in the lumbar spine and neck. This chapter details the assessment of UCM at the thoracic spine and describes retraining strategies.

DIAGNOSIS OF THE SITE AND DIRECTION OF UCM IN THE THORACIC SPINE

The diagnosis of the site and direction of UCM in the thoracic spine can be identified in terms of the *site* (being thoracic spine) and the *direction* of flexion, extension, rotation and respiratory movement (Table 7.1).

Linking the site of UCM to symptom presentation

A diagnosis of UCM requires evaluation of its clinical priority. This is based on the relationship between the UCM and the presenting symptoms. The therapist should look for a link between the direction of UCM and the direction of symptom provocation: i) Does the site of UCM relate to the site or joint that the patient complains of as the source of symptoms? ii) Does the direction of movement or load testing relate to the direction or position of provocation of symptoms? *This identifies the clinical priorities.*

Table 7.1 Site and direction of UCM in the thorax

SITE	DIRECTION
Thoracic	• Flexion • Extension • Rotation • Respiratory/ribs

The site and direction of UCM at the thoracic spine can link with different clinical presentations, and postures and activities which may aggravate symptoms. The typical assessment findings in the thoracic spine are identified in Table 7.2.

The following section will demonstrate the specific procedures for testing for UCM in the thoracic spine.

Table 7.2 The site and direction of UCM at the thoracic spine linked with different clinical presentations

SITE AND DIRECTION OF UCM	SYMPTOM PRESENTATION	PROVOCATIVE MOVEMENTS, POSTURES AND ACTIVITIES
THORACIC FLEXION UCM Can present as: • uncontrolled thoracic flexion (with or without hypermobile flexion range)	• Presents with symptoms in the posterior chest and/or lateral ribs • May present with a localised pain pattern • ± Radicular pain from myofascial and articular structures	Symptoms provoked by thoracic flexion movements and postures (especially if repetitive or sustained); for example, sustained sitting (especially if slouching at a desk), bending forwards, driving, looking down, reaching forwards
THORACIC EXTENSION UCM Can present as: • uncontrolled thoracic extension (with or without hypermobile extension range)	• Presents with symptoms in the posterior chest and/or lateral ribs • May present with a localised pain pattern • ± Radicular pain from myofascial and articular structures	Symptoms provoked by thoracic extension movements and postures (especially if repetitive or sustained); for example, sustained standing, arching backwards, looking up, reaching overhead, reaching backwards
THORACIC ROTATION UCM Can present as: • uncontrolled thoracic rotation (with or without hypermobile rotation range) • unilaterally or bilaterally	• Presents with symptoms in the posterior chest and/or lateral ribs • May present with a localised pain pattern • ± Radicular pain from myofascial and articular structures	Symptoms provoked by thoracic rotation movements and postures (especially if repetitive or sustained); for example, twisting to one side, looking over one shoulder, reaching forwards or backwards or out to the side with one arm, throwing, weight bearing on one arm or pushing with one arm
THORACIC/RIBS RESPIRATORY UCM Can present as: • uncontrolled thoracic or rib inspiratory or expiratory movement • unilaterally or bilaterally	• Presents with symptoms in the posterior chest and/or lateral ribs or anterior ribs and sternum • May present with a localised pain pattern • ± Radicular pain from myofascial and articular structures	Symptoms provoked by thoracic or rib respiratory movements (inspiration or expiration); for example, twisting or side-bending to one side, deep inspiration (breath in), full expiration (breath out), cough or sneeze, bracing ribcage to push, pull or lift a heavy load

THORACIC TESTS FOR UCM

Thoracic flexion control

THORACIC FLEXION CONTROL TESTS AND FLEXION CONTROL REHABILITATION

These flexion control tests assess the extent of flexion UCM in the thoracic spine and assess the ability of the dynamic stability system to adequately control flexion load or strain. It is a priority to assess for flexion UCM if the person complains of or demonstrates flexion-related symptoms or disability. The tests that identify dysfunction can also be used to guide and direct rehabilitation strategies.

Movement faults associated with thoracic flexion

Relative stiffness (restrictions)

- *Lumbopelvic restriction of flexion* – a lumbopelvic flexion restriction may contribute to compensatory increases in thoracic flexion range. This is confirmed with manual segmental assessment (e.g. Maitland PPIVMs or PAIVMs) of the lumbopelvic joints. There may also be a loss of lumbar-dorsal fascia extensibility if a lordotic posture is exaggerated.
- *Cervical restriction of flexion* – a cervical flexion restriction may contribute to compensatory increases in thoracic flexion range. This is not usually associated with articular restrictions of flexion. However, a chin poke neck posture may have an increased cervical lordosis and a loss of extensibility of the posterior cervical fascias and the ligamentum nuchae.
- *Scapular restriction of protraction* – recruitment overactivity or postural change may result in a loss of extensibility of the rhomboids. A subsequent myofascial restriction of scapular protraction may also contribute to compensatory increases in thoracic flexion range.

Relative flexibility (potential UCM)

- *Thoracic flexion* – the thoracic spine may initiate the movement into flexion and contribute more to producing forward bending while the lumbar spine and hip contributions start later and contribute less. At the limit of forward bending, excessive or hypermobile range of thoracic flexion may be observed. During the return to neutral the thoracic flexion persists and presents as an increased thoracic kyphosis.

Indications to test for thoracic flexion UCM

Observe or palpate for:
1. hypermobile thoracic flexion range
2. excessive initiation of bending or leaning forwards with thoracic flexion
3. symptoms (pain, discomfort, strain) associated with bending or reaching forwards with associated thoracic flexion.

The person complains of flexion-related symptoms in the thorax. Under flexion load, the thoracic spine has greater give *into flexion* relative to the lumbar spine, head and shoulders. The dysfunction is confirmed with motor control tests of flexion dissociation.

295

Tests of thoracic flexion control

T42 STANDING: BACK FLATTENING TEST (tests for thoracic flexion UCM)

This dissociation test assesses the ability to actively dissociate and control thoracic flexion then reverse the lumbar lordosis to the back flat position (i.e. flex the lumbar spine and posterior tilt the pelvis) while standing against a wall.

Test procedure

The person stands with the back of the pelvis, the upper thoracic spine and the back of the head resting against a wall with the shoulders and arms relaxed. The heels are positioned about 20 cm in front of the wall with the feet at least shoulder width apart and with the knees slightly flexed (hip flexors unloaded and wide base of support) (Figure 7.1). Then, keeping the thoracic spine and head stationary on the wall, the person is instructed to roll the pelvis backwards into posterior tilt to flatten the lumbar spine against the wall. The lumbar lordosis should reverse so that the whole lumbar spine is in full contact with the wall (Figure 7.2). There should be no flexion of the thorax, head or shoulders off the wall.

This test should be performed without any extra feedback (self-palpation, vision, etc.) or cueing for correction. When feedback is removed for testing, the therapist should use visual observation of the head and thorax relative to the wall to determine whether the control of thoracic flexion is adequate.

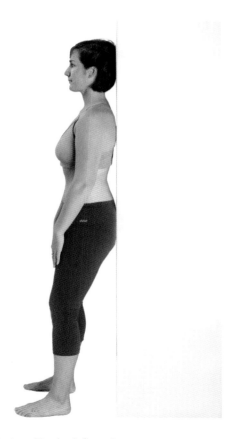

Figure 7.1 Start position back flattening test

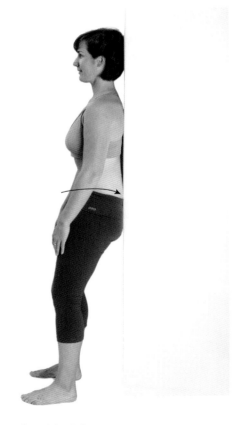

Figure 7.2 Benchmark back flattening test

Thoracic flexion UCM

The person complains of flexion-related symptoms in the thoracic spine. The thorax has UCM into flexion relative to the lumbar spine under flexion load. The head and thoracic spine start to flex off the wall before full back flattening and posterior tilt is achieved. During the attempt to dissociate the thoracic flexion from independent posterior pelvic tilt and lumbar flexion, the person either cannot control the UCM or has to concentrate and try hard to control the thoracic flexion.

Clinical assessment note for direction-specific motor control testing

If some other movement (e.g. a small amount of thoracic rotation) is observed during a motor control (dissociation) test of thoracic flexion, *do not* score this as uncontrolled thoracic flexion. The thoracic rotation motor control tests will identify if the observed unrelated movement is uncontrolled. *A test for thoracic flexion UCM is only positive if uncontrolled thoracic **flexion** is demonstrated.*

Rating and diagnosis of thoracic flexion UCM

(T42.1 and T42.2)

Correction

If control is poor, retraining is best started by allowing both the lumbar and thoracic spines to start in flexion, and then reverse the dysfunction by unrolling the thoracic spine back up the wall into extension. The person stands with the heels at least shoulder width apart and about 20 cm in front of a wall with the knees slightly flexed (hip flexors unloaded and wide base of support). Rest the pelvis against the wall and allow the whole spine to slump forwards into flexion, but roll the pelvis backwards into posterior tilt and flatten the lumbar spine against the wall (Figure 7.3). Once the pelvis and lumbar spine are in contact with the wall, slowly lift the head and chest to unroll the thoracic spine back up the wall (Figure 7.4). Only move as far as the thoracic extensor muscles can extend the thoracic spine while holding the lumbopelvic region flat on the wall.

The person should self-monitor the control of thoracic flexion UCM with a variety of feedback

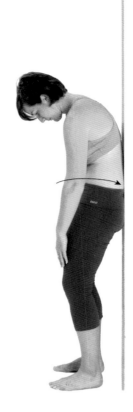

Figure 7.3 Correction start position

options (T42.3). There should be no provocation of any symptoms within the range that the flexion UCM can be controlled.

Once segmental unrolling and control of the thoracic flexion improves, the exercise can return to the original start position. The person stands with the back of the pelvis, the upper thoracic spine and the back of the head resting against a wall. Then, keeping the thoracic spine and head stationary on the wall, the person rolls the pelvis into posterior tilt to flatten the lumbar spine against the wall. They should only roll the pelvis into posterior tilt as far as the head and thoracic spine can stay on the wall (Figure 7.5). At the point in range that the head and thoracic spine begin to flex off the wall, the movement should stop.

T42.1 Assessment and rating of low threshold recruitment efficiency of the Back Flattening Test

BACK FLATTENING – STANDING (WALL)

ASSESSMENT

Control point:
- prevent thoracic flexion

Movement challenge: posterior pelvic tilt and lumbar flexion (standing – wall)

Benchmark range: independent posterior pelvic tilt to reverse the lumbar lordosis to fully flatten the back against a wall

RATING OF LOW THRESHOLD RECRUITMENT EFFICIENCY FOR CONTROL OF DIRECTION

	✓ or ✗		✓ or ✗
• Able to prevent UCM into the test direction. Correct dissociation pattern of movement	☐	• Looks easy, and in the opinion of the assessor, is performed with confidence	☐
Prevent thoracic UCM into:		• Feels easy, and the subject has sufficient awareness of the movement pattern that they confidently prevent UCM into the test direction	☐
• flexion			
and move posterior pelvic tilt and lumbar flexion			
• Dissociate movement through the benchmark range of: posterior pelvic tilt to fully flatten the back against the wall	☐	• The pattern of dissociation is smooth during concentric and eccentric movement	☐
If there is more available range than the benchmark standard, only the benchmark range needs to be actively controlled		• Does not (consistently) use *end-range* movement into the opposite direction to prevent the UCM	☐
• Without holding breath (though it is acceptable to use an alternate breathing strategy)	☐	• No extra feedback needed *(tactile, visual or verbal cueing)*	☐
• Control during eccentric phase	☐	• Without external support or unloading	☐
• Control during concentric phase	☐	• Relaxed natural breathing *(even if not ideal – so long as natural pattern does not change)*	☐
		• No fatigue	☐
CORRECT DISSOCIATION PATTERN		**RECRUITMENT EFFICIENCY**	

T42.2 Diagnosis of the site and direction of UCM from the Back Flattening Test

BACK FLATTENING TEST – STANDING (WALL)

Site	Direction	✗✗ or ✓✗
		(check box)
Thoracic	Flexion	☐

T42.3 Feedback tools to monitor retraining

FEEDBACK TOOL	PROCESS
Self-palpation	Palpation monitoring of joint position
Visual observation	Observe in a mirror or directly watch the movement
Adhesive tape	Skin tension for tactile feedback
Cueing and verbal correction	Listen to feedback from another observer

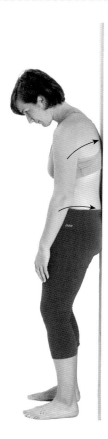
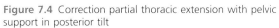
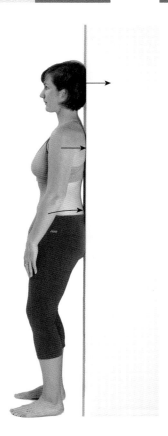

Figure 7.4 Correction partial thoracic extension with pelvic support in posterior tilt

Figure 7.5 Correction partial posterior tilt with head and thoracic support

T43 SITTING: HEAD HANG TEST (tests for thoracic flexion UCM)

This dissociation test assesses the ability to actively dissociate and control thoracic flexion then lower the head towards the chest to hang forwards (i.e. flex the cervical spine) while sitting upright and unsupported.

Test procedure

The person should have the ability to actively hang the head forwards towards the sternum (flexing the cervical spine) while controlling the thoracic spine and preventing thoracic flexion. The person sits tall with the feet off the floor and with the spine and head positioned in the neutral. Position the head directly over the shoulders without chin poke (Figure 7.6). Without letting the thoracic spine or shoulders move, lower the head forwards towards the sternum. Do not allow the sternum or shoulders to drop forwards. This is independent cervical flexion. Ideally, the person should have the ability to keep the thoracic spine neutral and prevent thoracic flexion while independently flexing the cervical spine region through full flexion so that the chin is within 2–3 cm of the upper sternum (Figure 7.7).

This test should be performed without any extra feedback (self-palpation, vision, etc.) or cueing for correction. The therapist should use visual observation of the head and thorax relative to the wall to determine whether the control of thoracic flexion is adequate when feedback is removed for testing.

Thoracic flexion UCM

The person complains of flexion-related symptoms in the thoracic spine. The thorax has UCM into flexion relative to the cervical spine under

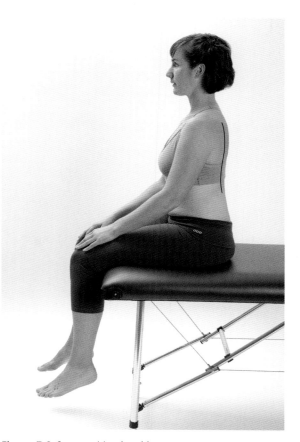

Figure 7.6 Start position head hang test

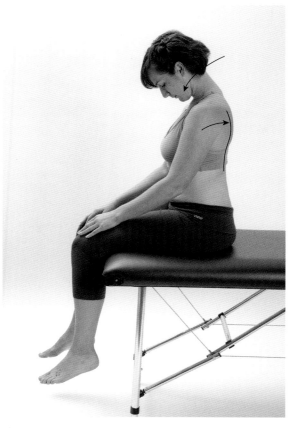

Figure 7.7 Benchmark head hang test

flexion load. The thoracic spine starts to flex before full cervical flexion (head hanging forwards and chin within 2–3 cm of the sternum) is achieved. During the attempt to dissociate the thoracic flexion from independent cervical flexion, the person either cannot control the UCM or has to concentrate and try hard to control the thoracic flexion.

Clinical assessment note for direction-specific motor control testing

If some other movement (e.g. a small amount of thoracic rotation) is observed during a motor control (dissociation) test of thoracic flexion, *do not* score this as uncontrolled thoracic flexion. The thoracic rotation motor control tests will identify if the observed unrelated movement is uncontrolled. *A test for thoracic flexion UCM is only positive if uncontrolled thoracic **flexion** is demonstrated.*

Rating and diagnosis of thoracic flexion UCM

(T43.1 and T43.2)

Correction

If control is poor, retraining is best started by supporting the thoracic spine against a wall and flexing the cervical spine through reduced range.

The person stands with the heels at least shoulder width apart and about 20 cm in front of a wall with the knees slightly flexed.

The thoracic spine and the back of the head are supported upright against a wall (Figure 7.8). The person should monitor the control of thoracic flexion by palpating the sternum or clavicles. Any forward or lowering movement of the sternum or clavicles indicates uncontrolled thoracic flexion. The person is instructed to slowly allow the head to flex forwards off the wall. Only allow the head to hang forwards as far as there is no thoracic flexion (monitored by the hand palpating the sternum). Using feedback from palpating the sternum, the person is trained to control and prevent thoracic flexion and perform independent lower cervical flexion (Figure 7.9).

The person should self-monitor the control of thoracic flexion UCM with a variety of feedback options (T43.3). There should be no provocation of any symptoms within the range that the flexion UCM can be controlled.

Once control of the thoracic flexion improves, the person should move away from the wall and the exercise can be performed with self-monitoring of thoracic flexion control by palpating the sternum, with the thoracic spine unsupported (no wall support).

T43.1 Assessment and rating of low threshold recruitment efficiency of the Head Hang Test

HEAD HANG – SITTING

ASSESSMENT

Control point:
- prevent thoracic flexion

Movement challenge: cervical flexion (sitting)

Benchmark range: independent cervical flexion (chin to within two finger-widths of sternum)

RATING OF LOW THRESHOLD RECRUITMENT EFFICIENCY FOR CONTROL OF DIRECTION

	✓ or ✗		✓ or ✗
• Able to prevent UCM into the test direction Correct dissociation pattern of movement Prevent thoracic UCM into: • flexion and move cervical flexion	☐	• Looks easy, and in the opinion of the assessor, is performed with confidence	☐
		• Feels easy, and the subject has sufficient awareness of the movement pattern that they confidently prevent UCM into the test direction	☐
• Dissociate movement through the benchmark range of: head hang to fully flex cervical spine to two finger-widths of sternum *If there is more available range than the benchmark standard, only the benchmark range needs to be actively controlled*	☐	• The pattern of dissociation is smooth during concentric and eccentric movement	☐
		• Does not (consistently) use *end-range* movement into the opposite direction to prevent the UCM	☐
• Without holding breath (though it is acceptable to use an alternate breathing strategy)	☐	• No extra feedback needed *(tactile, visual or verbal cueing)*	☐
		• Without external support or unloading	☐
• Control during eccentric phase	☐	• Relaxed natural breathing *(even if not ideal – so long as natural pattern does not change)*	☐
• Control during concentric phase	☐	• No fatigue	☐

CORRECT DISSOCIATION PATTERN   **RECRUITMENT EFFICIENCY**

T43.2 Diagnosis of the site and direction of UCM from the Head Hang Test

HEAD HANG TEST – SITTING

Site	Direction	✗✗ or &check✗ (check box)
Thoracic	Flexion	☐

T43.3 Feedback tools to monitor retraining

FEEDBACK TOOL	PROCESS
Self-palpation	Palpation monitoring of joint position
Visual observation	Observe in a mirror or directly watch the movement
Adhesive tape	Skin tension for tactile feedback
Cueing and verbal correction	Listen to feedback from another observer

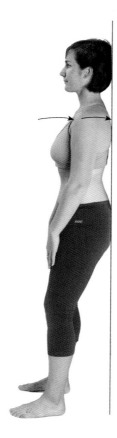

Figure 7.8 Correction start position on wall

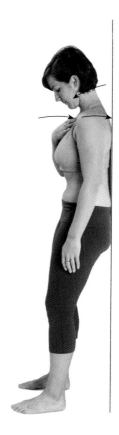

Figure 7.9 Correction partial head flexion with thoracic support on wall

T44 SITTING: PELVIC TAIL TUCK TEST (tests for thoracic flexion UCM)

This dissociation test assesses the ability to actively dissociate and control thoracic flexion then roll the pelvis backwards (i.e. 'tail tuck' or posterior pelvic tilt) while sitting upright and unsupported.

Test procedure

The person should have the ability to actively roll the pelvis backwards into posterior pelvic tilt while controlling and preventing thoracic flexion. The person sits tall with the feet off the floor and with the lumbar spine and pelvis positioned in the neutral. The therapist should passively support the thoracic spine and passively roll the pelvis backwards to assess the available range of posterior pelvic tilt that is independent of thoracic flexion. This also allows the person to experience and learn the movement pattern that will be tested.

The person is then instructed to make the spine as tall or as long as possible to position the normal curves in an elongated 'S'. Position the head directly over the shoulders without chin poke (Figure 7.10). Then, without letting the thoracic spine flex (sternum does not lower or move forwards), actively roll the pelvis backwards (tuck the tail under the pelvis) into full available posterior pelvic tilt. The person is required to produce the same range of posterior pelvic tilt that the therapist identified with passive assessment.

Ideally, the person should have the ability to dissociate the thoracic spine from posterior pelvic tilt as evidenced by the ability to prevent thoracic flexion while independently rolling the pelvis backwards (Figure 7.11). There must be no movement into thoracic flexion. There should be no provocation of any symptoms under posterior tilt

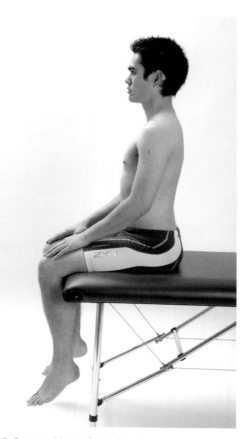

Figure 7.10 Start position pelvic tail tuck test

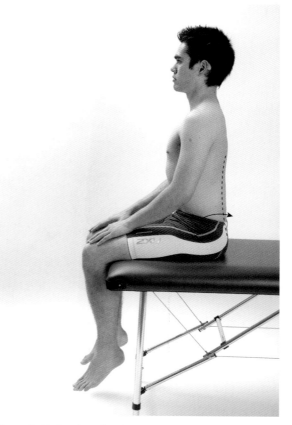

Figure 7.11 Benchmark pelvic tail tuck test

(flexion) load, so long as the thoracic flexion UCM can be controlled.

This test should be performed without any extra feedback (self-palpation, vision, etc.) or cueing for correction. When feedback is removed for testing the therapist should use visual observation of the thorax relative to the pelvis to determine whether the control of thoracic flexion is adequate.

Thoracic flexion UCM

The person complains of flexion-related symptoms in the thoracic spine. The thorax has UCM into flexion relative to posterior pelvic tilt under flexion load. The thoracic spine starts to flex before full independent posterior pelvic tilt ('tail tuck') is achieved. During the attempt to dissociate the thoracic flexion from independent posterior pelvic tilt, the person either cannot control the UCM or has to concentrate and try hard to control the thoracic flexion.

Clinical assessment note for direction-specific motor control testing

If some other movement (e.g. a small amount of thoracic rotation) is observed during a motor control (dissociation) test of thoracic flexion, *do not* score this as uncontrolled thoracic flexion. The thoracic rotation motor control tests will identify if the observed unrelated movement is uncontrolled. *A test for thoracic flexion UCM is only positive if uncontrolled thoracic* **flexion** *is demonstrated.*

Rating and diagnosis of thoracic flexion UCM

(T44.1 and T44.2)

Correction

Retraining is best started by supporting the thoracic spine against a wall for increased thoracic support and feedback and posterior tilting the pelvis through reduced range. The person stands with the back of the pelvis, the upper thoracic spine and the back of the head resting against a wall with the shoulders and arms relaxed. The pelvis is positioned in anterior tilt to start the training. This can also be performed with the person sitting on a low stool with the feet on the floor and the thoracic spine and head resting

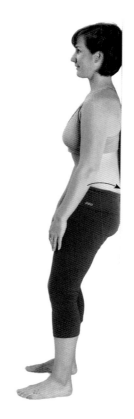

Figure 7.12 Correction partial posterior tilt with thoracic support

against a wall. Then, keeping the thoracic spine and head stationary on the wall, the person is instructed to roll the pelvis backwards into posterior pelvic tilt (Figure 7.12). It may be useful to visualise tucking an imaginary tail under the pelvis. Another visualisation cue is to visualise the pelvis as a bucket full of water and the thorax as the handle of the bucket. The aim is to visualise the ability to tip water out the back of the bucket but not allow the handle to swing forwards into thoracic flexion.

If control is poor, it is also recommended that the person use self-palpation to monitor the correct performance of the exercise. Monitor the control of thoracic flexion by placing one hand on the sternum or clavicles. Monitor lumbopelvic motion by placing the other hand on the sacrum (Figure 7.13). Without letting the thoracic spine flex (sternum does not lower or move forwards)

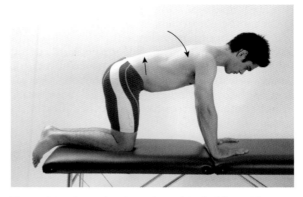

Figure 7.14 Correction (posterior pelvic tilt followed by thoracic extension)

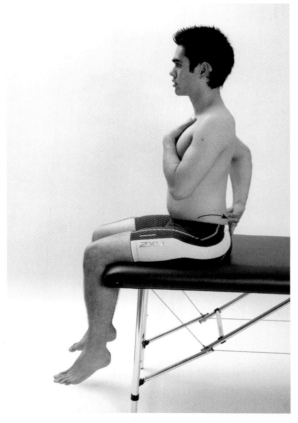

Figure 7.13 Correction partial posterior tilt with self-palpation

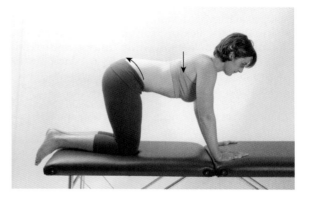

Figure 7.15 Correction (thoracic extension followed by posterior pelvic tilt)

actively roll the pelvis backwards (tuck the tail under the pelvis) into full available posterior pelvic tilt. Using feedback from palpating the sternum, the person is trained to control and prevent thoracic flexion and perform independent posterior pelvic tilt. Only allow posterior pelvic tilt (tail tuck) as far as there is no thoracic flexion (monitored by the hand palpating the sternum). There must be no UCM into thoracic flexion. There should be no provocation of any symptoms under flexion load, so long as the thoracic flexion UCM can be controlled.

The person should self-monitor the control of thoracic flexion UCM with a variety of feedback options (T44.3). There should be no provocation of any symptoms within the range that the flexion UCM can be controlled.

If control is very poor, rather than specific dissociation, for some patients it is easier to initially use a recruitment reversal exercise. The upper body and trunk weight can be supported on hands and knees. Position the pelvis in neutral pelvic tilt and the lumbar spine, the thoracic spine and head in neutral alignment (the back of the head touches an imaginary line connecting the sacrum and mid-thoracic spine). There are two recruitment reversal strategies that are appropriate:

1. First, actively posterior tilt the pelvis to end range, and then extend the thoracic spine as far as possible without losing the posterior tilt (Figure 7.14).
2. The reverse order of this same pattern may also be used. That is, first, actively extend the thoracic spine as far as possible and then posteriorly tilt the pelvis (Figure 7.15).

When the pattern of this recruitment reversal feels easy to perform, the person can progress back to the sitting dissociation exercise.

T44.1 Assessment and rating of low threshold recruitment efficiency of the Pelvic Tail Tuck Test

PELVIC TAIL TUCK – SITTING

ASSESSMENT

Control point:
• prevent thoracic flexion
Movement challenge: posterior pelvic tilt (sitting)
Benchmark range: active full independent posterior pelvic tilt (same range as passive assessment)

RATING OF LOW THRESHOLD RECRUITMENT EFFICIENCY FOR CONTROL OF DIRECTION

	✓ or ✗		✓ or ✗
• Able to prevent UCM into the test direction Correct dissociation pattern of movement Prevent thoracic UCM into: • flexion and move posterior pelvic tilt	☐	• Looks easy, and in the opinion of the assessor, is performed with confidence	☐
		• Feels easy, and the subject has sufficient awareness of the movement pattern that they confidently prevent UCM into the test direction	☐
• Dissociate movement through the benchmark range of: full range independent posterior pelvic tilt (as compared to passive assessment) *If there is more available range than the benchmark standard, only the benchmark range needs to be actively controlled*	☐	• The pattern of dissociation is smooth during concentric and eccentric movement	☐
		• Does not (consistently) use *end-range* movement into the opposite direction to prevent the UCM	☐
• Without holding breath (though it is acceptable to use an alternate breathing strategy)	☐	• No extra feedback needed *(tactile, visual or verbal cueing)*	☐
		• Without external support or unloading	☐
• Control during eccentric phase	☐	• Relaxed natural breathing *(even if not ideal – so long as natural pattern does not change)*	☐
• Control during concentric phase	☐	• No fatigue	☐

CORRECT DISSOCIATION PATTERN   **RECRUITMENT EFFICIENCY**

T44.2 Diagnosis of the site and direction of UCM from the Pelvic Tail Tuck Test

PELVIC TAIL TUCK TEST – SITTING

Site	Direction	✗✗ or ✗✓
		(check box)
Thoracic	Flexion	☐

T44.3 Feedback tools to monitor retraining

FEEDBACK TOOL	PROCESS
Self-palpation	Palpation monitoring of joint position
Visual observation	Observe in a mirror or directly watch the movement
Adhesive tape	Skin tension for tactile feedback
Cueing and verbal correction	Listen to feedback from another observer

T45 SITTING: BILATERAL FORWARD REACH TEST
(tests for thoracic flexion UCM)

This dissociation test assesses the ability to actively dissociate and control thoracic flexion then reach forwards in front of the body with both arms (i.e. bilateral scapular protraction) while sitting upright and unsupported.

Test procedure

The person should have the ability to actively reach forwards with both arms into full scapular protraction while controlling and preventing thoracic flexion. The person sits tall with the feet off the floor. The person is then instructed to sit upright with the spine in its neutral normal curves and the head directly over the shoulders without chin poke. Both arms are held at 90° of shoulder flexion, with the scapulae relaxed in a neutral mid-position (Figure 7.16). Then, without letting the thoracic spine flex (sternum does not lower or move forwards) or the head to move forwards, actively reach forwards with both hands into full available scapular protraction.

Ideally, the person should have the ability to dissociate the thoracic spine from scapular protraction as evidenced by the ability to prevent thoracic flexion while independently reaching forwards (Figure 7.17). There must be no movement into thoracic flexion. There should be no provocation of any symptoms under flexion load, so long as the thoracic flexion UCM can be controlled.

This test should be performed without any extra feedback (self-palpation, vision, etc.) or cueing for correction. When feedback is removed for testing the therapist should use visual

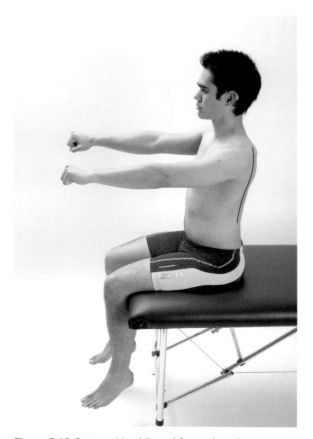

Figure 7.16 Start position bilateral forward reach test

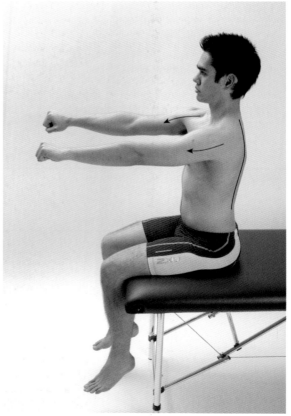

Figure 7.17 Benchmark bilateral forward reach test

observation of the head and thorax relative to the shoulders to determine whether the control of thoracic flexion is adequate.

Thoracic flexion UCM

The person complains of flexion-related symptoms in the thoracic spine. The thorax has UCM into flexion relative to scapular protraction. The thoracic spine starts to flex before full independent scapular protraction (forward reach) is achieved. During the attempt to dissociate the thoracic flexion from independent scapular protraction, the person either cannot control the UCM or has to concentrate and try hard to control the thoracic flexion.

Clinical assessment note for direction-specific motor control testing

If some other movement (e.g. a small amount of thoracic rotation) is observed during a motor control (dissociation) test of thoracic flexion, *do not* score this as uncontrolled thoracic flexion. The thoracic rotation motor control tests will identify if the observed unrelated movement is uncontrolled. *A test for thoracic flexion UCM is only positive if uncontrolled thoracic **flexion** is demonstrated.*

Rating and diagnosis of thoracic flexion uncontrolled movement

(T45.1 and T45.2)

Correction

If control is poor, retraining is best started by supporting the thoracic spine against a wall and reaching forwards (scapular protraction) through reduced range. The person stands with the heels at least shoulder width apart and about 20 cm in front of a wall with the knees slightly flexed.

The thoracic spine and the back of the head are supported upright against a wall. The person should monitor the control of thoracic flexion by palpating the sternum or clavicles with one hand. Any forward of lowering movement of the sternum or clavicles indicates uncontrolled thoracic flexion. The person is instructed to slowly reach forwards with the other arm. Only reach forwards as far as there is no thoracic flexion (monitored by the hand palpating the sternum) (Figure 7.18). Using feedback from palpating the sternum, the person is trained to control and prevent thoracic flexion and perform independent scapular protraction.

The person should self-monitor the control of thoracic flexion UCM with a variety of feedback options (T45.3). There should be no provocation of any symptoms within the range that the flexion UCM can be controlled.

Once control of the thoracic flexion improves, the person should reach forwards with both arms while using the wall for feedback and support of the thoracic spine (Figure 7.19). Eventually, they can move away from the wall and the exercise can be performed with the thoracic spine unsupported (no wall support).

Thoracic flexion UCM summary

(Table 7.3)

Table 7.3 Summary and rating of thoracic flexion tests		
UCM DIAGNOSIS AND TESTING		
SITE: THORACIC	**DIRECTION:** FLEXION	**CLINICAL PRIORITY** ☐
TEST	**RATING** (✓✓ or ✓✗ or ✗✗) and rationale	
Standing: back flattening		
Sitting: head hang		
Sitting: pelvic tail tuck		
Sitting: bilateral forward reach		

T45.1 Assessment and rating of low threshold recruitment efficiency of the Bilateral Forward Reach Test

BILATERAL FORWARD REACH – SITTING

ASSESSMENT

Control point:
- prevent thoracic flexion

Movement challenge: scapular protraction (sitting)

Benchmark range: active full independent scapular protraction

RATING OF LOW THRESHOLD RECRUITMENT EFFICIENCY FOR CONTROL OF DIRECTION

	✓ or ✗		✓ or ✗
• Able to prevent UCM into the test direction Correct dissociation pattern of movement Prevent thoracic UCM into: • flexion and move bilateral scapular protraction	☐	• Looks easy, and in the opinion of the assessor, is performed with confidence	☐
		• Feels easy, and the subject has sufficient awareness of the movement pattern that they confidently prevent UCM into the test direction	☐
• Dissociate movement through the benchmark range of: full range independent scapular protraction (reaching forwards at 90° bilateral shoulder flexion) *If there is more available range than the benchmark standard, only the benchmark range needs to be actively controlled*	☐	• The pattern of dissociation is smooth during concentric and eccentric movement	☐
		• Does not (consistently) use *end-range* movement into the opposite direction to prevent the UCM	☐
		• No extra feedback needed *(tactile, visual or verbal cueing)*	☐
• Without holding breath (though it is acceptable to use an alternate breathing strategy)	☐	• Without external support or unloading	☐
		• Relaxed natural breathing *(even if not ideal – so long as natural pattern does not change)*	☐
• Control during eccentric phase	☐	• No fatigue	☐
• Control during concentric phase	☐		

CORRECT DISSOCIATION PATTERN   **RECRUITMENT EFFICIENCY**

T45.2 Diagnosis of the site and direction of UCM from the Bilateral Forward Reach Test

BILATERAL FORWARD REACH TEST – SITTING

Site	Direction	✗✗ or ✗✓
		(check box)
Thoracic	Flexion	☐

T45.3 Feedback tools to monitor retraining

FEEDBACK TOOL	PROCESS
Self-palpation	Palpation monitoring of joint position
Visual observation	Observe in a mirror or directly watch the movement
Adhesive tape	Skin tension for tactile feedback
Cueing and verbal correction	Listen to feedback from another observer

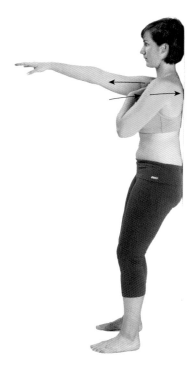

Figure 7.18 Correction unilateral forward reach with thoracic support on wall

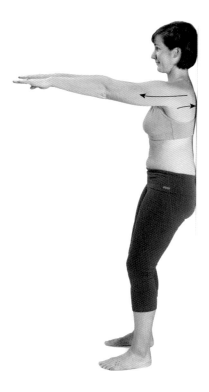

Figure 7.19 Correction bilateral forward reach with thoracic support on wall

Thoracic extension control

EXTENSION CONTROL TESTS AND EXTENSION CONTROL REHABILITATION

These extension control tests assess the extent of extension UCM in the thoracic spine and assess the ability of the dynamic stability system to adequately control extension load or strain. It is a priority to assess for extension UCM if the person complains of or demonstrates extension-related symptoms or disability. The tests that identify dysfunction can also be used to guide and direct rehabilitation strategies.

Indications to test for thoracic extension UCM

Observe or palpate for:

1. hypermobile thoracic extension range
2. excessive initiation of looking up or lifting with thoracic extension
3. symptoms (pain, discomfort, strain) associated with looking up or reaching overhead with associated thoracic extension.

The person complains of extension-related symptoms in the thorax. Under extension load, the thoracic spine has greater give *into extension* relative to the lumbar spine, head and shoulders. The dysfunction is confirmed with motor control tests of extension dissociation.

Tests of thoracic extension control

T46 STANDING: BILATERAL OVERHEAD REACH TEST
(tests for thoracic extension UCM)

This dissociation test assesses the ability to actively dissociate and control thoracic extension then reach overhead with both arms (i.e. bilateral shoulder flexion) while standing upright and unsupported.

Test procedure

The subject stands upright with the spine in its neutral normal curves, the head directly over the shoulders without chin poke and with the arms resting by the side with the shoulders in a neutral position (Figure 7.20). The person is then instructed to slowly lift both arms into flexion. Without letting the thoracic spine extend (sternum does not lift or move backwards) or the head move backwards, the person should be able to actively reach overhead with both hands into end-range shoulder flexion.

Ideally, the person should have the ability to dissociate the thoracic spine from overhead shoulder flexion as evidenced by the ability to prevent thoracic extension while independently reaching overhead to at least 160° bilateral shoulder flexion (Figure 7.21). There must be no movement into thoracic extension. There should be no provocation of any symptoms under overhead load, so long as the thoracic extension UCM can be controlled.

This test should be performed without any extra feedback (self-palpation, vision, etc.) or cueing for correction. When feedback is removed for testing the therapist should use visual observation of the head and thorax relative to the

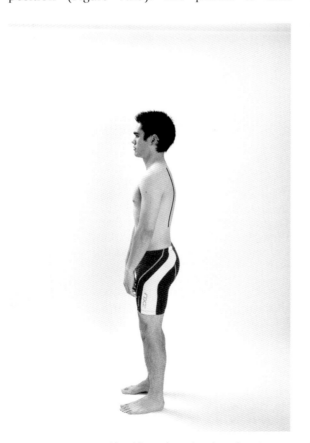

Figure 7.20 Start position bilateral overhead reach test

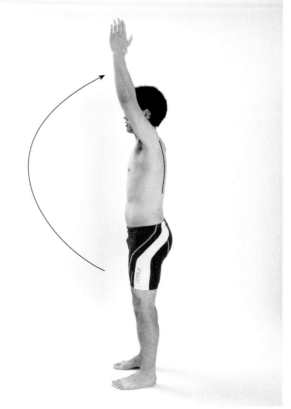

Figure 7.21 Benchmark bilateral overhead reach test

shoulders to determine whether the control of thoracic extension is adequate.

Thoracic extension UCM

The person complains of extension-related symptoms in the thoracic spine. The thorax has UCM into extension relative to overhead shoulder flexion. The thoracic spine starts to extend before 1600 of independent shoulder flexion (overhead reach) is achieved. During the attempt to dissociate the thoracic extension from independent overhead reach, the person either cannot control the UCM or has to concentrate and try hard to control the thoracic extension.

> ### Clinical assessment note for direction-specific motor control testing
>
> If some other movement (e.g. a small amount of thoracic rotation) is observed during a motor control (dissociation) test of thoracic extension, *do not* score this as uncontrolled thoracic extension. The thoracic rotation motor control tests will identify if the observed unrelated movement is uncontrolled. *A test for thoracic extension UCM is only positive if uncontrolled thoracic* **extension** *is demonstrated.*

Rating and diagnosis of thoracic extension UCM

(T46.1 and T46.2)

Correction

If control is poor, retraining is best started by supporting the thoracic spine against a wall and reaching overhead (shoulder flexion) with unilateral arm movement and through reduced range. The person stands with the thoracic spine and the back of the head supported upright against a wall. The person should flatten the lumbar spine against the wall to give additional feedback and support to the ability to prevent thoracic extension. If uncontrolled thoracic extension occurs the person will be aware of the thoracolumbar spine losing contact with the wall (arching into extension). Alternatively, the person may monitor the control of thoracic extension by palpating the sternum or clavicles with one hand. Any lifting movement of the sternum or clavicles also indicates uncontrolled thoracic extension.

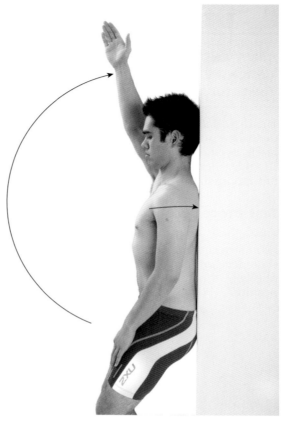

Figure 7.22 Correction partial unilateral overhead reach with thoracic support on wall

The person is instructed to slowly flex one arm through range to reach overhead. Only reach overhead as far as there is no thoracic extension (Figure 7.22). Using feedback from the back on the wall (or palpating the sternum), the person is trained to control and prevent thoracic extension and perform independent overhead shoulder flexion.

The person should self-monitor the control of thoracic extension UCM with a variety of feedback options (T46.3). There should be no provocation of any symptoms within the range that the extension UCM can be controlled.

Once control of the thoracic extension improves, the person should reach overhead with both arms while using the wall for feedback and support of the thoracic spine. Eventually, they can move away from the wall and the exercise can be performed with the thoracic spine unsupported (no wall support).

T46.1 Assessment and rating of low threshold recruitment efficiency of the Bilateral Overhead Reach Test

BILATERAL OVERHEAD REACH – STANDING

ASSESSMENT

Control point:
• prevent thoracic extension
Movement challenge: bilateral overhead shoulder flexion (standing)
Benchmark range: 160° active independent shoulder flexion

RATING OF LOW THRESHOLD RECRUITMENT EFFICIENCY FOR CONTROL OF DIRECTION

	✓ or ✗		✓ or ✗
• Able to prevent UCM into the test direction Correct dissociation pattern of movement Prevent thoracic UCM into: • extension and move bilateral overhead shoulder flexion	☐	• Looks easy, and in the opinion of the assessor, is performed with confidence	☐
		• Feels easy, and the subject has sufficient awareness of the movement pattern that they confidently prevent UCM into the test direction	☐
• Dissociate movement through the benchmark range of: 160° range independent bilateral shoulder flexion overhead *If there is more available range than the benchmark standard, only the benchmark range needs to be actively controlled*	☐	• The pattern of dissociation is smooth during concentric and eccentric movement	☐
		• Does not (consistently) use *end-range* movement into the opposite direction to prevent the UCM	☐
• Without holding breath (though it is acceptable to use an alternate breathing strategy)	☐	• No extra feedback needed *(tactile, visual or verbal cueing)*	☐
		• Without external support or unloading	☐
• Control during eccentric phase	☐	• Relaxed natural breathing *(even if not ideal – so long as natural pattern does not change)*	☐
• Control during concentric phase	☐	• No fatigue	☐

CORRECT DISSOCIATION PATTERN   **RECRUITMENT EFFICIENCY**

T46.2 Diagnosis of the site and direction of UCM from the Bilateral Overhead Reach Test

BILATERAL OVERHEAD REACH TEST – STANDING

Site	Direction	✗✗ or ✗✓
		(check box)
Thoracic	Extension	☐

T46.3 Feedback tools to monitor retraining

FEEDBACK TOOL	PROCESS
Self-palpation	Palpation monitoring of joint position
Visual observation	Observe in a mirror or directly watch the movement
Adhesive tape	Skin tension for tactile feedback
Cueing and verbal correction	Listen to feedback from another observer

T47 SITTING: HEAD RAISE TEST (tests for thoracic extension UCM)

This dissociation test assesses the ability to actively dissociate and control thoracic extension then move the low cervical spine into extension by raising the head backwards over the shoulders from a flexed position while sitting upright and unsupported.

Test procedure

The person should have the ability to actively extend the low cervical spine while controlling and preventing thoracic extension. The person sits upright with the feet off the floor and the spine in its neutral normal curves and the low cervical spine positioned in flexion by allowing the head to hang forwards (Figure 7.23). Without letting the sternum lift or the thoracic spine extend, the person is instructed to move the low cervical spine through extension by raising the head backwards over the shoulders.

Ideally, the person should have the ability to dissociate thoracic extension from low cervical extension as evidenced by the ability to prevent thoracic extension while independently raising the head from a flexed position so that the low cervical spine at least reaches the vertical position (Figure 7.24). There must be no movement into thoracic extension. There should be no provocation of any symptoms under extension load, so long as the thoracic extension UCM can be controlled.

This test should be performed without any extra feedback (self-palpation, vision, etc.) or cueing for correction. The therapist should use visual observation of the thorax relative to the head to determine whether the control of thoracic

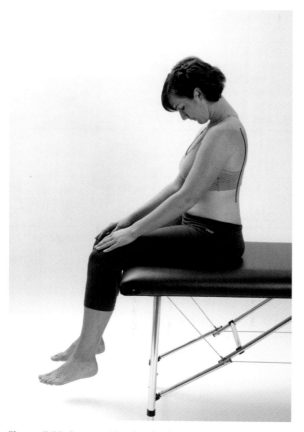

Figure 7.23 Start position head raise test

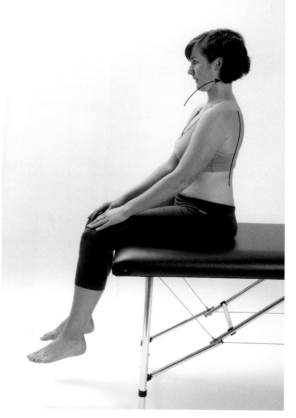

Figure 7.24 Benchmark head raise test

extension is adequate when feedback is removed for testing.

Thoracic extension UCM

The person complains of extension-related symptoms in the thoracic spine. The thorax has UCM into extension relative to raising the head from a flexed position. The thoracic spine starts to extend before low cervical extension reaches vertical. During the attempt to dissociate the thoracic extension from independent low cervical extension (head raise), the person either cannot control the UCM or has to concentrate and try hard to control the thoracic extension.

Clinical assessment note for direction-specific motor control testing

If some other movement (e.g. a small amount of thoracic rotation) is observed during a motor control (dissociation) test of thoracic extension, *do not* score this as uncontrolled thoracic extension. The thoracic rotation motor control tests will identify if the observed unrelated movement is uncontrolled. *A test for thoracic extension UCM is only positive if uncontrolled thoracic **extension** is demonstrated.*

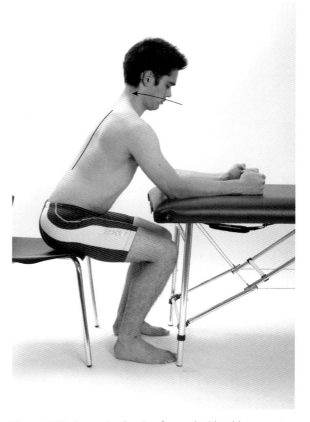

Figure 7.25 Correction leaning forward with table support

Rating and diagnosis of thoracic extension UCM

(T47.1 and T47.2)

Correction

If control is poor, retraining is best started by supporting the thoracic spine with weight bearing through the arms and raising the head backwards from a flexed position.

The person sits at a table and leans forwards to take weight through the elbows. The scapulae are positioned midway between elevation and depression with the head hanging forwards in neck flexion. Then the person pushes the chest away from the elbows to protract the scapula and use serratus anterior to help support the thorax and control thoracic extension.

Without letting the chest drop forwards towards the elbows or the sternum lift into thoracic extension, the person is instructed to slowly raise the head backwards over the shoulders. There should be no chin poke and the movement should be localised to the low cervical spine. They are to raise the head only as far as there is no thoracic extension (Figure 7.25). The person is trained to control and prevent thoracic extension and perform independent low cervical extension.

The person should self-monitor the control of thoracic extension UCM with a variety of feedback options (T47.3). There should be no provocation of any symptoms within the range that the extension UCM can be controlled.

Once control of the thoracic extension improves, the exercise can be performed with the thoracic spine unsupported (no weight bearing scapular support).

T47.1 Assessment and rating of low threshold recruitment efficiency of the Head Raise Test

HEAD RAISE – SITTING

ASSESSMENT

Control point:
• prevent thoracic extension
Movement challenge: low cervical extension (head raise backwards form flexion) (sitting)
Benchmark range: independent low cervical extension to the vertical position

RATING OF LOW THRESHOLD RECRUITMENT EFFICIENCY FOR CONTROL OF DIRECTION

	✓ or ✗		✓ or ✗
• Able to prevent UCM into the test direction Correct dissociation pattern of movement Prevent thoracic UCM into: • extension and move low cervical extension	☐	• Looks easy, and in the opinion of the assessor, is performed with confidence	☐
		• Feels easy, and the subject has sufficient awareness of the movement pattern that they confidently prevent UCM into the test direction	☐
• Dissociate movement through the benchmark range of: independent head raise to low cervical vertical alignment *If there is more available range than the benchmark standard, only the benchmark range needs to be actively controlled*	☐	• The pattern of dissociation is smooth during concentric and eccentric movement	☐
		• Does not (consistently) use *end-range* movement into the opposite direction to prevent the UCM	☐
• Without holding breath (though it is acceptable to use an alternate breathing strategy)	☐	• No extra feedback needed *(tactile, visual or verbal cueing)*	☐
		• Without external support or unloading	☐
• Control during eccentric phase	☐	• Relaxed natural breathing *(even if not ideal – so long as natural pattern does not change)*	☐
• Control during concentric phase	☐	• No fatigue	☐

CORRECT DISSOCIATION PATTERN   **RECRUITMENT EFFICIENCY**

T47.2 Diagnosis of the site and direction of UCM from the Head Raise Test

HEAD RAISE TEST – SITTING

Site	Direction	✗✗ or ✗✓
		(check box)
Thoracic	Extension	☐

T47.3 Feedback tools to monitor retraining

FEEDBACK TOOL	PROCESS
Self-palpation	Palpation monitoring of joint position
Visual observation	Observe in a mirror or directly watch the movement
Adhesive tape	Skin tension for tactile feedback
Cueing and verbal correction	Listen to feedback from another observer

T48 SITTING: PELVIC TAIL LIFT TEST (tests for thoracic extension UCM)

This dissociation test assesses the ability to actively dissociate and control thoracic extension then roll the pelvis forwards (i.e. 'tail lift' or anterior pelvic tilt) while sitting upright and unsupported.

Test procedure

The person should have the ability to actively roll the pelvis forwards into anterior pelvic tilt while controlling and preventing thoracic extension. The person sits tall with the feet off the floor and with the lumbar spine and pelvis positioned in the neutral. The therapist should passively support the thoracic spine and passively roll the pelvis forwards to assess the available range of anterior pelvic tilt that is independent of thoracic

extension. This also allows the person to experience and learn the movement pattern that will be tested.

The person is then instructed to make the spine as tall or as long as possible to position the normal curves in an elongated 'S'. Position the head directly over the shoulders without chin poke (Figure 7.26). Then, without letting the thoracic spine extend (sternum does not lift or move backwards), actively roll the pelvis forwards (lift the tail up from the pelvis) into full available anterior pelvic tilt. The person is required to produce the same range of anterior pelvic tilt that the therapist identified with passive assessment.

Ideally, the person should have the ability to dissociate the thoracic spine from anterior pelvic tilt as evidenced by the ability to prevent thoracic extension while independently rolling the pelvis forwards (Figure 7.27). There must be no movement into thoracic extension. There should be no provocation of any symptoms under anterior tilt

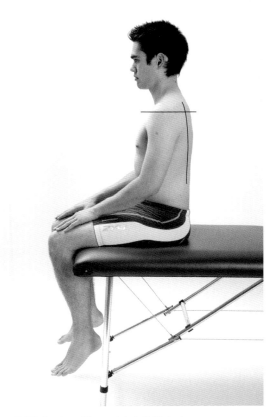

Figure 7.26 Start position pelvic tail lift test

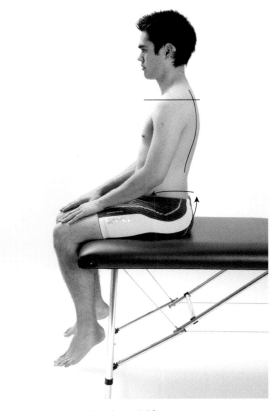

Figure 7.27 Benchmark pelvic tail lift test

(extension) load, so long as the thoracic extension UCM can be controlled.

This test should be performed without any extra feedback (self-palpation, vision, etc.) or cueing for correction. The therapist should use visual observation of the thorax relative to the pelvis to determine whether the control of thoracic extension is adequate when feedback is removed for testing.

Thoracic extension UCM

The person complains of extension-related symptoms in the thoracic spine. The thorax has UCM into extension relative to anterior pelvic tilt under extension load. The thoracic spine starts to extend before full independent anterior pelvic tilt ('tail lift') is achieved. During the attempt to dissociate the thoracic extension from independent anterior pelvic tilt, the person either cannot control the UCM or has to concentrate and try hard to control the thoracic extension.

Clinical assessment note for direction-specific motor control testing

If some other movement (e.g. a small amount of thoracic rotation) is observed during a motor control (dissociation) test of thoracic extension, *do not* score this as uncontrolled thoracic extension. The thoracic rotation motor control tests will identify if the observed unrelated movement is uncontrolled. *A test for thoracic extension UCM is only positive if uncontrolled thoracic **extension** is demonstrated.*

Rating and diagnosis of thoracic extension UCM

(T48.1 and T48.2)

Correction

Retraining is best started by supporting the thoracic spine against a wall for increased thoracic support and feedback and anterior tilting the pelvis through reduced range. The person stands with the back of the pelvis, the upper thoracic spine and the back of the head resting against a wall with the shoulders and arms relaxed. The pelvis is positioned in posterior tilt to start the training. This can also be performed with the person sitting on a low stool with the feet on the floor and the thoracic spine and head resting

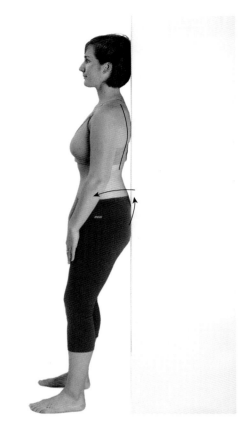

Figure 7.28 Correction partial anterior pelvic tilt with thoracic support on wall

against a wall. Then, keeping the thoracic spine and head stationary on the wall, the person is instructed to roll the pelvis forwards into anterior pelvic tilt (Figure 7.28). It may be useful to visualise lifting an imaginary tail up from behind the pelvis. Another visualisation cue is to visualise the pelvis as a bucket full of water and the thorax as the handle of the bucket. The aim is to visualise the ability to tip water out the front of the bucket but not allow the handle to swing backwards into thoracic extension.

If control is poor, it is also recommended that the person use self-palpation to monitor the correct performance of the exercise. Monitor the control of thoracic flexion by placing one hand on the sternum or clavicles. Monitor lumbopelvic motion by placing the other hand on the sacrum (Figure 7.29). Without letting the thoracic spine extend (sternum does not lift or move

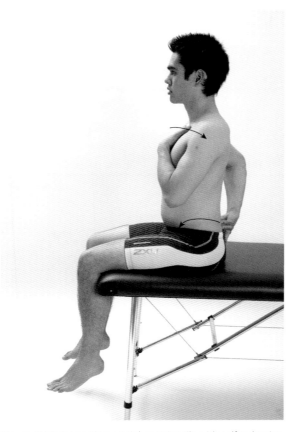

Figure 7.29 Correction partial anterior tilt with self-palpation

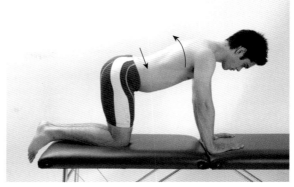

Figure 7.30 Correction (anterior pelvic tilt followed by thoracic flexion)

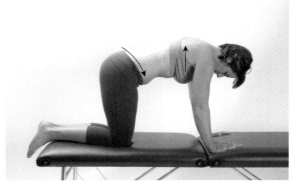

Figure 7.31 Correction (thoracic flexion followed by anterior pelvic tilt)

backwards), actively roll the pelvis forwards (lift the tail up from the pelvis) into full available anterior pelvic tilt. Using feedback from palpating the sternum, the person is trained to control and prevent thoracic extension and perform independent anterior pelvic tilt. Only allow anterior pelvic tilt (tail lift) as far as there is no thoracic extension (monitored by the hand palpating the sternum). There must be no UCM into thoracic extension. There should be no provocation of any symptoms under extension load, so long as the thoracic extension UCM can be controlled.

The person should self-monitor the control of thoracic extension UCM with a variety of feedback options (T48.3). There should be no provocation of any symptoms within the range that the extension UCM can be controlled.

If control is very poor, rather than specific dissociation, for some patients it is easier to initially use a recruitment reversal exercise. The upper body and trunk weight can be supported on hands and knees. Position the pelvis in neutral pelvic tilt and the lumbar spine, the thoracic spine and head in neutral alignment (the back of the head touches an imaginary line connecting the sacrum and mid-thoracic spine). There are two recruitment reversal strategies that are appropriate:

1. Actively anteriorly tilt the pelvis to end range, and then flex the thoracic spine as far as possible without losing the anterior tilt (Figure 7.30).
2. The reverse order of this same pattern may also be used. That is, first, actively flex the thoracic spine as far as possible and then anteriorly tilt the pelvis (Figure 7.31).

When the pattern of this recruitment reversal feels easy to perform, the person can progress back to the sitting dissociation exercise.

321

T48.1 Assessment and rating of low threshold recruitment efficiency of the Pelvic Tail Lift Test

PELVIC TAIL LIFT – SITTING

ASSESSMENT

Control point:
• prevent thoracic extension
Movement challenge: anterior pelvic tilt (sitting)
Benchmark range: active full independent anterior pelvic tilt (same range as passive assessment)

RATING OF LOW THRESHOLD RECRUITMENT EFFICIENCY FOR CONTROL OF DIRECTION

✓ or ✗		✓ or ✗	
• Able to prevent UCM into the test direction Correct dissociation pattern of movement	☐	• Looks easy, and in the opinion of the assessor, is performed with confidence	☐
Prevent thoracic UCM into:		• Feels easy, and the subject has sufficient awareness of the movement pattern that they confidently prevent UCM into the test direction	☐
• extension and move anterior pelvic tilt			
• Dissociate movement through the benchmark range of: full range independent anterior pelvic tilt (as compared to passive assessment) *If there is more available range than the benchmark standard, only the benchmark range needs to be actively controlled*	☐	• The pattern of dissociation is smooth during concentric and eccentric movement	☐
		• Does not (consistently) use *end-range* movement into the opposite direction to prevent the UCM	☐
		• No extra feedback needed *(tactile, visual or verbal cueing)*	☐
• Without holding breath (though it is acceptable to use an alternate breathing strategy)	☐	• Without external support or unloading	☐
		• Relaxed natural breathing *(even if not ideal – so long as natural pattern does not change)*	☐
• Control during eccentric phase	☐	• No fatigue	☐
• Control during concentric phase	☐		

CORRECT DISSOCIATION PATTERN   **RECRUITMENT EFFICIENCY**

T48.2 Diagnosis of the site and direction of UCM from the Pelvic Tail Lift Test

PELVIC TAIL LIFT TEST – SITTING

Site	Direction	✗✗ or ✗✓
		(check box)
Thoracic	Extension	☐

T48.3 Feedback tools to monitor retraining

FEEDBACK TOOL	PROCESS
Self-palpation	Palpation monitoring of joint position
Visual observation	Observe in a mirror or directly watch the movement
Adhesive tape	Skin tension for tactile feedback
Cueing and verbal correction	Listen to feedback from another observer

T49 STANDING: BILATERAL BACKWARD REACH TEST
(tests for thoracic extension UCM)

This dissociation test assesses the ability to actively dissociate and control thoracic extension then reach backwards with both arms (i.e. bilateral shoulder extension) while standing upright and unsupported.

Test procedure

The subject stands upright with the spine in its neutral normal curves, the head directly over the shoulders without chin poke and with the arms resting by the side with the shoulders in a neutral position (Figure 7.32). The person is then instructed to slowly reach backwards with both arms into shoulder extension. Without letting the thoracic spine extend (sternum does not lift or move backwards) or the head to move backwards, they should be able to actively reach backwards with both hands into shoulder extension.

Ideally, the person should have the ability to dissociate the thoracic spine from shoulder extension as evidenced by the ability to prevent thoracic extension while independently reaching backwards to at least 10–15° bilateral shoulder extension (Figure 7.33). There must be no movement into thoracic extension. There should be no provocation of any symptoms under shoulder extension load, so long as the thoracic extension UCM can be controlled.

This test should be performed without any extra feedback (self-palpation, vision, etc.) or cueing for correction. The therapist should use visual

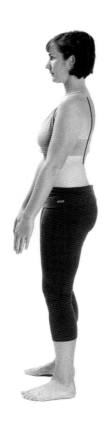

Figure 7.32 Start position bilateral reach back test

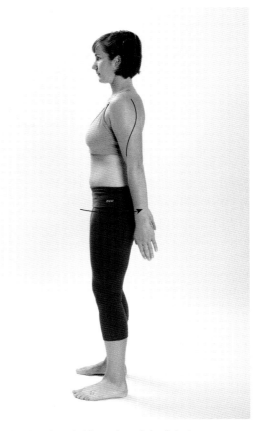

Figure 7.33 Benchmark bilateral reach back test

observation of the head and thorax relative to the shoulders to determine whether the control of thoracic extension is adequate when feedback is removed for testing.

Thoracic extension UCM

The person complains of extension-related symptoms in the thoracic spine. The thorax has UCM into extension relative to bilateral shoulder extension (reaching backwards). The thoracic spine starts to extend before 10–15° of independent shoulder extension is achieved. During the attempt to dissociate the thoracic extension from independent reaching backwards, the person either cannot control the UCM or has to concentrate and try hard to control the thoracic extension.

Clinical assessment note for direction-specific motor control testing

---

If some other movement (e.g. a small amount of thoracic rotation) is observed during a motor control (dissociation) test of thoracic extension, *do not* score this as uncontrolled thoracic extension. The thoracic rotation motor control tests will identify if the observed unrelated movement is uncontrolled. *A test for thoracic extension UCM is only positive if uncontrolled thoracic **extension** is demonstrated.*

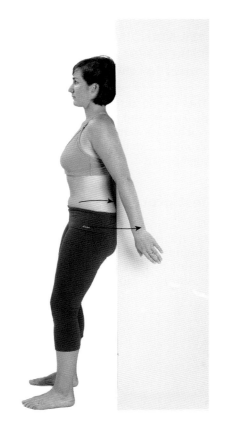

Figure 7.34 Correction unilateral arm extension with thoracic support on wall

Rating and diagnosis of thoracic extension UCM

(T49.1 and T49.2)

Correction

If control is poor, retraining is best started by supporting the thoracic spine against a wall and reaching backwards (shoulder flexion) with unilateral arm movement and through reduced range. The person stands with the thoracic spine and the back of the head supported upright against a wall. The person should flatten the lumbar spine against the wall to give additional feedback and support to the ability to prevent thoracic extension. If uncontrolled thoracic extension occurs the person will be aware of the thoracolumbar spine losing contact with the wall

(arching into extension). Alternatively, the person may monitor the control of thoracic extension by palpating the sternum or clavicles with one hand. Any lifting movement of the sternum or clavicles also indicates uncontrolled thoracic extension.

The person is instructed to slowly extend one arm through range to reach backwards. Only reach backwards as far as there is no thoracic extension (Figure 7.34). Using feedback from the back on the wall (or palpating the sternum), the person is trained to control and prevent thoracic extension and perform independent overhead shoulder extension.

The person should self-monitor the control of thoracic extension UCM with a variety of feedback options (T49.3). There should be no

T49.1 Assessment and rating of low threshold recruitment efficiency of the Bilateral Backward Reach Test

BILATERAL BACKWARD REACH – STANDING

ASSESSMENT

Control point:
• prevent thoracic extension
Movement challenge: bilateral shoulder extension (standing)
Benchmark range: 10–15° active independent shoulder extension

RATING OF LOW THRESHOLD RECRUITMENT EFFICIENCY FOR CONTROL OF DIRECTION

	✓ or ✗		✓ or ✗
• Able to prevent UCM into the test direction Correct dissociation pattern of movement Prevent thoracic UCM into: • extension and move bilateral shoulder extension	☐	• Looks easy, and in the opinion of the assessor, is performed with confidence	☐
		• Feels easy, and the subject has sufficient awareness of the movement pattern that they confidently prevent UCM into the test direction	☐
• Dissociate movement through the benchmark range of: 10–15° range independent bilateral shoulder extension (reaching backwards) *If there is more available range than the benchmark standard, only the benchmark range needs to be actively controlled*	☐	• The pattern of dissociation is smooth during concentric and eccentric movement	☐
		• Does not (consistently) use *end-range* movement into the opposite direction to prevent the UCM	☐
• Without holding breath (though it is acceptable to use an alternate breathing strategy)	☐	• No extra feedback needed (*tactile, visual or verbal cueing*)	☐
		• Without external support or unloading	☐
• Control during eccentric phase	☐	• Relaxed natural breathing (*even if not ideal – so long as natural pattern does not change*)	☐
• Control during concentric phase	☐	• No fatigue	☐

CORRECT DISSOCIATION PATTERN   **RECRUITMENT EFFICIENCY**

T49.2 Diagnosis of the site and direction of UCM from the Bilateral Backward Reach Test

BILATERAL BACKWARD REACH TEST – STANDING

Site	Direction	✗✗ or ✗✓
		(check box)
Thoracic	Extension	☐

T49.3 Feedback tools to monitor retraining

FEEDBACK TOOL	PROCESS
Self-palpation	Palpation monitoring of joint position
Visual observation	Observe in a mirror or directly watch the movement
Adhesive tape	Skin tension for tactile feedback
Cueing and verbal correction	Listen to feedback from another observer

provocation of any symptoms within the range that the extension UCM can be controlled.

Once control of thoracic extension improves the person should reach back with both arms while using a doorway or a pole for feedback and support of the thoracic spine. Eventually, they can move away from the wall and the exercise can be performed with the thoracic spine unsupported (no wall support).

Thoracic extension UCM summary

(Table 7.4)

Table 7.4 Summary and rating of thoracic extension tests		
UCM DIAGNOSIS AND TESTING		
SITE: **THORACIC**	**DIRECTION:** **EXTENSION**	**CLINICAL PRIORITY** ☐
TEST	**RATING** (✓✓ or ✓✗ or ✗✗) and rationale	
Standing: bilateral overhead reach		
Sitting: head backward raise		
Sitting: pelvic tail lift		
Standing: bilateral backward reach		

Thoracic rotation control

THORACIC ROTATION CONTROL TESTS AND ROTATION CONTROL REHABILITATION

These rotation control tests assess the extent of rotation UCM in the thoracic spine and assess the ability of the dynamic stability system to adequately control rotation load or strain. It is a priority to assess for rotation UCM if the person complains of or demonstrates rotation-related symptoms or disability. The tests that identify dysfunction can also be used to guide and direct rehabilitation strategies.

Indications to test for thoracic rotation UCM

Observe or palpate for:

1. hypermobile thoracic rotation range
2. excessive initiation of turning or twisting with thoracic rotation
3. symptoms (pain, discomfort, strain) associated with turning or twisting with associated thoracic rotation.

The person complains of rotation-related symptoms in the thorax. Under rotation load, the thoracic spine has greater give *into rotation* relative to the lumbar spine, head and shoulders. The dysfunction is confirmed with motor control tests of rotation dissociation.

Tests of thoracic rotation control

T50 SITTING: HEAD TURN TEST
(tests for thoracic rotation UCM)

This dissociation test assesses the ability to actively dissociate and control thoracic rotation and turn the head by rotating the neck through full range while sitting. During any asymmetrical or non-sagittal trunk or head movement a rotational force is transmitted to the thorax.

Test procedure

The person sits upright with feet unsupported and with the spine in its neutral normal curves; the head and neck in neutral alignment with the scapulae positioned in their neutral mid-range

alignment (Figure 7.35). The person is then instructed to fully rotate the head by turning to look over the shoulder, keeping the eyes and the shoulders horizontal. Without letting the thoracic spine rotate or lean to the side, they should be able to actively turn the head through approximately 70–80° of rotation.

Ideally, the person should have the ability to dissociate the thoracic spine from head rotation as evidenced by the ability to prevent thoracic rotation while independently turning the head to 70–80° of independent head rotation (Figure 7.36). There must be no movement into thoracic rotation. There should be no provocation of any symptoms under head rotation load, so long as the thoracic rotation UCM can be controlled.

This test should be performed without any extra feedback (self-palpation, vision, etc.) or cueing for correction. The therapist should use visual observation of the thorax relative to the head to

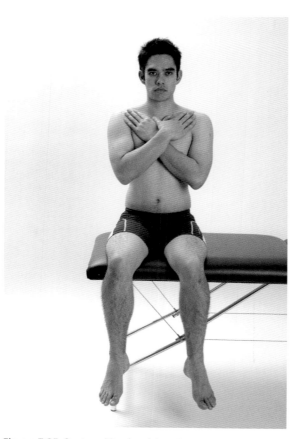

Figure 7.35 Start position head turn test

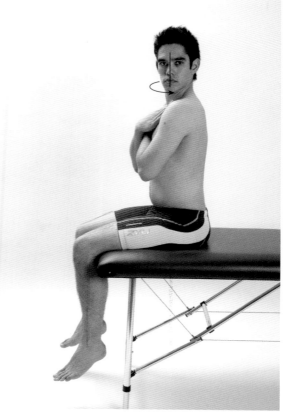

Figure 7.36 Benchmark head turn test

determine whether the control of thoracic rotation is adequate when feedback is removed for testing. Assess rotation to both sides separately.

Thoracic rotation UCM

The person complains of rotation-related symptoms in the thoracic spine. The thorax has UCM into rotation relative to cervical rotation (turning the head to look over the shoulder). The thoracic spine starts to rotate (or lean into lateral flexion) before 70–80° of independent head rotation is achieved. During the attempt to dissociate the thoracic rotation from independent head rotation, the person either cannot control the UCM or has to concentrate and try hard to control the thoracic rotation.

Clinical assessment note for direction-specific motor control testing

If some other movement (e.g. a small amount of thoracic flexion) is observed during a motor control (dissociation) test of thoracic rotation, *do not* score this as uncontrolled thoracic rotation. The thoracic flexion motor control tests will identify if the observed unrelated movement is uncontrolled. *A test for thoracic rotation UCM is only positive if uncontrolled thoracic **rotation** is demonstrated.*

Rating and diagnosis of thoracic rotation UCM

(T50.1 and T50.2)

Correction

Retraining is best started by supporting the thoracic spine against a wall for increased thoracic support and feedback and turning the head through reduced range. The person stands with the back of the pelvis, the upper thoracic spine and the back of the head resting against a wall with the shoulders neutral and the arms crossed in front of the chest. Both scapulae should contact the wall equally. This can also be performed with the person sitting on a low stool with the feet on the floor and the thoracic spine and head resting against a wall. Then, without letting the chest turn to follow the head (thoracic rotation) or allowing the shoulders to drop into lateral flexion, the person is instructed to slowly turn the head to

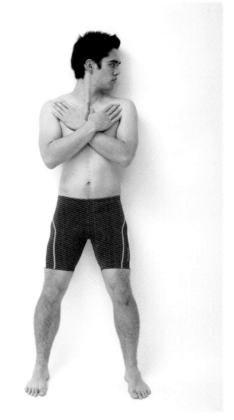

Figure 7.37 Correction partial head rotation with thoracic support on wall

look over the shoulder. They are to keep the occiput in contact with the wall to monitor that the head turns into rotation (axial movement) and does not roll (side-bend) into rotation. Both scapulae should actively maintain symmetrical contact on the wall and the thorax should not move. They are to turn the head only as far as there is no thoracic rotation (Figure 7.37). The person is trained to control and prevent thoracic rotation and perform independent cervical rotation.

The person should self-monitor the control of thoracic rotation UCM with a variety of feedback options (T50.3). There should be no provocation of any symptoms within the range that the rotation UCM can be controlled.

Once control of thoracic rotation improves, the exercise can be performed with the thoracic spine unsupported (no wall support).

T50.1 Assessment and rating of low threshold recruitment efficiency of the Head Turn Test

HEAD TURN – SITTING

ASSESSMENT

Control point:
• prevent thoracic rotation
Movement challenge: cervical rotation (sitting)
Benchmark range: 70–80° active independent head rotation

RATING OF LOW THRESHOLD RECRUITMENT EFFICIENCY FOR CONTROL OF DIRECTION

	✓ or ✗		✓ or ✗
• Able to prevent UCM into the test direction Correct dissociation pattern of movement Prevent thoracic UCM into: • rotation and move cervical rotation	☐	• Looks easy, and in the opinion of the assessor, is performed with confidence	☐
		• Feels easy, and the subject has sufficient awareness of the movement pattern that they confidently prevent UCM into the test direction	☐
• Dissociate movement through the benchmark range of: 70–80° independent head rotation (turn to look over shoulder) *If there is more available range than the benchmark standard, only the benchmark range needs to be actively controlled*	☐	• The pattern of dissociation is smooth during concentric and eccentric movement	☐
		• Does not (consistently) use *end-range* movement into the opposite direction to prevent the UCM	☐
• Without holding breath (though it is acceptable to use an alternate breathing strategy)	☐	• No extra feedback needed (*tactile, visual or verbal cueing*)	☐
		• Without external support or unloading	☐
• Control during eccentric phase	☐	• Relaxed natural breathing (*even if not ideal – so long as natural pattern does not change*)	☐
• Control during concentric phase	☐	• No fatigue	☐

CORRECT DISSOCIATION PATTERN   **RECRUITMENT EFFICIENCY**

T50.2 Diagnosis of the site and direction of UCM from the Head Turn Test

HEAD TURN TEST – SITTING

Site	Direction	Thorax to the left (L)	Thorax to the right (R)
		(check box)	(check box)
Thoracic	Rotation	☐	☐

T50.3 Feedback tools to monitor retraining

FEEDBACK TOOL	PROCESS
Self-palpation	Palpation monitoring of joint position
Visual observation	Observe in a mirror or directly watch the movement
Adhesive tape	Skin tension for tactile feedback
Cueing and verbal correction	Listen to feedback from another observer

T51 SITTING: PELVIC TWIST (SWIVEL CHAIR) TEST
(tests for thoracic rotation UCM)

This dissociation test assesses the ability to actively dissociate and control thoracic rotation and turn the pelvis by rotating the pelvis through full range while sitting on a swivel chair. During any asymmetrical or non-sagittal trunk or pelvic movement a rotational force is transmitted to the thorax.

Test procedure

The person sits upright on a swivel chair (height adjusted for feet clearance) with feet unsupported and with the spine in its neutral normal curves; the head and neck in neutral alignment with the scapulae positioned in their neutral midrange alignment. The finger tips touch a table in front of the body to provide a fixation point to turn the chair (Figure 7.38). The person is then instructed to rotate the chair to one side, but keep the upper thorax, shoulders and head facing the front. The eyes and the shoulders should maintain a horizontal alignment. Without letting the shoulders and upper chest rotate or lean to the side, they should be able to actively turn the chair through approximately 45° of rotation.

Ideally, the person should have the ability to dissociate the upper thoracic spine from pelvic rotation as evidenced by the ability to prevent upper thoracic rotation while independently turning the chair to 45° of independent pelvic rotation (Figure 7.39). There must be no movement into thoracic rotation. There should be no provocation of any symptoms under head rotation load, so long as the thoracic rotation UCM can be controlled.

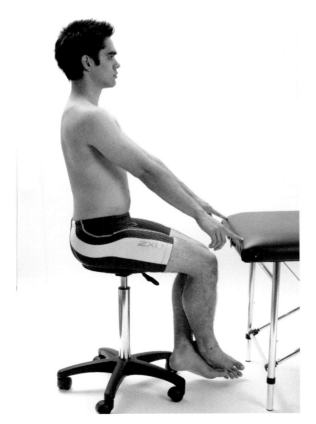

Figure 7.38 Start position pelvic twist test

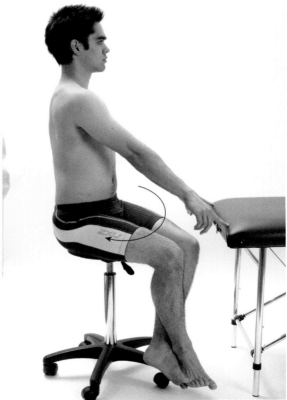

Figure 7.39 Benchmark pelvic twist test

This test should be performed without any extra feedback (self-palpation, vision, etc.) or cueing for correction. The therapist should use visual observation of the thorax relative to the pelvis to determine whether the control of thoracic rotation is adequate when feedback is removed for testing. Assess the pelvic twist to each side separately.

Thoracic rotation UCM

The person complains of rotation-related symptoms in the thoracic spine. The thorax has UCM into rotation relative to pelvic rotation (turning the chair to the side). The thoracic spine starts to rotate (or lean into lateral flexion) before 45° of independent chair rotation is achieved. During the attempt to dissociate the upper thoracic rotation from independent pelvic rotation, the person either cannot control the UCM or has to concentrate and try hard to control the thoracic rotation.

Clinical assessment note for direction-specific motor control testing

If some other movement (e.g. a small amount of thoracic flexion) is observed during a motor control (dissociation) test of thoracic rotation, *do not* score this as uncontrolled thoracic rotation. The thoracic flexion motor control tests will identify if the observed unrelated movement is uncontrolled. *A test for thoracic rotation UCM is only positive if uncontrolled thoracic rotation is demonstrated.*

Rating and diagnosis of thoracic rotation UCM

(T51.1 and T51.2)

Correction

Retraining is best started by supporting the thoracic spine with the shoulder girdle by holding the table with a firmer hand grip (increased fixation for thoracic support) and turning the chair through reduced range. The person sits upright on a swivel chair (height adjusted for feet clearance) with feet unsupported and the spine in its neutral normal curves. The head and shoulders are positioned in their neutral alignment and the hands firmly grip the table to provide a fixation point to turn the chair.

Then, without letting the chest turn to follow the pelvis or the shoulders drop into lateral flexion, the person is instructed to slowly turn the chair to the side. They are to keep the upper thorax, shoulders and head facing the front. They are to turn the chair and pelvis only as far as there is no upper thoracic rotation. The person is trained to control and prevent upper thoracic rotation and perform independent pelvic rotation.

The person should self-monitor the control of thoracic rotation UCM with a variety of feedback options (T51.3). There should be no provocation of any symptoms within the range that the rotation UCM can be controlled.

Once control of thoracic rotation improves, the exercise can be performed with the thoracic spine less supported (only finger tips for fixation support).

T51.1 Assessment and rating of low threshold recruitment efficiency of the Pelvic Twist Test

PELVIC TWIST – SITTING (SWIVEL CHAIR)

ASSESSMENT

Control point:
• prevent upper thoracic rotation
Movement challenge: pelvic rotation (sitting – swivel chair)
Benchmark range: 45° active independent pelvic/chair rotation

RATING OF LOW THRESHOLD RECRUITMENT EFFICIENCY FOR CONTROL OF DIRECTION

	✓ or ✗		✓ or ✗
• Able to prevent UCM into the test direction Correct dissociation pattern of movement Prevent thoracic UCM into: • rotation and move pelvic rotation	☐	• Looks easy, and in the opinion of the assessor, is performed with confidence	☐
		• Feels easy, and the subject has sufficient awareness of the movement pattern that they confidently prevent UCM into the test direction	☐
• Dissociate movement through the benchmark range of: 45° independent pelvic rotation (turn swivel chair the side) *If there is more available range than the benchmark standard, only the benchmark range needs to be actively controlled*	☐	• The pattern of dissociation is smooth during concentric and eccentric movement	☐
		• Does not (consistently) use *end-range* movement into the opposite direction to prevent the UCM	☐
• Without holding breath (though it is acceptable to use an alternate breathing strategy)	☐	• No extra feedback needed *(tactile, visual or verbal cueing)*	☐
		• Without external support or unloading	☐
• Control during eccentric phase	☐	• Relaxed natural breathing *(even if not ideal – so long as natural pattern does not change)*	☐
• Control during concentric phase	☐	• No fatigue	☐
CORRECT DISSOCIATION PATTERN		**RECRUITMENT EFFICIENCY**	

T51.2 Diagnosis of the site and direction of UCM from the Pelvic Twist Test

PELVIC TWIST TEST – SITTING (SWIVEL CHAIR)

Site	Direction	Thorax to the left (L)	Thorax to the right (R)
		(check box)	(check box)
Thoracic	Rotation	☐	☐

T51.3 Feedback tools to monitor retraining

FEEDBACK TOOL	PROCESS
Self-palpation	Palpation monitoring of joint position
Visual observation	Observe in a mirror or directly watch the movement
Adhesive tape	Skin tension for tactile feedback
Cueing and verbal correction	Listen to feedback from another observer

T52 STANDING: PELVIC SIDE-SHIFT TEST (tests for thoracic rotation UCM)

This dissociation test assesses the ability to actively dissociate and control thoracic rotation and side-shift the pelvis through full range of lateral pelvic shift while standing unsupported. During any asymmetrical or non-sagittal trunk or pelvic movement, a rotational force is transmitted to the thorax.

Test procedure

The person stands upright (unsupported), the feet at least shoulder width apart and with the knees slightly flexed (hip flexors unloaded and wide base of support). The arms are crossed in front of the chest with the shoulders and the pelvis level (horizontal) (Figure 7.40). Then,

keeping the shoulders level and stationary, they are instructed to side-shift the pelvis laterally to one side. Without letting the thoracic spine rotate, lean to the side, or move laterally, the person should be able to actively side-shift the pelvis at least 5 cm (Figure 7.41).

Ideally, the person should have the ability to dissociate the thoracic spine from lateral pelvic side-shift as evidenced by the ability to prevent thoracic rotation or lateral flexion while independently laterally shifting the pelvis to the side. There must be no movement into thoracic rotation. There should be no provocation of any symptoms under pelvic side-shift load, so long as the thoracic rotation UCM can be controlled.

This test should be performed without any extra feedback (self-palpation, vision, etc.) or cueing for correction. The therapist should use visual observation of the thorax relative to the pelvis to determine whether the control of thoracic

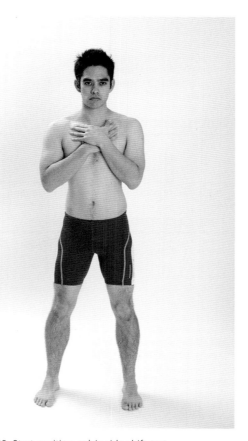

Figure 7.40 Start position pelvic side shift test

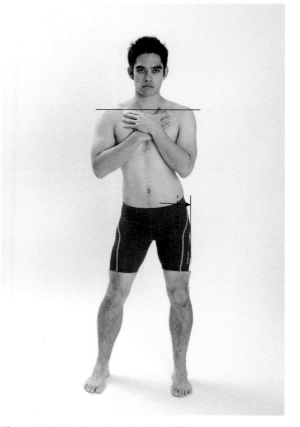

Figure 7.41 Benchmark pelvic side shift test

rotation is adequate when feedback is removed for testing. Assess side-shift to each side separately. There should also be good symmetry to each side.

Thoracic rotation UCM

The person complains of rotation-related symptoms in the thoracic spine. The thorax has UCM into rotation relative to lateral pelvic side-shift. The thoracic spine starts to rotate (or lean into lateral flexion) before 5 cm of independent side-shift is achieved. During the attempt to dissociate the thoracic rotation from independent pelvic side-shift, the person either cannot control the UCM or has to concentrate and try hard to control the thoracic rotation.

Clinical assessment note for direction-specific motor control testing

If some other movement (e.g. a small amount of thoracic flexion) is observed during a motor control (dissociation) test of thoracic rotation, *do not* score this as uncontrolled thoracic rotation. The thoracic flexion motor control tests will identify if the observed unrelated movement is uncontrolled. *A test for thoracic rotation UCM is only positive if uncontrolled thoracic **rotation** is demonstrated.*

Rating and diagnosis of thoracic rotation UCM

(T52.1 and T52.2)

Correction

Retraining is best started by supporting the thoracic spine against a wall for increased thoracic support and feedback and turning the head through reduced range. The person stands with the back of the pelvis, the upper thoracic spine and the back of the head resting against a wall with the shoulders neutral and the arms crossed in front of the chest. Both scapulae should contact the wall equally. This can also be performed with the person sitting on a low stool with the feet on the floor and the thoracic spine and head resting against a wall.

Then, without letting the chest turn to follow the pelvis (thoracic rotation) or allowing the

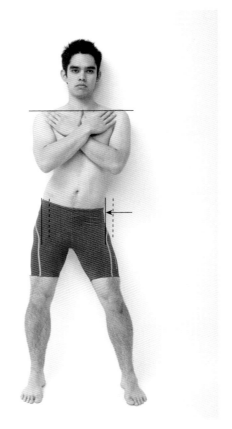

Figure 7.42 Correction partial pelvic side shift with thoracic support on wall

shoulders to drop into lateral flexion, the person is instructed to slowly slide the pelvis laterally on the wall. Both scapulae should actively maintain symmetrical contact on the wall and the thorax should not move. They are to side-shift the pelvis only as far as there is no thoracic rotation (Figure 7.42). The person is trained to control and prevent thoracic rotation and perform independent lateral pelvic side-shift.

The person should self-monitor the control of thoracic rotation UCM with a variety of feedback options (T52.3). There should be no provocation of any symptoms within the range that the rotation UCM can be controlled.

Once control of thoracic rotation improves, the exercise can be performed with the thoracic spine unsupported (no wall support).

T52.1 Assessment and rating of low threshold recruitment efficiency of the Pelvic Side-Shift Test

PELVIC SIDE-SHIFT – STANDING

ASSESSMENT

Control point:
• prevent thoracic rotation
Movement challenge: lateral pelvic side-shift (standing)
Benchmark range: 5 cm active independent lateral pelvic side-shift

RATING OF LOW THRESHOLD RECRUITMENT EFFICIENCY FOR CONTROL OF DIRECTION

	✓ or ✗		✓ or ✗
• Able to prevent UCM into the test direction Correct dissociation pattern of movement Prevent thoracic UCM into: • rotation and move lateral pelvic side-shift	☐	• Looks easy, and in the opinion of the assessor, is performed with confidence	☐
		• Feels easy, and the subject has sufficient awareness of the movement pattern that they confidently prevent UCM into the test direction	☐
• Dissociate movement through the benchmark range of: 5 cm independent lateral side-shift *If there is more available range than the benchmark standard, only the benchmark range needs to be actively controlled*	☐	• The pattern of dissociation is smooth during concentric and eccentric movement	☐
		• Does not (consistently) use *end-range* movement into the opposite direction to prevent the UCM	☐
• Without holding breath (though it is acceptable to use an alternate breathing strategy)	☐	• No extra feedback needed *(tactile, visual or verbal cueing)*	☐
• Control during eccentric phase	☐	• Without external support or unloading	☐
• Control during concentric phase	☐	• Relaxed natural breathing *(even if not ideal – so long as natural pattern does not change)*	☐
		• No fatigue	☐

CORRECT DISSOCIATION PATTERN   **RECRUITMENT EFFICIENCY**

T52.2 Diagnosis of the site and direction of UCM from the Pelvic Side-Shift Test

PELVIC SIDE-SHIFT TEST – STANDING

Site	Direction	Thorax to the left (L)	Thorax to the right (R)
		(check box)	(check box)
Thoracic	Rotation	☐	☐

T52.3 Feedback tools to monitor retraining

FEEDBACK TOOL	PROCESS
Self-palpation	Palpation monitoring of joint position
Visual observation	Observe in a mirror or directly watch the movement
Adhesive tape	Skin tension for tactile feedback
Cueing and verbal correction	Listen to feedback from another observer

T53 STANDING: ONE ARM WALL PUSH TEST
(tests for thoracic rotation UCM)

This dissociation test assesses the ability to actively dissociate and control thoracic rotation and perform a one arm 'push up' against a wall while standing. During any unilateral or asymmetrical upper limb movement, a rotational force is transmitted to the thorax.

Test procedure

The person stands upright facing a wall, with one arm held horizontal (90° shoulder flexion) with the wrist extended and the palm facing forwards. The shoulders are held neutral (midway between elevation and depression). The body is positioned arm's length from the wall with the palm resting on the wall at shoulder height and the fingers vertical (Figure 7.43).

The person is then instructed to lean their body weight onto the hand and slowly bend the elbow to lower the forearm to the wall. The forearm should stay vertically aligned under the hand (not out to the side). The body should maintain a straight line from the ankles through the hips and back to the head and shoulders as the body leans in towards the wall in the 'one arm wall push'. Without allowing the thoracic spine to rotate or the scapula to 'wing' off the thorax, the person should be able to actively lean in to the wall and take full weight on the vertical forearm and then push off the wall to return to the start position.

Ideally, the person should have the ability to dissociate the thoracic spine from unilateral arm loading as evidenced by the ability to prevent thoracic rotation while independently performing the one arm wall push (Figure 7.44). There

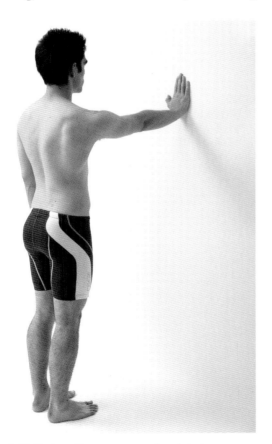

Figure 7.43 Start position one arm wall push test

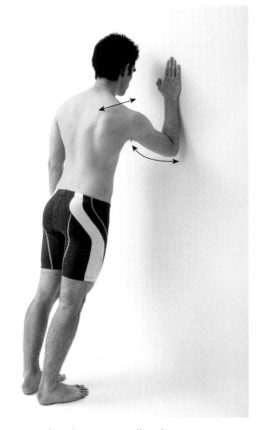

Figure 7.44 Benchmark one arm wall push test

must be no movement into thoracic rotation. There should be no provocation of any symptoms under unilateral arm load, so long as the thoracic rotation UCM can be controlled.

This test should be performed without any extra feedback (self-palpation, vision, etc.) or cueing for correction. When feedback is removed for testing the therapist should use visual observation of the thorax relative to the shoulder and arm to determine whether the control of thoracic rotation is adequate. Assess one arm wall push to each side separately. Performance to right and left sides should be symmetrical.

Thoracic rotation UCM

The person complains of rotation-related symptoms in the thoracic spine. The thorax has UCM into rotation relative to unilateral arm weight bearing. The thoracic spine starts to rotate (or the scapula wings) before the forearm lowers body weight to the wall and pushes off again. During the attempt to dissociate the thoracic rotation from independent unilateral arm loading, the person either cannot control the UCM or has to concentrate and try hard to control the thoracic rotation.

Clinical assessment note for direction-specific motor control testing

If some other movement (e.g. a small amount of thoracic flexion) is observed during a motor control (dissociation) test of thoracic rotation, *do not* score this as uncontrolled thoracic rotation. The thoracic flexion motor control tests will identify if the observed unrelated movement is uncontrolled. *A test for thoracic rotation UCM is only positive if uncontrolled thoracic **rotation** is demonstrated.*

Rating and diagnosis of thoracic rotation UCM

(T53.1 and T53.2)

Correction

Retraining is best started by standing closer to the wall to reduce body load during the one arm wall push. The person stands upright facing a wall, with the palm resting on the wall horizontally in front of the shoulder (fingers vertical). The body is positioned less than arm's length from the wall. At this point the elbow will be partially flexed.

The person is then instructed to lean their body weight onto the hand and slowly lower the forearm to the wall, keeping the forearm vertically aligned under the hand. The body should maintain a straight line from the ankles to the head. Then, without letting the thoracic spine rotate (or the scapula 'wing' of the thorax), the person is instructed to slowly lower the forearm to the wall. They are to lean in towards the wall only as far as there is no thoracic rotation. The person is trained to control and prevent thoracic rotation and perform independent one arm wall push.

The person should self-monitor the control of thoracic rotation UCM with a variety of feedback options (T53.3). There should be no provocation of any symptoms within the range that the rotation UCM can be controlled.

Once control of thoracic rotation improves, the exercise can be performed standing further away from the wall (increased body load in unilateral weight bearing).

T53.1 Assessment and rating of low threshold recruitment efficiency of the One Arm Wall Push Test

ONE ARM WALL PUSH – STANDING (WALL)

ASSESSMENT

Control point:
- prevent thoracic rotation

Movement challenge: independent unilateral arm weight bearing with sagittal elbow and shoulder movement (standing – wall)

Benchmark range: standing at arm's length from wall, lower the forearm vertically to the wall (supporting body weight on one hand) and return without thoracic compensation

RATING OF LOW THRESHOLD RECRUITMENT EFFICIENCY FOR CONTROL OF DIRECTION

	✓ or ✗		✓ or ✗
• Able to prevent UCM into the test direction Correct dissociation pattern of movement Prevent thoracic UCM into: • rotation and move unilateral arm weight bearing + sagittal elbow and shoulder movement	☐	• Looks easy, and in the opinion of the assessor, is performed with confidence	☐
		• Feels easy, and the subject has sufficient awareness of the movement pattern that they confidently prevent UCM into the test direction	☐
• Dissociate movement through the benchmark range of lower the forearm vertically to the wall with body weight on one hand (arm's length from wall) *If there is more available range than the benchmark standard, only the benchmark range needs to be actively controlled*	☐	• The pattern of dissociation is smooth during concentric and eccentric movement	☐
		• Does not (consistently) use *end-range* movement into the opposite direction to prevent the UCM	☐
		• No extra feedback needed *(tactile, visual or verbal cueing)*	☐
• Without holding breath (though it is acceptable to use an alternate breathing strategy)	☐	• Without external support or unloading	☐
		• Relaxed natural breathing *(even if not ideal – so long as natural pattern does not change)*	☐
• Control during eccentric phase	☐	• No fatigue	☐
• Control during concentric phase	☐		

CORRECT DISSOCIATION PATTERN	**RECRUITMENT EFFICIENCY**

T53.2 Diagnosis of the site and direction of UCM from the One Arm Wall Push Test

ONE ARM WALL PUSH TEST – STANDING (WALL)

Site	Direction	Thorax to the left (L)	Thorax to the right (R)
		(check box)	(check box)
Thoracic	Rotation	☐	☐

T53.3 Feedback tools to monitor retraining	
FEEDBACK TOOL	**PROCESS**
Self-palpation	Palpation monitoring of joint position
Visual observation	Observe in a mirror or directly watch the movement
Adhesive tape	Skin tension for tactile feedback
Cueing and verbal correction	Listen to feedback from another observer

T54 4 POINT: ONE ARM LIFT TEST
(tests for thoracic rotation UCM)

This dissociation test assesses the ability to actively dissociate and control thoracic rotation and actively lift one arm forward of the body while in 4 point kneeling (hands and knees). During any unilateral or asymmetrical upper limb movement, a rotational force is transmitted to the thorax.

Test procedure

The person should have the ability to actively lift one arm forward of the body while weight bearing on the other arm and controlling the thoracic rotation. The person positions themselves in 4 point kneeling (hands and knees) with the spine and scapulae in neutral (mid-position) alignment and hands under the shoulders (weight bearing at 90° of flexion) (Figures 7.45 and 7.46). The person is then instructed to lean body weight onto one hand and slowly lift the other arm into shoulder flexion to reach forwards of the body. Without allowing the thoracic spine to rotate or the scapulae to 'wing' off the thorax or to hitch into elevation, the person should be able to actively reach forwards with the non-weight bearing arm to 150° flexion while maintaining weight bearing control with the other (weight bearing) arm.

Ideally, the person should have the ability to dissociate the thoracic spine from asymmetrical shoulder loading as evidenced by the ability to prevent thoracic rotation while independently weight bearing on one arm and lifting the other arm forwards to 150° flexion (Figure 7.47). There must be no movement into thoracic rotation. There should be no provocation of any symptoms under asymmetrical arm load, so long as the thoracic rotation UCM can be controlled.

This test should be performed without any extra feedback (self-palpation, vision, etc.) or cueing

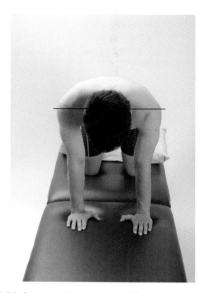

Figure 7.46 Start position one arm lift test (front view)

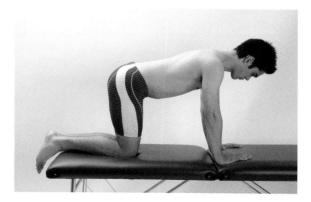

Figure 7.45 Start position one arm lift test (lateral view)

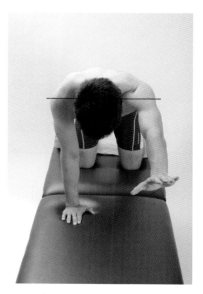

Figure 7.47 Benchmark one arm lift test

for correction. The therapist should use visual observation of the thorax relative to the shoulders to determine whether the control of thoracic rotation is adequate when feedback is removed for testing. Assess the unilateral arm lift to each side separately. Performance to right and left sides should be symmetrical.

Thoracic rotation UCM

The person complains of rotation-related symptoms in the thoracic spine. The thorax has UCM into rotation relative to asymmetrical arm loading. The thoracic spine starts to rotate (or the scapula wings or elevates on the thorax) before the arm lifts forwards to 150° flexion while weight bearing on the other arm. During the attempt to dissociate the thoracic rotation from independent asymmetrical arm loading, the person either cannot control the UCM or has to concentrate and try hard to control the thoracic rotation.

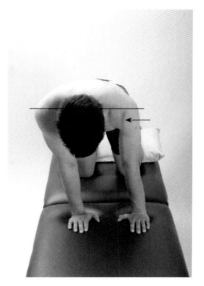

Figure 7.48 Correction lateral weight shift

Clinical assessment note for direction-specific motor control testing

If some other movement (e.g. a small amount of thoracic flexion) is observed during a motor control (dissociation) test of thoracic rotation, *do not* score this as uncontrolled thoracic rotation. The thoracic flexion motor control tests will identify if the observed unrelated movement is uncontrolled. *A test for thoracic rotation UCM is only positive if uncontrolled thoracic rotation is demonstrated.*

Rating and diagnosis of thoracic rotation UCM

(T54.1 and T54.2)

Correction

Retraining is best started by controlling thoracic rotation during weight shift movement without full weight transfer to one arm.

The person positions themselves in 4 point kneeling (hands and knees) with the spine and scapulae in neutral (mid-position) alignment and hands under the shoulders (weight bearing at 90° of flexion). Then, without allowing the thoracic spine to rotate, the person is instructed to slowly lean body weight laterally onto one hand but not to shift full weight onto that hand. The other arm maintains some partial weight bearing load.

They are to shift weight laterally only as far as there is no thoracic rotation. The person is trained to control and prevent thoracic rotation and perform independent partial weight transfer from one arm to the other (Figure 7.48).

An alternative progression is to start in a push-up position off elbows and knees (Figure 7.49). Keep the scapula and chest in mid-position and slowly shift upper body weight onto one arm (Figure 7.50) only so far as there is thoracic rotation can be controlled.

The person should self-monitor the control of thoracic rotation UCM with a variety of feedback options (T54.3). There should be no provocation of any symptoms within the range that the rotation UCM can be controlled.

Once control of thoracic rotation improves, the exercise can be performed with full weight transfer and one arm lift into flexion.

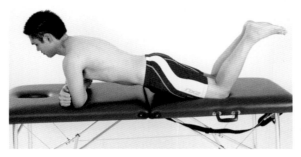

Figure 7.49 Correction – push up position off elbows: start position

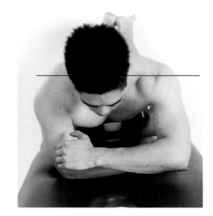

Figure 7.50 Correction – lateral weight shift off elbows

T54.1 Assessment and rating of low threshold recruitment efficiency of the One Arm Lift Test

ARM LIFT – 4 POINT KNEELING

ASSESSMENT

Control point:
- prevent thoracic rotation

Movement challenge: independent asymmetrical shoulder load: unilateral arm weight bearing with opposite arm non-weight bearing flexion (4 point)

Benchmark range: weight bearing on one arm at 90° flexion + non-weight bearing flexion of other arm to 150° forward of body without thoracic compensation

RATING OF LOW THRESHOLD RECRUITMENT EFFICIENCY FOR CONTROL OF DIRECTION

	✓ or ✗		✓ or ✗
• Able to prevent UCM into the test direction Correct dissociation pattern of movement Prevent thoracic UCM into: • rotation and move asymmetrical arm load: unilateral weight bearing + opposite non-weight bearing	☐	• Looks easy, and in the opinion of the assessor, is performed with confidence	☐
		• Feels easy, and the subject has sufficient awareness of the movement pattern that they confidently prevent UCM into the test direction	☐
• Dissociate movement through the benchmark range of 150° independent forward flexion of 1 arm + weight bearing at 90° flexion with other arm *If there is more available range than the benchmark standard, only the benchmark range needs to be actively controlled*	☐	• The pattern of dissociation is smooth during concentric and eccentric movement	☐
		• Does not (consistently) use *end-range* movement into the opposite direction to prevent the UCM	☐
		• No extra feedback needed (*tactile, visual or verbal cueing*)	☐
• Without holding breath (though it is acceptable to use an alternate breathing strategy)	☐	• Without external support or unloading	☐
		• Relaxed natural breathing (*even if not ideal – so long as natural pattern does not change*)	☐
• Control during eccentric phase	☐	• No fatigue	☐
• Control during concentric phase	☐		

CORRECT DISSOCIATION PATTERN   **RECRUITMENT EFFICIENCY**

T54.2 Diagnosis of the site and direction of UCM from the One Arm Lift Test

ONE ARM LIFT TEST – 4 POINT KNEELING

Site	Direction	Thorax to the left (L)	Thorax to the right (R)
		(check box)	(check box)
Thoracic	Rotation	☐	☐

T54.3 Feedback tools to monitor retraining

FEEDBACK TOOL	PROCESS
Self-palpation	Palpation monitoring of joint position
Visual observation	Observe in a mirror or directly watch the movement
Adhesive tape	Skin tension for tactile feedback
Cueing and verbal correction	Listen to feedback from another observer

T55 SIDE-LYING: LATERAL ARM LIFT TEST (tests for thoracic rotation UCM)

This dissociation test assesses the ability to actively dissociate and control thoracic rotation and lift one arm laterally backwards (unilateral horizontal abduction in the axial plane) while side-lying. During any unilateral or asymmetrical upper limb movement, a rotational force is transmitted to the thorax.

Test procedure

The person lies on one side with the hips and knees flexed and the spine in neutral alignment. The pelvis, thorax and head should be positioned in neutral rotation (all facing forwards). The uppermost (top) arm should be held horizontal to the floor in 90° of flexion (Figure 7.51). The person is instructed to maintain the neutral thoracic position and lift the uppermost arm backwards (towards the ceiling in the axial plane). This movement is often referred to as 'horizontal abduction' when performed in standing.

Ideally, the person should have the ability to dissociate the thoracic spine from unilateral shoulder 'horizontal' abduction, as evidenced by the ability to prevent thoracic rotation while independently lifting the arm backwards. The scapula should independently retract and the arm should be able to lift backwards to the vertical position (abduction in the axial plane) without any thoracic rotation following the arm movement (Figure 7.52). There should be no provocation of any symptoms under asymmetrical arm load, so long as the thoracic rotation UCM can be controlled.

This test should be performed without any extra feedback (self-palpation, vision, etc.) or cueing

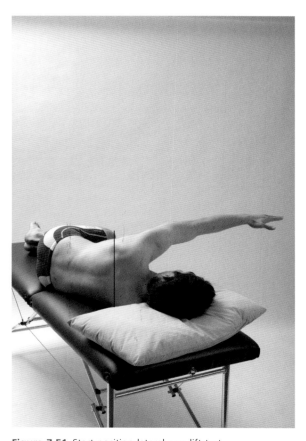

Figure 7.51 Start position lateral arm lift test

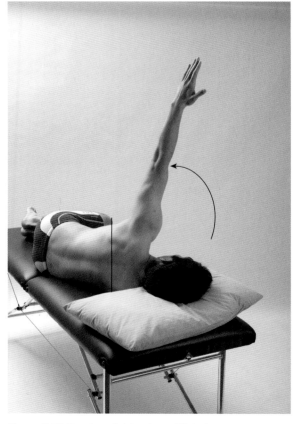

Figure 7.52 Benchmark lateral arm lift test

for correction. The therapist should use visual observation of the thorax relative to the shoulder to determine whether the control of thoracic rotation is adequate when feedback is removed for testing. Assess the lateral arm lift to each side separately. Performance to right and left sides should be symmetrical.

Thoracic rotation UCM

The person complains of rotation-related symptoms in the thoracic spine. The thorax has UCM into rotation relative to asymmetrical arm loading. The thoracic spine starts to rotate before the arm lifts backwards in the axial plane (abduction to the vertical position). During the attempt to dissociate the thoracic rotation from independent unilateral arm abduction, the person either cannot control the UCM or has to concentrate and try hard to control the thoracic rotation.

Clinical assessment note for direction-specific motor control testing

If some other movement (e.g. a small amount of thoracic flexion) is observed during a motor control (dissociation) test of thoracic rotation, *do not* score this as uncontrolled thoracic rotation. The thoracic flexion motor control tests will identify if the observed unrelated movement is uncontrolled. *A test for thoracic rotation UCM is only positive if uncontrolled thoracic* **rotation** *is demonstrated.*

Rating and diagnosis of thoracic rotation UCM

(T55.1 and T55.2)

Correction

Retraining is best started by supporting the thoracic spine against a wall for increased thoracic support and feedback and lifting the arm through reduced range. The person lies on one side on the floor, with the hips and knees flexed and the spine in neutral alignment and the back supported flat against a wall. The pelvis, thorax and head should be positioned in neutral rotation (all facing forwards). The uppermost (top) arm should be held horizontal to the floor in 90° of flexion.

Using the wall for support and feedback, the person is instructed to maintain the neutral thoracic position and lift the uppermost arm backwards (towards the ceiling in the axial plane). They are to lift the arm only as far as there is no thoracic rotation. The person is trained to control and prevent thoracic rotation and perform independent lateral arm lift.

The person should self-monitor the control of thoracic rotation UCM with a variety of feedback options (T55.3). There should be no provocation of any symptoms within the range that the rotation UCM can be controlled.

Once control of thoracic rotation improves, the exercise can be performed with the thoracic spine unsupported (no wall support).

T55.1 Assessment and rating of low threshold recruitment efficiency of the Lateral Arm Lift Test

LATERAL ARM LIFT – SIDE-LYING

ASSESSMENT

Control point:
- prevent thoracic rotation

Movement challenge: unilateral arm 'horizontal' abduction in the axial plane (scapular retraction) (side-lying)

Benchmark range: independent scapular retraction and shoulder abduction in the axial plane to vertical alignment without thoracic compensation

RATING OF LOW THRESHOLD RECRUITMENT EFFICIENCY FOR CONTROL OF DIRECTION

	✓ or ✗		✓ or ✗
• Able to prevent UCM into the test direction Correct dissociation pattern of movement Prevent thoracic UCM into: • rotation and move unilateral scapular retraction and arm abduction in the axial plane	☐	• Looks easy, and in the opinion of the assessor, is performed with confidence	☐
		• Feels easy, and the subject has sufficient awareness of the movement pattern that they confidently prevent UCM into the test direction	☐
• Dissociate movement through the benchmark range of independent 'horizontal' abduction – backwards to the arm vertical position *If there is more available range than the benchmark standard, only the benchmark range needs to be actively controlled*	☐	• The pattern of dissociation is smooth during concentric and eccentric movement	☐
		• Does not (consistently) use *end-range* movement into the opposite direction to prevent the UCM	☐
		• No extra feedback needed (*tactile, visual or verbal cueing*)	☐
• Without holding breath (though it is acceptable to use an alternate breathing strategy)	☐	• Without external support or unloading	☐
		• Relaxed natural breathing (*even if not ideal – so long as natural pattern does not change*)	☐
• Control during eccentric phase	☐	• No fatigue	☐
• Control during concentric phase	☐		

CORRECT DISSOCIATION PATTERN   **RECRUITMENT EFFICIENCY**

T55.2 Diagnosis of the site and direction of UCM from the Lateral Arm Lift Test

LATERAL ARM LIFT TEST – SIDE-LYING

Site	Direction	Thorax to the left (L)	Thorax to the right (R)
		(check box)	(check box)
Thoracic	Rotation	☐	☐

T55.3 Feedback tools to monitor retraining

FEEDBACK TOOL	PROCESS
Self-palpation	Palpation monitoring of joint position
Visual observation	Observe in a mirror or directly watch the movement
Adhesive tape	Skin tension for tactile feedback
Cueing and verbal correction	Listen to feedback from another observer

T56 SIDE-LYING: SIDE BRIDGE TEST (tests for thoracic rotation UCM)

This dissociation test assesses the ability to actively dissociate and control thoracic rotation and weight bear laterally on one arm in a 'side bridge' or 'side plank' position (unilateral abduction) while side-lying. During any unilateral or asymmetrical upper limb movement, a rotational force is transmitted to the thorax.

Test procedure

The person lies on one side with the spine in neutral alignment and the legs straight (in line with the trunk). The pelvis, thorax and head should be positioned in neutral rotation (all facing forwards). Body weight is supported on the lowermost (underneath) elbow with that elbow positioned under the shoulder and the forearm facing forwards. The uppermost (top) hand rests on the lateral pelvis (Figure 7.53). The person is instructed to maintain the neutral thoracic position and lift the pelvis and hips (away from the floor) so that the head, spine and legs are all in the same line. Body weight is supported between the feet and the weight bearing elbow. The weight bearing shoulder should be at 90° of abduction. This movement is often referred to as a 'side bridge' or a 'side plank'.

Ideally, the person should have the ability to dissociate the thoracic spine from weight bearing unilateral shoulder abduction as evidenced by the ability to support body weight and prevent thoracic rotation (and scapular winging) while independently lifting the pelvis into a 'side bridge'

(Figure 7.54). There should be no provocation of any symptoms under unilateral shoulder abduction in weight bearing, so long as the thoracic rotation UCM can be controlled.

This test should be performed without any extra feedback (self-palpation, vision, etc.) or cueing for correction. When feedback is removed for testing the therapist should use visual observation of the thorax relative to the shoulder to determine whether the control of thoracic rotation is adequate. Assess the side bridge to each side separately. Performance to right and left sides should be symmetrical.

Thoracic rotation UCM

The person complains of rotation-related symptoms in the thoracic spine. The thorax has UCM into rotation relative to unilateral weight bearing shoulder abduction. The thoracic spine starts to rotate before body weight is supported at 90° shoulder abduction in the side plank position. During the attempt to dissociate the thoracic rotation from independent unilateral weight bearing abduction, the person either cannot control the UCM or has to concentrate and try hard to control the thoracic rotation.

Clinical assessment note for direction-specific motor control testing

If some other movement (e.g. a small amount of thoracic flexion) is observed during a motor control (dissociation) test of thoracic rotation, *do not* score this as uncontrolled thoracic rotation. The thoracic flexion motor control tests will identify if the observed unrelated movement is uncontrolled. *A test for thoracic rotation UCM is only positive if uncontrolled thoracic **rotation** is demonstrated.*

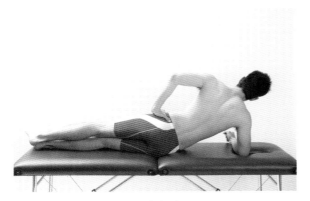

Figure 7.53 Start position side bridge test

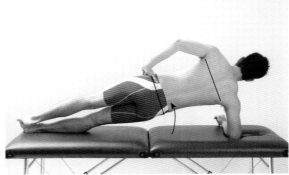

Figure 7.54 Benchmark side bridge test

Rating and diagnosis of thoracic rotation UCM

(T56.1 and T56.2)

Correction

Retraining is best started using reduced body load by bending the knees and performing the side bridge between the knees and the weight bearing elbow (instead of feet and elbow). The person lies on one side with the spine in neutral alignment and the hips straight (in line with the trunk) but with the knees bent to 90° of flexion. The pelvis, thorax and head should be positioned in neutral rotation (all facing forwards). Body weight is supported on the lowermost (underneath) elbow with that elbow positioned under the shoulder and the forearm facing forwards.

Using reduced body load, the person is instructed to maintain the neutral thoracic position and lift the pelvis and hips (away from the floor) so that the head, spine and thighs are all in the same line. Body weight is supported between the knees and the weight bearing elbow (Figure 7.55). They are to lift the pelvis only as far as there is no thoracic rotation. The person is trained to control and prevent thoracic rotation and perform independent side bridge of the knees.

The person should self-monitor the control of thoracic rotation UCM with a variety of feedback options (T56.3). There should be no provocation of any symptoms within the range that the rotation UCM can be controlled.

If control is very poor, the uppermost (top) hand can be used for support and balance by contact with the floor. Once control of thoracic rotation improves, the exercise can be performed with full body load (long lever side-bridge off the feet).

Thoracic rotation UCM summary

(Table 7.5)

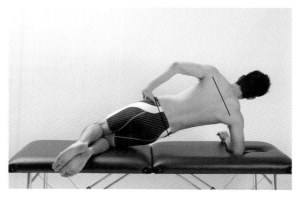

Figure 7.55 Correction reduced load side bridge off knees

Table 7.5 Summary and rating of thoracic rotation tests

UCM DIAGNOSIS AND TESTING		
SITE: THORACIC	DIRECTION: ROTATION	CLINICAL PRIORITY ☐
TEST	RATING (✓✓ or ✓✗ or ✗✗) and rationale Thorax to (L)	Thorax to (R)
Sitting: head turn		
Sitting: pelvic twist (swivel chair)		
Standing: pelvic side-shift		
Standing: one arm wall push		
4 point: one arm lift		
Side-lying: lateral arm lift		
Side-lying: side bridge		

T56.1 Assessment and rating of low threshold recruitment efficiency of the Side Bridge Test

SIDE BRIDGE – SIDE-LYING

ASSESSMENT

Control point:
• prevent thoracic rotation

Movement challenge: unilateral arm 'horizontal' abduction in the axial plane (scapular retraction) (side-lying)

Benchmark range: independent scapular retraction and shoulder abduction in the axial plane to vertical alignment without thoracic compensation

RATING OF LOW THRESHOLD RECRUITMENT EFFICIENCY FOR CONTROL OF DIRECTION

	✓ or ✗		✓ or ✗
• Able to prevent UCM into the test direction Correct dissociation pattern of movement Prevent thoracic UCM into: • rotation and move unilateral arm weight bearing in shoulder abduction	☐	• Looks easy, and in the opinion of the assessor, is performed with confidence	☐
		• Feels easy, and the subject has sufficient awareness of the movement pattern that they confidently prevent UCM into the test direction	☐
• Dissociate movement through the benchmark range of 90° independent shoulder abduction in side bridge (weight bearing: body weight supported at feet and one elbow) *If there is more available range than the benchmark standard, only the benchmark range needs to be actively controlled*	☐	• The pattern of dissociation is smooth during concentric and eccentric movement	☐
		• Does not (consistently) use *end-range* movement into the opposite direction to prevent the UCM	☐
		• No extra feedback needed (*tactile, visual or verbal cueing*)	☐
		• Without external support or unloading	☐
• Without holding breath (though it is acceptable to use an alternate breathing strategy)	☐	• Relaxed natural breathing (*even if not ideal – so long as natural pattern does not change*)	☐
• Control during eccentric phase	☐	• No fatigue	☐
• Control during concentric phase	☐		

CORRECT DISSOCIATION PATTERN   **RECRUITMENT EFFICIENCY**

T56.2 Diagnosis of the site and direction of UCM from the Side Bridge Test

SIDE BRIDGE TEST – SIDE-LYING

Site	Direction	Thorax to the left (L)	Thorax to the right (R)
		(check box)	(check box)
Thoracic	Rotation	☐	☐

T56.3 Feedback tools to monitor retraining

FEEDBACK TOOL	PROCESS
Self-palpation	Palpation monitoring of joint position
Visual observation	Observe in a mirror or directly watch the movement
Adhesive tape	Skin tension for tactile feedback
Cueing and verbal correction	Listen to feedback from another observer

Thoracic and rib respiratory control

THORACIC AND RIB RESPIRATORY CONTROL TESTS AND RESPIRATORY CONTROL REHABILITATION

These respiratory control tests assess the extent of respiratory UCM in the thoracic spine and ribcage and assess the ability of the dynamic stability system to adequately control respiratory load or strain. It is a priority to assess for respiratory UCM if the person complains of or demonstrates respiratory or ribcage-related symptoms or disability. The tests that identify dysfunction can also be used to guide and direct rehabilitation strategies.

Indications to test for thoracic respiratory UCM

Observe or palpate for:

1. hypermobile rib movement
2. excessive initiation or dominant ribcage elevation or depression associated with either costal, apical or abdominal movement
3. symptoms (pain, discomfort, strain) associated with inspiration or expiration or rib pain associated with thoracic or ribcage movement.

The person complains of respiratory or rib-related symptoms in the thorax. Under respiratory load, the thoracic spine and ribcage has greater give *into ribcage elevation or depression* relative to inspiration or expiration. The dysfunction is confirmed with motor control tests of respiratory dissociation.

Tests of thoracic and ribcage respiratory control

T57 STANDING: APICAL DROP + INSPIRATION TEST
(tests for thoracic respiratory UCM)

This dissociation test assesses the ability to actively dissociate and control apical ribcage elevation then breathe in while standing upright and unsupported.

Test procedure

The person stands upright with the spine in its neutral normal curves; the head directly over the shoulders and the arms resting by the side with the shoulders in a neutral position. The person

takes a relaxed breath in and then is asked to fully exhale (breathe out) to ensure that the apical ribcage has been fully depressed (Figure 7.56). They are then to hold this position as the start position for the test. Then, keeping the apical ribcage held down in depression, the person is instructed to slowly start to breathe in (slow inspiration). During normal inspiration the ribcage naturally elevates. However, excessive elevation of the apical ribcage is often associated with upper thoracic, upper rib, arm pain and neck pain. The ability to control this excessive apical ribcage elevation may be useful in managing these symptoms.

Ideally, the person should have the ability to dissociate the apical ribcage elevation from inspiration as evidenced by the ability to prevent apical elevation (from a fully depressed position) while independently breathing in to about ½ normal inspiratory volume (Figure 7.57). There must be

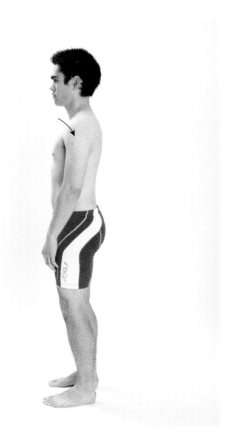

Figure 7.56 Start position apical drop + inspiration test

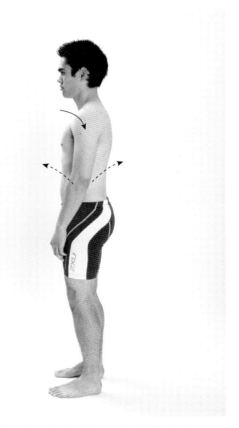

Figure 7.57 Benchmark apical drop + inspiration test

no movement into apical ribcage elevation. There is usually an observed increase in costal or posterolateral basal ribcage expansion associated with correct performance of this test. There should be no provocation of any symptoms under inspiratory effort, so long as the apical elevation UCM can be controlled.

This test should be performed without any extra feedback (self-palpation, vision, etc.) or cueing for correction. When feedback is removed for testing the therapist should use visual observation of the thorax relative to the respiratory movement to determine whether the control of thoracic respiration is adequate.

Thoracic respiratory (apical ribcage elevation) UCM

The person complains of respiratory or ribcage-related symptoms in the thorax. The apical ribcage has UCM into elevation relative to inspiratory movement. The apical ribcage starts to elevate before adequate respiratory inspiration is achieved. During the attempt to dissociate the apical ribcage elevation from independent inspiration, the person either cannot control the UCM or has to concentrate and try hard to control the apical ribcage.

Clinical assessment note for direction-specific motor control testing

If some other movement (e.g. a small amount of thoracic rotation) is observed during a motor control (dissociation) test of thoracic respiration, *do not* score this as uncontrolled thoracic respiration. The thoracic rotation motor control tests will identify if the observed unrelated movement is uncontrolled. *A test for thoracic respiration UCM is only positive if uncontrolled thoracic **respiration** is demonstrated.*

Rating and diagnosis of thoracic respiratory UCM

(T57.1 and T57.2)

Correction

Retraining is best started using a reduced amount of inspiration and self-palpation of the upper ribcage for feedback. The person stands upright with the spine in its neutral normal curves, and palpates the upper ribcage. They take a relaxed breath in and then fully exhale (breathe out) to ensure that the apical ribcage has fully depressed. Then, keeping the apical ribcage held down in depression, the person is instructed to slowly start to breathe in (slow inspiration). They are to breathe in only as far as there is no apical ribcage elevation. The person is trained to control and prevent apical elevation and perform independent inspiration.

The person should self-monitor the control of thoracic respiration UCM with a variety of feedback options (T57.3). There should be no provocation of any symptoms within the range that the apical ribcage elevation UCM can be controlled.

Once control of apical ribcage elevation improves, the exercise can be performed with greater volume of inspiration.

T57.1 Assessment and rating of low threshold recruitment efficiency of the Apical Drop + Inspiration Test

APICAL DROP + INSPIRATION – STANDING

ASSESSMENT

Control point:
• prevent apical ribcage elevation
Movement challenge: inspiration (breathe in) (standing)
Benchmark range: full independent apical ribcage depression + ½ inspiration without apical elevation

RATING OF LOW THRESHOLD RECRUITMENT EFFICIENCY FOR CONTROL OF DIRECTION

	✓ or ✗		✓ or ✗
• Able to prevent UCM into the test direction Correct dissociation pattern of movement	☐	• Looks easy, and in the opinion of the assessor, is performed with confidence	☐
Prevent thoracic (apical ribcage) UCM into:		• Feels easy, and the subject has sufficient awareness of the movement pattern that they confidently prevent UCM into the test direction	☐
• elevation and move inspiration (breathe in)			
• Dissociate movement through the benchmark range of full independent apical ribcage depression + ½ inspiration	☐	• The pattern of dissociation is smooth during concentric and eccentric movement	☐
If there is more available range than the benchmark standard, only the benchmark range needs to be actively controlled		• Does not (consistently) use *end-range* movement into the opposite direction to prevent the UCM	☐
• Without holding breath (though it is acceptable to use an alternate breathing strategy)	☐	• No extra feedback needed (*tactile, visual or verbal cueing*)	☐
		• Without external support or unloading	☐
• Control during eccentric phase	☐	• Relaxed natural breathing (*even if not ideal – so long as natural pattern does not change*)	☐
• Control during concentric phase	☐	• No fatigue	☐

CORRECT DISSOCIATION PATTERN   **RECRUITMENT EFFICIENCY**

T57.2 Diagnosis of the site and direction of UCM from the Apical Drop + Inspiration Test

APICAL DROP + INSPIRATION TEST – STANDING

Site	Direction	✗✗ or ✗✓
		(check box)
Apical ribcage (Thoracic)	Depression (Respiration)	☐

T57.3 Feedback tools to monitor retraining

FEEDBACK TOOL	PROCESS
Self-palpation	Palpation monitoring of joint position
Visual observation	Observe in a mirror or directly watch the movement
Adhesive tape	Skin tension for tactile feedback
Cueing and verbal correction	Listen to feedback from another observer

T58 STANDING: ANTERIOR COSTAL LIFT + EXPIRATION TEST (tests for thoracic respiratory UCM)

This dissociation test assesses the ability to actively dissociate and control anterior costal ribcage and sternal depression then breathe out while standing upright and unsupported.

Test procedure

The person stands upright with the spine in its neutral normal curves and the head directly over the shoulders. The person is asked to have a relaxed breath out and then fully inhale (breathe in) to ensure that the anterior costal ribcage and sternum has fully elevated (Figure 7.58). They are to hold this position as the start position for the test. Then, keeping the anterior costal ribcage and sternum held up in elevation, the person is instructed to slowly start to breathe out (slow expiration). During normal expiration the ribcage naturally depresses. However, excessive depression of the anterior costal ribcage is often observed associated with lower thoracic, lumbar and pelvic pain. The ability to control this excessive anterior costal ribcage depression may be useful in managing these symptoms.

Ideally, the person should have the ability to dissociate the anterior costal ribcage depression from expiration as evidenced by the ability to prevent anterior costal depression (from a fully elevated position) while independently breathing out to about $\frac{1}{2}$ normal expiratory volume (Figure 7.59). There must be no movement into anterior costal ribcage depression. There should be no

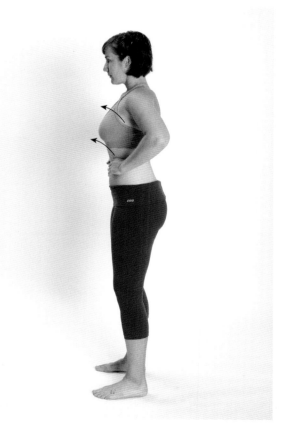

Figure 7.58 Start position anterior costal lift + expiration test

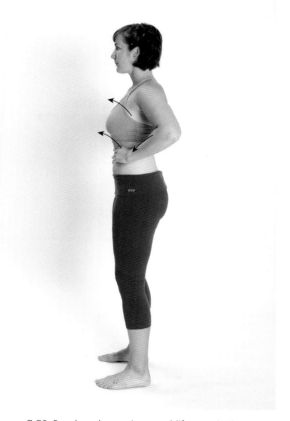

Figure 7.59 Benchmark anterior costal lift + expiration test

provocation of any symptoms under expiratory effort, so long as the anterior costal depression UCM can be controlled.

This test should be performed without any extra feedback (self-palpation, vision, etc.) or cueing for correction. When feedback is removed for testing the therapist should use visual observation of the thorax relative to the respiratory movement to determine whether the control of thoracic respiration is adequate.

Thoracic respiratory (costal ribcage depression) UCM

The person complains of respiratory or ribcage-related symptoms in the thorax. The anterior costal ribcage has UCM into depression relative to expiratory movement. The ribcage or thorax starts to depress before adequate respiratory expiration is achieved. During the attempt to dissociate the anterior costal ribcage depression from independent expiration, the person either cannot control the UCM or has to concentrate and try hard to control the anterior costal ribcage.

Clinical assessment note for direction-specific motor control testing

If some other movement (e.g. a small amount of thoracic rotation) is observed during a motor control (dissociation) test of thoracic respiration, *do not* score this as uncontrolled thoracic respiration. The thoracic rotation motor control tests will identify if the observed unrelated movement is uncontrolled. *A test for thoracic respiration UCM is only positive if uncontrolled thoracic **respiration** is demonstrated.*

Rating and diagnosis of thoracic respiratory UCM

(T58.1 and T58.2)

Correction

Retraining is best started using a reduced amount of expiration combined with self-palpation of the lower anterior costal ribcage for feedback. The person stands upright with the spine in its neutral normal curves, and palpates the anterior costal ribcage. They fully inhale (breathe in) and ensure that the anterior costal ribcage has fully elevated. Then, keeping the anterior costal ribcage held up in elevation, the person is instructed to slowly start to breathe out (slow expiration). They are to breathe out only as far as there is no anterior costal ribcage depression. The person is trained to control and prevent anterior costal depression and perform independent expiration.

The person should self-monitor the control of thoracic respiration UCM with a variety of feedback options (T58.3). There should be no provocation of any symptoms within the range that the anterior costal ribcage depression UCM can be controlled.

Once control of anterior costal ribcage depression improves, the exercise can be performed with greater volume of expiration.

T58.1 Assessment and rating of low threshold recruitment efficiency of the Anterior Costal Lift + Expiration Test

ANTERIOR COSTAL LIFT + EXPIRATION – STANDING

ASSESSMENT

Control point:
- prevent anterior costal ribcage depression

Movement challenge: expiration (breathe out) (standing)

Benchmark range: full independent costal ribcage and sternal elevation + $\frac{1}{2}$ expiration without anterior costal depression

RATING OF LOW THRESHOLD RECRUITMENT EFFICIENCY FOR CONTROL OF DIRECTION

	✓ or ✗		✓ or ✗
• Able to prevent UCM into the test direction Correct dissociation pattern of movement Prevent thoracic (anterior costal ribcage) UCM into: • depression and move expiration (breathe out)	☐	• Looks easy, and in the opinion of the assessor, is performed with confidence	☐
		• Feels easy, and the subject has sufficient awareness of the movement pattern that they confidently prevent UCM into the test direction	☐
• Dissociate movement through the benchmark range of full independent anterior costal ribcage elevation + $\frac{1}{2}$ expiration *If there is more available range than the benchmark standard, only the benchmark range needs to be actively controlled*	☐	• The pattern of dissociation is smooth during concentric and eccentric movement	☐
		• Does not (consistently) use *end-range* movement into the opposite direction to prevent the UCM	☐
• Without holding breath (though it is acceptable to use an alternate breathing strategy)	☐	• No extra feedback needed (*tactile, visual or verbal cueing*)	☐
		• Without external support or unloading	☐
• Control during eccentric phase	☐	• Relaxed natural breathing (*even if not ideal – so long as natural pattern does not change*)	☐
• Control during concentric phase	☐	• No fatigue	☐

CORRECT DISSOCIATION PATTERN **RECRUITMENT EFFICIENCY**

T58.2 Diagnosis of the site and direction of UCM from the Anterior Costal Lift + Expiration Test

ANTERIOR COSTAL LIFT + EXPIRATION TEST – STANDING

Site	Direction	✗✗ or ✗✓
		(check box)
Anterior costal ribcage (Thoracic)	Elevation (Respiration)	☐

T58.3 Feedback tools to monitor retraining

FEEDBACK TOOL	PROCESS
Self-palpation	Palpation monitoring of joint position
Visual observation	Observe in a mirror or directly watch the movement
Adhesive tape	Skin tension for tactile feedback
Cueing and verbal correction	Listen to feedback from another observer

T59 STANDING: ABDOMINAL HOLLOWING + EXPIRATION TEST (tests for thoracic respiratory UCM)

This dissociation test assesses the ability to actively dissociate and control abdominal bracing (bulge) and lateral basal ribcage depression then breathe out while standing upright and unsupported.

Test procedure

The person stands upright with the spine in its neutral normal curves and the head directly over the shoulders. The person has a relaxed breath out. They are then instructed to inhale (breathe in) and ensure that the lateral basal ribcage has fully elevated. At the same time as inhaling, they are to 'hollow' (pull in) the upper and lower abdominal wall (Figure 7.60). They are then to hold this position as the start position for the test. Keeping the abdominal wall hollowed (pulled in) and the lateral basal ribcage held up in elevation, the person is then instructed to slowly start to breathe out (slow expiration). They are to exhale without loss of the abdominal hollowing and no lateral basal ribcage depression.

During normal expiration the ribcage naturally depresses. However, excessive depression of the lateral basal ribcage and abdominal bracing is often observed associated with lower thoracic and back pain. The ability to control this excessive lateral basal ribcage depression and abdominal bracing (bulge) may be useful in managing these symptoms. Ideally, the person should have the ability to dissociate the abdominal bracing and lateral basal ribcage depression from expiration as evidenced by the ability to prevent lateral basal depression (from a fully elevated position) while independently breathing out to about ½ normal expiratory volume (Figure 7.61).

There must be no movement into abdominal bracing or lateral basal ribcage depression. There is usually an observed increase in apical ribcage depression associated with correct performance of this test. There should be no provocation of any symptoms under expiratory effort, so long as the lateral costal depression UCM can be controlled.

This test should be performed without any extra feedback (self-palpation, vision, etc.) or cueing for correction. When feedback is removed for

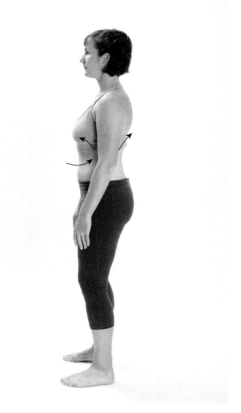

Figure 7.60 Start position abdominal hollowing + expiration test

testing the therapist should use visual observation of the abdominal wall and thorax relative to the respiratory movement to determine whether the control of thoracic respiration is adequate.

Thoracic respiratory (costal ribcage depression) UCM

The person complains of respiratory or ribcage-related symptoms in the thorax. The lateral basal ribcage has UCM into depression relative to expiratory movement. The lateral basal ribcage or thorax starts to depress and the abdominal wall bulges out into a bracing action before adequate respiratory expiration is achieved. During the attempt to dissociate the lateral basal ribcage depression from independent expiration, the person either cannot control the UCM or has to concentrate and try hard to control the abdominal bracing and lateral basal ribcage.

357

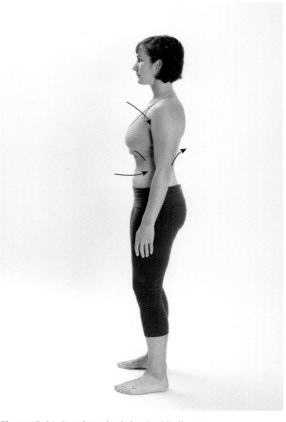

Figure 7.61 Benchmark abdominal hollowing + expiration test

Rating and diagnosis of thoracic respiratory UCM

(T59.1 and T59.2)

Correction

Retraining is best started using a reduced volume of expiration combined with self-palpation of the lower lateral basal ribcage for feedback. The person stands upright with the spine in its neutral normal curves, and palpates the lateral basal ribcage. They take a relaxed breath out and then fully inhale (breathe in) to ensure that the lateral basal ribcage has fully elevated and concurrently pull in (hollow) the abdominal wall. Then, keeping the abdominal hollowing and the lateral basal ribcage held up in elevation, the person is instructed to slowly start to breathe out (slow expiration). They are to breathe out only as far as there is no loss of the abdominal hollowing or no lateral basal ribcage depression. The person is trained to control and prevent lateral basal depression and perform independent expiration.

The person should self-monitor the control of thoracic respiration UCM with a variety of feedback options (T59.3). There should be no provocation of any symptoms within the range that the lateral basal ribcage depression UCM can be controlled.

Once control of lateral basal ribcage depression improves, the exercise can be performed with greater volume of expiration.

Clinical assessment note for direction-specific motor control testing

If some other movement (e.g. a small amount of thoracic rotation) is observed during a motor control (dissociation) test of thoracic respiration, *do not* score this as uncontrolled thoracic respiration. The thoracic rotation motor control tests will identify if the observed unrelated movement is uncontrolled. *A test for thoracic respiration UCM is only positive if uncontrolled thoracic **respiration** is demonstrated.*

T59.1 Assessment and rating of low threshold recruitment efficiency of the Abdominal Hollowing + Expiration Test

ABDOMINAL HOLLOWING + EXPIRATION – STANDING

ASSESSMENT

Control point:
- prevent abdominal bracing and lateral basal ribcage depression

Movement challenge: expiration (breathe out) (standing)

Benchmark range: independent abdominal hollowing and lateral basal ribcage elevation + ½ expiration without abdominal bulge or lateral basal depression

RATING OF LOW THRESHOLD RECRUITMENT EFFICIENCY FOR CONTROL OF DIRECTION

	✓ or ✗		✓ or ✗
• Able to prevent UCM into the test direction Correct dissociation pattern of movement Prevent thoracic (lateral basal ribcage) UCM into: • depression • abdominal bracing and move expiration (breathe out)	☐	• Looks easy, and in the opinion of the assessor, is performed with confidence	☐
		• Feels easy, and the subject has sufficient awareness of the movement pattern that they confidently prevent UCM into the test direction	☐
• Dissociate movement through the benchmark range of independent abdominal hollowing and basal ribcage elevation + ½ expiration *If there is more available range than the benchmark standard, only the benchmark range needs to be actively controlled*	☐	• The pattern of dissociation is smooth during concentric and eccentric movement	☐
		• Does not (consistently) use *end-range* movement into the opposite direction to prevent the UCM	☐
		• No extra feedback needed *(tactile, visual or verbal cueing)*	☐
• Without holding breath (though it is acceptable to use an alternate breathing strategy)	☐	• Without external support or unloading	☐
		• Relaxed natural breathing *(even if not ideal – so long as natural pattern does not change)*	☐
• Control during eccentric phase	☐	• No fatigue	☐
• Control during concentric phase	☐		
CORRECT DISSOCIATION PATTERN		**RECRUITMENT EFFICIENCY**	

T59.2 Diagnosis of the site and direction of UCM from the Abdominal Hollowing + Expiration Test

ABDOMINAL HOLLOWING + EXPIRATION TEST – STANDING

Site	Direction	✗✗ or ✗✓
		(check box)
Lateral basal ribcage (Thoracic)	Elevation (Respiration)	☐

T59.3 Feedback tools to monitor retraining

FEEDBACK TOOL	PROCESS
Self-palpation	Palpation monitoring of joint position
Visual observation	Observe in a mirror or directly watch the movement
Adhesive tape	Skin tension for tactile feedback
Cueing and verbal correction	Listen to feedback from another observer

Thoracic respiratory UCM summary

(Table 7.6)

Table 7.6 Summary and rating of thoracic respiratory tests		
UCM DIAGNOSIS AND TESTING		
SITE: **THORACIC/RIBS**	**DIRECTION:** **RESPIRATORY** ☐	**CLINICAL PRIORITY**
TEST	**RATING** (✓✓ or ✓✗ or ✗✗) and rationale	
Standing: apical drop + inspiration (prevent apical ribcage elevation)		
Standing: anterior costal lift + expiration (prevent anterior costal ribcage depression)		
Standing: abdominal hollowing + expiration (prevent lateral basal ribcage depression)		

REFERENCES

Carrière, B., 1996. Therapeutic exercise and self correction. In: Flynn, T.W. (Ed.), The thoracic spine and rib cage: musculoskeletal evaluation and treatment. Butterworth-Heinemann, Boston.

Edmondston, S.J., Singer, K.P., 1997. Thoracic spine: anatomical and biomechanical considerations for manual therapy. Manual Therapy 2 (3), 132–143.

Lee, D., 2003. The thorax: an integrated approach. In: Diane, G. (Ed.), Lee Physiotherapist Corporation. Surrey, Canada.

Lee, D.G., 1996. Rotational stability of the mid-thoracic spine: assessment and management. Manual Therapy 1 (5), 234–241.

Lee, L.J., Coppieters, M.W., Hodges, P.W., 2005. Differential activation of the thoracic multifidus and longissimus thoracic during trunk rotation. Spine 30 (8), 870–876.

Maitland, G., Hengeveld, E., Banks, K., English, K., 2005. Maitland's vertebral manipulation. Butterworth Heinemann, Oxford.

Watkins 4th, R., Watkins 3rd, R., Williams, L., Ahlbrand, S., Garcia, R., Karamanian, A., et al., 2005. Stability provided by the sternum and ribcage in the thoracic spine. Spine 30 (11), 1283–1286.

CHAPTER 8
THE SHOULDER GIRDLE

Chapter | **8** |

The shoulder girdle

The complexity of shoulder girdle dysfunction makes diagnosis difficult, with definitions for common diagnoses, such as impingement and frozen shoulder, being unclear, inconsistent and unreliable (Schellingerhout et al 2008). An epidemiological study examining 1960 people successfully identified current and past shoulder problems, but was unable to discriminate between discrete shoulder pathologies (Walker-Bone et al 2004). Therapy for shoulder girdle pain and disability is predominantly concerned with restoration of optimal movement and function rather than applying diagnostic labels, with traditional approaches to clinical diagnosis at the shoulder girdle frequently neglecting to assess dynamic movement faults, a significant factor associated with shoulder dysfunction (Lukasiewicz et al 1999; Ludewig & Cook 2000; Lin et al 2006; Tate et al 2008). Classification of movement control faults at the shoulder girdle is gaining recognition, with Kibler & McMullen (2003) describing a clinical classification of scapular dyskinesis (scapular movement control faults). A classification of dysfunction in terms of site and direction of uncontrolled movement (UCM) has been proposed (Mottram 2003; Mottram et al 2009a; Comerford & Mottram 2011), and diagnosis based on movement impairment (Sahrmann 2002; Caldwell et al 2007) encouraged. The consensus statement at a recent scapular summit (Kibler et al 2009) agreed that the observation of scapular dyskinesis and clinical tests that alter symptoms (UCM in this text) should form the basis for the scapular evaluation.

This chapter sets out to explore the assessment and retraining of UCM in the shoulder. Before details of the assessment and retraining of UCM in the shoulder region are explained, a brief review of function, changes in muscle function and movement and postural control in the region is presented.

Scapula function and glenohumeral joint stability

The ability to control the orientation and movement of the scapula is essential for optimal arm function. The bony, capsular and ligamentous restraints are minimal at the scapulothoracic 'joint' so stability is dependent on active muscular control. Movement faults and changes in muscle function of the scapula are associated with shoulder symptoms (Lukasiewicz et al 1999; Ludewig & Cook 2000; Lin et al 2006; Roy et al 2008; Tate et al 2008).

The glenohumeral joint has the greatest range of motion of any human joint. This mobility is necessary for upper limb functions, which range from weight bearing to high-speed acceleration and deceleration at the extremes of its range. Stability is sacrificed to a significant degree to achieve this mobility function. The scapula provides the base for attachment of muscles that move the glenohumeral joint. The scapula should be orientated to optimise the length–tension relationship of these muscles (van der Helm 1994) and provides the proximal articular surface of the glenohumeral joint (glenoid) and orientates the glenoid, to increase the range available to the upper limb. The scapula facilitates optimal contact with the humeral head – increasing joint congruency and stability (Saha 1971). Abnormal scapular kinematics have been identified in people with multidirectional instability (Ogston & Ludewig 2007). Full upward rotation of the glenoid enhances mechanical stability of the joint by bringing the glenoid fossa directly under the head of the humerus (Lucas 1973) and prevents impingement under the subacromial and coracoacromial arch. Glenohumeral function is influenced to a large extent by the position and orientation of the glenoid and hence scapula stability; however, the glenohumeral joint exhibits a number of mechanisms to retain joint congruency during functional movement which include passive stability mechanisms and active stability mechanisms. Passive stability mechanisms include the capsular and ligamentous restraints, labrum and mechanisms such as the creation on negative intra-articular pressure to resist translation.

Changes in shoulder muscle function

Muscle stiffness is required at the scapula-thoracic and glenohumeral to enhance stability. It has been shown that moderate levels of muscle contraction can significantly increase glenohumeral joint stiffness and stability (Huxel et al 2008). A non-specific pre-setting action of the rotator cuff and biceps is seen prior to rotation of the shoulder joint, and this recruitment is aimed mainly at enhancing the joint 'stiffness' and hence its stability (David et al 2000). A similar action is seen in upper trapezius (Wadsworth & Bullock-Saxton 1997), suggesting it has a pre-setting role at the scapula. Evidence suggests that muscle function around the shoulder girdle can be impaired by

pain and pathology. Altered timing (latency) of electromyographic (EMG) activity has been identified in muscles of the scapula (Wadsworth & Bullock-Saxton 1997; Cools et al 2003; Lin et al 2005; Falla et al 2007; Moraes et al 2008) and the glenohumeral joint (Hess et al 2005). Interestingly, muscle function (or dysfunction) has been associated with movement faults; for example, decreased serratus anterior activity has been associated with an increase in forward tilt of the scapula (Ludewig & Cook 2000; Lin et al 2005). This literature supports the need for specific assessment of movement faults so individual rehabilitation strategies can be implemented. Further research is needed to explore the relationship between movement abnormalities and symptoms and muscle function.

Identifying UCM at the shoulder girdle

Motion analysis studies have identified abnormal movements of the scapula which include scapula internal rotation (Ludewig & Cook 2000; Nawoczenski et al 2003; Tsai et al 2003; Borstad & Ludewig 2005; Borstad 2006); scapular downward rotation (Ludewig & Cook 2000; Tsai et al 2003; Lin et al 2006); scapula anterior tilt (Lukasiewicz et al 1999; Ludewig & Cook 2000; Nawoczenski et al 2003; Borstad & Ludewig 2005; Lin et al 2005; Morrissey 2005); and elevation (Lukasiewicz et al 1999; Tsai et al 2003; Lin et al 2005). UCM of the glenohumeral joint has been identified and includes translation (Baeyens et al 2001; Ruediger et al 2002; von Eisenhart-Rothe et al 2002, Ludewig and Cook 2002) and external rotation (Baeyens et al 2001).

In the current literature it is clear that alterations in dynamic control of the glenohumeral and scapula-thoracic joints are important factors in shoulder pathology (Ludewig and Cook 2000; Morrissey 2005; Alexander 2007; Ogston & Ludewig 2007). Although these studies demonstrated clear differences in movement patterns for symptomatic shoulders, they do not describe test manoeuvres that could be used specifically to detect the abnormalities in the clinical environment, therefore neglecting a significant component of assessment. This chapter details the assessment of UCM at the shoulder region and describes retraining strategies.

Table 8.1 Site and direction of UCM at the shoulder girdle

SITE	SCAPULA	GLENOHUMERAL
Direction	• Downward rotation • Forward tilt • Winging • Elevation • Retraction • Protraction	• Anterior translation • Inferior translation • Posterior translation • Medial rotation

DIAGNOSIS OF THE SITE AND DIRECTION OF UCM AT THE SHOULDER GIRDLE

The diagnosis of site and direction of UCM at the shoulder girdle can be observed at the scapula in terms of downward rotation, forward tilt, winging (internal rotation), elevation, retraction and protraction (abduction) and the glenohumeral joint in terms of anterior, inferior, posterior translation and medial rotation (Table 8.1).

Linking the site of UCM to symptom presentation

A diagnosis of UCM requires evaluation of its clinical priority. This is based on the relationship between the UCM and the presenting symptoms. The therapist should look for a link between the direction of UCM and the direction of symptom provocation: a) Does the site of UCM relate to the site or joint that the patient complains of as the source of symptoms? b) Does the direction of movement or load testing relate to the direction or position of provocation of symptoms? *This identifies the clinical priorities.*

The site and direction of UCM at the scapula and the glenohumeral joint can be linked to different clinical presentations and postures and activities that provoke or produce symptoms (Table 8.2).

In a shoulder with signs and symptoms of impingement and instability, control of movement needs to be effective to manage symptoms and dysfunction. These mechanisms are highlighted in Table 8.3 and the assessment of these

mechanisms is an important aspect of a comprehensive shoulder girdle assessment.

The site and direction of uncontrolled movement at the shoulder girdle can be linked to different clinical presentations of shoulder impingement syndrome and glenohumeral instability. Table 8.4 illustrates the clinical guidelines for impingement and instability.

IDENTIFYING SITE AND DIRECTION OF UCM AT THE SCAPULOTHORACIC AND GLENOHUMERAL JOINTS

The key principles for assessment and classification of UCM are described in Chapter 3. All dissociation tests are performed with the scapula and glenohumeral in the neutral training region. This can be passively positioned by the therapist prior to each test. The subject needs to clearly understand the test and appropriate facilitation strategies employed, including cognitive awareness, tactile, visual and technological feedback, and proprioceptive input.

Scapula and glenohumeral joint neutral training region

The natural resting position of the shoulder girdle is often displaced from an optimal training position. If there is poor antigravity postural control the scapula often rests in a downwardly rotated or forward tilted position. If there is a restriction (e.g. a stiffer pectoralis minor), the scapula will rest in relatively more forward tilt than is ideal. The therapist should passively position the shoulder girdle into its 'neutral training region' and then palpate reference landmarks to ensure optimal neutral alignment for testing and retraining movement control.

As a useful guide to repositioning the scapula in the *neutral training region,* the therapist stands to the side of the patient's shoulder and places the pisiform and ulnar border of one hand on the medial side of the patient's inferior scapular angle. The therapist then places the ulnar border of the other hand on the patient's coracoid with the hollow of the palm over the humeral head (Figure 8.1). With the fingers of both hands pointing to the ceiling, the therapist lifts both their elbows so that both forearms are in line. The therapist then gently 'squeezes' both hands

Table 8.2 The link between the site and direction of UCM at the shoulder and different clinical presentations

SITE AND DIRECTION OF UCM	CLINICAL EXAMPLES OF SYMPTOMS PRESENTATIONS	PROVOCATIVE MOVEMENTS, POSTURES AND ACTIVITIES
SCAPULA • Downward rotation • Forward tilt • Winging • Elevation • Retraction • Protraction Can present as: • uncontrolled movement of the scapular into any of these directions resulting in an increased inferior–anterior orientation of the glenoid (IAG) (± hypermobile range)	• Symptoms of subacromial or coracoacromial impingement; that is, pain at the point of the shoulder, in the region of the coracoid and anterior and lateral deltoid region • ± Referral from myofascial, articular and neural structures	Symptoms provoked by arm movements and postures into elevation above 60° (if especially sustained or loaded); for example, lifting, reaching forwards, reaching overhead, pushing or pulling with the arm above shoulder height, sustained static postures with the scapula dropped
GLENOHUMERAL Medial rotation Can present as: • uncontrolled range of the humerus into medial rotation (± hypermobile medial rotation range)	• Symptoms of coracoacromial impingement; that is, pain at the point of the shoulder, in the region of the coracoid and anterior and lateral deltoid region • ± Referral from myofascial, articular and neural structures	Symptoms provoked by arm movements and postures into forward elevation above 60° (if especially sustained or loaded); for example, lifting, reaching forwards, reaching overhead, pushing or pulling with the arm above shoulder height, sustained static postures with the scapula dropped
GLENOHUMERAL • Anterior translation • Inferior translation • Posterior translation Can present as • uncontrolled translation of the humeral head into any of the above directions (anterior is most common) (± hypermobile translation)	• Symptoms of glenohumeral instability; that is, pain in the anterior and posterior shoulder, at the point of the shoulder and deep axillary pain • ± Referral from myofascial, articular and neural structures	Symptoms provoked by arm movements and postures into end range positions (especially if end-range rotation is combined); for example, lifting, reaching forwards, reaching overhead, pushing or pulling with the arm above shoulder height, sustained static postures with the scapula dropped

Table 8.3 Normal mechanisms to minimise impingement and instability during arm elevation

IMPINGEMENT	INSTABILITY
• Upward rotation of glenoid • Glenohumeral lateral rotation timing • Inferior humeral head glide	• Passive capsular and ligamentous restraints • Dynamic (active) control of translation • Ideal length and recruitment of glenohumeral rotator muscles • A stable scapula to provide a biomechanically sound platform for glenohumeral movement

Table 8.4 Clinical guidelines for impingement and instability

IMPINGEMENT	INSTABILITY
<ul><li>Palpable tenderness ++</li><li>Mid-range arc or catch of pain</li><li>Pain on static isolated muscle loading</li><li>Associated weakness/inhibition</li><li>Positive impingement tests</li><li>Positive manual therapy stress tests to implicate pain-sensitive compression of subacromial or coracoacromial structures</li><li>Movement dysfunction indicates impingement; that is, positive kinetic medial rotation test (scapula)</li></ul>	<ul><li>Full or hypermobile range</li><li>Pain (if any) at the limits of range (often only at stress points)</li><li>Symptoms of instability, subluxation, dislocation, clicking, dysfunction and disability (loss of performance)</li><li>Resisted rotation often pain-free</li><li>Good strength (mid-range)</li><li>Positive instability tests</li><li>Positive manual therapy stress tests to implicate pain-sensitive capsular strain and ligamentous laxity</li><li>Movement dysfunction indicates instability; that is, positive kinetic medial rotation test (glenohumeral)</li></ul>

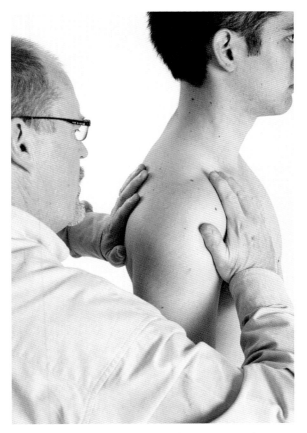

Figure 8.1 Therapist hand position for positioning the scapula 'neutral' orientation

together so that the acromion rises up, the humeral head moves backwards and the inferior scapular angle moves laterally around the chest wall (Figure 8.2). While the therapist passively supports the shoulder here, the person is asked to relax the shoulder and then is asked to use 'minimal' effort to actively maintain this position (Figure 8.3). With the scapula being actively maintained in this position, the therapist should palpate a series of landmarks (Box 8.1) and make any minor adjustments required.

A useful guide is to passively position the shoulder and, using visual and palpation feedback, the person feels the neutral position as a mid-position between elevation and depression, forward and backward tilt, upward and downward rotation and protraction and retraction. They are then instructed to move away from neutral and actively return to neutral using this feedback to ensure accurate repositioning.

Inferior anterior glenoid (IAG)

A common dysfunction pattern seen with loss of scapula neutral is the orientation of the glenoid in an inferior anterior direction, termed the inferior anterior glenoid (IAG) (Figure 8.4). This can be corrected by rotation of the scapula in the coronal plane – observed by the acromion moving superiorly while the inferior angle moves laterally (upward rotation of the scapula in the sagittal plane). The scapula also moves upward and backward (posterior or backward tilt) (Mottram et al 2009b) away from the IAG position.

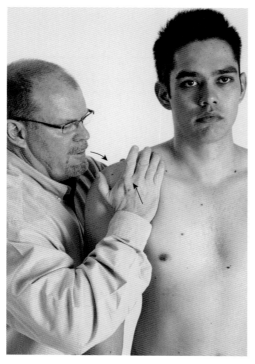

Figure 8.2 Passive positioning into scapula neutral

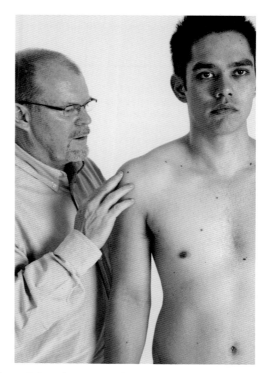

Figure 8.3 Active control of scapula neutral

Box 8.1 **Palpation reference guidelines for a neutral shoulder girdle**

Palpation guidelines for shoulder girdle neutral

- Superior-medial corner of scapula is level with T2.
- Medial edge of the spine of the scapula is level with T3.
- Spine of the scapula projects to T4.
- Inferior scapular angle level with T7.
- Acromion should be higher than the superior-medial scapular corner, with the spine of the scapula angled upwards (i.e. no downward rotation).
- Plane of the spine of the scapula is orientated between 15 and 30° forward of the coronal plane.
- Acromions are level or horizontal.
- Coracoids are symmetrical.
- Clavicles are symmetrical and inclined slightly upwards.

- Inferior scapular angle is in contact with ribcage (i.e. no forward tilt/'pseudo-winging').
- Medial border of scapula is in contract with ribcage (i.e. no winging).
- Medial border of spine of the scapula is approximately 5–6 cm lateral from the vertebral spinous processes.
- No more than $\frac{1}{3}$ of the humeral head should protrude forward of the acromion.
- Scapula must be positioned in neutral alignment prior to assessing humeral rotation and the humerus must be positioned in neutral alignment to assess forearm position.
- Elbow olecranon faces posteriorly and the elbow cubital fossa faces anteriorly (differentiate from forearm pronation.

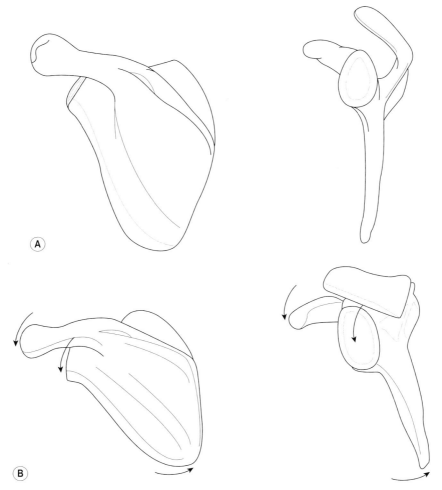

Figure 8.4 A. Neutral scapula orientation. B. Scapula inferior – anterior glenoid (IAG)

Segmental translatatory and global range specific UCM

When direction-specific UCM is observed at the shoulder, it can present in two ways. The UCM can present as either a segmental translatatory UCM (primarily of the humeral head) or a global range UCM (of either the scapula or the glenohumeral joint).

Segmental translatatory UCM

This is a segmental UCM in which the humeral head appears to 'glide forwards' into excessive anterior, inferior or posterior translatatory displacement associated with medial rotation, lateral rotation, flexion, abduction or extension motion testing. Uncontrolled humeral head anterior translation can be identified in motion testing. In medial rotation, lateral rotation and extension movements of the shoulder, palpation of the anterior prominence of the humeral head is used to identify excessive anterior translation. The ability to maintain the neutral axis and prevent excessive forward glide of the anterior prominence of the humeral head during active medial rotation, lateral rotation and extension is evaluated.

Global range-specific UCM

A global range-specific UCM demonstrates UCM (± hypermobile range) of the scapula or the glenohumeral joint. This is observed as either excessive

369

or dominant scapular or glenohumeral motion at the initiation of the movement or hypermobile range of motion to complete the movement.

A global range specific *scapular* UCM can be identified in motion testing. In any functional movement of the arm, observe or palpate for uncontrolled scapular:

- downward rotation
- forward tilt
- winging
- elevation
- protraction/abduction
- retraction/adduction.

A global range-specific *glenohumeral* UCM can be identified in motion testing. In any functional movement of the arm, observe or palpate for uncontrolled glenohumeral medial rotation.

The following section will demonstrate the specific procedures for testing for UCM in the shoulder girdle.

SHOULDER GIRDLE TESTS FOR UCM

Shoulder medial rotation control

OBSERVATION AND ANALYSIS OF SHOULDER MEDIAL ROTATION

Description of ideal pattern

While supine or standing, with the shoulder in 90° of abduction (scapular plane), there is 60° of medial rotation of the humerus without significant scapula-thoracic movement or glenohumeral anterior translation.

The therapist passively stabilises the scapula and glenohumeral joint and assesses the passive range of glenohumeral rotation without compensation (Figure 8.5).

Movement faults associated with glenohumeral medial rotation

Relative stiffness (restrictions)

- *Restrictions – reduced glenohumeral medial rotation with the arm abducted.* When the scapula and humeral head are passively supported to control scapula-thoracic

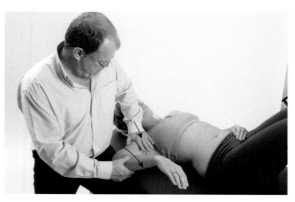

Figure 8.5 Assessment of glenohumeral medial rotation range with passive stabilisation

movement or glenohumeral anterior translation, a significant loss of glenohumeral medial rotation is often observed. Ideal passive range of medial rotation is 60°. Loss of medial rotation range may be due to several reasons:

- *Capsular restriction.* Capsular shortening may contribute to a loss of medial rotation, though this is not the most common cause. If capsular shortening is present then there is usually a significant loss of lateral rotation first observed as less than 90° lateral rotation in abduction.
- *Myofascial restriction.* Over-activity, dominance and relative stiffness of the glenohumeral lateral rotator muscles: a common presentation-related to the loss of medial rotation is over-activity and shortening of the lateral rotator muscles (infraspinatus and teres minor). Assessment of both the contractile and connective tissue shortening needs to be made and appropriate soft tissue work applied.
- *Co-contraction rigidity.* Occasionally, active medial rotation range at the glenohumeral joint may be limited by co-contraction rigidity. In the attempt to medially rotate, all glenohumeral muscles co-contract excessively and seem to 'splint' the shoulder from achieving full rotation. This is often a guarding response associated with instability or acute pathology or a protective 'spasm' in an acute inflammatory episode.

Relative flexibility (potential UCM)

- *UCM – compensatory strategies associated with restriction of glenohumeral joint medial rotation.* A variety of compensation strategies for restrictions can be employed to maintain functional range of motion. If glenohumeral medial rotation is restricted, compensatory movement can be made at both the scapula and the humeral head (Sahrmann 2002; Morrissey 2005).

  - *Uncontrolled scapula forward tilt, downward rotation or elevation.* The scapula may forward tilt, downwardly rotate or elevate to compensate for the loss of medial rotation. The accuracy of this palpation has been validated with three-dimensional ultrasound and motion analysis measures (Morrissey et al 2008). A positive test (scapula movement) has been linked with risk of impingement and symptoms (Morrissey 2005). The test is useful for diagnosis, especially for impingement, particularly when used with other impingement tests (Morrissey 2005).
  - *Uncontrolled glenohumeral translation control.* Excessive anterior translation of the humeral head compensates for a lack of glenohumeral medial rotation. A positive test (glenohumeral movement) has been linked with instability symptoms and risk (Morrissey 2005).

Indications to test for shoulder medial rotation UCM

Observe or palpate for:
1. hypermobile medial rotation range
2. discrepancies of shoulder medial rotation range in different positions of arm elevation
3. excessive initiation of scapular compensation during shoulder medial rotation
4. excessive glenohumeral translation during medial rotation
5. symptoms (pain, discomfort, strain) associated with shoulder medial rotation movements.

The person complains of rotation-related symptoms in the shoulder. During shoulder medial rotation load or movements, the scapula or glenohumeral joint has greater 'give' or compensation relative to the trunk or arm. The dysfunction is confirmed with motor control tests of shoulder medial rotation dissociation.

Test of shoulder medial rotation control

T60 KINETIC MEDIAL ROTATION TEST (KMRT) (tests for scapula and glenohumeral UCM)

This dissociation test assesses the ability to actively dissociate and control scapula movement and glenohumeral translation during glenohumeral medial rotation.

Test procedure

Start supine and with the humerus in 90° abduction (hand to the ceiling), and the humerus supported in the plane of the scapula. The therapist palpates the coracoid and humeral head during the procedure (Figure 8.6). The accuracy of this palpation has been measured (Morrissey et al 2008). Medial rotation of the humerus should occur without compensation at the scapula or glenohumeral joint. The scapula should not move into forward tilt, downward rotation or elevation and the humeral head should not translate anteriorly (Morrissey 2005). There should be 60° of active medial rotation (Figure 8.7). An alternative

test position is in standing with or without wall support of the scapula.

Rating and diagnosis of shoulder girdle UCM

(T60.1 and T60.2)
These UCMs have been linked to pathology. The scapula may forward tilt, downwardly rotate or elevate to compensate for the loss of medial rotation. A positive test (scapula UCM) has been linked with risk of impingement and symptoms (Morrissey 2005). The test is useful for diagnosis, especially for impingement, particularly when used with other impingement tests (Morrissey 2005). Uncontrolled anterior translation of the humeral head compensates for a lack of glenohumeral medial rotation. A positive test (glenohumeral UCM) has been linked with instability symptoms and risk (Morrissey 2005) (T60.3).

Correction

With visual, auditory and kinaesthetic cues the person becomes familiar with the task of medially rotating the glenohumeral joint to 60° without scapula movement or glenohumeral translation. Some useful clinical cues are illustrated in Box 8.2.

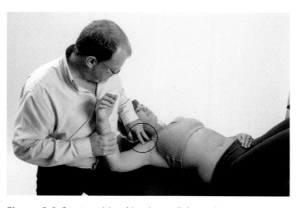

Figure 8.6 Start position kinetic medial rotation test

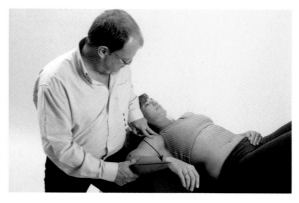

Figure 8.7 Benchmark kinetic medial rotation test – ideal movement

T60.1 Assessment and rating of low threshold recruitment efficiency of the Kinetic Medial Rotation Test

KINETIC MEDIAL ROTATION TEST

ASSESSMENT

Control point:
- prevent scapula forward tilt, downward rotation and elevation
- prevent glenohumeral anterior translation

Movement challenge: glenohumeral medial rotation (supine – arm 90° abduction)

Benchmark range: 60° glenohumeral medial rotation

RATING OF LOW THRESHOLD RECRUITMENT EFFICIENCY

	✓ or ✗		✓ or ✗
• Able to prevent 'give' into the test direction Correct dissociation pattern of movement	☐	• Looks easy, and in the opinion of the assessor, is performed with confidence	☐
Prevent scapula 'give' into:		• Feels easy, and the subject has sufficient awareness of the movement pattern that they confidently prevent 'give' into the test direction	☐
• forward tilt			
• downward rotation			
• elevation		• The pattern of dissociation is smooth during concentric and eccentric movement	☐
Prevent glenohumeral 'give' into:			
• anterior translation		• Does not (consistently) use *end-range* movement into the opposite direction to prevent the give	☐
and move glenohumeral medial rotation			
• Dissociate movement through the benchmark range of 60° glenohumeral medial rotation (arm abducted 90°) *If there is more available range than the benchmark standard, only the benchmark range needs to be actively controlled*	☐	• No extra feedback needed (*tactile, visual or verbal cueing*)	☐
		• Without external support or unloading	☐
		• Relaxed natural breathing (*even if not ideal – so long as natural pattern does not change*)	☐
• Without holding breath (though it is acceptable to use an alternate breathing strategy)	☐	• No fatigue	☐
• Control during eccentric phase	☐		
• Control during concentric phase	☐		
CORRECT DISSOCIATION PATTERN		**RECRUITMENT EFFICIENCY**	

T60.2 Diagnosis of the site and direction of UCM from the Kinetic Medial Rotation Test

KINETIC MEDIAL ROTATION TEST

Site	Direction	(L)	(R)
Scapula	Forward tilt	☐	☐
	Downward rotation	☐	☐
	Elevation	☐	☐
Glenohumeral	Anterior translation	☐	☐

T60.3 Relating the site and direction of UCM to impingement and instability

RISK ASSOCIATED WITH THE KINETIC MEDIAL ROTATION TEST

Ideal	60° glenohumeral medial rotation without scapula movement or humeral anterior translation. No anterior displacement of coracoid or humeral head (Figure 8.7)
Impingement risk	Scapular forward tilt, downward rotation or elevation occurs before 60° glenohumeral medial rotation is achieved. Note anterior displacement of coracoid with (stable) humeral head 'tagging along' in proportion (Figure 8.8) • Confirm the impingement risk with impingement tests and palpation
Instability risk	Humeral head anterior translation occurs before 60° glenohumeral medial rotation is achieved. Note anterior displacement of humeral head with (stable) coracoid maintaining stable position (Figure 8.9) • Confirm the direction(s) of instability with instability tests
Combined impingement and instability risk	Scapular forward tilt, downward rotation or elevation occurs before 60° glenohumeral medial rotation is achieved. However, excessive humeral head anterior translation also occurs before 60° glenohumeral medial rotation is achieved. Note anterior displacement of coracoid with the humeral head moving even further forward of the (unstable) coracoid • Differentiate to determine whether symptoms are primarily due to impingement or instability

---

Box 8.2 **Useful clinical facilitation and retraining cues**

Cues for facilitation and feedback to enhance teaching and retraining movement

- Palpate the scapula or glenohumeral joint to monitor the UCM.
- Imagery of rotating the glenohumeral joint about a coronal axis (proprioceptive feedback can be given through olecranon).
- Keep the coracoids open and wide.
- Palpate acromion/coracoid.
- Visualise a string holding the acromion up.
- Unload passively.
- Tape (proprioceptive skin tension).
- Keep same distance between coracoid and ear.
- Keep shoulder blades wide.

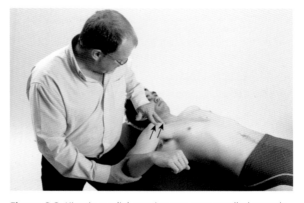

Figure 8.8 Kinetic medial rotation test uncontrolled scapula movement

An alternative position for retraining the KMRT

Lean against a wall with the wall supporting the shoulder blade position. The upper body has to turn 15–30° off the wall so that the shoulder blade and upper arm can be supported flat on the wall. Only rotate the shoulder forwards as far as the neutral scapula can be controlled (Figure 8.10). When rotation control on the wall is efficient progress to the same movement unsupported away from the wall (Figure 8.11).

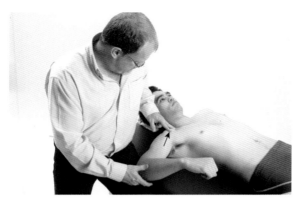

Figure 8.9 Kinetic medial rotation test uncontrolled glenohumeral movement

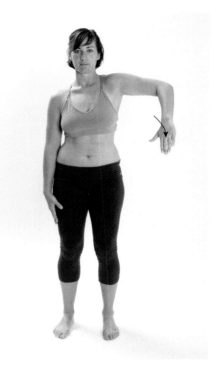

Figure 8.11 Correction standing – unsupported

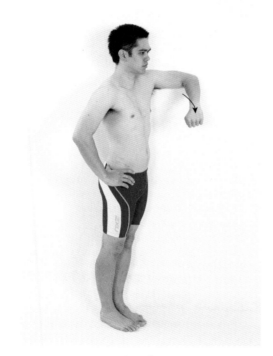

Figure 8.10 Correction with wall support

Shoulder lateral rotation control

OBSERVATION AND ANALYSIS OF SHOULDER LATERAL ROTATION

Description of ideal pattern

This can be observed in standing or supine. While standing with the humerus by the side in the scapular plane (elbow forward of the anterior axillary line) and the elbow flexed to 90° (hand pointing forwards, palm in) there should be approximately 60° range of functional lateral turn out of the arm – at least 45° being gleno-humeral lateral rotation and about 15° coming from scapular retraction. The glenohumeral lateral rotation should be the dominant movement early in the movement with the scapula contributing later in range.

The therapist assesses the passive range of glenohumeral lateral rotation. There should be 45° of independent passive lateral rotation. It should be relatively easy to independently dissociate the 45° glenohumeral lateral rotation from the scapular movement (Figure 8.12).

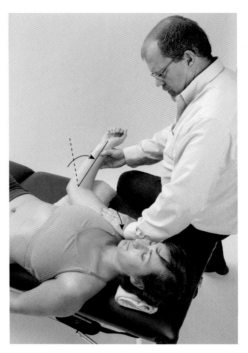

Figure 8.12 Assessment of glenohumeral lateral rotation range with passive stabilisation

Movement faults associated with glenohumeral lateral rotation

Scapular retraction initiates or dominates the early range of functional arm turn out. This indicates either a restriction (relative stiffness) of glenohumeral lateral rotation or compensation (relative flexibility) of scapular retraction.

Relative stiffness (restriction)

- *Reduced glenohumeral lateral rotation with the elbow by side.* Functional restrictions of glenohumeral lateral rotation are identified with the scapula stabilised and the arm by the side. A significant loss of glenohumeral lateral rotation with the arm by the side is frequently identified. This restriction of functional lateral rotation range may be due to several reasons:
  - ▪ *Capsular restriction.* A capsular restriction may cause a loss of lateral rotation with the arm by the side but there will be significant (if not greater) loss of lateral rotation with the arm elevated to 90°.

Examination of the shoulder 'quadrant' test (Maitland et al 2005) would be positive for a capsular restriction. If at 90° of arm abduction the lateral rotation range is normal then the capsule is a very unlikely source of restriction.

- ▪ *Loss of posterior translation of the humerus at limit of lateral rotation.* At the limit of active or passive glenohumeral lateral rotation the capsule tensions anteriorly and the humeral head is forced to translate posteriorly in order to achieve full range (Moseley et al 1992; Wilk et al 1997). A loss of this posterior translation of the humeral head at the limit of lateral rotation can significantly reduce the ability to achieve full active or passive lateral rotation at the shoulder when the arm is by the side. This is identified by a decreased range of joint play and a restricted end feel on posterior translation of the humeral head at end range lateral rotation. Appropriate mobilisation of this articular restriction (e.g. with glenohumeral accessory anteroposterior glides at the limit of physiological lateral rotations) is often appropriate here.

- *Loss of extensibility of myofascial structures.* It may be possible that excessive shortening of myofascial structures may limit lateral rotation range. Pectoralis major and latissimus dorsi may limit lateral rotation with the arm high overhead but for lateral rotation to be limited when the arm is by the side, subscapularis and teres major are likely to be very short. Clinically, this is uncommon but may be associated with a prolonged period of immobilisation, surgery and capsular shortening.
- *Co-contraction rigidity.* Occasionally, active lateral rotation range at the glenohumeral joint may be limited by co-contraction rigidity. This is often a guarding response associated with instability or acute pathology or protective 'spasm' in an acute inflammatory episode.

- UCM – compensatory strategies associated with restriction of glenohumeral joint lateral rotation. If lateral rotation is restricted, different compensation strategies can be seen:
  - *Uncontrolled scapula retraction (scapular retraction initiating or dominating glenohumeral lateral rotation).* This can be assessed in standing with the arm by the side. This is most frequently associated with a functional loss of glenohumeral lateral rotation range and the development of greater relative flexibility at the scapulothoracic joint. Instead of scapular retraction providing extra movement after the glenohumeral joint has completed lateral rotation, scapular retraction increases to compensate for the inefficient glenohumeral movement. In extreme cases the recruitment of scapular retraction even precedes the recruitment of glenohumeral lateral rotation.
  - *Uncontrolled scapula downward rotation.* The apparent loss of lateral rotation is very commonly due to a lack of ability to position the glenoid in neutral alignment. If the glenoid is downwardly rotated then lateral rotation can be limited. This is confirmed by passively positioning the scapula in correct alignment. When the scapula (and glenoid) is in neutral

alignment the active lateral rotation movement returns to normal.
- *Uncontrolled scapula forward tilt.* This is similar to the above. If the glenoid is orientated antero-inferiorly, lateral rotation can be limited. This is confirmed by passively positioning the scapula in correct alignment. When the scapula (and glenoid) is in neutral alignment the active lateral rotation movement returns to normal.
- *Uncontrolled glenohumeral anterior translation.* The apparent loss of lateral rotation may be related to an unstable glenohumeral joint. If the glenohumeral joint has excessive anterior translation (due to anterior capsular laxity or instability) then the axis of rotation is displaced and normal lateral rotation cannot be achieved. If the humeral head is palpated with the shoulder resting at end range lateral rotation it is observed to be prominent anteriorly. Upon assessment of a posterior translational glide in this position, a significantly increased range of joint play and a lax soft end feel is identified. This cause of dysfunction is confirmed if full lateral rotation range returns when the humeral head is passively glided posteriorly and maintained in its neutral position.

Indications to test for shoulder lateral rotation UCM

Observe or palpate for:

1. hypermobile lateral rotation range
2. discrepancies of shoulder lateral rotation range in different positions of arm elevation
3. excessive initiation of scapular compensation during shoulder lateral rotation
4. excessive glenohumeral translation during lateral rotation
5. symptoms (pain, discomfort, strain) associated with shoulder lateral rotation movements.

The person complains of rotation-related symptoms in the shoulder. During shoulder lateral rotation load or movements, the scapula or glenohumeral joint has greater 'give' or compensation relative to the trunk or arm. The dysfunction is confirmed with motor control tests of shoulder lateral rotation dissociation.

Test of shoulder lateral rotation control

T61 KINETIC LATERAL ROTATION TEST (KLRT)
(tests for scapula and glenohumeral UCM)

This dissociation test assesses the ability to actively dissociate and control scapula movement and glenohumeral translation from the glenohumeral lateral rotation.

Test procedure

This is a two-part test.

KLRT Part 1

Start standing, with the elbow by the side in the scapular plane (elbow forward of the anterior axillary line) and the elbow flexed to 90° (hand pointing forwards, palm in (Figure 8.13). The therapist palpates the corocoid/acromion (or inferior angle of scapula) and humeral head during the procedure. The person is instructed to maintain a neutral position of the scapula and turn the arm out into lateral rotation. The scapula should not move into forward tilt, downward rotation or retraction and the humeral head should not translate anteriorly. There should be 45° of active lateral rotation of the humerus without compensation at the scapula or glenohumeral joint (Figures 8.14 and 8.15).

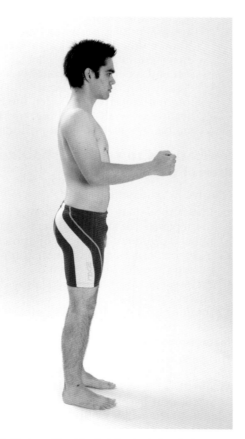

Figure 8.13 Start position kinetic lateral rotation test

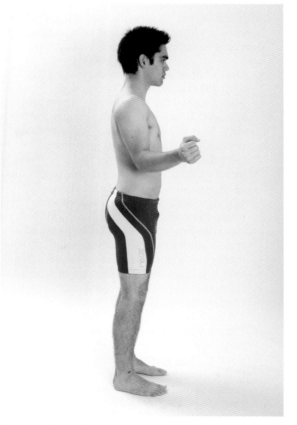

Figure 8.14 Benchmark kinetic lateral rotation test

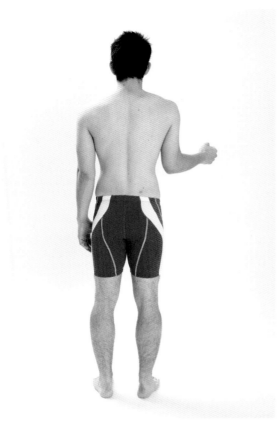

Figure 8.15 Kinetic lateral rotation test demonstrating good scapula control

KLRT Part 2

Position the person supine, with the elbow by the side in the scapular plane (elbow forward of the anterior axillary line) and the elbow flexed to 90° (hand pointing forwards, palm in). There should be 45° of active lateral rotation of the humerus when the scapula is stabilised by lying on it. If there is a restriction of lateral rotation in this position the therapist must determine if the restriction is real or if it is the result of uncontrolled scapula or glenohumeral movement.

Differentiation between scapular and glenohumeral contributions to apparent restricted range

Scapular UCM

The apparent loss of lateral rotation is very commonly due to a lack of ability to position the glenoid in neutral alignment. This is confirmed by passively positioning the scapula in upward rotation and observing that when the scapula (and glenoid) is in correct alignment the active lateral rotation movement returns to normal (Figure 8.16).

Glenohumeral UCM

The apparent loss of lateral rotation may be related to an unstable glenohumeral joint. If the glenohumeral joint has excessive anterior translation (due to anterior capsular laxity or instability) then the axis of rotation is displaced and normal lateral rotation cannot be achieved. This cause of dysfunction is confirmed if full lateral rotation range returns when the humeral head is passively glided posteriorly and maintained in its correct position (Figure 8.17).

Shoulder girdle control dysfunction

During active glenohumeral lateral rotation to 45° benchmark range, the subject is unable to maintain control of either:

- scapula forward tilt, downward rotation or retraction
- glenohumeral anterior translation.

Rating and diagnosis of shoulder girdle UCM

(T61.1 and T61.2)

These UCMs may be linked to pathology. A positive test for scapula UCM may be linked with risk of impingement and symptoms. The test is useful for diagnosis, especially for impingement, particularly when used with other impingement tests. A positive test of glenohumeral UCM may be linked with instability symptoms and risk (T61.3).

Correction

Initial correction can be performed lying in supine with the arm supported by the side. Active lateral rotation is performed through partial range with the scapula stabilised in upward rotation (lying on scapula) and the humeral head stabilised in posterior glide (self-palpation)

T61.1 Assessment and rating of low threshold recruitment efficiency of the Kinetic Lateral Rotation Test

KINETIC LATERAL ROTATION TEST

ASSESSMENT

Control point:
- prevent scapula forward tilt, downward rotation and retraction
- prevent glenohumeral anterior translation

Movement challenge: glenohumeral lateral rotation (standing – arm by side)

Benchmark range: 45° glenohumeral lateral rotation

RATING OF LOW THRESHOLD RECRUITMENT EFFICIENCY

	✓ or ✗		✓ or ✗

• Able to prevent 'give' into the test direction. Correct dissociation pattern of movement
Prevent scapula 'give' into:
    forward tilt
    downward rotation
    retraction
Prevent glenohumeral 'give' into:
    anterior translation
and move glenohumeral lateral rotation
	☐	• Looks easy, and in the opinion of the assessor, is performed with confidence	☐

		• Feels easy, and the subject has sufficient awareness of the movement pattern that they confidently prevent 'give' into the test direction	☐
• Dissociate movement through the benchmark range of 45° glenohumeral lateral rotation (arm by side) *If there is more available range than the benchmark standard, only the benchmark range needs to be actively controlled*	☐	• The pattern of dissociation is smooth during concentric and eccentric movement	☐
		• Does not (consistently) use *end-range* movement into the opposite direction to prevent the give	☐
		• No extra feedback needed *(tactile, visual or verbal cueing)*	☐
• Without holding breath (though it is acceptable to use an alternate breathing strategy)	☐	• Without external support or unloading	☐
		• Relaxed natural breathing *(even if not ideal – so long as natural pattern does not change)*	☐
• Control during eccentric phase	☐	• No fatigue	☐
• Control during concentric phase	☐		

CORRECT DISSOCIATION PATTERN   **RECRUITMENT EFFICIENCY**

T61.2 Diagnosis of the site and direction of UCM from the Kinetic Lateral Rotation Test

KINETIC LATERAL ROTATION TEST

Site	Direction	(L)	(R)
Scapula	Forward tilt	☐	☐
	Downward rotation	☐	☐
	Retraction	☐	☐
Glenohumeral	Anterior translation	☐	☐

T61.3 Relating the site and direction of UCM to impingement and instability

RISK ASSOCIATED WITH THE KINETIC LATERAL ROTATION TEST

Ideal	45° glenohumeral lateral rotation without scapula movement or humeral anterior translation. No anterior displacement of coracoid or humeral head (Figure 8.18)
Impingement risk	A significant restriction of shoulder lateral rotation is noted (Figure 8.19). Manual passive repositioning of the scapula in upward rotation and backward tilt (correction of resting position of excessive downward rotation/forward tilt) results in ability to actively produce the full benchmark range of 45° lateral rotation (Figure 8.20) • Confirm scapular control dysfunction by passively positioning the scapula back into downward rotation and forward tilt and observe a significant reduction in active shoulder lateral rotation range • Confirm the impingement risk with impingement tests and palpation
Instability risk	A significant restriction of shoulder lateral rotation is noted (Figure 8.21). Manual passive repositioning of the humeral head into posterior translation with light manual posterior pressure from two fingers (correction of resting position of excessive anterior translation) results in ability to actively produce the full benchmark range of 45° lateral rotation (Figure 8.22) • Confirm glenohumeral translation control dysfunction by passively positioning the humeral head back into anterior translation and observe a significant reduction in active shoulder lateral rotation range • Confirm the direction(s) of instability with instability tests

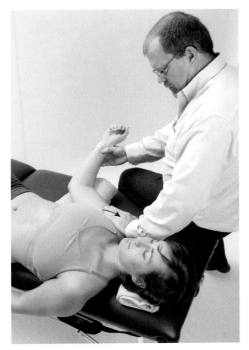

Figure 8.16 Passive restabilisation of scapula into upward rotation to confirm if uncontrolled movement contributes to restricted functional range

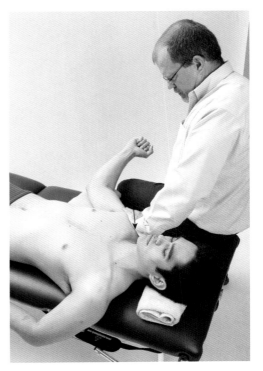

Figure 8.17 Passive restabilisation of humeral head with posterior glide to confirm if uncontrolled movement contributes to restricted functional range

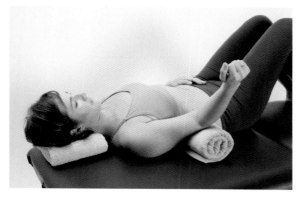

Figure 8.18 Kinetic lateral rotation test – ideal active control

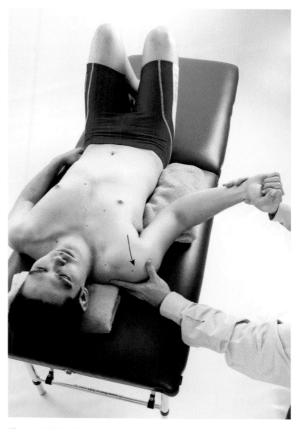

Figure 8.20 Kinetic lateral rotation test (scapular UCM) – increased lateral rotation with scapular repositioning

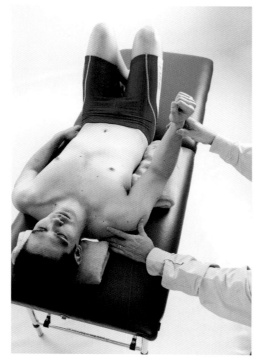

Figure 8.19 Kinetic lateral rotation test (scapular UCM) – restricted lateral rotation with scapular downward rotation

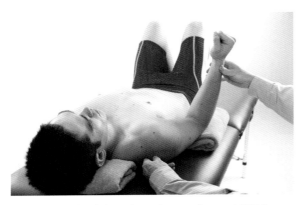

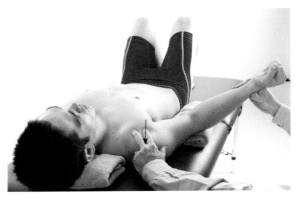

Figure 8.21 Kinetic lateral rotation test (humeral UCM) – restricted lateral rotation with humeral head forward displacement

Figure 8.22 Kinetic lateral rotation test (humeral UCM) – increased lateral rotation with humeral head repositioning

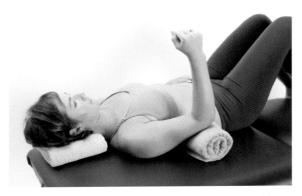

Figure 8.23 Correction partial range lateral rotation with scapula and glenohumeral support

(Figure 8.23). An alternative position for retraining the KMLT is to lean against a wall with the wall supporting the shoulder blade position. The upper body has to turn 15–30° off the wall so that the shoulder blade and upper arm can be supported flat on the wall. Only rotate the shoulder backwards as far as the neutral scapula can be controlled (Figure 8.24). As control improves, the active lateral rotation is performed in standing with the scapula and humeral head unsupported (Figure 8.25). With visual, auditory and kinaesthetic cues the person becomes familiar with the task of laterally rotating the glenohumeral joint to 45° without scapula movement or glenohumeral translation. Some useful clinical cues are illustrated in Box 8.3.

Box 8.3 Useful clinical facilitation and retraining cues

Cues for facilitation and feedback to enhance teaching and retraining movement

- Palpate the scapula or glenohumeral joint to monitor the UCM.
- Imagery of rotating the glenohumeral joint about a coronal axis (proprioceptive feedback can be given through olecranon).
- Keep the coracoids open and wide.
- Palpate acromion/coracoid/inferior angle.
- Visualise a string holding the acromion up.
- Unload passively.
- Tape (proprioceptive skin tension).
- Keep same distance between coracoid and ear.
- Keep shoulder blades wide.

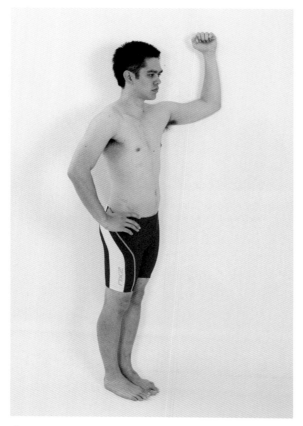

Figure 8.24 Correction with wall support

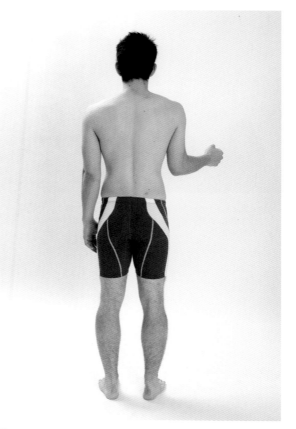

Figure 8.25 Correction partial range lateral rotation with unsupported shoulder girdle

Shoulder flexion control

OBSERVATION AND ANALYSIS OF SHOULDER FLEXION

Description of ideal pattern

Throughout arm elevation overhead, the normal scapulohumeral rhythm is approximately humzzeral: scapula movement of a ratio 2:1 or 3:2. During elevation three distinct processes should occur:

1. glenohumeral elevation
2. upward rotation of the glenoid and slight scapular elevation
3. slight trunk movement.

Although both glenohumeral and scapular movement should occur simultaneously, the first phase predominantly consists of glenohumeral elevation with the scapula relatively stable. This should occur through approximately the first 90° of flexion. Medial rotation of the arm should not be excessive during flexion. Humeral head inferior translation should start in this phase. The second phase is dominated by upward rotation of the glenoid of the scapula (associated with slight scapular elevation) with concurrent glenohumeral rolling into arm elevation. Clavicular rotation is necessary for full and appropriate scapular rotation. The head of the humerus should continue to glide inferiorly on the glenoid during this phase. There should not be excessive elevation or protraction of the scapula during flexion. After 160° of arm elevation some slight trunk movement may occur, but this should be minimal and should only occur towards the end of glenohumeral and scapular movement. Thoracic extension occurs during arm flexion and thoracic lateral flexion occurs during unilateral arm flexion. The scapula should not wing during concentric or eccentric movement and any protraction should be minimal. In full arm elevation/flexion the inferior angle of the scapula should not protrude any further than 1.5 cm laterally from the chest wall but should rotate around the chest wall to reach the mid-axillary line (Figures 8.26 and 8.27).

Movement faults associated with arm flexion

These faults can be observed with the natural pattern of thoraco-scapulohumeral motion through the full range of arm flexion overhead.

Dysfunctions of scapulothoracic control

- *Uncontrolled scapula downward rotation.* This presents as dominance of scapular downward rotation and/or inefficient upward rotation and may be observed in several ways:
  - At the initial part of the scapular movement phase the scapula downwardly rotates instead of upwardly rotating. This is observed with medial movement of the inferior angle before it moves laterally.
  - Reduced upward rotation of the scapula at the completion of the scapular movement phase. This is observed as a lack of lateral movement of scapular inferior angle – it

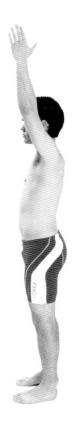

Figure 8.26 Shoulder flexion overhead – lateral view

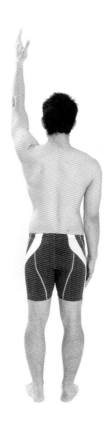

Figure 8.27 Shoulder flexion overhead – back view

does not reach the mid-axillary line in elevation. This is often associated with shortness and relative stiffness in the rhomboids and pectoralis minor (which restrict upward rotation) and inefficient serratus anterior (which cannot upwardly rotate the scapula).

- During eccentric lowering of the arm and the scapula there is uncontrolled downward rotation of the scapula. This is observed as either the scapula in a downwardly rotated position by 90° flexion or the inferior angle travelling medially beyond the 'normal resting position' of the scapula as the arm returns to the side (Mottram et al 2009a).

Uncontrolled downward rotation of the scapula is associated with either length or recruitment changes in the scapular rotator muscles. There is

noticeable dominance or shortening of the downward rotators (rhomboids, pectoralis minor and levator scapula) and poor stabilisation and control of upward rotation (poor stability function of trapezius and serratus anterior).

- *Uncontrolled scapular elevation (overhead) – scapular elevation is uncontrolled or initiates movement during flexion.* This is associated with inefficient lower trapezius activity to counterbalance the scapular elevators (particularly rhomboids and levator scapula) during arm flexion. Elevation of the scapula is the dominant motion instead of upward rotation. This is most evident at the limit of overhead flexion.
- *Uncontrolled scapular protraction during flexion.* This is associated with inefficient scapular stabiliser (middle and lower trapezius) activity to counterbalance the scapular protractors (serratus anterior and an overactive pectoralis minor) during arm flexion. Protraction (and elevation) of the scapula is the dominant motion instead of upward rotation. This is most evident during eccentric lowering when the scapula is held forwards in protraction throughout most of the movement and suddenly 'flicks' back in the last 45° of lowering.
- *Uncontrolled scapular winging (prominence of the entire medial border of the scapula off the rib cage):*
  - During concentric elevation of the arm and at rest in static posture: associated with an inefficient of serratus anterior.
  - During eccentric lowering of the arm: timing problem associated with the scapulohumeral muscles not relaxing as quickly as the scapulo-trunk muscles. The scapulohumeral muscles are relatively stiffer and the glenohumeral muscles relatively more flexible.
  - During upper limb weight bearing: associated with 'long' and inefficient medial scapular stabilisers and serratus anterior.
- *Uncontrolled scapular forward tilt.* Observe prominence of the inferior angle of the scapula or protrusion off the lower rib cage, often with concurrent downward rotation of the scapula. This is associated with excessive shortness of pectoralis minor and downward rotation of the scapula with a concurrent

loss of upward rotation position and poor control by lower trapezius and serratus anterior.

Dysfunctions of glenohumeral control

- *Uncontrolled glenohumeral medial rotation during arm flexion.* During flexion uncontrolled medial rotation occurs. As a rough guide, the arm should be in neutral rotation (thumb forwards) when the hand rests by the side, and as the arm flexes it should stay neutral and not medially rotate. Medial rotation is associated with over-activity and dominance of the medial rotator muscles (pectoralis major or latissimus dorsi) or shortness of latissimus dorsi resulting in the arm being forced into medial rotation to achieve the full overhead position.
- *Uncontrolled glenohumeral inferior translation – excessive inferior translational glide of the humerus during overhead elevation.* Inadequate upward rotation of the scapula and poor glenohumeral rotation timing often result in increased compensatory glenohumeral inferior translation. Observe deep posterior acromial depression or 'dimple' instead of a small skin crease when the arm is in full elevation and a 'bulge' of the humeral head is in the axilla.

Indications to test for shoulder flexion UCM

Observe or palpate for:

1. hypermobile flexion range
2. excessive initiation of scapular compensation during shoulder flexion
3. excessive glenohumeral translation during shoulder flexion
4. symptoms (pain, discomfort, strain) associated with shoulder flexion movements.

The person complains of flexion-related symptoms in the shoulder. During shoulder flexion load or movements, the scapula or glenohumeral joint has greater 'give' or compensation relative to the trunk or arm. The dysfunction is confirmed with motor control tests of shoulder flexion dissociation.

Test of shoulder flexion control

T62 ARM FLEXION TEST
(tests for scapula and glenohumeral UCM)

This dissociation assesses the ability to actively dissociate and control scapula movement and glenohumeral medial rotation during glenohumeral flexion.

Test procedure

The subject stands with the arm resting by the side with the scapula in a neutral position and the glenohumeral joint in neutral rotation (palm in) (Figure 8.28). The subject is instructed to keep the scapula in the neutral position and lift the arm through 90° of shoulder flexion and lower the arm back to the side (Figure 8.29). Ideally, the scapula should maintain the neutral position and not elevate during lifting into 90° flexion or drop into downward rotation, forward tilt or depression during lowering back to the side.

There should be no winging. The neutral rotation (palm in, thumb up) should be maintained. UCM can be monitored by observation or palpation: dropping of the acromion (downward rotation); the coracoid moving inferiorly and the inferior angle moving posteriorly (forward tilt); the medial border of the scapula lifting off the chest (winging); and hitching of the acromion (elevation).

Rating and diagnosis of shoulder girdle UCM

(T62.1 and T62.2)

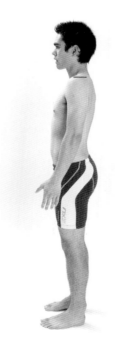

Figure 8.28 Start position arm flexion test

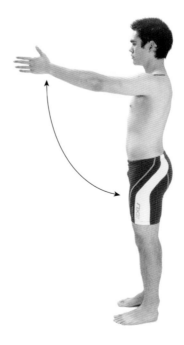

Figure 8.29 Benchmark arm flexion test

T62.1 Assessment and rating of low threshold recruitment efficiency of the Arm Flexion Test

ARM FLEXION TEST

ASSESSMENT

Control point:
- prevent downward rotation, scapula forward tilt, winging, elevation, and protraction
- prevent glenohumeral medial rotation

Movement challenge: glenohumeral flexion (standing – arm horizontal in front)

Benchmark range: 90° glenohumeral flexion

RATING OF LOW THRESHOLD RECRUITMENT EFFICIENCY

	✓ or ✗		✓ or ✗

• Able to prevent 'give' into the test direction. Correct dissociation pattern of movement
 Prevent scapula 'give' into:
   downward rotation
   forward tilt
   winging
   elevation
   protraction/abduction
 Prevent glenohumeral 'give' into:
   medial rotation
 and move glenohumeral flexion
	☐	• Looks easy, and in the opinion of the assessor, is performed with confidence	☐

		• Feels easy, and the subject has sufficient awareness of the movement pattern that they confidently prevent 'give' into the test direction	☐
		• The pattern of dissociation is smooth during concentric and eccentric movement	☐
		• Does not (consistently) use *end-range* movement into the opposite direction to prevent the give	☐
• Dissociate movement through the benchmark range of 90° glenohumeral flexion (arm horizontal in front) *If there is more available range than the benchmark standard, only the benchmark range needs to be actively controlled*	☐	• No extra feedback needed (*tactile, visual or verbal cueing*)	☐
		• Without external support or unloading	☐
		• Relaxed natural breathing (*even if not ideal – so long as natural pattern does not change*)	☐
• Without holding breath (though it is acceptable to use an alternate breathing strategy)	☐	• No fatigue	☐
• Control during eccentric phase	☐		
• Control during concentric phase	☐		
CORRECT DISSOCIATION PATTERN		**RECRUITMENT EFFICIENCY**	

T62.2 Diagnosis of the site and direction of UCM from the Arm Flexion Test

ARM FLEXION TEST

Site	Direction	(L)	(R)
Scapula	Downward rotation	☐	☐
	Forward tilt	☐	☐
	Winging	☐	☐
	Elevation	☐	☐
	Protraction/abduction	☐	☐
Glenohumeral	Medial rotation	☐	☐

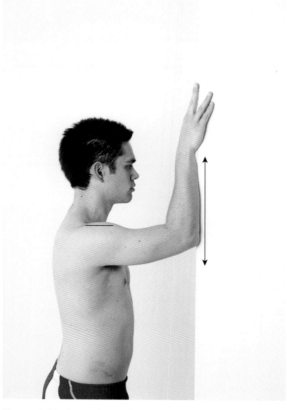

Figure 8.30 Correction with wall support

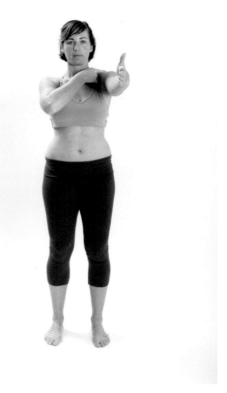

Figure 8.31 Correction arm flexion with self-palpation

Correction

Initial correction can be performed standing with the elbow flexed to reduce the arm lever length and decrease load and the scapula supported by leaning against a wall (Figure 8.30). As control improves, the arm flexion is performed unsupported through the partial range that can be controlled well with self-palpation. This is eventually progressed throughout the full benchmark range with the elbow straight (Figure 8.31). With visual, auditory and kinaesthetic cues the person becomes familiar with the task of flexing the glenohumeral joint to 90° without scapula movement or glenohumeral translation. Some useful clinical cues are illustrated in Box 8.4.

Box 8.4 Useful clinical facilitation and retraining cues

Cues for facilitation and feedback to enhance teaching and retraining movement

- Palpate the scapula or glenohumeral joint to monitor the UCM.
- Imagery of lifting the shoulder blade as the arm lowers.
- Turn the hand (palm in) and follow the thumb overhead.
- Keep the coracoids open and wide.
- Palpate acromion/coracoid/inferior angle.
- Visualise a string holding the acromion up.
- Unload passively.
- Tape (proprioceptive skin tension).
- Keep same distance between coracoid and ear.
- Keep shoulder blades wide.

Shoulder abduction control

OBSERVATION AND ANALYSIS OF SHOULDER ABDUCTION

Description of ideal pattern

Observe the natural patterns of thoraco-scapulohumeral motion through the full range of arm abduction overhead in the scapular plane. The ideal pattern is similar for flexion (see previous section) but there are a few points specific to abduction. Although both glenohumeral and scapula movement should occur simultaneously, the first phase should predominantly consist of glenohumeral elevation with the scapula relatively stable through the first 60° of movement in abduction. During abduction, glenohumeral lateral rotation is initiated early in this phase and should continue throughout range. Slight thoracic lateral flexion occurs during unilateral arm abduction (Figures 8.32, 8.33, 8.34).

Movement faults associated with arm abduction

These faults can be observed with the natural pattern of thoraco-scapulohumeral motion through the full range of arm abduction overhead.

Dysfunctions of scapulothoracic control

- *Uncontrolled scapular downward rotation.* This presents as dominance of scapular downward rotation and/or inefficient upward rotation and is described above in the flexion pattern.

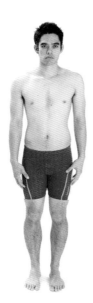

Figure 8.32 Shoulder resting position

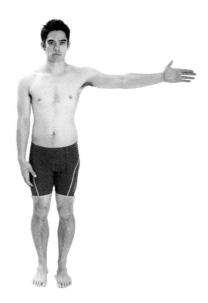

Figure 8.33 Shoulder abduction mid-range with glenohumeral lateral rotation

Dysfunctions of glenohumeral control

- *Uncontrolled glenohumeral rotation – late or absent glenohumeral lateral rotation during arm abduction.* During abduction the required lateral rotation movement is absent or late. The arm should be in neutral rotation (thumb forwards) when the hand rests by the side and should actively laterally rotate the greater tuberosity posteriorly throughout the range of abduction. As a rough guide, by 60° the thumb should start to turn upwards. By at least 120° the thumb should point to the ceiling and by 180° the thumb should point posteriorly and the palms face in towards each other. If the palms face down to the floor and the thumbs point forwards at 90° the lateral rotation timing is late.
- *Uncontrolled glenohumeral inferior translation – excessive inferior translational glide of the humerus during overhead elevation.* Inadequate upward rotation of the scapula and poor glenohumeral rotation timing often result in increased compensatory glenohumeral inferior translation. Observe deep posterior acromial dimple instead of a small skin crease when the arm is in full elevation and there is a 'bulge' of the humeral head in the axilla.

Indications to test for shoulder abduction UCM

Observe or palpate for:

1. hypermobile abduction rotation range
2. excessive initiation of scapular compensation during shoulder abduction
3. excessive glenohumeral translation during shoulder abduction
4. symptoms (pain, discomfort, strain) associated with shoulder abduction movements.

The person complains of abduction-related symptoms in the shoulder. During shoulder abduction load or movements, the scapula or glenohumeral joint has greater 'give' or compensation relative to the trunk or arm. The dysfunction is confirmed with motor control tests of shoulder abduction dissociation.

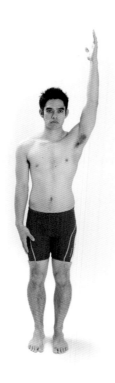

Figure 8.34 Shoulder abduction overhead with glenohumeral lateral rotation

- *Uncontrolled scapular elevation (overhead) – scapular elevation is excessive or initiates movement during abduction.* This presents more consistently in the full overhead position (above 140°). With the arms fully overhead, when the person is asked to relax their shoulders but keep their hands fully overhead, the scapula drops from an excessively elevated position.
- *Uncontrolled scapular winging (prominence of the entire medial border of the scapula off the rib cage).* This presents most consistently during eccentric lowering of the arm from overhead.
- *Uncontrolled scapular forward tilt ('tipping' of the scapula).* This presents most consistently during eccentric lowering of the arm from overhead.

Test of shoulder abduction control

T63 ARM ABDUCTION TEST (tests for scapula and glenohumeral UCM)

This dissociation assesses the ability to actively dissociate and control scapula movement and glenohumeral medial rotation during glenohumeral flexion.

Test procedure

The subject stands with the arm resting by the side in neutral rotation (palm in towards the side) and with the scapula in a neutral position. The subject is instructed to keep the scapula in the neutral position and lift the arm through 90° of shoulder abduction (in the scapula plane) and lower the arm back to the side (Figure 8.35).

Ideally, the scapula should maintain the neutral position and not elevate during lifting into 90° abduction or drop into downward rotation or depression during lowering back to the side. The arm should start active lateral rotation through this range (palm starting to turn forwards should be maintained (Figure 8.36).

Rating and diagnosis of shoulder girdle UCM

(T63.1 and T63.2)

Correction

Initial correction can be performed standing with the elbow flexed to reduce the arm lever length and decrease load and the scapula supported by leaning against a wall (Figure 8.37). As control improves the arm abduction is performed unsupported through the partial range that can be controlled well with self-palpation (Figure 8.38). This is eventually progressed throughout the full benchmark range with the elbow straight.

With visual, auditory and kinaesthetic cues the person becomes familiar with the task of abducting the glenohumeral joint to 90° without scapula movement or glenohumeral translation. Some useful clinical cues are illustrated in Box 8.5.

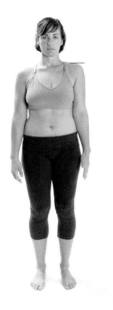

Figure 8.35 Start position arm abduction test

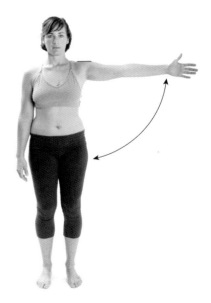

Figure 8.36 Benchmark arm abduction test

T63.1 Assessment and rating of low threshold recruitment efficiency of the Arm Abduction Test

ARM ABDUCTION TEST

ASSESSMENT

Control point:
- prevent downward rotation, scapula forward tilt, winging and elevation
- prevent glenohumeral medial rotation

Movement challenge: glenohumeral abduction (standing – arm horizontal in the scapula plane)

Benchmark range: 90° glenohumeral abduction

RATING OF LOW THRESHOLD RECRUITMENT EFFICIENCY

	✓ or ✗		✓ or ✗

• Able to prevent 'give' into the test direction. Correct dissociation pattern of movement
Prevent scapula 'give' into:
  downward rotation
  forward tilt
  winging
  elevation
Prevent glenohumeral 'give' into:
  medial rotation
and move glenohumeral abduction
	☐	• Looks easy, and in the opinion of the assessor, is performed with confidence	☐

		• Feels easy, and the subject has sufficient awareness of the movement pattern that they confidently prevent 'give' into the test direction	☐
		• The pattern of dissociation is smooth during concentric and eccentric movement	☐
• Dissociate movement through the benchmark range of 90° glenohumeral abduction (arm horizontal in the scapula plane) *If there is more available range than the benchmark standard, only the benchmark range needs to be actively controlled*	☐	• Does not (consistently) use *end-range* movement into the opposite direction to prevent the give	☐
		• No extra feedback needed *(tactile, visual or verbal cueing)*	☐
		• Without external support or unloading	☐
• Without holding breath (though it is acceptable to use an alternate breathing strategy)	☐	• Relaxed natural breathing *(even if not ideal – so long as natural pattern does not change)*	☐
• Control during eccentric phase	☐	• No fatigue	☐
• Control during concentric phase	☐		

CORRECT DISSOCIATION PATTERN   **RECRUITMENT EFFICIENCY**

T63.2 Diagnosis of the site and direction of UCM from the Arm Abduction Test

ARM ABDUCTION TEST

Site	Direction	(L)	(R)
Scapula	Downward rotation	☐	☐
	Forward tilt	☐	☐
	Winging	☐	☐
	Elevation	☐	☐
Glenohumeral	Medial rotation	☐	☐

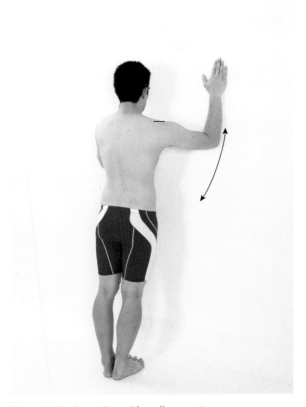

Figure 8.37 Correction with wall support

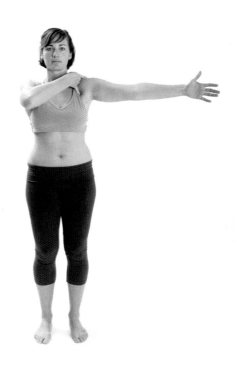

Figure 8.38 Correction arm abduction with self-palpation

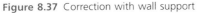

Box 8.5 **Useful clinical facilitation and retraining cues**

Cues for facilitation and feedback to enhance teaching and retraining movement

- Palpate the scapula or glenohumeral joint to monitor the UCM.
- Imagery of lifting the shoulder blade as the arm lowers.
- Turn the hand to ensure lateral rotation throughout range.

- Keep the coracoids open and wide.
- Palpate acromion/coracoid/inferior angle.
- Visualise a string holding the acromion up.
- Unload passively.
- Tape (proprioceptive skin tension).
- Keep same distance between coracoid and ear.
- Keep shoulder blades wide.

Shoulder extension control

OBSERVATION AND ANALYSIS OF SHOULDER EXTENSION

Description of ideal pattern

Observe the natural patterns of thoraco-scapulohumeral motion through the full range of arm extension. Although both glenohumeral and scapula movement should occur simultaneously, the first phase should predominantly consist of glenohumeral extension with the scapula relatively stable through the first 15° of movement in extension. Medial rotation should not be excessive during extension. Some humeral anterior translation should start in this phase, but should not be excessive.

The second phase is dominated by retraction of the scapula. Thoracic flexion occurs towards the end of bilateral arm extension and thoracic rotation occurs towards the end of unilateral arm extension.

The scapula should not rotate downwardly or tilt forwards during concentric or eccentric movement and retraction should occur later in range. In full extension, no more than one-third of the anterior humeral head should protrude forward of the anterior edge of the acromion (Sahrmann 2002). Thoracic movement should not initiate or dominate arm extension (Figure 8.39).

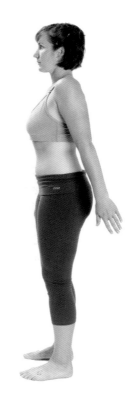

Figure 8.39 Shoulder extension

Movement faults associated with extension

Dysfunction of scapula-thoracic control

- *Uncontrolled scapular downward rotation.* Uncontrolled downward rotation may occur before the end of arm extension. This is observed with medial movement of the inferior angle as the arm moves behind midline trunk. This is associated with either length or recruitment changes in the scapular rotator muscles. There is noticeable dominance or shortening of the downward rotators (rhomboids, pectoralis minor and levator scapula) and poor stabilisation control of upward rotation (inefficient function of trapezius and serratus anterior).

- *Uncontrolled scapular retraction –* scapular retraction initiating or dominating glenohumeral extension. This is most frequently associated with a functional loss of extensibility of the posterior shoulder muscle (infraspinatus and teres minor) and the development of greater relative flexibility at the scapulothoracic joint. Instead of scapular retraction providing extra movement after the glenohumeral joint has completed extension, scapular retraction increases to compensate for the inefficient glenohumeral movement. In some instances the recruitment of scapular retraction is observed before the arm extends past the neutral midline of the trunk.

- *Uncontrolled scapular winging – true winging of the scapula.* Winging is observed with prominence of the entire medial border of the scapula lifting off the rib cage:

- During concentric elevation of the arm and at rest in static posture: associated with poor function of serratus anterior.
- During extension from a flexed position of the arm: timing problem associated with the scapulohumeral muscles not relaxing as quickly as the scapulothoracic muscles.
- During upper limb weight bearing in extension (e.g. push off the armrests of a chair): associated with inefficient medial scapular stabilisers and serratus anterior.

- *Uncontrolled scapular forward tilt – forward tilt of the scapula (or 'tipping' of the scapula).* Forward tilt is observed as prominence of the inferior angle of the scapula lifting off the lower rib cage and often combined with downward rotation of the scapula taking the glenoid into an anterior inferior position. This is most frequently associated with excessive shortness of pectoralis minor and downward rotation of the scapula with a concurrent loss of upward rotation position and poor control by lower trapezius and serratus anterior; and the development of greater relative flexibility at the scapulothoracic joint. Instead of scapular retraction providing extra movement after the glenohumeral joint has completed extension, scapular retraction increases to compensate for the inefficient glenohumeral movement.

Dysfunctions of glenohumeral control

- *Uncontrolled glenohumeral medial rotation.* During extension, uncontrolled medial rotation may occur. As a rough guide, the arm should be in neutral rotation (thumb forwards) when the hand rests by the side, and as the arm extends it should stay neutral and not medially rotate. Uncontrolled or excessive medial rotation is often associated with dominance of the latissimus dorsi.
- *Uncontrolled glenohumeral anterior translation.* Uncontrolled anterior translation of the humeral head often develops to compensate for a lack of glenohumeral extension or restricted glenohumeral lateral rotation during extension.

Indications to test for shoulder extension UCM

Observe or palpate for:

1. hypermobile extension range
2. excessive initiation of scapular compensation during shoulder extension
3. excessive glenohumeral translation during shoulder extension
4. symptoms (pain, discomfort, strain) associated with shoulder extension movements.

The person complains of extension-related symptoms in the shoulder. During shoulder extension load or movements, the scapula or glenohumeral joint has greater 'give' or compensation relative to the trunk or arm. The dysfunction is confirmed with motor control tests of shoulder extension dissociation.

Test of shoulder extension control

T64 ARM EXTENSION TEST (tests for scapula and glenohumeral UCM)

This dissociation test assesses the ability to actively dissociate and control scapula movement and glenohumeral translation and rotation during glenohumeral extension.

Test procedure

The subject stands with the arm resting by the side in neutral rotation (palm in towards the side) and with the scapula in a neutral position (Figure 8.40). The subject is instructed to keep the scapula and glenohumeral joint in the neutral position and move the arm through 15° of shoulder extension and return the arm back to the side (Figure 8.41). Ideally, the scapula should maintain the neutral position and not elevate or forward tilt during extension or drop into downward rotation or retract during the return back to the side. The glenohumeral joint should not demonstrate palpable anterior translation. The arm should increase medial rotation. It should start in neutral rotation (palm in) and should stay in neutral rotation throughout this movement.

Rating and diagnosis of shoulder girdle UCM

(T64.1 and T64.2)

Correction

Initial correction can be performed standing with the elbow flexed to reduce the arm lever length and decrease load, and with the scapula

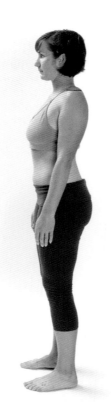

Figure 8.40 Start position arm extension test

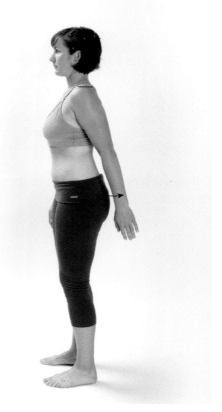

Figure 8.41 Benchmark arm extension test

T64.1 Assessment and rating of low threshold recruitment efficiency of the Arm Extension Test

ARM EXTENSION TEST

ASSESSMENT

Control point:
- prevent downward rotation, scapula forward tilt, winging, and retraction
- prevent glenohumeral anterior translation and medial rotation

Movement challenge: glenohumeral extension (standing – arm behind body)

Benchmark range: 15° glenohumeral extension

RATING OF LOW THRESHOLD RECRUITMENT EFFICIENCY

	✓ or ✗		✓ or ✗
• Able to prevent 'give' into the test direction. Correct dissociation pattern of movement Prevent scapula 'give' into: downward rotation forward tilt winging retraction Prevent glenohumeral 'give' into: anterior translation medial rotation and move glenohumeral extension	☐	• Looks easy, and in the opinion of the assessor, is performed with confidence	☐
		• Feels easy, and the subject has sufficient awareness of the movement pattern that they confidently prevent 'give' into the test direction	☐
• Dissociate movement through the benchmark range of 15° glenohumeral extension (arm behind body) *If there is more available range than the benchmark standard, only the benchmark range needs to be actively controlled*	☐	• The pattern of dissociation is smooth during concentric and eccentric movement	☐
		• Does not (consistently) use *end-range* movement into the opposite direction to prevent the give	☐
		• No extra feedback needed *(tactile, visual or verbal cueing)*	☐
• Without holding breath (though it is acceptable to use an alternate breathing strategy)	☐	• Without external support or unloading	☐
		• Relaxed natural breathing *(even if not ideal – so long as natural pattern does not change)*	☐
• Control during eccentric phase	☐	• No fatigue	☐
• Control during concentric phase	☐		

CORRECT DISSOCIATION PATTERN   **RECRUITMENT EFFICIENCY**

T64.2 Diagnosis of the site and direction of UCM from the Arm Extension Test

ARM EXTENSION TEST

Site	Direction	(L)	(R)
Scapula	Downward rotation	☐	☐
	Forward tilt	☐	☐
	Winging	☐	☐
	Retraction	☐	☐
Glenohumeral	Anterior translation	☐	☐
	Medial rotation	☐	☐

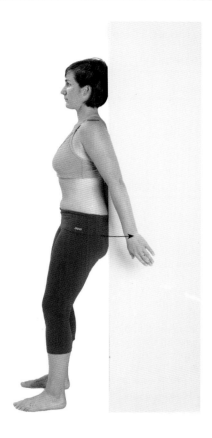

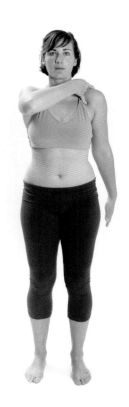

Figure 8.42 Correction with wall support at corner

Figure 8.43 Correction unsupported arm extension with self-palpation

supported by leaning against the corner of a wall (Figure 8.42). As control improves, the arm extension is performed unsupported through the partial range that can be controlled well with self-palpation. This is eventually progressed throughout the full benchmark range with the elbow straight (Figure 8.43).

An alternative progression is to use unilateral horizontal arm extension, initially with the scapula supported against a wall (Figure 8.44) and finally unsupported (Figure 8.45).

With visual, auditory and kinaesthetic cues the person becomes familiar with the task of extending the glenohumeral joint to 15° without scapula movement or glenohumeral translation. Some useful clinical cues are illustrated in Box 8.6.

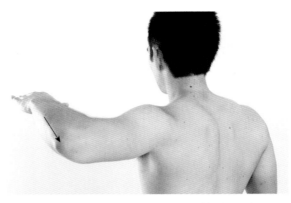

Figure 8.45 Correction using unsupported horizontal arm extension

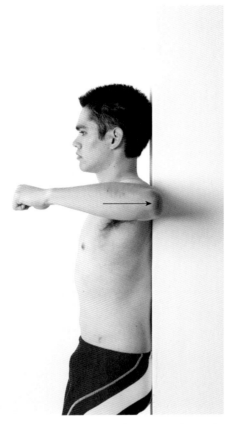

Figure 8.44 Correction using horizontal arm extension and wall support

Box 8.6 **Useful clinical facilitation and retraining cues**

Cues for facilitation and feedback to enhance teaching and retraining movement

- Palpate the scapula or glenohumeral joint to monitor the UCM.
- Imagery of lifting the shoulder blade as the arm lowers.
- Turn the hand (palm in) and keep palm in.
- Keep the coracoids open and wide.
- Palpate acromion/coracoid/inferior angle.
- Visualise a string holding the acromion up.
- Unload passively.
- Tape (proprioceptive skin tension).
- Keep same distance between coracoid and ear.
- Keep shoulder blades wide.

OTHER USEFUL DISSOCIATION MOVEMENTS FOR THE SHOULDER GIRDLE

As with all other regions, the principles of dissociation can be applied. The scapula and glenohumeral joint can be maintained in neutral and movement occurs above or below or in the same region, but in a different direction. Other tests, and subsequent retraining exercises, can be useful for individual cases and Table 8.5 illustrates some additional dissociation tests.

At this stage there is no definitive measurement or consistent peer consensus as to the benchmark ranges for these dissociation tests of UCM. The authors recommend that if symptoms are associated with these functional movements and the ability to control (or prevent) the site and direction of the UCM is poor, then retraining through the range that can be controlled is a useful clinical option.

Table 8.5 Potential additional tests for shoulder UCM

TEST (LINKED TO SYMPTOMATIC FUNCTION)	MOVEMENT CHALLENGE	CONTROL POINT – OBSERVE FOR AND PREVENT UCM (SITE AND DIRECTION)
Shoulder overhead reach	Arm flexion/abduction 90° to full overhead position (standing) (Figure 8.46)	• Scapula elevation • Glenohumeral inferior translation • Glenohumeral medial rotation
Shoulder forward reach	Protraction of scapula with arm in horizontal flexion (standing) (Figure 8.47)	• Scapula forward tilt • Scapula downward rotation • Glenohumeral medial rotation
Shoulder press off elbows	Shoulder protraction (prone weight bearing on elbows) (Figure 8.48)	• Scapula winging • Scapula forward tilt
Elbow straightening	Elbow flexion and extension with the upper arm by the side (standing)	• Glenohumeral anterior translation • Glenohumeral medial rotation
Forearm twist	Forearm supination (from a pronated position) with the upper arm by the side	• Scapula retraction • Scapula downward rotation
Neck flexion	Cervicothoracic flexion with the arms by the side (standing)	• Scapula downward rotation • Scapula forward tilt
Full head turn	Neck rotation with arms by side (sitting)	• Scapula elevation (ipsilateral shoulder) • Scapula retraction (ipsilateral shoulder) • Scapula forward tilt (ipsilateral shoulder) • Scapula downward rotation (ipsilateral shoulder)
Full chest turn	Thoracic rotation with arms by side (sitting)	• Scapula retraction (ipsilateral shoulder) • Scapula elevation (ipsilateral shoulder) • Scapula forward tilt (contralateral shoulder) • Scapula downward rotation (contralateral shoulder)

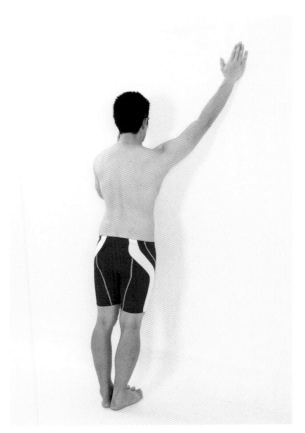

Figure 8.46 Correction with overhead arm abduction on wall

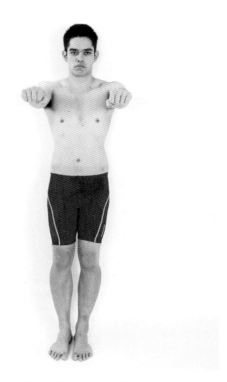

Figure 8.47 Correction with horizontal flexion

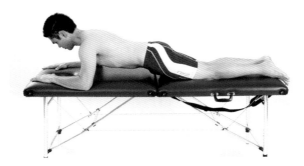

Figure 8.48 Correction with push-up off elbows

UCM AND PRESENTATION WITH IMPINGEMENT AND INSTABILITY

The primary site of UCM needs to be established with the tests. The UCM can present predominantly at glenohumeral or scapulothoracic joints. This can be identified with the kinetic medial rotation test. There are characteristic movement faults which are related to impingement and instability and these are described in Boxes 8.7 and 8.8. The rehabilitation of impingement is usually targeted at improving dynamic control of the scapula and control of glenohumeral medial rotation. The rehabilitation of instability is usually targeted at dynamic control of translation of the humerus and rotation control of the humerus.

Correction

Rehabilitation strategies directed at correcting the movement faults of the shoulder following evidence-based assessment, rather than diagnostic category of pathology alone, is gaining recognition as patients may present with a common diagnostic label but differing kinematic mechanisms. Altering movement patterns can influence shoulder signs (Caldwell et al 2007; Tate et al 2008), but it is important to establish a clear diagnosis of the movement faults and from this base implement an appropriate rehabilitation strategy.

Evidence shows physiotherapy does influence pain and disability around the shoulder and includes many differing modalities – ultrasound, acupuncture, manual therapy, and stretching to name a few (Ginn et al 1997; Johansson et al 2005; Nawoczenski et al 2006). There is substantial support for the effectiveness of exercise treatment programs emphasising scapula retraining (Ginn et al 1997; Nawoczenski et al 2006). It is clear that 'scapula stabilising' helps but therapists need to identify specific motor control deficits of the scapula. This can only be enhanced with a more thorough understanding of, and assessment of, movement faults so therapy can focus on individual needs. This can be classified as the diagnosis of mechanical shoulder dysfunction based on identifying the site and direction of UCM. The tests have been described in this chapter and, from these strategies for retraining, motor control of the shoulder girdle can be implemented. Based

---

Box 8.7 Movement faults related to impingement of the shoulder

Impingement assessment priorities

- Scapula UCM:
  - downward rotation
  - forward tilt
  - elevation
  - protraction
  - winging.
- Glenohumeral rotation timing UCM:
  - medial rotation (late or absent lateral rotation during abduction)
  - medial rotation (excessive medial rotation during eccentric flexion).
- Glenohumeral inferior translation – restriction:
  - restricted or limited inferior humeral head glide during abduction.

Box 8.8 Movement faults related to instability of the shoulder

Instability assessment priorities

- Glenohumeral UCM:
  - anterior translation
  - inferior translation
  - posterior translation
  - medial rotation.
  Passive:
  - damage or insidious laxity of capsular, ligamentous and labral restraints.
- Scapula UCM contributing to inappropriate orientation of the glenoid for optimal glenohumeral stability:
  - downward rotation
  - forward tilt
  - elevation
  - protraction
  - winging.

---

on the results of testing, the retraining needs to be prescriptive.

Retraining suggestions and options

There are many retraining strategies available to address UCM around the shoulder girdle. Critical to success is the patient understanding the movement fault and the therapist facilitating the

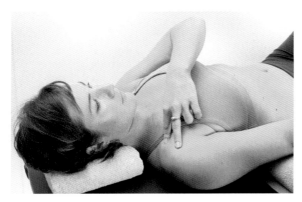

Figure 8.49 Feedback: self-palpation

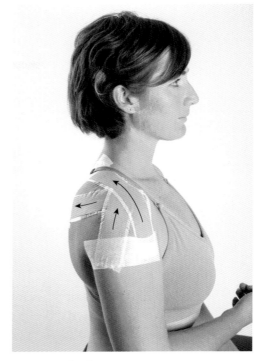

Figure 8.51 Feedback: tape

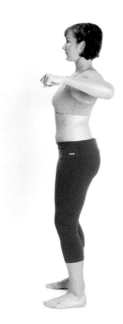

Figure 8.50 Feedback: short lever

appropriate pattern of control. Useful strategies for the shoulder include:

- palpation of the fault for feedback (e.g. Figure 8.49)
- shortening the lever (e.g. Figure 8.50)
- tape to enhance control of the movement fault (e.g. Figure 8.51)
- changing the start position to reduce limb load against gravity (e.g. Figure 8.52)
- using a wall for feedback and support (e.g. Figure 8.53).

Useful exercise options for retraining control of the scapula and glenohumeral joint movement are described in Boxes 8.9 and 8.10. Integrating control into functional tasks is essential. Principles and strategies to enhance functional integration are described in Chapter 4.

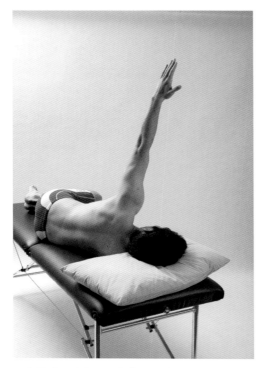

Figure 8.52 Retraining: reducing gravity moment arm

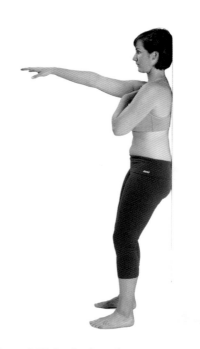

Figure 8.53 Feedback: wall support

Box 8.9 **Useful retraining exercises for scapular control**

- Dissociate flexion to 90° (Figure 8.54).
- Dissociate abduction to 90°+ rotation timing (Figure 8.55).
- Dissociate medial rotation – supine arm abducted 90° (Figure 8.56).
- Dissociate lateral rotation – standing arm by side (Figure 8.57).
- Dissociate extension to 15° + rotation timing (Figure 8.58).
- Dissociate lateral rotation – prone arm overhead (wrist lift) (Figure 8.59).
- Dissociate medial rotation – prone arm overhead (elbow lift) (Figure 8.60).
- Full range overhead movement – flexion and abduction (Figure 8.61).

Box 8.10 **Useful retraining exercise for glenohumeral control**

- Dissociate lateral rotation – standing arm by side (Figure 8.62).
- Dissociate medial rotation – supine arm abducted 90° (Figure 8.63).
- Dissociate extension to 15° (Figure 8.64).
- Dissociate lateral rotation – prone wrist lift (Figure 8.65).
- Dissociate medial rotation – prone elbow lift (Figure 8.66).
- Full range overhead movement – flexion and abduction (Figure 8.67).

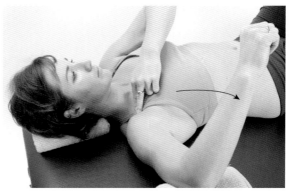

Figure 8.56 Dissociation medial rotation with palpation feedback of scapula

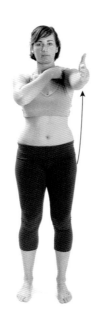

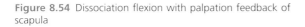

Figure 8.54 Dissociation flexion with palpation feedback of scapula

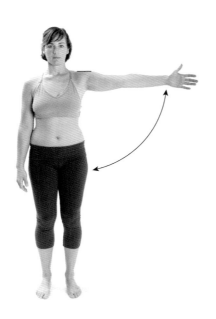

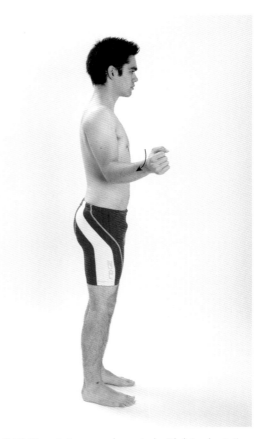

Figure 8.57 Dissociation scapula control with lateral rotation

Figure 8.55 Dissociation abduction with palpation feedback of scapula

407

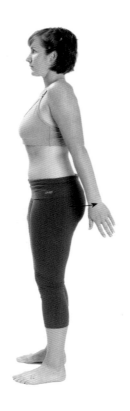

Figure 8.58 Dissociation scapula control with extension

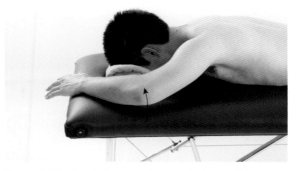

Figure 8.60 Dissociation scapula control with medial rotation overhead

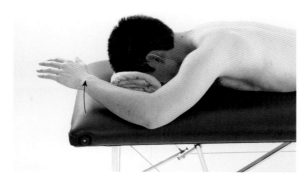

Figure 8.59 Dissociation scapula control with lateral rotation overhead

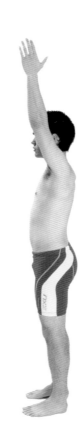

Figure 8.61 Dissociation scapula control with full range overhead flexion or abduction

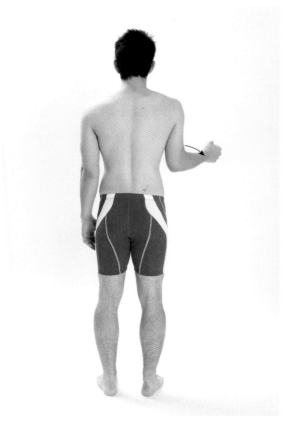

Figure 8.62 Dissociate lateral rotation standing

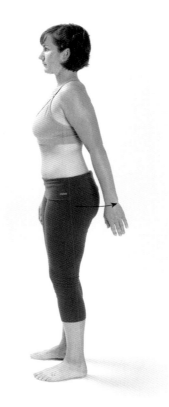

Figure 8.64 Dissociate extension standing

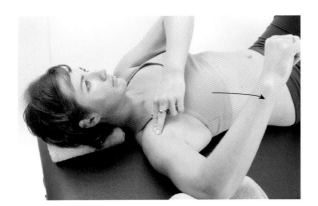

Figure 8.63 Dissociation medial rotation with palpation feedback of humeral head

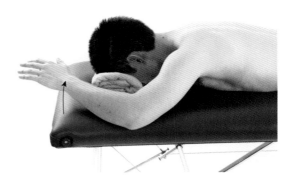

Figure 8.65 Dissociation lateral rotation overhead with humeral head control

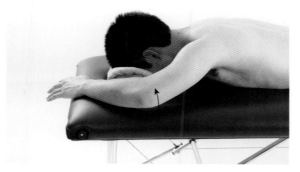

Figure 8.66 Dissociation medial rotation overhead with humeral head control

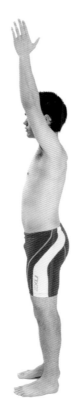

Figure 8.67 Dissociate full overhead flexion or abduction with humeral head control

Table 8.6 Summary and rating of shoulder girdle tests

UCM DIAGNOSIS AND TESTING

SITE	DIRECTION	CLINICAL PRIORITY ☐
TEST of stability control	**RATING** (✓✓ or ✓✗ or ✗✗) and rationale	
Scapula	Downward rotation	
Kinetic medial rotation test	(L)	(R)
Kinetic lateral rotation test		
Arm flexion test		
Arm abduction test		
Arm extension test		
Scapula	Forward tilt	
Kinetic medial rotation test	(L)	(R)
Kinetic lateral rotation test		
Arm flexion test		
Arm abduction test		
Arm extension test		
Scapula	Winging	
Arm flexion test	(L)	(R)
Arm abduction test		
Arm extension test		
Scapula	Elevation	
Kinetic medial rotation test	(L)	(R)
Arm flexion test		
Arm abduction test		
Scapula	Retraction	
Kinetic lateral rotation test	(L)	(R)
Arm extension test		
Scapula	Protraction/abduction	
Arm flexion test	(L)	(R)
Glenohumeral	Anterior translation	
Kinetic medial rotation test	(L)	(R)
Kinetic lateral rotation test		
Arm extension test		
Glenohumeral	Medial rotation	
Arm flexion test	(L)	(R)
Arm abduction test		
Arm extension test		

REFERENCES

Alexander, C.M., 2007. Altered control of the trapezius muscle in subjects with non-traumatic shoulder instability. Clinical Neurophysiology 118, 2664–2671.

Baeyens, J., Roy, P.V., Schepper, A.D., Declercq, G., Clarijs, J., 2001. Glenohumeral joint kinematics related to minor anterior instability of the shoulder at the end of the late preparatory phase of throwing. Clinical Biomechanics 16, 752–757.

Borstad, J.D., 2006. Resting position variables at the shoulder: evidence to support a posture-impairment association. Physical Therapy 86 (4), 549–557.

Borstad, J.D., Ludewig, P.M., 2005. The effects of long versus short pectoralis minor resting length on scapular kinematics in healthy individuals. Journal of Orthopaedic and Sports Physical Therapy 35, 227–238.

Caldwell, C., Sahrmann, S., Van Dillen, L., 2007. Use of a movement system impairment diagnosis for physical therapy in the management of a patient with shoulder pain. Journal of Orthopaedic and Sports Physical Therapy 37 (9), 551–563.

Comerford, M.J., Mottram, S.L., 2011. Diagnosis, subgroup classification and motor control retraining of the shoulder girdle. Kinetic Control, UK.

Cools, A.M., Witvrouw, E.E., Declercq, G.A., Danneels, L.A., Cambier, D.C., 2003. Scapular muscle recruitment patterns: trapezius muscle latency with and without impingement symptoms. American Journal of Sports Medicine 31, 542–549.

David, G., Magarey, M., Jones, M.A., Dvir, Z., Turker, K.S., Sharpe, M., 2000. EMG and strength correlates of selected shoulder muscles during rotations of the glenohumeral joint. Clinical Biomechanics 15, 95–102.

Falla, D., Farina, D., Graven-Nielsen, T., 2007. Experimental muscle pain results in reorganization of coordination among trapezius muscle subdivisions during repetitive shoulder flexion. Experimental Brain Research 178 (3), 385–393.

Ginn, K.A., Herbert, R.D., Khouw, W., Lee, R., 1997. A randomized, controlled clinical trial of a treatment for shoulder pain. Physical Therapy 77, 802–809.

Hess, S.A., Richardson, C., Darnell, R., Friis, P., Lisle, D., Myers, P., 2005. Timing of rotator cuff activation during shoulder external rotation in throwers with and without symptoms of pain. Journal of Orthopaedic and Sports Physical Therapy 35 (12), 812–820.

Huxel, K.C., Swanik, C.B., Swanik, K.A., Bartolozzi, A.R., Hillstrom, H.J., Sitler, M.R., et al., 2008. Stiffness regulation and muscle-recruitment strategies of the shoulder in response to external rotation perturbations. Journal of Bone and Joint Surgery. American volume 90 (1), 154–162.

Johansson, K.M., Adolfsson, L.E., Foldevi, M.O., 2005. Effects of acupuncture versus ultrasound in patients with impingement syndrome: randomized clinical trial. Physical Therapy 85, 490–501.

Kibler, B.W., Ludewig, P.M., McClure, P., Uhl, T.L., Sciascia, A., 2009. Scapular summit 2009. Journal of Orthopaedic and Sports Physical Therapy 39 (11), A1–A8.

Kibler, W.B., McMullen, J., 2003. Scapular dyskinesis and its relation to shoulder pain. Journal of the American Academy of Orthopedic Surgeons 11, 142–151.

Lin, J.J., Hanten, W.P., Olson, S.L., Roddey, T.S., Soto-quijano, D.A., Lim, H.K., et al., 2005. Functional activity characteristics of individuals with shoulder dysfunctions. Journal of Electromyography and Kinesiology 15, 576–586.

Lin, J., Hanten, W.P., Olson, S.L., Roddey, T.S., Soto-quijano, D.A., Lim, H.K., et al., 2006. Shoulder dysfunction, assessment: self-report and impaired scapular movements. Physical Therapy 86, 1065–1074.

Lucas, D., 1973. Biomechanics of the shoulder joint. Archives of Surgery 107, 425–432.

Ludewig, P.M., Cook, T.M., 2000. Alterations in shoulder kinematics and associated muscle activity in people with symptoms of shoulder impingement. Physical Therapy 80, 276–291.

Ludewig, P.M., Cook, T.A., 2002. Translations of the humerus in persons with shoulder impingement symptoms. Journal of Orthopaedic and Sports Physical Therapy 32, 248–259.

Lukasiewicz, A.C., McClure, P., Michener, L., Pratt, N.A., Sennett, B., 1999. Comparison of 3-dimensional scapular position and orientation between subjects with and without shoulder impingement. Journal of Orthopaedic and Sports Physical Therapy 29, 574–583.

Maitland, G., Hengeveld, E., Banks, K., English, K., 2005. Maitland's vertebral manipulation. Butterworth Heinemann, Oxford.

Moseley, J.B., Jobe, F.W., Pink, M., Perry, J., Tibone, J., 1992. EMG analysis of the scapula muscles during a shoulder rehabilitation program. American Journal of Sports Medicine 20 (2), 128–134.

Moraes, G.F., Faria, C.D., Teixeira-Salmela, L.F., 2008. Scapular muscle recruitment patterns and isokinetic strength ratios of the shoulder rotator muscles in individuals with and without impingement syndrome. Journal of Shoulder and Elbow Surgery 17, 48S–53S.

Morrissey, D., 2005. Development of the kinetic medial rotation test of the shoulder: a dynamic clinical test of shoulder instability and impingement. PhD thesis, University of London.

Morrissey, D., Morrissey, M.C., Driver, W., King, J.B., Woledge, R.C., 2008. Manual landmark identification and tracking during the medial rotation test of the shoulder: an accuracy study using three-dimensional ultrasound and motion analysis measures. Manual Therapy 13 (6), 529–535.

Mottram, S.L., 2003. Dynamic stability of the scapula. In: Beeton, K.S. (Ed.), Manual therapy masterclasses – the peripheral joints. Churchill Livingstone, Edinburgh, pp. 3–17.

Mottram, S., Warner, M., Chappell, P., Morrissey, D., Stokes, M., 2009a.

Impaired control of scapular rotation during a clinical dissociation test in people with a history of shoulder pain. 2009 3rd International Conference on Movement Dysfunction, Edinburgh, UK.

Mottram, S.L., Wolege, R., Morrissey, D., 2009b. Motion analysis study of a scapular orientation exercise and subjects' ability to learn the exercise. Manual Therapy 14 (1), 13–18.

Ogston, J.B., Ludewig, P.M., 2007. Differences in 3-dimensional shoulder kinematics between persons with multidirectional instability and asymptomatic controls. American Journal of Sports Medicine 35 (8), 1361–1370.

Nawoczenski, D.A., Clobes, S.M., Gore, S.L., Neu, J.L., Olsen, J.E., Borstad, J.D., et al., 2003. Three-dimensional shoulder kinematics during a pressure relief technique and wheelchair transfer. Archives of Physical Medicine and Rehabilitation 84, 1293–1300.

Nawoczenski, D.A., Ritter-Soronen, J.M., Wilson, C.M., Howe, B.A., Ludewig, P.M., 2006. Clinical trial of exercise for shoulder pain in chronic spinal injury. Physical Therapy 86 (12), 1604–1618.

Roy, J.-S., Moffet, H., McFadyen, B.J., 2008. Upper limb motor strategies in persons with and without shoulder impingement syndrome across different speeds of movement. Clinical Biomechanics 23 (10), 1227–1236.

Ruediger, M.O., von Eisenhart-Rothe, R.M., Jäger, A., Englmeier, K., Vogl, T., Graichen, H., 2002. Relevance of arm position and muscle activity on three-dimensional glenohumeral translation in patients with traumatic and atraumatic shoulder instability. American Journal of Sports Medicine 30, 514–522.

Saha, A.K., 1971. Dynamic stability of the glenohumeral joint. Acta Orthopaedica Scaninavica 42, 491–495.

Sahrmann, S.A., 2002. Diagnosis and treatment of movement impairment syndromes. Mosby, St Louis.

Schellingerhout, J.M., Verhagen, P.A., Thomas, S., Koes, B.W., 2008. Lack of uniformity in diagnostic labeling of shoulder pain: time for a different approach. Manual Therapy 13 (6), 478–483.

Tate, A.R., McClure, P., Kareha, S., Irwin, D., 2008. Effect of the scapula reposition test on shoulder impingement symptoms and elevation in overhead athletes. Journal of Orthopaedic and Sports Physical Therapy 38 (1), 4–11.

Tsai, N.-T., McClure, P.W., Karduna, A.R., 2003. Effects of muscle fatigue on 3-dimensional scapular kinematics. Archives of Physical Medicine and Rehabilitation 84, 1000–1005.

van der Helm, F.C.T., 1994. Analysis of the kinematic and dynamic behaviour of the shoulder mechanism. Journal of Biomechanics 27 (5), 527–550.

von Eisenhart-Rothe, R.M., Jäger, A., Englmeier, K.H., Vogl, T.J., Graichen, H., 2002. Relevance of arm position and muscle activity on three-dimensional glenohumeral translation in patients with traumatic and atraumatic shoulder instability. American Journal of Sports Medicine 30 (4), 514–522.

Wadsworth, D.J., Bullock-Saxton, J.E., 1997. Recruitment patterns of the scapular rotator muscles in freestyle swimmers with subacromial impingement. International Journal of Sports Medicine 18 (8), 618–624.

Walker-Bone, K., Palmer, K.T., Reading, I. Coggon, D. Cooper, C., 2004. Prevalence and impact of musculoskeletal disorders of the upper limb in the general population. Arthritis and Rheumatism 51, 642–651.

Wilk, K.E., Arrigo, C.A., Andrews, J.R., 1997. Current concepts: the stabilizing structures of the glenohumeral joint. Journal of Orthopaedic and Sports Physical Therapy 25 (6), 364–379.

CHAPTER 9
THE HIP

Chapter | 9 |

The hip

INTRODUCTION

The vast majority of hip pain referred to in the research and clinical literature primarily relates this pain to degenerative osteoarthritis (OA) of the hip. This pain usually originates from the groin with inconsistent patterns of radiation and referral of symptoms towards the trochanteric region and presents with varying degrees of movement restriction and loss of function. Simms (1999) states that hip pain is usually related to particular movements or sustained positions of the hip joint. Hip pain related to non-degenerative causes is largely under-reported in the literature. Hip pain from non-degenerative causes is often poorly diagnosed and frequently attributed to potential lumbar and sacroiliac referral mechanisms.

A clinical reasoning process is required to differentiate groin, trochanteric and buttock pain arising from the hip as opposed to that arising from the lumbar spine or sacroiliac joint (Sahrmann 2002; Lee 2011). Sahrmann (2002) and Lee (2001) both describe patterns of altered muscle function (or 'muscle imbalances') to classify hip dysfunction. They argue that the presence of these patterns of altered muscle function, when linked to painful or dysfunctional hip movements, can be used to diagnose and differentiate hip-related pain from lumbar or sacroiliac sources. A study comparing manual therapy (manipulation and mobilisation) with exercise therapy in osteoarthritis of the hip showed the manual

therapy program to be superior to the exercise therapy program (Hoeksma et al 2004). However, motor control issues were not specifically identified or addressed in this paper.

This chapter sets out to explore the assessment and retraining of uncontrolled movement (UCM) in the hip. Before details of the assessment and retraining of UCM in hip region are explained, a brief review of changes in muscle function and movement and control in the region is presented.

Changes in muscle function around the hip

Hardcastle & Nade (1985) state that one of the most consistent markers of hip dysfunction is the lack of lateral control of the hip and pelvis in single leg stance. Several studies have attempted to make links between hip joint pain and altered function of the gluteal muscles. The majority of these studies have focused on measuring weakness during strength tests. Strength deficits are commonly reported. Some studies have evaluated changes in muscle size and appearance with pain or altered muscle function. Arokoski et al (2002) showed that subjects with hip osteoarthritis (OA) had a decrease in abduction strength by as much as 31% compared to controls. The cross-sectional area (CSA) of the pelvic and thigh muscles, however, did not show significant differences between the two groups. Those with hip OA demonstrated a 13% decrease in the CSA of the gluteals and the adductors on the more severely affected hip as compared to the better hip. Interestingly, the decrease in CSA in the abductor and adductor muscles was not a direct indicator of muscle strength deficits.

Robinson et al (2005) presented a series of eight case reports of subjects with hip pain. All cases presented with a decrease of CSA in the piriformis, gemelli inferior, obturator externus or a combination of one or more of these muscles. Grimaldi et al (2009) evaluated changes in gluteus maximus and tensor fasciae latae (TFL) muscle volumes in subjects with unilateral hip joint pathology. Twelve subjects with hip joint pain ranging from labral pathology to advanced OA were evaluated by magnetic resonance imaging (MRI), in order to achieve a volume measurement, and compared to 12 control subjects. The MRI evaluation of gluteus maximus identified two functionally differentiated compartments within gluteus maximus: an upper (superficial lateral) compartment (UGM) and a lower (deep medial) compartment (LGM). Their results demonstrated the LGM had a significant decrease in volume related to pain and OA while the TFL and UGM, which insert into the iliotibial band, both maintained muscle bulk in the presence of OA hip pain. Findings such as this suggest that assessment of gross strength deficits per se may not adequately identify hip dysfunction.

Variations in the timing and sequencing of activation of various hip muscles have been reported by several authors. Many authors (Janda 1983; Long et al 1993; Sahrmann 2002) report changes in the neuromuscular coordination between TFL and gluteus medius (GMD). They demonstrate increased activity, earlier recruitment and loss of extensibility in TFL in some subjects. During a prone hip extension movement a delay in the activation of GMD or failure to maintain efficient holding tension in inner range has been reported (Janda 1983; Richardson & Sims 1991; Bullock-Saxton et al 1994; Sahrmann 2002; Lehman et al 2004).

UCM at the hip

Abnormal control of femoral translation and femoral rotation has been linked to anterior hip pain and pathologies of the labrum and associated hip capsule and anterior muscles (Sahrmann 2002; Lee 2001; Shindle et al 2006; Lewis et al 2007). The authors postulate that tissue loading and pathology results from a variety of biomechanical mechanisms, which include mechanical impingement, rotational strain and instability. Lewis et al (2007) developed a biomechanical model that found that decreased force contributions from the gluteal muscles (during hip extension) and decreased iliopsoas force (during hip flexion) resulted in an increase in anterior hip loading. They also reported that the hip loading was greater if the hip was positioned in extension to initiate these movements.

Sahrmann (2002) describes clinical tests to palpate for the presence of excessive or uncontrolled femoral head anterior glide during hip flexion and hip extension movements. Sahrmann (2002) postulates that the development of excessive hip medial rotation leads to abnormal loading on the anterior hip structures, which in turn results in hip pain and pathology. Levinger et al (2007) demonstrate excessive and uncontrolled hip medial rotation during a single leg squat. Lewis et al (2007) report that the hip demonstrates increased medial rotation if the iliopsoas force decreases and the TFL force increases, and that this 'imbalance' produces an excessive increase in anterior hip loading.

Mechanical dysfunctions of the hip commonly present as combinations of impingement, instability and rotational strain dysfunctions – all of which can develop into degenerative conditions. Motor control dysfunction within the hip local and global musculature contributes significantly to insidious onset, chronicity and recurrence of these hip problems. When symptoms arise from mechanical dysfunction in the regional tissues, consistent patterns of altered motor recruitment are evident. These recruitment patterns present as motor control inhibition of muscle function and motor imbalance. This chapter details the assessment of UCM at the hip region and describes retraining strategies.

DIAGNOSIS OF THE SITE AND DIRECTION OF UCM IN THE HIP

The diagnosis of the site and direction of UCM at the hip can be identified in terms of the *site* (being hip) and the *direction* of medial rotation, lateral rotation, flexion, extension and forwards glide (Box 9.1). As with all UCM, the motor control deficit can present as uncontrolled translational movement (e.g. forwards glide) or uncontrolled range of functional movement (e.g. hip flexion) (Sahrmann 2002).

Linking the site of UCM to symptom presentation

A diagnosis of UCM requires evaluation of its clinical priority. This is based on the relationship between the UCM and the presenting symptoms. The therapist should look for a link between the direction of UCM and the direction of symptom provocation: a) Does the site of UCM relate to the site or joint that the patient complains of as the source of symptoms? b) Does the direction of movement or load testing relate to the direction or position of provocation of symptoms? *This identifies the clinical priorities.*

The site and direction of UCM at the hip can be linked with different clinical presentations and postures and activities that provoke or produce symptoms (Table 9.1).

IDENTIFYING SITE AND DIRECTION OF UCM AT THE HIP

The key principles for assessment and classification of UCM are described in Chapter 3. All dissociation tests are performed with the hip in a mid-range neutral training region. However, this may be closer to end range but not at end range (e.g. close to extension while attempting to prevent flexion).

Segmental translatatory and global range-specific uncontrolled motion

When direction-specific, uncontrolled motion is observed at the hip, it can present in two ways. The uncontrolled motion can present as either a segmental translatatory UCM or a global range-specific UCM.

Segmental translatatory UCM

A segmental UCM occurs when the femoral head appears to 'glide forwards' into excessive anterior or anteroinferior translatatory displacement associated with flexion, extension or lateral rotation/abduction motion testing.

A segmental translatatory *femoral forwards glide* UCM (uncontrolled femoral head anterior translation) can be identified in motion testing in several ways:

- In sagittal plane movements (flexion or extension), palpation of the trochanter during passive hip movement is used to identify the location of the neutral axis of hip motion. The ability to maintain the neutral axis and prevent excessive forwards glide of the trochanter during active unassisted flexion or extension is compared with the passive evaluation.
- In axial plane movements (lateral rotation and abduction), palpation of the anterior prominence of the femoral head during passive movement with manual stabilisation is used to identify the location of the neutral axis of hip motion. The ability to maintain the neutral axis and prevent excessive forwards glide of the anterior prominence of the femoral head during active unassisted lateral rotation and abduction is compared with the passive evaluation.

Global range-specific UCM

A global range-specific UCM demonstrates uncontrolled motion (±hypermobile range) into hip flexion or into hip extension. This is observed as either excessive or dominant hip motion at the initiation of the movement or hypermobile range of hip motion to complete the movement.

A global range-specific *hip flexion* UCM can be identified in motion testing in several ways:

- Observe or palpate excessive or hypermobile range of hip flexion. During the test movement, the therapist relies on visual observation or manual palpation to identify if the subject cannot control (prevent or eliminate) additional hip flexion. The subject demonstrates an

417

Table 9.1 The link between the site and direction of UCM at the hip and different clinical presentations

SITE AND DIRECTION OF UCM	SYMPTOM PRESENTATION	PROVOCATIVE MOVEMENTS, POSTURES AND ACTIVITIES
HIP FLEXION UCM Can present as: • uncontrolled hip flexion (with or without hypermobile range) • uncontrolled forward glide of the femoral head (segmental anterior translation) during open chain hip flexion • unilaterally or bilaterally	• Presents with symptoms in the groin, lateral hip (trochanteric region) or posterior lateral buttock • May present with a segmental localised pain pattern • ± Radicular pain from myofascial and articular structures	Symptoms provoked by hip flexion movements and postures (especially if repetitive or sustained); for example, sustained sitting (especially if leaning forwards at a desk), bending forwards, driving, squatting, knee lift activities (e.g. stair climbing and walking up hills)
HIP EXTENSION UCM Can present as: • uncontrolled hip extension (with or without hypermobile range) • uncontrolled forward glide of the femoral head (segmental anterior translation) during hip extension • unilaterally or bilaterally	• Presents with symptoms in the groin, lateral hip (trochanteric region) or posterior lateral buttock • May present with a segmental localised pain pattern • ± Radicular pain from myofascial and articular structures	Symptoms provoked by hip extension movements and postures (especially if repetitive or sustained); for example, sustained standing arching backwards, lifting, lying prone, walking or running (especially down hills)
HIP ROTATION UCM Can present as: • uncontrolled hip medial rotation or lateral rotation/abduction (with or without hypermobile range) • uncontrolled forward glide of the femoral head (segmental anterior translation) during hip lateral rotation • unilaterally or bilaterally	• Presents with symptoms in the groin, lateral hip (trochanteric region) or posterior lateral buttock • May present with a segmental localised pain pattern • ± Radicular pain from myofascial and articular structures	Symptoms provoked by hip rotation movements and postures (especially if repetitive or sustained); for example, sustained standing (especially if weight shift onto leg in adduction and medial rotation), jumping or stepping down onto one leg, sustained sitting (especially if cross-legged), bending forwards or squatting with knees jammed together
HIP ADDUCTION UCM Can present as: • uncontrolled hip adduction (with or without hypermobile range) • uncontrolled forward glide of the femoral head (segmental anterior translation) during hip adduction • unilaterally or bilaterally	• Presents with symptoms in the groin, lateral hip (trochanteric region) or posterior lateral buttock • May present with a segmental localised pain pattern • ± Radicular pain from myofascial and articular structures	Symptoms provoked by hip adduction movements and postures (especially if repetitive or sustained); for example, sustained sitting (especially if legs are crossed), sustained standing (especially if weight shift onto leg in adduction), stepping down onto one leg

inability to prevent movement into further hip flexion when instructed to prevent flexion.
• Observe or palpate that during a functional multi-joint movement into flexion, hip flexion dominates the initiation of the movement pattern. The subject demonstrates an inability to reverse this pattern. They cannot easily initiate the movement with thoracolumbar flexion or lower leg flexion when instructed to do so.
• Place a long piece of adhesive strapping tape across the posterior hip (e.g. from the posterior superior iliac spine (PSIS) to the upper portion of the posterior thigh), with the hip positioned in an extension position relevant to the specific test. By skin tensioning from the lowermost attachment

(below) to the uppermost attachment, if the subject cannot prevent or control hip flexion, the tape pulls off the skin when uncontrolled flexion motion is produced.

A global range-specific *hip extension* UCM can be identified in motion testing in several ways:

- Observe or palpate excessive or hypermobile range of hip extension. During the test movement, the therapist relies on visual observation or manual palpation to identify if the subject cannot control (prevent or eliminate) additional hip extension. The subject demonstrates an inability to prevent movement into further hip extension when instructed to prevent extension.
- Observe or palpate that during a functional multi-joint movement into extension, hip extension dominates the initiation of the movement pattern. The subject demonstrates an inability to reverse this pattern. They cannot easily initiate the movement with thoracolumbar extension or lower leg extension when instructed to do so.
- Place a long piece of adhesive strapping tape across the anterior hip (e.g. from the anterior superior iliac spine (ASIS) to the upper portion of the anterior thigh) with the hip positioned in a flexion position relevant to the specific test. By skin tensioning from the lowermost attachment (below) to the uppermost attachment, if the subject cannot prevent or control hip extension, the tape pulls off the skin when uncontrolled extension motion is produced.

A global range-specific *hip medial rotation* UCM can be identified in motion testing in several ways:

- Observe or palpate excessive or hypermobile range of hip medial rotation. During the test movement, the therapist relies on visual observation or manual palpation to identify if the subject cannot control (prevent or eliminate) additional hip medial rotation. The subject demonstrates an inability to prevent movement into further hip medial rotation when instructed to prevent rotation.
- Observe or palpate that during a functional multi-joint movement into rotation, hip medial rotation dominates the initiation of

the movement pattern. The subject demonstrates an inability to reverse this pattern. They cannot easily initiate the movement with thoracolumbar rotation or lower leg rotation when instructed to do so.

- Place a long piece of adhesive strapping tape across the lateral hip (e.g. from the posterior iliac crest to the medial portion of the anterior thigh) with the hip positioned in a lateral rotation position relevant to the specific test. By skin tensioning from the lowermost attachment (below) to the uppermost attachment, if the subject cannot prevent or control hip medial rotation, the tape pulls off the skin when uncontrolled motion is produced.

A global range-specific *hip lateral rotation/ abduction* UCM can be identified in motion testing in several ways:

- Observe or palpate excessive or hypermobile range of hip lateral rotation or abduction. During the test movement, the therapist relies on visual observation or manual palpation to identify if the subject cannot control (prevent or eliminate) additional hip lateral rotation or abduction. The subject demonstrates an inability to prevent movement into further hip lateral rotation/ abduction when instructed to prevent this movement.
- Observe or palpate that during a functional multi-joint movement into rotation, hip lateral rotation or abduction dominates the initiation of the movement pattern. The subject demonstrates an inability to reverse this pattern. They cannot easily initiate the movement with thoracolumbar rotation or lower leg rotation when instructed to do so.
- Place a long piece of adhesive strapping tape across the medial hip (e.g. from the inguinal ligament and anterior iliac crest to the lateral portion of the posterior thigh) with the hip positioned in a medial rotation and adduction position (relevant to the specific test). By skin tensioning from the lowermost attachment (below) to the uppermost attachment, if the subject cannot prevent or control hip lateral rotation and abduction, the tape pulls off the skin when uncontrolled motion is produced.

419

Occasionally, both segmental translatatory forwards glide and global range-specific dysfunctions can present together.

Examples

Hip flexion UCM

The patient complains of flexion-related symptoms in the hip region (groin, lateral hip or posterolateral buttock). The hip demonstrates UCM *into flexion* relative to the lower leg or thoracolumbar spine under flexion load. During a motor control test of active lower leg or thoracolumbar flexion where the instruction is to prevent hip flexion (dissociation), the hip demonstrates UCM into either:

- *global hip flexion* – uncontrolled flexion during active lower leg flexion or thoracolumbar flexion dissociation tests

or

- *segmental hip forwards glide* – uncontrolled segmental anterior translation of the femoral head during active hip flexion.

Hip extension UCM

The patient complains of extension-related symptoms in the hip region (groin, lateral hip or posterolateral buttock). The hip demonstrates UCM *into extension* relative to the lower leg or thoracolumbar spine under extension load. During a motor control test of active lower leg or thoracolumbar extension where the instruction is to prevent hip extension (dissociation), the hip demonstrates UCM into either:

- *global hip extension* – uncontrolled extension during active lower leg extension or thoracolumbar extension dissociation tests

or

- *segmental hip forwards glide* – uncontrolled segmental anterior translation of the femoral head during active hip extension.

Hip medial rotation UCM

The patient complains of rotation-related symptoms in the hip region (groin, lateral hip or posterolateral buttock). The hip demonstrates UCM *into medial rotation* relative to the lower leg or thoracolumbar spine under rotation load. During a motor control test of active lower leg or thoracolumbar rotation where the instruction is to

prevent hip medial rotation (dissociation), the hip demonstrates UCM into either:

- *global hip medial rotation* – uncontrolled medial rotation during active unilateral lower leg movement or thoracolumbar rotation dissociation tests

or

- *segmental hip forwards glide* – uncontrolled segmental anterior translation of the femoral head during active hip medial rotation.

Hip lateral rotation/abduction UCM

The patient complains of rotation-related symptoms in the hip region (lateral hip or posterolateral buttock ± groin). The hip demonstrates UCM *into lateral rotation or abduction* relative to the lower leg or thoracolumbar spine under rotation load. During a motor control test of active lower leg or thoracolumbar rotation where the instruction is to prevent hip lateral rotation and abduction (dissociation), the hip demonstrates UCM into either:

- *global hip lateral rotation/abduction* – uncontrolled lateral rotation or abduction during active unilateral lower leg movement or thoracolumbar rotation dissociation tests

or

- *segmental hip forwards glide* – uncontrolled segmental anterior translation of the femoral head during active hip lateral rotation/ abduction or 'turnout' movements.

Hip adduction UCM

The patient complains of adduction-related symptoms in the hip region (groin, lateral hip or posterolateral buttock). The hip demonstrates UCM *into adduction* relative to the lower leg or thoracolumbar spine under rotation load. During a motor control test of active lower leg weight bearing or thoracolumbar side-bend where the instruction is to prevent hip adduction (dissociation), the hip demonstrates UCM into either:

- *global hip adduction* – uncontrolled medial rotation during active unilateral lower leg weight bearing or thoracolumbar side-bend dissociation tests

or

- *segmental hip forwards glide* – uncontrolled segmental anterior translation of the femoral head during active adduction rotation.

HIP TESTS FOR UCM

Hip sagittal motion control

OBSERVATION AND ANALYSIS OF SAGITTAL HIP FLEXION AND BENDING

Several functional movement patterns can identify movement faults associated with hip flexion. These include observing and analysing the relative hip contributions to:

1. natural or 'automatic' forwards bending
2. natural rocking backwards on to hips in 4 point kneeling
3. supine passive hip flexion
4. natural small knee bend.

Description of ideal pattern of forwards bending

The subject is instructed to stand with the feet in a natural stance and bend forwards in a normal relaxed pattern. Ideally, there should be even flexion throughout the lumbar and thoracic regions with the hips flexing to approximately to 70°. The spinal flexion and hip flexion should occur concurrently. The fingertips should reach the floor without the need to bend the knees (Figure 9.1).

There should be good symmetry of movement without any lateral deviation, tilt or rotation of the trunk or pelvis. The pelvis and hips should lead the return to standing with the spine unrolling on the way back to the upright posture.

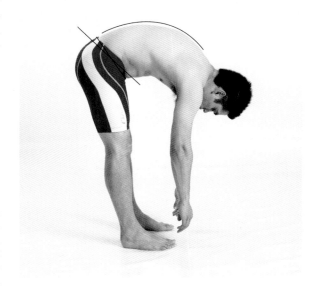

Figure 9.1 Ideal pattern of forward bending

Movement faults associated with hip UCM in forwards bending

Relative stiffness (restrictions)

- *Thoracolumbar restriction of flexion*: thoracic or lumbar flexion restriction may also contribute to compensatory increases in hip flexion range. This is confirmed with manual assessment of hip flexion range.
- *Gastrocnemius or talocrural joint restriction of ankle dorsiflexion*: the ankle lacks normal range of dorsiflexion in standing forwards bending. The hip frequently may increase flexion to compensate for the lack of ankle mobility. Gastrocnemius extensibility can be tested passively and dynamically with manual muscle extensibility examination and restrictions of talocrural joint dorsiflexion can be confirmed with manual assessment of joint mobility.

Relative flexibility (potential UCM)

- *Hip flexion*: the hip may initiate the movement into flexion; contribute more to producing forward bending while the thoracolumbar contributions start later and contribute less. At the limit of forwards bending, excessive or hypermobile range of hip flexion may be observed. During the return to neutral the hip flexion persists and unrolls late.

421

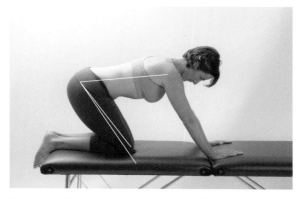

Figure 9.2 Ideal pattern of backward rocking

Description of ideal pattern of backward rocking (hands and knees 4 point kneeling)

With the subject on hands and knees and the spine and pelvis in neutral alignment, place the knees hip width apart. The subject is instructed to rock backwards towards their heels. Monitor pelvic motion with one hand placed on the sacrum to identify the point of initiation of posterior pelvic tilt. This point identifies the limit of hip flexion range as the posterior hip structures are tensioned and pull the pelvis into posterior tilt. Ideally, the person should have the ability to dissociate the lumbar spine and pelvis from hip flexion as evidenced by 120° of hip flexion during backward rocking while preventing lumbar flexion or posterior pelvic tilt (Figure 9.2). After 120° hip flexion the pelvis should start to tilt posteriorly and the spine should start to flex as the pelvis moves towards the heels.

Movement faults associated with hip UCM in backward rocking

Relative stiffness (restrictions)

* *Thoracolumbar restriction of flexion*: thoracic or lumbar flexion restriction may also contribute to compensatory increases in hip flexion range. Soleus extensibility can be tested passively and dynamically with manual muscle extensibility examination, and restrictions of talocrural joint dorsiflexion can be confirmed with manual assessent of joint mobility.

Relative flexibility (potential UCM)

* *Hip flexion*: the hip may initiate the movement into flexion; contribute more to producing rocking backwards while the thoracolumbar contributions start later and contribute less. Greater than 120° of hip flexion range is observed during backward rocking before any posterior pelvic tilt or lumbar flexion is produced. The person can almost sit back onto their heels using excessive hip flexion while maintaining a straight lumbar spine.

Description of ideal pattern of supine passive hip flexion

With the person lying supine, place one hand under the lumbar lordosis to monitor pelvic tilt. Flex one hip and knee up in the neutral sagittal plane. Ideally, the person should have 120° of hip flexion independently of pelvic tilt and spinal motion. After 120° hip flexion the pelvis should start to tilt posteriorly and the spine should start to flex. Greater than 120° of hip flexion range before any posterior pelvic tilt or lumbar flexion is produced, indicates excessive relative hip flexion.

Description of ideal pattern of small knee bend (SKB)

The person stands upright with the feet hip width apart (heels approximately 10–15 cm apart) with the inside borders of the feet parallel (not turned out) and the 2nd metatarsal aligned along the 'neutral line' of weight transfer (a line that is 10° lateral to the sagittal plane). Perform a bilateral small knee bend (SKB) by flexing at the knees and dorsiflexing the ankles while keeping the heels on the floor. Hold the knee out over the foot to orientate the line of the femur out over the 2nd toe (on the 'neutral line') (Figure 9.3).

The knees are to bend as far as the heels can stay on the floor and correct rotational alignment is maintained. Ideally, the trunk should stay vertical (as if sliding down a wall) and the knees flex so that a vertical plumb line dropped from the front of the knees should fall 3–8 cm past the longest toes, without any hip medial rotation or midfoot pronation (Figure 9.4). Body weight should stay equally distributed on each foot and there should be no lateral shift of the pelvis.

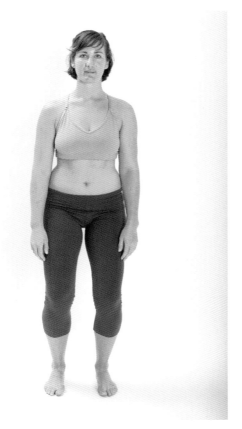

Figure 9.3 Ideal small knee bend front view

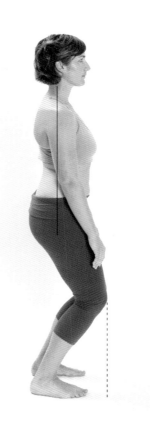

Figure 9.4 Ideal small knee bend side view

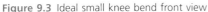

Sagittal movement faults associated with hip UCM in the SKB

Relative stiffness (restrictions)

- *Knee and ankle restriction of flexion/dorsiflexion*: a restriction of ankle dorsiflexion or knee flexion may contribute to compensatory increases in hip flexion range. This is confirmed with manual assessment of hip flexion range.

Relative flexibility (potential UCM)

- *Hip flexion*: the natural pattern of movement is that the hips initiate the movement and contribute more to producing the SKB while the ankle and knee contributions start later and contribute less. Observe that the trunk leans forwards into hip flexion. With a SKB

on correct rotational alignment the knees do not move sufficiently past the toes.

Hip and lower quadrant sagittal alignment evaluation

- Stand in neutral foot alignment with correct tibial rotational alignment (2nd metatarsal on the neutral line of weight transfer).
- Perform a SKB (in weight bearing, flex the knees and dorsiflex the ankles while keeping both heels on the floor).
- Control femoral rotational alignment (femurs of neutral line of weight transfer).
- Knee bend as far as the heels can stay on the floor.

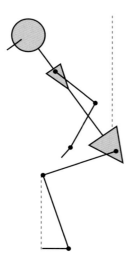

Figure 9.5 Sagittal alignment group 2 – hip flexion dysfunction: excessive hip flexion relative to limited knee and ankle movement

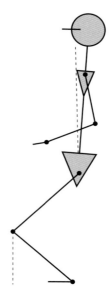

Figure 9.6 Sagittal alignment group 3 – lower leg flexion dysfunction: limited hip flexion relative to excessive knee and ankle movement

- Observe the relative sagittal alignment of hip, knee and ankle in the natural pattern (without cueing and alignment correction).

IDEAL SAGITTAL ALIGNMENT

The long axis of the femur and the 2nd metatarsal are both aligned to the lower limb neutral line (a line 10° lateral to the sagittal plane) (Figure 9.4).

Dysfunction

- With a SKB on correct alignment the knees do not move sufficiently past the toes. The knee alignment is less than 3 cm past the toe. It is common for the knees to only move as far as the metatarsal heads. To maintain functional ability to bend down, hip flexion significantly increases as uncontrolled compensation. The subject cannot correct the pattern or finds it very difficult to correct. Many do not realise that the hips are 'hanging out the back' and often believe that the trunk is vertical when it is obviously inclined forwards.
- With a SKB on correct alignment the knees do not move sufficiently past the toes. The knee alignment is greater than 8 cm past

the toes. Hip flexion significantly decreases. The subject cannot correct the pattern or finds it very difficult to correct. The trunk is often inclined backwards to maintain balance.

Sagittal alignment can be classified into one of three groups:

1. Ideal (Figure 9.4):
   a. plumb line dropped from the front of knee falls between 3 and 8 cm in front of toes.
2. Hip flexion dysfunction (Figure 9.5):
   a. plumb line dropped from the front of the knee falls less than 3 cm in front of the toes
   b. relatively restricted knee flexion and ankle dorsiflexion
   c. relatively excessive or uncontrolled hip flexion
   d. the trunk leans forwards from vertical (more hip flexion than ideal) to keep the centre of mass balanced over the midfoot.
3. Lower leg flexion dysfunction (Figure 9.6):
   a. plumb line dropped from the front of the knee falls more than 8 cm in front of the toes
   b. relatively restricted hip flexion

c. relatively excessive or uncontrolled hip flexion and ankle dorsiflexion

d. the trunk leans backwards from vertical (more hip extension than ideal) to keep the centre of mass balanced over the midfoot.

HIP FLEXION CONTROL TESTS AND FLEXION CONTROL REHABILITATION

These flexion control tests assess the extent of flexion UCM in the hip and assess the ability of the dynamic stability system to adequately control flexion load or strain. It is a priority to assess for flexion UCM if the patient complains of or demonstrates flexion-related symptoms or disability.

The tests that identify dysfunction can also be used to guide and direct rehabilitation strategies.

Indications to test for hip flexion UCM

Observe or palpate for:

1. hypermobile hip flexion range
2. excessive initiation of bending or leaning forwards with hip flexion
3. symptoms (pain, discomfort, strain) associated with bending or leaning forwards or sustained hip flexion postures.

The person complains of flexion-related symptoms in the hip. Under flexion load, the hip has greater give *into flexion* relative to the trunk and lower leg. The dysfunction is confirmed with motor control tests of flexion dissociation.

425

Hip flexion control tests

T65 STANDING: VERTICAL TRUNK SINGLE LEG ¼ SQUAT TEST (tests for hip flexion UCM)

This dissociation test assesses the ability to actively dissociate and control hip flexion and perform a single leg ¼ squat – small knee bend (SKB) by flexing the knee and dorsiflexing the ankle while in single leg standing.

Test procedure

The person stands with the feet hip width apart (heels approximately 10–15 cm apart) with the inside borders of the feet parallel (not turned out). The upper body should be vertical and the weight balanced over the midfoot. The person is asked to shift full weight onto one foot and lift the other foot just clear of the floor. In this position, the person is standing on one leg with the 2nd metatarsal aligned along the 'neutral line' of weight transfer (a line that is 10° lateral to the sagittal plane). The pelvis should be level and the trunk upright (vertical). There should be no lateral deviation, tilt or rotation of the trunk or pelvis. The head, sternum and pubic symphysis should be vertically aligned above the inside edge of the stance foot with the shoulders level in an upright posture (Figure 9.7).

From this start position, the person then performs a single leg small knee bend (SKB) by flexing at the knee and dorsiflexing the ankle while keeping the heel on the floor. The body weight should be on the heel, not the ball, of the foot and the trunk kept vertical (as if sliding the back down a wall). Do not lean the trunk forwards. Hold the knee out over the foot to orientate the line of the femur out over the 2nd toe (on the 'neutral line') (Figures 9.8 and 9.9). The trunk should stay vertical (as if sliding down a wall) and the knee should move past the toes. If a plumb line were dropped from the front of the knee it should fall between 3 and 8 cm in front of the longest toe. Ideally, there should be approximately 3–8 cm of independent SKB past the toes, without any forwards lean of the trunk or posterior shift of the hips and pelvis into increased hip flexion.

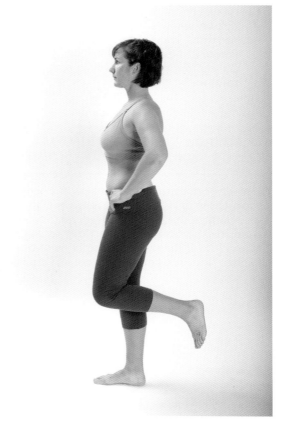

Figure 9.7 Start position vertical trunk single leg ¼ squat test

This test should be performed without any feedback (self-palpation, vision, etc.) or cueing for correction. When feedback is removed for testing the therapist should use visual observation of the femur and trunk to determine whether the control of hip flexion is adequate. Assess both legs separately.

Hip flexion UCM

The person complains of pain in the hip (groin impingement, lateral trochanteric or posterolateral buttock pain) associated with hip flexion activities. During the vertical trunk ¼ squat test, the hip demonstrates UCM into flexion (the trunk leans forwards and the hips move backwards into excessive hip flexion) before the knee reaches 3–8 cm past the toes. Under weight

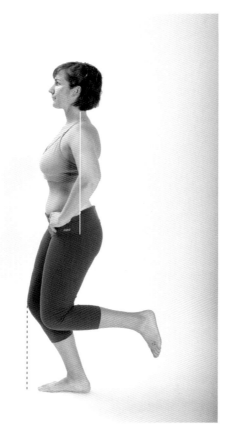
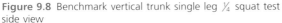

Figure 9.8 Benchmark vertical trunk single leg ¼ squat test side view

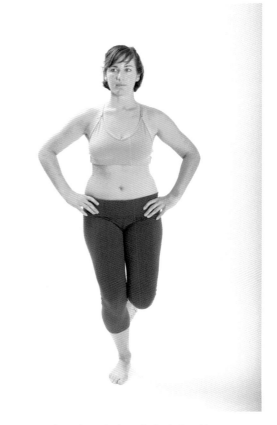

Figure 9.9 Benchmark vertical trunk single leg ¼ squat test front view

bearing knee flexion and ankle dorsiflexion, the hip has UCM *into flexion* relative to the knee and ankle. Hip flexion control is poor if the subject is unable to prevent or resist the excessive hip flexion.

The uncontrolled hip flexion is often associated with inefficiency of the stability function of the gluteal extensor muscles (especially deep gluteus maximus) which provide isometric or eccentric control of hip flexion. During the attempt to dissociate the hip flexion from knee flexion and ankle dorsiflexion, the person either cannot control the UCM or has to concentrate and try hard to control the hip flexion. The movement must be assessed on both sides. If hip flexion UCM presents bilaterally, one side may be better or worse than the other.

Clinical assessment note for direction-specific motor control testing

If some other movement (e.g. a small amount of rotation) is observed during a motor control (dissociation) test of flexion control, *do not* score this as uncontrolled flexion. The rotation motor control tests will identify whether the observed movement is uncontrolled. *A test for hip flexion UCM is only positive if uncontrolled hip flexion is demonstrated.*

Rating and diagnosis of hip flexion UCM

(T65.1 and T65.2)

Correction

Initial retraining is best started with the trunk supported against a wall. The person stands with the back against a wall and the feet hip width apart (heels approximately 10–15 cm apart) with the inside borders of the feet parallel. The person is asked to stand upright with the upper body vertical and the weight balanced over the midfoot. The heels should be approximately 5–10 cm from the wall. The pelvis should be level and the trunk upright (vertical against the wall) (Figure 9.10). If control is poor, perform a SKB by sliding the trunk down the wall to a ¼ squat position. The person should keep the back on the wall and weight balanced equally on both feet. Only slide down the wall as far as the trunk can stay on the wall and do not lean forwards into increased hip flexion.

As control improves, the person is instructed to shift their weight to stand on one leg and perform a single leg SKB to the ¼ squat position. Keep the trunk vertical on the wall and the knee should move past the toes. Only slide down the wall as far as the trunk can stay on the wall and do not lean forwards into increased hip flexion (Figure 9.11). At the point in range that the trunk starts to lean forwards into hip flexion or the knee moves medially to allow compensation at the foot and ankle, the movement should stop and return to the start position. The person should self-monitor the hip and trunk alignment and control hip flexion UCM with a variety of feedback options (T65.3). There should be no provocation of any symptoms within the range that the hip flexion UCM can be controlled.

As the ability to control hip flexion and forwards lean of the trunk gets easier and the pattern of dissociation feels less unnatural, the exercise can be progressed to performing this same movement unsupported, without the wall, in single leg stance.

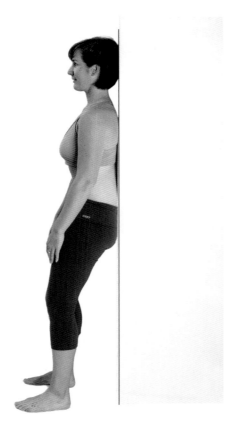

Figure 9.10 Correction bilateral small knee bend with wall support

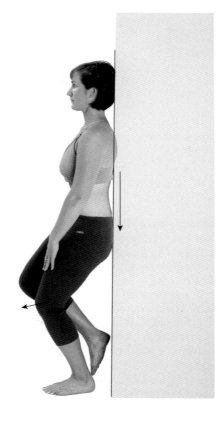

Figure 9.11 Correction unilateral small knee bend with wall support

T65.1 Assessment and rating of low threshold recruitment efficiency of the Vertical Trunk Single Leg ¼ Squat Test

VERTICAL TRUNK SINGLE LEG ¼ SQUAT – STANDING

ASSESSMENT

Control point:
- prevent hip flexion

Movement challenge: unilateral knee flexion and ankle dorsiflexion (standing)

Benchmark range: knee flexion 3–8 cm past toes with trunk upright

RATING OF LOW THRESHOLD RECRUITMENT EFFICIENCY FOR CONTROL OF DIRECTION

	✓ or ✗		✓ or ✗
• Able to prevent UCM into the test direction Correct dissociation pattern of movement Prevent hip UCM into: • flexion and move single leg knee flexion and ankle dorsiflexion	☐	• Looks easy, and in the opinion of the assessor, is performed with confidence	☐
		• Feels easy, and the subject has sufficient awareness of the movement pattern that they confidently prevent UCM into the test direction	☐
• Dissociate movement through the benchmark range of: knee flexion to 3–8 cm past toes with trunk upright in ¼ squat *If there is more available range than the benchmark standard, only the benchmark range needs to be actively controlled*	☐	• The pattern of dissociation is smooth during concentric and eccentric movement	☐
		• Does not (consistently) use *end-range* movement into the opposite direction to prevent the UCM	☐
		• No extra feedback needed *(tactile, visual or verbal cueing)*	☐
• Without holding breath (though it is acceptable to use an alternate breathing strategy)	☐	• Without external support or unloading	☐
		• Relaxed natural breathing *(even if not ideal – so long as natural pattern does not change)*	☐
• Control during eccentric phase	☐	• No fatigue	☐
• Control during concentric phase	☐		

CORRECT DISSOCIATION PATTERN   **RECRUITMENT EFFICIENCY**

T65.2 Diagnosis of the site and direction of UCM from the Vertical Trunk Single Leg ¼ Squat Test

VERTICAL TRUNK SINGLE LEG ¼ SQUAT TEST – STANDING

Site	Direction	(L) leg	(R) leg
		(check box)	(check box)
Hip	Flexion	☐	☐

T65.3 Feedback tools to monitor retraining

FEEDBACK TOOL	PROCESS
Self-palpation	Palpation monitoring of joint position
Visual observation	Observe in a mirror or directly watch the movement
Adhesive tape	Skin tension for tactile feedback
Cueing and verbal correction	Listen to feedback from another observer

T66 STANDING: SINGLE FOOT LIFT TEST (tests for hip flexion UCM)

This dissociation test assesses the ability to actively dissociate and control hip flexion in single leg standing and maintain weight bearing hip control in a small knee bend (SKB) position and perform hip flexion on the other leg.

Test procedure

The person should stand upright with the upper body vertical, the weight balanced over the feet and the pelvis centred over the heels (Figure 9.12). The person is instructed to shift full weight onto one leg and, keeping the shoulders and pelvis level, slowly lift the other foot off the floor to 90° hip flexion (Figure 9.13). There should be no increase in hip flexion on the weight bearing stance leg. Movement of the buttocks backwards

by more than 2 cm indicates uncontrolled hip flexion.

As soon as any movement indicating a loss of control into increased hip flexion is observed, the movement must stop and return back to the start position. The unilateral single foot lift (non-weight bearing hip flexion) must be independent of any hip flexion on the weight bearing stance leg. This test should be performed without any feedback (self-palpation, vision, flexicurve, etc.) or cueing for correction. The therapist should use visual observation of the pelvis and leg to determine whether the control of hip flexion is adequate when feedback is removed for testing. Assess both sides.

Hip flexion UCM

The person complains of pain in the hip (groin impingement, lateral trochanteric or posterolateral buttock pain) associated with hip flexion

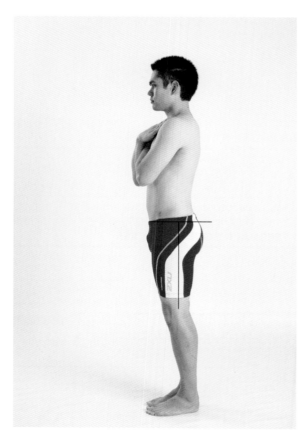

Figure 9.12 Start position single foot lift test

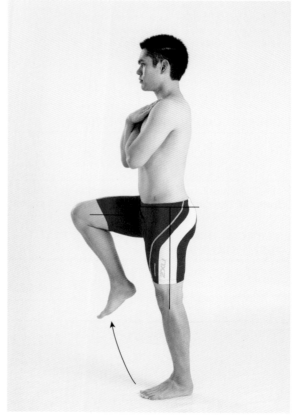

Figure 9.13 Benchmark single foot lift test

activities. During the single foot lift test, the weight bearing hip demonstrates UCM into flexion (the trunk leans forwards and the hips flex moving the buttocks backwards as the foot lifts). The hip has UCM *into flexion* relative to the contralateral hip flexion. Hip flexion control is poor if the subject is unable to prevent or resist the increased hip flexion on the stance leg.

The uncontrolled hip flexion is often associated with inefficiency of the stability function of the gluteal extensor muscles (especially deep gluteus maximus), which provide isometric or eccentric control of hip flexion. During the attempt to dissociate the weight bearing hip flexion from contralateral hip flexion, the person either cannot control the UCM or has to concentrate and try hard to control the hip flexion. The movement must be assessed on both sides. If hip flexion UCM presents bilaterally, one side may be better or worse than the other.

Clinical assessment note for direction-specific motor control testing

---

If some other movement (e.g. a small amount of rotation) is observed during a motor control (dissociation) test of flexion control, *do not* score this as uncontrolled flexion. The rotation motor control tests will identify whether the observed movement is uncontrolled. *A test for hip flexion UCM is only positive if uncontrolled hip flexion is demonstrated.*

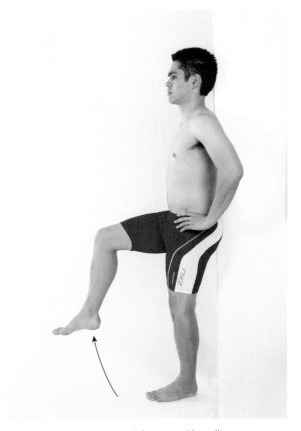

Figure 9.14 Correction partial range with wall support

Rating and diagnosis of hip flexion UCM

(T66.1 and T66.2)

Correction

Initial retraining is best started with the trunk supported against a wall. The person stands with the back against a wall, the feet hip width apart and the weight balanced over the feet. The heels should be approximately 5–10 cm from the wall. The pelvis should be level and the trunk upright (vertical against the wall). The person should be instructed to perform a SKB by sliding the trunk down the wall to a $\frac{1}{4}$ squat position with weight balanced equally on both feet. This is followed by a shift of full weight onto one leg, allowing the pelvis and shoulders to move laterally to keep body weight centred over the weight bearing foot.

The shoulders and pelvis should stay level. The person should then slowly lift the other foot 15–20 cm off the floor (as if stepping up onto a step) (Figure 9.14). There should be no increase in hip flexion on the weight bearing stance leg. Only lift the foot as far as the trunk can stay on the wall and do not lean forwards into increased hip flexion.

The person should self-monitor the hip and trunk alignment and control hip flexion UCM with a variety of feedback options (T66.3). There should be no provocation of any symptoms within the range that the hip flexion UCM can be controlled.

As the ability to control hip flexion and forwards lean of the trunk gets easier and the pattern of dissociation feels less unnatural, the exercise can be progressed to performing this same movement unsupported, without the wall, in single leg stance.

431

T66.1 Assessment and rating of low threshold recruitment efficiency of the Single Foot Lift Test

SINGLE FOOT LIFT – STANDING

ASSESSMENT

Control point:
- prevent hip flexion (weight bearing leg)

Movement challenge: contralateral hip flexion (standing)

Benchmark range: lift contralateral foot 15–20 cm

RATING OF LOW THRESHOLD RECRUITMENT EFFICIENCY FOR CONTROL OF DIRECTION

	✓ or ✗		✓ or ✗
• Able to prevent UCM into the test direction Correct dissociation pattern of movement Prevent hip UCM into: • flexion and move contralateral hip flexion	☐	• Looks easy, and in the opinion of the assessor, is performed with confidence	☐
		• Feels easy, and the subject has sufficient awareness of the movement pattern that they confidently prevent UCM into the test direction	☐
• Dissociate movement through the benchmark range of: contralateral foot lift to 90° hip flexion *If there is more available range than the benchmark standard, only the benchmark range needs to be actively controlled*	☐	• The pattern of dissociation is smooth during concentric and eccentric movement	☐
		• Does not (consistently) use *end-range* movement into the opposite direction to prevent the UCM	☐
• Without holding breath (though it is acceptable to use an alternate breathing strategy)	☐	• No extra feedback needed *(tactile, visual or verbal cueing)*	☐
		• Without external support or unloading	☐
• Control during eccentric phase	☐	• Relaxed natural breathing *(even if not ideal – so long as natural pattern does not change)*	☐
• Control during concentric phase	☐	• No fatigue	☐

CORRECT DISSOCIATION PATTERN   **RECRUITMENT EFFICIENCY**

T66.2 Diagnosis of the site and direction of UCM from the Single Foot Lift Test

SINGLE FOOT LIFT TEST – STANDING

Site	Direction	(L) leg	(R) leg
		(check box)	(check box)
Hip	Flexion	☐	☐

T66.3 Feedback tools to monitor retraining

FEEDBACK TOOL	PROCESS
Self-palpation	Palpation monitoring of joint position
Visual observation	Observe in a mirror or directly watch the movement
Adhesive tape	Skin tension for tactile feedback
Cueing and verbal correction	Listen to feedback from another observer

T67 STANDING: SPINAL ROLL DOWN TEST (tests for hip flexion UCM)

This dissociation test assesses the ability to actively dissociate and control hip flexion and perform spinal flexion by rolling the spine down into flexion while standing.

Test procedure

The person stands with pelvis and upper back supported against the wall, the feet at least shoulder width apart and the knees slightly flexed (hip flexors unloaded and wide base of support). The heels are positioned about 15–20 cm in front of the wall (Figure 9.15). Then, they are instructed to actively lower the sternum towards the pelvis by flexing the thoracic spine while rolling the pelvis backwards (posterior pelvic tilt) to flatten the back onto the wall. The person should monitor that they can feel the sacrum flattened against the wall. They should then continue to flex the spine by slowly letting the head and chest drop towards the pelvis. The spine should unroll into flexion, but the pelvis and sacrum should stay firmly flattened against the wall.

The person should have the ability to dissociate the hip flexion from spinal flexion as evidenced by preventing the pelvis rolling off the wall, while rolling the spine down from the wall into spinal flexion. Ideally, the person should be able to roll down into full spinal flexion and maintain the pelvis posteriorly tilted against the wall (Figure 9.16). There should be no forwards pelvic tilt off the wall (i.e. hip flexion) as the spine rolls forwards off the wall into spinal flexion. The spinal flexion must be independent of any hip flexion

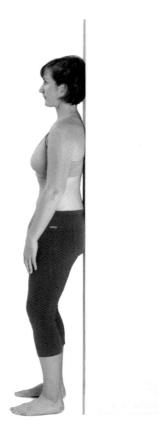

Figure 9.15 Start position spinal roll down test

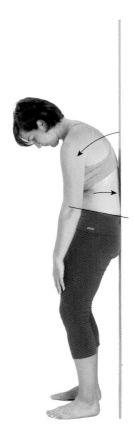

Figure 9.16 Benchmark spinal roll down test

or movement of the pelvis. Note any uncontrolled hip flexion under spinal flexion load. This test should be performed without any feedback (self-palpation, vision, etc.) or cueing for correction. The therapist should use visual observation of the femur and pelvis to determine whether the control of hip flexion is adequate.

Hip flexion UCM

The person complains of pain in the hip (groin impingement, lateral trochanteric or lateral buttock pain) associated with hip flexion activities. During the spinal roll down test, the hip demonstrates UCM into flexion (the pelvis rolls forwards off the wall to follow the spinal roll down). The hip has UCM *into flexion* relative to the spine. Hip flexion control is poor if the subject is unable to prevent or resist the excessive hip flexion or the top of the pelvis rolling forwards off the wall.

The uncontrolled hip flexion is often associated with inefficiency of the stability function of the gluteal extensor muscles (especially deep gluteus maximus), which provide isometric or eccentric control of hip flexion. During the attempt to dissociate the hip flexion from spinal flexion, the person either cannot control the UCM or has to concentrate and try hard to control the hip flexion.

Clinical assessment note for direction-specific motor control testing

If some other movement (e.g. a small amount of rotation) is observed during a motor control (dissociation) test of flexion control, *do not* score this as uncontrolled flexion. The rotation motor control tests will identify whether the observed movement is uncontrolled. *A test for hip flexion UCM is only positive if uncontrolled hip flexion is demonstrated.*

Rating and diagnosis of hip flexion UCM

(T67.1 and T67.2)

Correction

Retraining is best started with the trunk supported against a wall, the feet at least shoulder width apart and the knees slightly flexed (hip flexors

unloaded and wide base of support). If control is poor, the heels are initially positioned about 30–40 cm in front of the wall. Then they are instructed to actively lower the sternum towards the pelvis by flexing the thoracic spine while rolling the pelvis backwards (posterior pelvic tilt) to flatten the back onto the wall. The person should monitor that they can feel the sacrum flattened against the wall. Only roll the spine down off the wall through partial flexion range (Figure 9.17). Ensure that the sacrum and upper pelvis can stay firmly in contact with the wall and not roll forwards into increased hip flexion.

As control improves, the person is instructed to shift their feet closer to the wall and to increase the range of spinal roll down. At the point in range that the pelvis starts to roll forwards into hip flexion the movement should stop and return to the start position. The person should

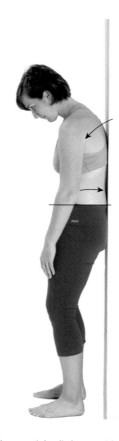

Figure 9.17 Correction partial roll down with wall support

self-monitor the hip and pelvis alignment and control hip flexion UCM with a variety of feedback options (T67.3). There should be no provocation of any symptoms within the range that the hip flexion UCM can be controlled.

As the ability to control hip flexion and forwards lean of the trunk gets easier and the pattern of dissociation feels less unnatural, the exercise can be progressed to performing this same movement unsupported, without the wall.

T67.1 Assessment and rating of low threshold recruitment efficiency of the Spinal Roll Down Test

SPINAL ROLL DOWN – STANDING (WALL)

ASSESSMENT

Control point:
• prevent hip flexion
Movement challenge: spinal flexion (standing – wall)
Benchmark range: independent full range spinal flexion without pelvic or hip movement

RATING OF LOW THRESHOLD RECRUITMENT EFFICIENCY FOR CONTROL OF DIRECTION

	✓ or ✗		✓ or ✗
• Able to prevent UCM into the test direction Correct dissociation pattern of movement	☐	• Looks easy, and in the opinion of the assessor, is performed with confidence	☐
Prevent hip UCM into: • flexion and move spinal flexion		• Feels easy, and the subject has sufficient awareness of the movement pattern that they confidently prevent UCM into the test direction	☐
• Dissociate movement through the benchmark range of: full end range spinal flexion with sacrum flat on wall *If there is more available range than the benchmark standard, only the benchmark range needs to be actively controlled*	☐	• The pattern of dissociation is smooth during concentric and eccentric movement	☐
		• Does not (consistently) use *end-range* movement into the opposite direction to prevent the UCM	☐
• Without holding breath (though it is acceptable to use an alternate breathing strategy)	☐	• No extra feedback needed *(tactile, visual or verbal cueing)*	☐
		• Without external support or unloading	☐
• Control during eccentric phase	☐	• Relaxed natural breathing *(even if not ideal – so long as natural pattern does not change)*	☐
• Control during concentric phase	☐	• No fatigue	☐

CORRECT DISSOCIATION PATTERN **RECRUITMENT EFFICIENCY**

T67.2 Diagnosis of the site and direction of UCM from the Spinal Roll Down Test

SPINAL ROLL DOWN TEST – STANDING

Site	Direction	
		(check box)
Hip	Flexion	☐

T67.3 Feedback tools to monitor retraining

FEEDBACK TOOL	PROCESS
Self-palpation	Palpation monitoring of joint position
Visual observation	Observe in a mirror or directly watch the movement
Adhesive tape	Skin tension for tactile feedback
Cueing and verbal correction	Listen to feedback from another observer

T68 SIDE-LYING: SINGLE LEG ABDUCTION TEST
(tests for hip flexion UCM)

This dissociation test assesses the ability to actively dissociate and control hip flexion and perform a single leg hip abduction and lateral rotation.

Test procedure

The person lies on one side with uppermost (top) leg extended in line with the trunk and the other (bottom leg) hip flexed to 45° and the knees flexed to 90° (Figure 9.18). The pelvis should be positioned in neutral rotation. The person is instructed to maintain the neutral pelvis position and turn the uppermost foot outwards (hip lateral rotation). Then they should slowly lift the uppermost leg vertically up and out to the side while keeping the leg and foot turned out into lateral rotation. Ideally, the top leg should be able to maintain the hip extension and turnout and lift into at least 35° (above horizontal) of hip abduction and lateral rotation (Figure 9.19) and return, without associated loss of neutral extension into any flexion of the hip.

The unilateral hip abduction must be independent of any hip flexion. Note any excessive hip flexion under hip abduction load. This test should be performed without any feedback (self-palpation, vision, flexicurve, etc.) or cueing for correction. The therapist should use visual observation of the pelvis to determine whether the control of hip flexion is adequate when feedback is removed for testing. Assess both sides.

Hip flexion UCM

The person complains of flexion-related symptoms in the hip. During the single leg abduction test, the leg moves forwards of the body (hip flexion UCM) before the abduction reaches 35° above horizontal). Under unilateral hip loading, the hip has UCM *into flexion*.

The uncontrolled hip flexion is often associated with inefficiency of the stability function of the gluteal extensor muscles (especially deep gluteus maximus), which provide isometric or eccentric control of hip flexion. During the attempt to dissociate the hip flexion from spinal flexion, the person either cannot control the UCM or has to concentrate and try hard to control the hip flexion. The movement must be assessed on both sides. If hip flexion UCM presents bilaterally, one side may be better or worse than the other.

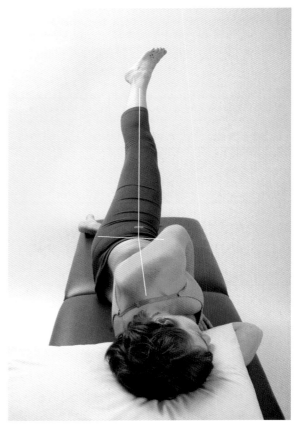

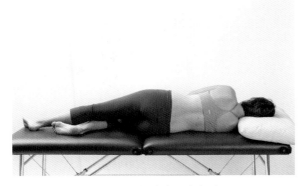

Figure 9.18 Start position single leg abduction test

Figure 9.19 Benchmark single leg abduction test

Clinical assessment note for direction-specific motor control testing

If some other movement (e.g. a small amount of rotation) is observed during a motor control (dissociation) test of flexion control, *do not* score this as uncontrolled flexion. The rotation motor control tests will identify whether the observed movement is uncontrolled. *A test for hip flexion UCM is only positive if uncontrolled hip flexion is demonstrated.*

Rating and diagnosis of hip flexion UCM

(T68.1 and T68.2)

Correction

If control is poor, retraining can initially begin with reduced leg load. With the person side-lying and the hips extended to neutral (0° extension), the knees flexed to 60° and the feet together, the pelvis should be positioned in neutral rotation. Keeping the heels together the person is instructed to lift the top leg up and out to the side. Hold this position, and lift the heel of the top foot 2–3 cm away from the bottom heel. Ensure that, as the heel lifts, the leg does not move forwards into hip flexion. At the point in range that the hip starts to lose control of flexion, the movement should stop. The hip position is restabilised (lift the knee and keep the heel down), then hold this position for a few seconds and return to the start position.

The unilateral hip abduction must be independent of any hip flexion. The person should self-monitor the hip alignment and control flexion UCM with a variety of feedback options (T68.3). There should be no provocation of any symptoms within the range that the rotation UCM can be controlled.

As the ability to control hip flexion gets easier and the pattern of dissociation feels less unnatural, the exercise can be progressed to performing the hip abduction and lateral rotation with the leg fully extended.

Hip flexion UCM summary

(Table 9.2)

Table 9.2 Summary and rating of hip flexion tests

UCM DIAGNOSIS AND TESTING

SITE: HIP	DIRECTION: FLEXION	CLINICAL PRIORITY ☐
TEST	RATING (✓✓ or ✓✗ or ✗✗) and rationale	
Standing: vertical trunk single leg ¼ squat		
Standing: single foot lift		
Standing: spinal roll down		
Side-lying: single leg abduction		

T68.1 Assessment and rating of low threshold recruitment efficiency of the Single Leg Abduction Test

SINGLE LEG ABDUCTION TEST – SIDE-LYING

ASSESSMENT

Control point:
- prevent hip flexion

Movement challenge: unilateral hip abduction and lateral rotation (side-lying)

Benchmark range: 35° independent hip abduction and lateral rotation without compensation

RATING OF LOW THRESHOLD RECRUITMENT EFFICIENCY FOR CONTROL OF DIRECTION

	✓ or ✗		✓ or ✗
• Able to prevent UCM into the test direction Correct dissociation pattern of movement	☐	• Looks easy, and in the opinion of the assessor, is performed with confidence	☐
Prevent hip UCM into:		• Feels easy, and the subject has sufficient awareness of the movement pattern that they confidently prevent UCM into the test direction	☐
• medial flexion and move hip abduction and lateral rotation (turnout)			
• Dissociate movement through the benchmark range of: 35° hip abduction and lateral rotation *If there is more available range than the benchmark standard, only the benchmark range needs to be actively controlled*	☐	• The pattern of dissociation is smooth during concentric and eccentric movement	☐
		• Does not (consistently) use *end-range* movement into the opposite direction to prevent the UCM	☐
		• No extra feedback needed *(tactile, visual or verbal cueing)*	☐
• Without holding breath (though it is acceptable to use an alternate breathing strategy)	☐	• Without external support or unloading	☐
		• Relaxed natural breathing *(even if not ideal – so long as natural pattern does not change)*	☐
• Control during eccentric phase	☐	• No fatigue	☐
• Control during concentric phase	☐		

CORRECT DISSOCIATION PATTERN   **RECRUITMENT EFFICIENCY**

T68.2 Diagnosis of the site and direction of UCM from the Single Leg Abduction Test

SINGLE LEG ABDUCTION TEST – STANDING

Site	Direction	(L) leg	(R) leg
		(check box)	(check box)
Hip	Flexion	☐	☐

T68.3 Feedback tools to monitor retraining

FEEDBACK TOOL	PROCESS
Self-palpation	Palpation monitoring of joint position
Visual observation	Observe in a mirror or directly watch the movement
Adhesive tape	Skin tension for tactile feedback

Hip extension control

Movement faults associated with hip extension

The modified Thomas test can be used to further identify the origin and nature of movement faults associated with hip extension.

Modified Thomas test

The person sits on the end of a plinth or table, holds onto one knee and rolls backwards onto their back keeping both legs flexed. With the lower thoracic spine and sacrum flat on the table, the subject pulls one knee up towards the chest until the lumbar spine flattens onto the table, but not so far that the sacrum rolls off the table into lumbopelvic flexion. The subject uses both hands holding one knee to support this flat back position. The therapist then passively lowers the test leg down towards the table (hip extension), keeping the hip adducted to the midline and knee flexed to 90° while monitoring maintenance of the lumbopelvic position (Figures 9.20 and 9.21).

Relative stiffness (restrictions of hip extension)

If the thigh hangs above horizontal some hip flexor structure lacks extensibility. Further assessment can differentiate the origin of relative stiffness to short tensor fasciae latae/iliotibial band, rectus femoris or anterior capsule:

- *Rectus femoris.* From the lowered position (leg hanging above the table) while the

lumbar spine remains in neutral and the thigh adducted to the midline, the knee is passively extended to unload tension from rectus femoris. If rectus femoris is one of the short hip flexors, the hip is able to extend further and the leg drops closer to the table (Figure 9.22).

- *Tensor fasciae latae and iliotibial band.* From the lowered position (leg hanging above the table) while the lumbar spine remains in neutral and the knee flexed to 80°, the thigh is passively abducted to unload tension from the iliotibial band. If the iliotibial band is one of the short hip flexors, the hip is able to extend further and the leg drops closer to the table (Figure 9.23).

- *Anterior capsule or (iliacus).* From the lowered position (leg hanging above the table) while the lumbar spine remains in neutral, the thigh is passively abducted to unload tension

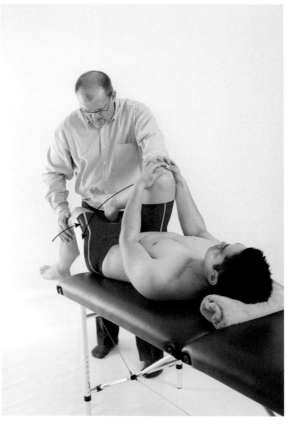

Figure 9.21 Modified Thomas test final position

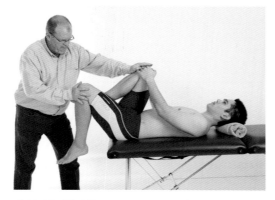

Figure 9.20 Modified Thomas test start position

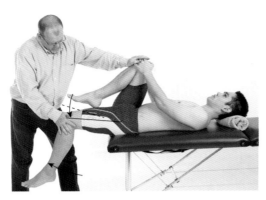

Figure 9.22 Modified Thomas test rectus femoris contribution

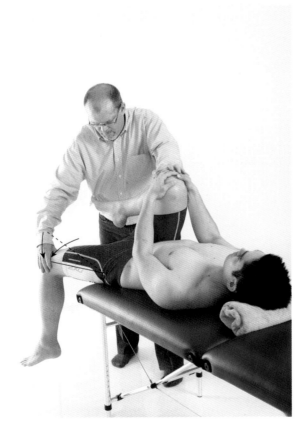

Figure 9.23 Modified Thomas test tensor fasciae latae – iliotibial band contribution

from the iliotibial band and the knee is passively extended to unload tension from rectus femoris. If the anterior capsule is short, the hip still hangs above the table and cannot extend fully.

Relative flexibility (potential UCM)

• *Excessive hip extension.* Unload the myofascial structures by slightly extending the knee and abducting the hip. If the thigh hangs more than 10° below the horizontal there is excessive range of hip extension with laxity of the anterior restraints (elongated iliacus and anterior hip capsule). If excessive hip extension is noted it is important to test further for uncontrolled anterior femoral head translation (hip forwards glide) as well as uncontrolled extension.

HIP EXTENSION CONTROL TESTS AND EXTENSION CONTROL REHABILITATION

These extension control tests assess the amount of extension UCM in the hip and assess the ability of the dynamic stability system to adequately control extension load or strain. It is a priority to assess for extension UCM if the patient complains of or demonstrates extension-related symptoms or disability. The tests that identify dysfunction can also be used to guide and direct rehabilitation strategies.

Indications to test for hip extension UCM

Observe or palpate for:

1. hypermobile hip extension range
2. excessive initiation of leaning backwards or knee extension with hip extension
3. symptoms (pain, discomfort, strain) associated with hip extension or sustained extension postures.

The person complains of extension-related symptoms in the hip. Under extension load, the hip has greater give *into extension* relative to the trunk and lower leg. The dysfunction is confirmed with motor control tests of extension dissociation.

441

Hip extension control tests

T69 STANDING: THORACOLUMBAR EXTENSION TEST
(tests for hip extension UCM)

This dissociation test assesses the ability to actively control hip extension while actively lifting the sternum up and forwards into thoracolumbar extension in standing.

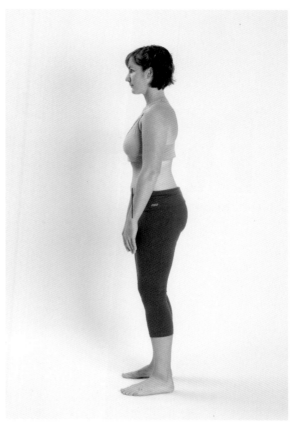

Figure 9.24 Start position thoracolumbar extension test

Test procedure

The person initially stands tall with the upper thighs against the edge of a plinth, bench or table and with the feet as far under the table as balance can be maintained. Position the head directly over the shoulders without chin poke. Demonstrate or manually assist the movement of thoracolumbar extension. The sternum, clavicles and acromions should all move up and forwards. There should be no hip extension or forwards sway of the pelvis (the table provides feedback and support). The normal anterior pelvic should be present (with slight concurrent hip flexion) and all of the lumbar spine and the lower thoracic vertebrae should contribute to the thoracolumbar extension initiated from the thoracic region.

For testing, feedback and the support of the table are taken away. The person stands tall and unsupported with legs straight and the lumbar spine and pelvis positioned in the neutral. The head is positioned directly over the shoulders without chin poke (Figure 9.24). Without letting the lumbopelvic region move into forwards sway, the person should have the ability to actively lift the sternum and chest up and forwards through the full available range of thoracolumbar extension.

Ideally, the person should have the ability to prevent hip extension and forwards sway of the pelvis while independently extending the thoracolumbar region from a position of relaxed flexion through to full extension (Figure 9.25). The available range of dissociated thoracolumbar extension is small. This test should be performed without any feedback (self-palpation, vision, tape, etc.) or cueing for correction.

Hip extension UCM

The person complains of extension-related symptoms in the hip. The hip has UCM into hip extension and forwards pelvic sway relative to the spine under extension load. During active hip extension, the hip starts to move into extension before achieving thoracolumbar extension. The upper lumbar spine and thoracic spine may only contribute (if at all) to extension at the completion of hip extension. During the attempt to dissociate the hip extension from independent thoracolumbar extension (while allowing normal slight anterior pelvic tilt) the person either cannot control the UCM or has to concentrate and try hard.

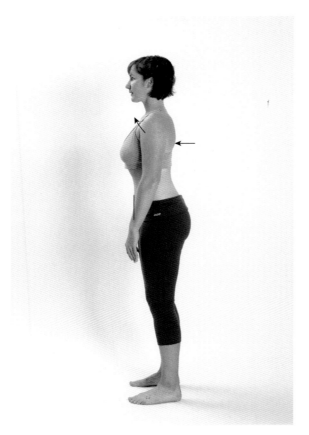

Figure 9.25 Benchmark thoracolumbar extension test

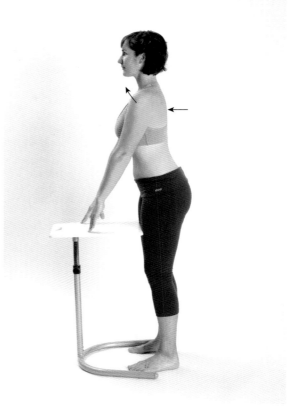

Figure 9.26 Correction thoracic extension with hip support

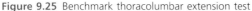

Clinical assessment note for direction-specific motor control testing

If some other movement (e.g. a small amount of rotation) is observed during a motor control (dissociation) test of extension control, *do not* score this as uncontrolled extension. The rotation motor control tests will identify whether the observed movement is uncontrolled. *A test for hip extension UCM is only positive if uncontrolled hip extension is demonstrated.*

Rating and diagnosis of hip extension UCM

(T69.1 and T69.2)

Correction

The person stands tall and unsupported with legs straight and the spine, pelvis and hips positioned in the neutral. Without letting the hips move into extension or forwards sway of the pelvis, the person actively lifts the chest up and forwards into thoracolumbar extension only as far as hip extension and forwards sway of the pelvis can be actively controlled or prevented. The normal anterior pelvic tilt should be present (with slight concurrent hip flexion) and all of the lumbar spine and the lower thoracic vertebrae should contribute to the spinal extension initiated from the thoracolumbar region.

If control is poor, start retraining with additional feedback and support. The person stands with the upper thighs against the edge of a bench or table and with the feet as far under the table as balance can be maintained. With the table preventing hip extension and forwards sway of the pelvis, the chest should move up and forwards. Also, the upper body and trunk weight can be supported by weight bearing through the arms to decrease the load that must be controlled (Figure 9.26). Train by moving into thoracolumbar

443

extension only as far as the hip extension can be prevented.

The person should monitor the hip alignment and control with a variety of feedback options (T69.3). There should be no provocation of any symptoms under thoracolumbar extension load, within the range that the hip extension UCM can be controlled.

As the ability to control the UCM gets easier, and the pattern of dissociation feels less unnatural, the exercise can be progressed to the unsupported position without a bench or table and then it should be integrated into various functional postures and positions.

T69.1 Assessment and rating of low threshold recruitment efficiency of the Thoracolumbar Extension Test

THORACOLUMBAR EXTENSION TEST – STANDING

ASSESSMENT

Control point:
- prevent hip extension (forward pelvic sway)

Movement challenge: thoracolumbar extension (standing)

Benchmark range: full available dissociated thoracolumbar extension without compensation

RATING OF LOW THRESHOLD RECRUITMENT EFFICIENCY FOR CONTROL OF DIRECTION

	✓ or ✗		✓ or ✗
• Able to prevent UCM into the test direction Correct dissociation pattern of movement Prevent hip UCM into: • extension (forward pelvic sway) and move thoracolumbar extension	☐	• Looks easy, and in the opinion of the assessor, is performed with confidence	☐
		• Feels easy, and the subject has sufficient awareness of the movement pattern that they confidently prevent UCM into the test direction	☐
• Dissociate movement through the benchmark range of: full available thoracolumbar extension *If there is more available range than the benchmark standard, only the benchmark range needs to be actively controlled*	☐	• The pattern of dissociation is smooth during concentric and eccentric movement	☐
		• Does not (consistently) use *end-range* movement into the opposite direction to prevent the UCM	☐
• Without holding breath (though it is acceptable to use an alternate breathing strategy)	☐	• No extra feedback needed (*tactile, visual or verbal cueing*)	☐
• Control during eccentric phase	☐	• Without external support or unloading	☐
• Control during concentric phase	☐	• Relaxed natural breathing (*even if not ideal – so long as natural pattern does not change*)	☐
		• No fatigue	☐

CORRECT DISSOCIATION PATTERN   **RECRUITMENT EFFICIENCY**

T69.2 Diagnosis of the site and direction of UCM from the Thoracolumbar Extension Test

THORACOLUMBAR EXTENSION TEST – STANDING

Site	Direction	(L) leg	(R) leg
		(check box)	(check box)
Hip	Extension	☐	☐

T69.3 Feedback tools to monitor retraining

FEEDBACK TOOL	PROCESS
Self-palpation	Palpation monitoring of joint position
Visual observation	Observe in a mirror or directly watch the movement
Adhesive tape	Skin tension for tactile feedback
Cueing and verbal correction	Listen to feedback from another observer

T70 STANDING: SINGLE KNEE LIFT + ANTERIOR TILT TEST (tests for hip extension UCM)

This dissociation test assesses the ability to actively dissociate and control hip extension and maintain unilateral hip flexion while actively extending the spine and anteriorly tilting the pelvis.

Test procedure

The person stands on one leg and, keeping the shoulders and pelvis level, slowly lifts the other foot off the ground to lift the thigh to 90° hip flexion with the lower leg relaxed and the heel hanging vertically under the knee. The thigh should be horizontal and the lumbopelvic region should maintain a neutral relaxed shallow lordosis (Figure 9.27). The person is then instructed to hold the hip flexed position (thigh horizontal) and slowly start to tilt the pelvis forwards (anterior pelvic tilt) and extend the lumbar spine. The subject should maintain the hip flexed position to prevent any increase in hip extension (lowering of the thigh) as the pelvis tilts and the lumbar spine extends.

Ideally, the pelvis should be able to achieve full anterior pelvic tilt independently of any hip extension (keep the thigh horizontal) (Figure 9.28). As soon as any movement indicating a loss of control into hip extension is observed, or swaying the pelvis forwards to maintain the leg position, the movement must stop and return back to the start position. Anterior pelvic tilt must be demonstrated with the hip flexion maintained at 90° (thigh horizontal) and with shoulders and pelvis level.

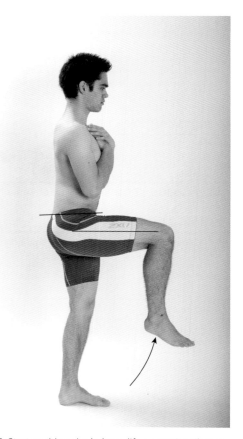

Figure 9.27 Start position single knee lift + anterior tilt test

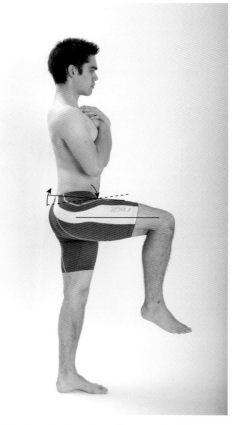

Figure 9.28 Benchmark single knee lift + anterior tilt test

The anterior pelvic tilt must be independent of any hip extension. Note any uncontrolled hip extension under pelvic tilt load. This test should be performed without any feedback (self-palpation, vision, flexicurve, etc.) or cueing for correction. When feedback is removed for testing the therapist should use visual observation of the pelvis and leg to determine whether the control of hip extension is adequate. Assess both sides.

Hip extension UCM

The person complains of pain in the hip (groin impingement or lateral buttock pain) associated with hip extension activities. During the single knee lift + anterior tilt test, the person lacks the ability to prevent the thigh from lowering and the hip from extending as the pelvis tilts forwards and the spine extends. The thigh lowers from horizontal before the pelvis achieves full anterior tilt. Under anterior pelvic tilt loading, the hip has UCM *into extension*. Swaying the pelvis forwards to hold the thigh horizontal is a common substitution strategy for inefficient control.

The uncontrolled hip extension is often associated with inefficiency of the stability function of the anterior hip stabilisers (especially iliacus and pectineus) providing isometric or eccentric control of hip extension. During the attempt to dissociate the hip extension from spinal extension and anterior pelvic tilt, the person either cannot control the UCM or has to concentrate and try hard to control the hip extension. The movement must be assessed on both sides. If hip extension UCM presents bilaterally, one side may be better or worse than the other.

Clinical assessment note for direction-specific motor control testing

If some other movement (e.g. a small amount of rotation) is observed during a motor control (dissociation) test of extension control, *do not* score this as uncontrolled extension. The rotation motor control tests will identify whether the observed movement is uncontrolled. *A test for hip extension UCM is only positive if uncontrolled hip extension is demonstrated.*

Rating and diagnosis of hip extension UCM

(T70.1 and T70.2)

Correction

If control is poor, initial retraining is best started in a ½ lunge position. The person stands in a shallow ½ lunge with the trunk and the rear thigh vertical and the front thigh weight bearing and held flexed to about 60°. The lumbopelvic region should maintain a neutral relaxed shallow lordosis. If needed, the person can hold onto a table or chair for balance or to support body load. The person is then instructed to hold the front hip flexed (60°) position and slowly start to tilt the pelvis forwards (anterior pelvic tilt) and extend the lumbar spine (Figure 9.29).

The person should maintain the hip flexed position to prevent any increase in hip extension (lifting the body and straightening up) as the pelvis tilts and the lumbar spine extends. They are to extend the spine and tilt the pelvis only as far as the front thigh position is maintained

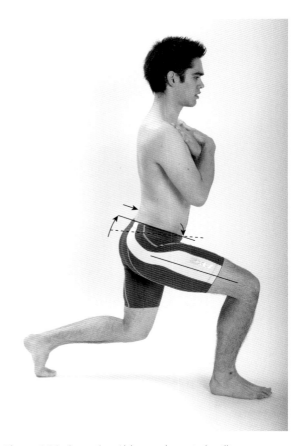

Figure 9.29 Correction ½ lunge plus anterior tilt

(monitored with feedback). At the point in range that the body starts to lift or straighten at the front hip, the movement should stop.

The person should self-monitor the hip alignment and control extension UCM with a variety of feedback options (T70.3). There should be no provocation of any symptoms withzin the range that the rotation UCM can be controlled.

As the ability to control hip extension gets easier and the pattern of dissociation feels less unnatural, the exercise can be progressed to performing this spinal extension in a lower or deeper lunge (front thigh horizontal at 90° hip flexion). Finally, the exercise is progressed to a non-weight bearing exercise position, as in the test position (i.e. standing upright with the hip held unsupported in hip flexion).

T70.1 Assessment and rating of low threshold recruitment efficiency of the Single Knee Lift + Anterior Tilt Test

SINGLE KNEE LIFT + ANTERIOR TILT TEST – STANDING

ASSESSMENT

Control point:
• prevent hip extension

Movement challenge: unilateral hip flexion + spinal extension and anterior pelvic tilt (standing)

Benchmark range: full independent anterior pelvic tilt and maintain 90° hip flexion without compensation of hip extension

RATING OF LOW THRESHOLD RECRUITMENT EFFICIENCY FOR CONTROL OF DIRECTION

	✓ or ✗		✓ or ✗
• Able to prevent UCM into the test direction Correct dissociation pattern of movement Prevent hip UCM into: • extension and move spinal extension and anterior pelvic tilt	☐	• Looks easy, and in the opinion of the assessor, is performed with confidence	☐
		• Feels easy, and the subject has sufficient awareness of the movement pattern that they confidently prevent UCM into the test direction	☐
• Dissociate movement through the benchmark range of: full anterior pelvic tilt + 90° unilateral hip flexion *If there is more available range than the benchmark standard, only the benchmark range needs to be actively controlled*	☐	• The pattern of dissociation is smooth during concentric and eccentric movement	☐
		• Does not (consistently) use *end-range* movement into the opposite direction to prevent the UCM	☐
• Without holding breath (though it is acceptable to use an alternate breathing strategy)	☐	• No extra feedback needed (*tactile, visual or verbal cueing*)	☐
		• Without external support or unloading	☐
• Control during eccentric phase	☐	• Relaxed natural breathing (*even if not ideal – so long as natural pattern does not change*)	☐
• Control during concentric phase	☐	• No fatigue	☐

CORRECT DISSOCIATION PATTERN | **RECRUITMENT EFFICIENCY**

T70.2 Diagnosis of the site and direction of UCM from the Single Knee Lift + Anterior Tilt Test

SINGLE KNEE LIFT + ANTERIOR TILT TEST – STANDING

Site	Direction	(L) leg	(R) leg
		(check box)	(check box)
Hip	Extension	☐	☐

T70.3 Feedback tools to monitor retraining

FEEDBACK TOOL	PROCESS
Self-palpation	Palpation monitoring of joint position
Visual observation	Observe in a mirror or directly watch the movement
Adhesive tape	Skin tension for tactile feedback
Cueing and verbal correction	Listen to feedback from another observer

T71 STANDING: SINGLE KNEE LIFT + KNEE EXTENSION TEST (tests for hip extension UCM)

This dissociation test assesses the ability to actively dissociate and control hip extension and maintain unilateral hip flexion while actively extending the knee.

Test procedure

The person stands on one leg and, keeping the shoulders and pelvis level, slowly lifts the other foot off the ground to lift the thigh to 90° of hip flexion with the lower leg relaxed and the heel hanging vertically under the knee. The thigh should be horizontal and the lumbopelvic region should maintain a neutral relaxed shallow lordosis (Figure 9.30). The person is then instructed to hold the non-weight bearing hip flexed position (thigh horizontal) and slowly start to straighten the knee (knee extension). The subject should maintain the hip flexed position to prevent any increase in non-weight bearing hip extension (lowering of the thigh) as the knee extends.

Ideally, the knee should be able to straighten to within 20° of full extension independently of any hip extension on the non-weight bearing side (keep the thigh horizontal) (Figure 9.31). As soon as any movement indicating a loss of control into hip extension is observed, or swaying the pelvis forwards to maintain the leg position is noted, the movement must stop and return back to the start position. Knee extension must be demonstrated with the hip flexion maintained at 90°

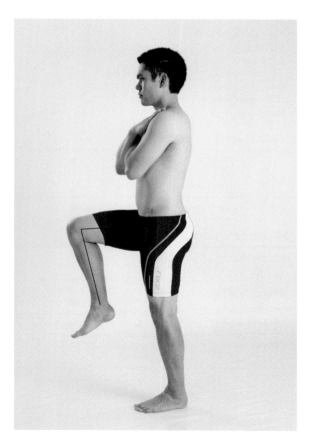

Figure 9.30 Start position single knee lift + knee extension test

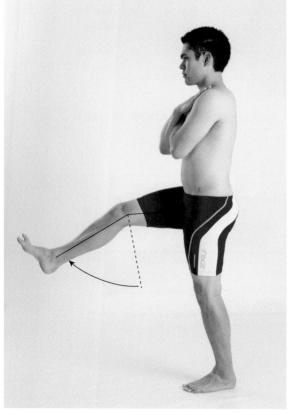

Figure 9.31 Benchmark single knee lift + knee extension test

(thigh horizontal) and with shoulders and pelvis level.

The knee extension must be independent of any hip extension. Note any uncontrolled hip extension under knee extension load. This test should be performed without any feedback (self-palpation, vision, flexicurve, etc.) or cueing for correction. The therapist should use visual observation of the pelvis and leg to determine whether the control of hip extension is adequate when feedback is removed for testing. Assess both sides.

Hip extension UCM

The person complains of pain in the hip (groin impingement or lateral buttock pain) associated with hip extension activities. During the single knee lift + knee extension test, the person lacks the ability to prevent the thigh from lowering and the hip from extending as the knee extends. The thigh lowers from horizontal before the knee reaches 20° from full extension. Under knee extension loading, the hip has UCM *into extension*.

The uncontrolled hip extension is often associated with inefficiency of the stability function of the anterior hip stabilisers (especially iliacus and pectineus), providing isometric or eccentric control of hip extension. During the attempt to dissociate the hip extension from knee extension, the person either cannot control the UCM or has to concentrate and try hard to control the hip extension. The movement must be assessed on both sides. If hip extension UCM presents bilaterally, one side may be better or worse than the other.

Clinical assessment note for direction-specific motor control testing

If some other movement (e.g. a small amount of rotation) is observed during a motor control (dissociation) test of extension control, *do not* score this as uncontrolled extension. The rotation motor control tests will identify whether the observed movement is uncontrolled. *A test for hip extension UCM is only positive if uncontrolled hip extension is demonstrated.*

Rating and diagnosis of hip extension UCM

(T71.1 and T71.2)

Correction

If control is poor, initial retraining is best started with the hip held in less than 90° of hip flexion. The lumbopelvic region should maintain a neutral relaxed shallow lordosis. If needed, the person can support the back against a wall or hold onto a table or chair for balance or to support body load. The person is then instructed to stand on one leg and to hold the other hip flexed to 60° and slowly start to extend the knee (Figure 9.32).

The person should maintain the hip flexed position (at 60°) and prevent any increase in hip extension (further lowering of the thigh) as the knee extends. They are to extend the knee only as far as the thigh position is maintained (monitored with feedback). At the point in range that the thigh starts to lower into increased hip flexion, the movement should stop.

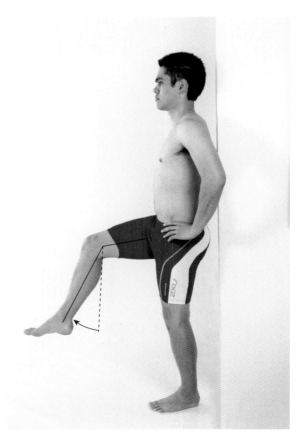

Figure 9.32 Correction on wall

The person should self-monitor the hip alignment and control extension UCM with a variety of feedback options (T71.3). There should be no provocation of any symptoms within the range that the rotation UCM can be controlled.

As the ability to control hip extension gets easier and the pattern of dissociation feels less unnatural, the exercise can be progressed to maintaining the thigh horizontal (at 90° hip flexion).

Hip extension UCM summary

(Table 9.3)

Table 9.3 Summary and rating of hip extension tests		
UCM DIAGNOSIS AND TESTING		
SITE: **HIP**	**DIRECTION:** **EXTENSION**	**CLINICAL PRIORITY** ☐
TEST	**RATING** (✓✓ or ✓✗ or ✗✗) and rationale	
Standing: thoracolumbar extension		
Standing: single knee lift + anterior tilt		
Standing: single knee lift + knee extension		

T71.1 Assessment and rating of low threshold recruitment efficiency of the Single Knee Lift + Knee Extension Test

SINGLE KNEE LIFT + KNEE EXTENSION TEST – STANDING

ASSESSMENT

Control point:
• prevent hip extension
Movement challenge: unilateral hip flexion + knee extension (standing)
Benchmark range: 20° from full knee extension and maintain 90° hip flexion without compensation of hip extension

RATING OF LOW THRESHOLD RECRUITMENT EFFICIENCY FOR CONTROL OF DIRECTION

	✓ or ✗		✓ or ✗
• Able to prevent UCM into the test direction Correct dissociation pattern of movement Prevent hip UCM into: • extension and move knee extension	☐	• Looks easy, and in the opinion of the assessor, is performed with confidence	☐
		• Feels easy, and the subject has sufficient awareness of the movement pattern that they confidently prevent UCM into the test direction	☐
• Dissociate movement through the benchmark range of: 20° from full knee extension + 90° unilateral hip flexion *If there is more available range than the benchmark standard, only the benchmark range needs to be actively controlled*	☐	• The pattern of dissociation is smooth during concentric and eccentric movement	☐
		• Does not (consistently) use *end-range* movement into the opposite direction to prevent the UCM	☐
• Without holding breath (though it is acceptable to use an alternate breathing strategy)	☐	• No extra feedback needed (*tactile, visual or verbal cueing*)	☐
		• Without external support or unloading	☐
• Control during eccentric phase	☐	• Relaxed natural breathing (*even if not ideal – so long as natural pattern does not change*)	☐
• Control during concentric phase	☐	• No fatigue	☐

CORRECT DISSOCIATION PATTERN   **RECRUITMENT EFFICIENCY**

T71.2 Diagnosis of the site and direction of UCM from the Single Knee Lift + Knee Extension Test

SINGLE KNEE LIFT + KNEE EXTENSION TEST – STANDING

Site	Direction	(L) leg	(R) leg
		(check box)	(check box)
Hip	Extension	☐	☐

T71.3 Feedback tools to monitor retraining

FEEDBACK TOOL	PROCESS
Self-palpation	Palpation monitoring of joint position
Visual observation	Observe in a mirror or directly watch the movement
Adhesive tape	Skin tension for tactile feedback
Cueing and verbal correction	Listen to feedback from another observer

Hip rotation control

OBSERVATION AND ANALYSIS OF HIP ROTATION AND TRUNK TURNING

Description of ideal pattern

The subject is instructed to stand with the feet in a natural stance and shift weight to stand on one leg by lifting the foot of one leg just clear of the floor. The subject is instructed to turn to each side as far as comfortably possible. Ideally, the shoulders and upper body (measured by a line across both acromions) should be able to turn at least 90° from the stance foot. The pelvis should be able to turn at least 45° from the stance foot. Rotation should occur concurrently below the pelvis (at the ankle, knee, hip) and above the pelvis (lumbar spine, thoracic spine, scapulae), with approximately one-half of the contribution coming from above and one-half from below the pelvis (Figure 9.33).

There should be good symmetry of movement without any lateral deviation, tilt or rotation of the trunk or pelvis. The head, sternum and pubic symphysis should be aligned above the stance foot with the shoulders level in an upright posture.

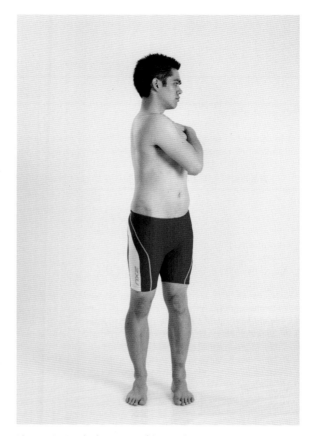

Figure 9.33 Ideal pattern of hip and trunk rotation

Movement faults associated with hip rotation

Relative stiffness (restrictions)

- *Thoracolumbar restriction of rotation* – the upper body lacks 45° of normal range of turning towards the stance leg (i.e. <45° of upper body rotation to the right when standing on the right foot). A thoracolumbar rotation restriction may contribute to compensatory increases in hip rotation range. This is confirmed with motion assessment and manual segmental joint assessment (e.g. Maitland PPIVMs or PAIVMs).
- *Restriction of hip lateral rotation* – the pelvis lacks 45° of normal range of turning away from the stance leg (i.e. <45° of pelvis rotation to the left when standing on the right foot). Hip medial rotation may increase to compensate for the lack of hip lateral rotation. This is a common presentation.

- *Restriction of hip medial rotation* – the pelvis lacks 45° of normal range of turning towards the stance leg (i.e. <45° of pelvis rotation to the right when standing on the right foot). Hip lateral rotation may increase to compensate for the lack of hip medial rotation.

Relative flexibility (potential UCM)

- *Hip medial rotation.* The hip may initiate the movement into turning, and contribute more to producing rotation while the upper body starts later and contributes less. At the limit of turning, excessive or hypermobile range of hip rotation may be observed. During the return to neutral, the hip rotation persists and returns late. Increased range or uncontrolled hip medial rotation is a common compensation for reduced thoracolumbar rotation and reduced hip lateral rotation.

- *Hip lateral rotation.* The hip may initiate the movement into turning, contribute more to producing rotation while the upper body starts later and contributes less. Excessive or hypermobile range of hip rotation may be observed. During the return to neutral, the hip rotation persists and returns late. Increased range or uncontrolled hip lateral rotation is a compensation for reduced thoracolumbar rotation and reduced hip medial rotation.

Assessment of relative hip rotation range

Assess relative hip rotation range in hip extension (prone). This is where hip rotation is used functionally. The majority of textbook measurements of hip rotation are performed with the hip flexed to 90° (medial rotation 35–40°, lateral rotation 45–60°). This is not particularly relevant to the weight bearing hip where functional loading usually occurs in an extended or neutral position.

In a prone position, with the knees together and the hip in neutral based on Craig's test, assess rotation range. Ideally, there should be 35° of active lateral rotation and 35° of active medial rotation from neutral. A difference of less than 10° between medial and lateral rotation is not clinically significant (Sahrmann 2002).

Movement faults

- *Excessive medial rotation of hip (common).* Poor stability function or excessive length of the capsule or lateral rotator stability muscles (posterior gluteus medius and intrinsic hip lateral rotators) may be noted. This can be clarified by further assessment of the stability function for specific muscles, and determination if muscle active shortening matches joint passive range. This is retrained using low threshold (non-fatiguing) active recruitment training in shortened range positions (inner range hold).
- *Excessive lateral rotation of hip.* Poor stability function or excessive length of the medial rotator stability muscles (anterior gluteus medius and minimus) may be noted. This

can be clarified by further assessment of stability function for specific muscles and determination if muscle active shortening matches joint passive range. This is retrained using low threshold (non-fatiguing) active recruitment training in shortened range positions (inner range hold).

- *Decreased lateral rotation of hip (common).* This may arise due to shortening of capsule or myofascial structures (TFL/ITB). Differentiate by end feel; also take leg into abduction by 5 cm, and if the restricted range of lateral rotation increased, TFL/ITB is limiting movement (no change capsule). Specific muscle length tests can confirm myofascial shortening. This is best recovered using a combination of active inhibitory lengthening techniques and passive myofascial mobilisation techniques.
- *Decreased medial rotation of hip.* This may arise due to shortening of capsule or myofascial structures (e.g. piriformis or superficial fibres of gluteus maximus). Differentiate by end feel. Specific muscle length tests can confirm myofascial shortening. However, in this hip extended position the piriformis or superficial fibres of gluteus maximus are unloaded and could not contribute to decreased medial rotation. The restriction is more likely to be articular or capsular. This is best recovered using a combination of passive articular and capsular mobilisation techniques and active exercise to maintain mobility.

Assessment of rotation dysfunction at the hip

Lower quadrant rotational alignment evaluation

- Stand in *natural* stance.
- Do a SKB. (In weight bearing, flex the knees and dorsiflex the ankles while keeping both heels on the floor.)
- Knee bend as far as the heels can stay on the floor.
- Observe the relative rotational alignment of hip, knee and foot in the natural pattern (without cueing and alignment correction) (Figure 9.34).

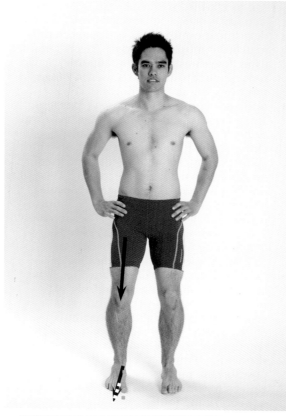

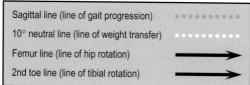

Sagittal line (line of gait progression) ··········
10° neutral line (line of weight transfer) ▪▪▪▪▪▪▪▪▪▪
Femur line (line of hip rotation) ⟶
2nd toe line (line of tibial rotation) ⟶

Figure 9.34 Ideal rotation (axial) alignment

Ideal rotational alignment

The long axis of the femur and the 2nd metatarsal are both aligned to the lower limb neutral line (a line 10° lateral to the sagittal plane – starting at the heel of each foot).

Dysfunctions

The long axis (line) of femur falls medial to the neutral 10° sagittal line *or* the 2nd metatarsal aligns lateral to the neutral 10° sagittal line

suggesting either a structural or functional problem:

- Femoral medial rotation indicates a loss of femoral rotation control (poor stability of posterior gluteus medius or overactivity of tensor fasciae latae). Observe that the femur medially rotates and the long axis of the femur moves medial to the neutral 10° sagittal line (and medial to the 2nd metatarsal).
- Lateral tibial rotation indicates a loss of tibial rotation control (poor stability of popliteus and overactivity of tensor fasciae latae/anterior iliotibial band, superficial gluteus maximus/posterior iliotibial band or biceps femoris). Observe that the heel pulls in or the foot turns out so that the line of the 2nd metatarsal moves lateral to the neutral 10° sagittal line and is more than 10° lateral to the sagittal plane (and lateral to the long axis of the femur).
- Once proximal stability has been lost (loss of femoral or tibial rotation control) the rearfoot or midfoot loses functional stability and the medial longitudinal arch is forced to collapse. This is often associated with a lack of closed chain stability control by tibialis posterior. Observe substitution with overactivity of the toe flexors.

'Natural' (uncorrected) rotational alignment can be classified into one of four groups:

1. Ideal (Figure 9.34):
   a. femur and tibia (foot) correctly aligned on the neutral line (=10°).
2. Hip (femoral) medial rotation dysfunction (Figure 9.35):
   a. femur aligned inside the neutral line (<10°)
   b. tibia (foot) correctly aligned on the neutral line (=10°).
3. Tibial lateral rotation dysfunction (Figure 9.36):
   a. tibia (foot) aligned outside the neutral line (>10°)
   b. femur correctly aligned on the neutral line (=10°).
4. Femoral medial rotation + tibial lateral rotation dysfunction (Figure 9.37):
   a. femur aligned inside the neutral line (<10°)
   b. tibia (foot) aligned outside the neutral line (>10°).

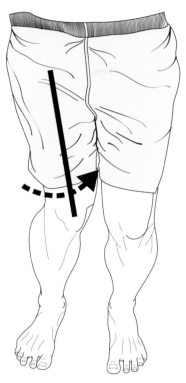

Figure 9.35 Rotation (axial) alignment group 2 – hip medial rotation dysfunction: excessive hip medial rotation (knee turned in) relative to a neutral foot (tibial) alignment

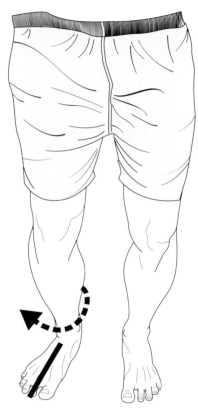

Figure 9.36 Rotation (axial) alignment group 3 – tibial lateral rotation dysfunction: excessive tibial lateral rotation (foot turned out) relative to neutral hip and knee alignment

Correcting neutral rotational alignment of the small knee bend (SKB)

Correct neutral alignment is often required as a start position for many of the dissociation tests for UCM. Correct the foot position (place the feet hip width apart with the 2nd metatarsal aligned along the 'neutral line' of weight transfer (a line that is 10° lateral to the sagittal plane) and perform a SKB, by flexing the knees and dorsiflexing the ankles while keeping both heels on the floor (Figure 9.34). Visualise resting the back against a wall and then bend the knees to slide the back down the wall. The line of the femur should also be on the 10° neutral line (the knees should be further apart than the feet). The trunk should stay vertical and the knees should move past the toes.

In weight bearing, with correct alignment, the line of the femur should be over and parallel to the line of the 2nd metatarsal. Note whether correction can be achieved with ease or only with difficulty, or if it cannot be corrected. When correcting the SKB to neutral, note if there is a sensation of strain. This often indicates a site of restriction. Assess that area for articular of myofascial restrictions.

Progress to performing this same movement without the wall, with both feet. The final progression is to perform the SKB unsupported in single leg stance.

HIP MEDIAL ROTATION CONTROL TESTS AND MEDIAL ROTATION CONTROL REHABILITATION

These rotation control tests assess the extent of medial rotation UCM in the hip and assess the ability of the dynamic stability system to

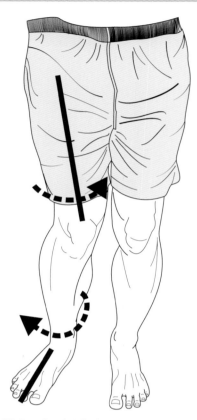

Figure 9.37 Rotation (axial) alignment group 4 – hip medial rotation dysfunction: excessive hip medial rotation (knee turned in) as well as tibial lateral rotation dysfunction: excessive tibial lateral rotation (foot turned out)

adequately control medial rotation load or strain. It is a priority to assess for rotation UCM if the patient complains of or demonstrates medial rotation-related symptoms or disability. The tests that identify dysfunction can also be used to guide and direct rehabilitation strategies.

Indications to test for hip medial rotation UCM

Observe or palpate for:

1. hypermobile hip medial rotation range
2. excessive initiation of turning with hip medial rotation
3. symptoms (pain, discomfort, strain) associated with turning into hip medial rotation.

The person complains of rotation-related symptoms in the hip. Under unilateral or rotation load, the hip has greater give *into medial rotation* relative to the trunk or lower leg. The dysfunction is confirmed with motor control tests of medial rotation dissociation.

Hip medial rotation control tests

T72 STANDING: SINGLE LEG SKB TEST (tests for hip medial rotation UCM)

This dissociation test assesses the ability to actively dissociate and control hip medial rotation and perform a single leg ¼ squat – SKB by moving one hip and knee through flexion while in single leg standing. During any unilateral or asymmetrical lower limb movement, a rotational force is transmitted to the pelvic and hip region.

Test procedure

The person stands with the feet hip width apart (heels approximately 10–15 cm apart) with the inside borders of the feet parallel (not turned out). Stance is upright with the upper body vertical and the weight balanced over the midfoot. The person is instructed to shift full weight onto one foot and lift the other foot just clear of the floor. The person should stand on one leg with the 2nd metatarsal aligned along the 'neutral line' of weight transfer (a line that is 10° lateral to the sagittal plane). The pelvis should be level and the trunk upright (vertical). There should be no lateral deviation, tilt or rotation of the trunk or pelvis. The head, sternum and pubic symphysis should be vertically aligned above the inside edge of the stance foot with the shoulders level in an upright posture (Figure 9.38).

In this position, the person performs a single leg SKB by flexing at the knee and dorsiflexing the ankle while keeping the heel on the floor. The body weight is kept on the heel, not the ball of the foot, and the trunk is vertical (as if sliding the back down a wall) with no forwards lean. The knee is held out over the foot to orientate the line of the femur out over the 2nd toe (on the 'neutral line') (Figure 9.39). The trunk should stay vertical and the knees should move 3–8 cm past the toes.

Some people may experience a sensation of a lack of the required knee bend range. This test requires that during testing for UCM the knees bend to move at least 5 cm past the longest toe so that the compensation and UCM can be identified.

Ideally, there should be approximately 3–8 cm of independent SKB, without any hip medial

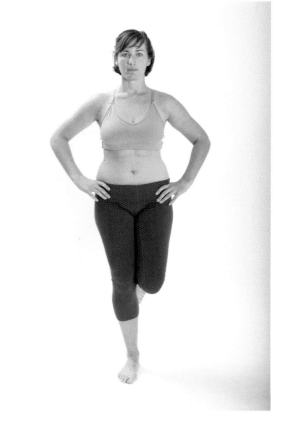

Figure 9.38 Start position single leg small knee bend test

rotation or midfoot pronation. Body weight should stay balanced over the foot and there should be no lateral shift of the pelvis. This test should be performed without any feedback (self-palpation, vision, etc.) or cueing for correction. The therapist should use visual observation of the femur and foot to determine whether the control of hip medial rotation is adequate when feedback is removed for testing. Assess both legs separately.

Hip medial rotation UCM

The person complains of rotation-related symptoms in the hip. During the single leg SKB the hip demonstrates UCM into medial rotation (the knee moves medially) before the knee reaches 3–8 cm past the toes. As the knee moves medial to the foot, the medial longitudinal arch collapses

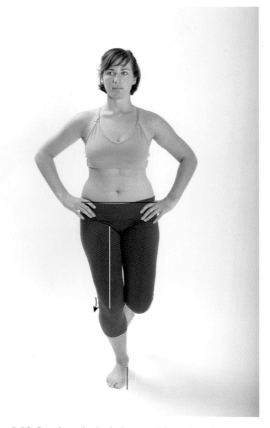

Figure 9.39 Benchmark single leg small knee bend test

Rating and diagnosis of hip rotation UCM

(T72.1 and T72.2)

Correction

If control is poor, the uncontrolled hip medial rotation presents in bilateral weight bearing. Initial retraining is best started in bilateral stance with the trunk supported against a wall. The person stands with the back against a wall and the feet hip width apart (heels approximately 10–15 cm apart), with the inside borders of the feet parallel (not turned out) so that the 2nd toe (both feet) is aligned to the neutral line of weight transfer. The person should stand upright with the upper body vertical and the weight balanced over the midfoot. The heels should be approximately 5–10 cm from the wall. The pelvis should be level and the trunk upright (vertical).

The person is instructed to perform a bilateral SKB. This is achieved by sliding the trunk down the wall by flexing at the knees and dorsiflexing the ankles while keeping the heels down with no forwards trunk lean. The person should be instructed to keep the knees out over the foot to orientate the line of the femur out over the neutral line (along with the 2nd toe) (Figure 9.40). The trunk slides down the wall and the knee flexes only as far as neutral hip rotation can be controlled (monitored with feedback). At the point in range that the hip starts to lose control of medial rotation the movement should stop. The hip is restabilised (move the knee out over the 2nd toe) and returns to the start position with control of the hip rotation UCM.

The person should self-monitor the hip alignment and control medial rotation UCM with a variety of feedback options (T72.3). There

into midfoot pronation. Under unilateral hip and knee weight bearing, the hip has UCM *into medial rotation* relative to the knee and foot.

The uncontrolled hip medial rotation is often associated with inefficiency of the stability function of the gluteal lateral rotators (especially posterior gluteus medius and deep gluteus maximus) providing isometric or eccentric control of hip medial rotation and for popliteus to control rotation at the knee. During the attempt to dissociate the hip medial rotation from unilateral leg movement, the person either cannot control the UCM or has to concentrate and try hard to control the hip medial rotation. The movement must be assessed on both sides. If hip medial rotation UCM presents bilaterally, one side may be better or worse than the other.

T72.1 Assessment and rating of low threshold recruitment efficiency of the Single Leg SKB Test

SINGLE LEG SMALL KNEE BEND TEST – STANDING

ASSESSMENT

Control point:
• prevent hip medial rotation
Movement challenge: unilateral hip and knee flexion (standing)
Benchmark range: unilateral knee flexion without compensation

RATING OF LOW THRESHOLD RECRUITMENT EFFICIENCY FOR CONTROL OF DIRECTION

	✓ or ✗		✓ or ✗
• Able to prevent UCM into the test direction Correct dissociation pattern of movement Prevent hip UCM into: • medial rotation and move unilateral knee and hip flexion	☐	• Looks easy, and in the opinion of the assessor, is performed with confidence	☐
		• Feels easy, and the subject has sufficient awareness of the movement pattern that they confidently prevent UCM into the test direction	☐
• Dissociate movement through the benchmark range of: knee flexion to 3–8 cm past toes with trunk upright in ¼ squat *If there is more available range than the benchmark standard, only the benchmark range needs to be actively controlled*	☐	• The pattern of dissociation is smooth during concentric and eccentric movement	☐
		• Does not (consistently) use *end-range* movement into the opposite direction to prevent the UCM	☐
• Without holding breath (though it is acceptable to use an alternate breathing strategy)	☐	• No extra feedback needed (*tactile, visual or verbal cueing*)	☐
		• Without external support or unloading	☐
• Control during eccentric phase	☐	• Relaxed natural breathing (*even if not ideal – so long as natural pattern does not change*)	☐
• Control during concentric phase	☐	• No fatigue	☐

CORRECT DISSOCIATION PATTERN   **RECRUITMENT EFFICIENCY**

T72.2 Diagnosis of the site and direction of UCM from the Single Leg SKB Test

SINGLE LEG SKB TEST – STANDING

Site	Direction	(L) leg	(R) leg
		(check box)	(check box)
Hip	Medial rotation	☐	☐

T72.3 Feedback tools to monitor retraining

FEEDBACK TOOL	PROCESS
Self-palpation	Palpation monitoring of joint position
Visual observation	Observe in a mirror or directly watch the movement
Adhesive tape	Skin tension for tactile feedback
Cueing and verbal correction	Listen to feedback from another observer

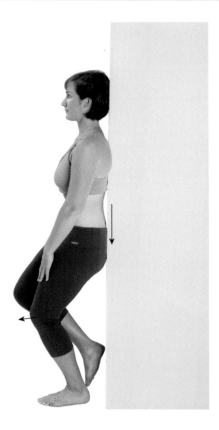

Figure 9.40 Partial small knee bend with wall support

should be no provocation of any symptoms within the range that the rotation UCM can be controlled.

As the ability to control hip medial rotation gets easier and the pattern of dissociation feels less unnatural, the exercise can be progressed to performing this same movement without the wall for support, with both feet. The final progression is to perform the SKB unsupported in single leg stance.

Note whether correction can be achieved with ease or only with difficulty, or if it cannot be corrected at all. When trying to correct the SKB to neutral, note if there is a sensation of 'strain'. This often indicates a site of restriction. Assess that area for articular or myofascial restrictions.

T73 STANDING: ONE LEG SKB + TRUNK ROTATION AWAY TEST (tests for hip medial rotation UCM)

This dissociation test assesses the ability to actively dissociate and control hip medial rotation and perform a single leg ¼ squat – SKB and rotate the trunk and pelvis away from the stance leg. During any asymmetrical or non-sagittal trunk movement a rotational force is transmitted to the pelvic and hip region.

Test procedure

The person stands with the feet hip width apart (heels approximately 10–15 cm apart), with the inside borders of the feet parallel (not turned out). The person is instructed to stand upright with the upper body vertical and the weight balanced over the midfoot. They then shift full weight onto one foot and lift the other foot just clear of the floor. A single leg SKB is then performed by flexing at the knee and dorsiflexing the ankle while keeping the heel on the floor. The person is instructed to keep body weight on the heel, not the ball of the foot, and keep the trunk vertical (as if sliding the back down a wall) without allowing forwards trunk lean. Hold the knee out over the foot to orientate the line of the femur out over the 2nd toe (on the 10° 'neutral line' of weight transfer) (Figure 9.41).

Then, while standing on one leg, the person is instructed to rotate the trunk and pelvis away from the stance leg (i.e. if standing on the right leg, turn the trunk and pelvis to the left). Keep the knee aligned to the neutral line. They should have the ability to actively rotate the trunk and pelvis (hip lateral rotation relative to the pelvis) without the knee moving medially to follow the pelvis. Ideally, there should be approximately 35° of independent trunk and pelvis rotation (Figure 9.42). As soon as any medial movement of the knee occurs, the movement must stop and return to the start position. This test should be performed without any feedback (self-palpation, vision, etc.) or cueing for correction. When feedback is removed for testing the therapist should use visual observation of the pelvis to determine whether the control of hip medial rotation is adequate. Assess both sides.

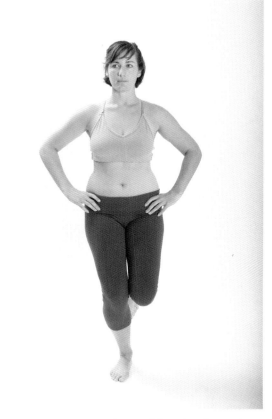

Figure 9.41 Start position 1 leg small knee bend + trunk rotation away test

Hip medial rotation UCM

The person complains of rotation-related symptoms in the hip. During the single leg SKB the knee moves medially before the knee reaches 5–10 cm past the toes. During the one leg SKB + trunk rotation away test, the hip demonstrates UCM into medial rotation (the knee moves medially) before the trunk and pelvis rotation reaches 35° lateral rotation away from the stance leg. As the knee moves medial to the foot, the medial longitudinal arch collapses into midfoot pronation. Under unilateral hip and knee weight bearing, the hip has UCM *into medial rotation* relative to the knee and foot.

The uncontrolled hip medial rotation is often associated with inefficiency of the stability function of the gluteal lateral rotators (especially posterior gluteus medius and deep gluteus maximus) providing isometric or eccentric control of hip

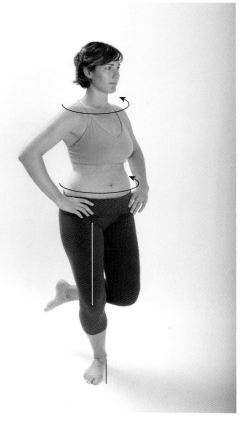

Figure 9.42 Benchmark 1 leg small knee bend + trunk rotation away test

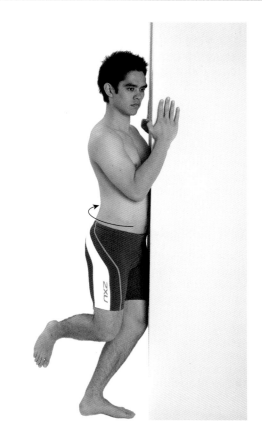

Figure 9.43 Correction partial range with wall support

medial rotation and for popliteus to control rotation at the knee. During the attempt to dissociate the hip medial rotation from unilateral leg movement, the person either cannot control the UCM or has to concentrate and try hard to control the hip medial rotation. The movement must be assessed on both sides. If hip medial rotation UCM presents bilaterally, one side may be better or worse than the other.

Clinical assessment note for direction-specific motor control testing

If some other movement (e.g. a small amount of flexion or extension) is observed during a motor control (dissociation) test of medial rotation control, *do not* score this as uncontrolled medial rotation. The flexion and extension motor control tests will identify whether the observed movement is uncontrolled. *A test for hip medial rotation UCM is only positive if uncontrolled hip medial rotation is demonstrated.*

Rating and diagnosis of hip rotation UCM

(T73.1 and T73.2)

Correction

The person stands facing the frame of a doorway or a corner section of wall, with the toes approximately 5 cm from the wall/doorframe. They should stand on one leg with the inside border of the foot perpendicular to the wall. The person first performs a SKB to position the thigh and trunk against the wall/doorframe. They are then instructed to turn the trunk and pelvis away from the stance leg. The wall or doorframe provides support and feedback for the subject to monitor and control the knee from moving medially while the trunk and pelvis laterally rotate (Figure 9.43). The trunk and pelvis rotate only as far as the thigh position can be controlled (monitored with feedback). At the point in range that the knee moves medially to the neutral line, the movement should stop. The hip is restabilised (move the knee out over the 2nd toe) and returns to the start position with control of the hip rotation UCM.

The person should self-monitor the hip alignment and control medial rotation UCM with a variety of feedback options (T73.3). There should be no provocation of any symptoms within the range that the rotation UCM can be controlled.

As the ability to control hip medial rotation gets easier and the pattern of dissociation feels less unnatural, the exercise can be progressed to performing this same movement unsupported, without the wall, in single leg stance.

T73.1 Assessment and rating of low threshold recruitment efficiency of the One Leg SKB + Trunk Rotation Away Test

ONE LEG SMALL KNEE BEND + TRUNK ROTATION AWAY TEST – STANDING

ASSESSMENT

Control point:
- prevent hip medial rotation

Movement challenge: unilateral SKB + trunk/pelvis rotation away from stance leg (standing)

Benchmark range: 35° independent trunk/pelvis lateral rotation (unilateral SKB) with knee aligned on the 2nd toe (neutral line) without compensation of hip medial rotation

RATING OF LOW THRESHOLD RECRUITMENT EFFICIENCY FOR CONTROL OF DIRECTION

	✓ or ✗		✓ or ✗
• Able to prevent UCM into the test direction Correct dissociation pattern of movement Prevent hip UCM into: • medial rotation and move trunk and pelvis lateral rotation away from stance leg	☐	• Looks easy, and in the opinion of the assessor, is performed with confidence	☐
		• Feels easy, and the subject has sufficient awareness of the movement pattern that they confidently prevent UCM into the test direction	☐
• Dissociate movement through the benchmark range of: 35° trunk/pelvis lateral rotation *If there is more available range than the benchmark standard, only the benchmark range needs to be actively controlled*	☐	• The pattern of dissociation is smooth during concentric and eccentric movement	☐
		• Does not (consistently) use *end-range* movement into the opposite direction to prevent the UCM	☐
• Without holding breath (though it is acceptable to use an alternate breathing strategy)	☐	• No extra feedback needed (*tactile, visual or verbal cueing*)	☐
		• Without external support or unloading	☐
• Control during eccentric phase	☐	• Relaxed natural breathing (*even if not ideal – so long as natural pattern does not change*)	☐
• Control during concentric phase	☐	• No fatigue	☐

CORRECT DISSOCIATION PATTERN　　　　**RECRUITMENT EFFICIENCY**

T73.2 Diagnosis of the site and direction of UCM from the One Leg SKB + Trunk Rotation Away Test

ONE LEG SMALL KNEE BEND + TRUNK ROTATION AWAY TEST – STANDING

Site	Direction	(L) leg	(R) leg
		(check box)	(check box)
Hip	Medial rotation	☐	☐

T73.3 Feedback tools to monitor retraining

FEEDBACK TOOL	PROCESS
Self-palpation	Palpation monitoring of joint position
Visual observation	Observe in a mirror or directly watch the movement
Adhesive tape	Skin tension for tactile feedback
Cueing and verbal correction	Listen to feedback from another observer

T74 SIDE-LYING: TOP LEG TURNOUT LIFT TEST
(tests for hip medial rotation UCM)

This dissociation test assesses the ability to actively dissociate and control hip medial rotation and perform a single leg hip abduction and lateral rotation. During any unilateral or asymmetrical lower limb movement, a rotational force is transmitted to the pelvic and hip region.

Test procedure

The person lies on one side with uppermost (top) leg extended in line with the trunk, the other (bottom leg) hip flexed to 45° and the knees flexed to 90° (Figure 9.44). The pelvis should be positioned in neutral rotation. The person is instructed to maintain the neutral pelvis position and turn the uppermost foot outwards (hip lateral rotation). Then they should slowly lift the uppermost leg vertically up and out to the side while keeping the leg and foot turned out into lateral rotation. Ideally, the top leg should be able to maintain the hip extension and turnout and lift into at least 35° (above horizontal) of hip abduction and lateral rotation (Figure 9.45) and return, without associated loss of full turnout into any medial rotation of the hip.

The unilateral hip abduction must be independent of any hip medial rotation. Note any excessive hip medial rotation under hip abduction load. This test should be performed without any feedback (self-palpation, vision, flexicurve, etc.) or cueing for correction. The therapist should use visual observation of the pelvis to determine whether the control of hip medial rotation is adequate when feedback is removed for testing. Assess both sides.

Hip medial rotation UCM

The person complains of rotation-related symptoms in the hip. During the top leg turnout lift test, the foot begins to rotate down (hip medial rotation UCM) before the abduction lift reaches 35° above horizontal. Under unilateral hip loading, the hip has UCM *into medial rotation*.

The uncontrolled hip medial rotation is often associated with inefficiency of the stability function of the gluteal lateral rotators (especially posterior gluteus medius and deep gluteus maximus) providing isometric or eccentric control of hip medial rotation. During the attempt to dissociate the hip medial rotation from unilateral leg

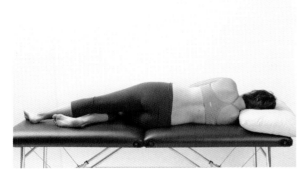

Figure 9.44 Start position top leg turnout lift test

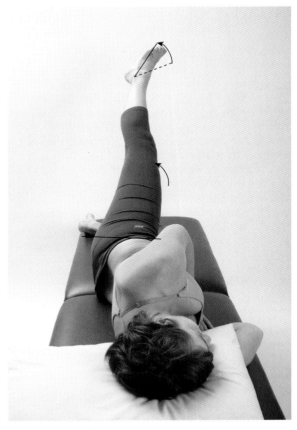

Figure 9.45 Benchmark top leg turnout lift test

467

movement, the person either cannot control the UCM or has to concentrate and try hard to control the hip medial rotation. The movement must be assessed on both sides. If hip medial rotation UCM presents bilaterally, one side may be better or worse than the other.

Clinical assessment note for direction-specific motor control testing

If some other movement (e.g. a small amount of flexion or extension) is observed during a motor control (dissociation) test of medial rotation control, *do not* score this as uncontrolled medial rotation. The flexion and extension motor control tests will identify whether the observed movement is uncontrolled. *A test for hip medial rotation UCM is only positive if uncontrolled hip medial rotation is demonstrated.*

Rating and diagnosis of hip rotation UCM

(T74.1 and T74.2)

Correction

If control is poor, retraining can initially begin with reduced leg load. With the person side-lying and the hips flexed to 45°, the knees flexed to 90° and the feet together, the pelvis should be positioned in neutral rotation. Keeping the heels together the person is instructed to lift the top leg up and out to the side (Figure 9.46). Hold this position, and lift the heel of the top leg 2–3 cm away from the bottom heel. Ensure that, as the heel lifts, the knee does not drop down into hip

medial rotation. At the point in range that the hip starts to lose control of rotation, the movement should stop. The hip position is restabilised (lift the knee and keep the heel down), then hold this position for a few seconds and return to the start position.

The unilateral hip abduction must be independent of any hip medial rotation. The person should self-monitor the hip alignment and control medial rotation UCM with a variety of feedback options (T74.3). There should be no provocation of any symptoms within the range that the rotation UCM can be controlled.

As the ability to control hip medial rotation gets easier and the pattern of dissociation feels less unnatural, the exercise can be progressed to performing the hip abduction and lateral rotation with the leg fully extended.

Hip medial rotation UCM summary

(Table 9.4)

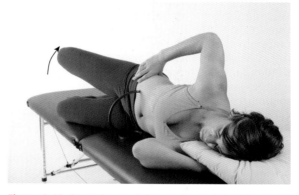

Figure 9.46 Correction partial range turnout short lever

Table 9.4 Summary and rating of hip medial rotation tests		
UCM DIAGNOSIS AND TESTING		
SITE: HIP	**DIRECTION:** MEDIAL ROTATION	**CLINICAL PRIORITY** ☐
TEST	**RATING** (✓✓ or ✓✗ or ✗✗) and rationale (L)	(R)
Standing: single leg small knee bend		
Standing: one leg knee bend + trunk rotation away		
Side-lying: top leg turnout lift		

T74.1 Assessment and rating of low threshold recruitment efficiency of the Top Leg Turnout Lift Test

TOP LEG TURNOUT LIFT TEST – SIDE-LYING

ASSESSMENT

Control point:
- prevent hip medial rotation

Movement challenge: unilateral hip abduction and lateral rotation (side-lying)

Benchmark range: 35° independent hip abduction and lateral rotation without compensation

RATING OF LOW THRESHOLD RECRUITMENT EFFICIENCY FOR CONTROL OF DIRECTION

	✓ or ✗		✓ or ✗
• Able to prevent UCM into the test direction Correct dissociation pattern of movement Prevent hip UCM into: • medial rotation and move hip abduction and lateral rotation (turnout)	☐	• Looks easy, and in the opinion of the assessor, is performed with confidence	☐
		• Feels easy, and the subject has sufficient awareness of the movement pattern that they confidently prevent UCM into the test direction	☐
• Dissociate movement through the benchmark range of: 35° hip abduction and lateral rotation *If there is more available range than the benchmark standard, only the benchmark range needs to be actively controlled*	☐	• The pattern of dissociation is smooth during concentric and eccentric movement	☐
		• Does not (consistently) use *end-range* movement into the opposite direction to prevent the UCM	☐
• Without holding breath (though it is acceptable to use an alternate breathing strategy)	☐	• No extra feedback needed *(tactile, visual or verbal cueing)*	☐
		• Without external support or unloading	☐
• Control during eccentric phase	☐	• Relaxed natural breathing *(even if not ideal – so long as natural pattern does not change)*	☐
• Control during concentric phase	☐	• No fatigue	☐

CORRECT DISSOCIATION PATTERN | **RECRUITMENT EFFICIENCY**

T74.2 Diagnosis of the site and direction of UCM from the Top Leg Turnout Lift Test

TOP LEG TURNOUT LIFT TEST – STANDING

Site	Direction	(L) leg	(R) leg
		(check box)	(check box)
Hip	Medial rotation	☐	☐

T74.3 Feedback tools to monitor retraining

FEEDBACK TOOL	PROCESS
Self-palpation	Palpation monitoring of joint position
Visual observation	Observe in a mirror or directly watch the movement
Adhesive tape	Skin tension for tactile feedback
Cueing and verbal correction	Listen to feedback from another observer
Flexicurve positional marker	Visual and sensory feedback of positional alignment

HIP LATERAL ROTATION/ABDUCTION CONTROL TESTS AND LATERAL ROTATION/ABDUCTION CONTROL REHABILITATION

These rotation control tests assess the extent of lateral rotation/abduction UCM in the hip and assess the ability of the dynamic stability system to adequately control lateral rotation and abduction load or strain. It is a priority to assess for lateral rotation/abduction UCM if the patient complains of or demonstrates lateral rotation or abduction-related symptoms or disability. The tests that identify dysfunction can also be used to guide and direct rehabilitation strategies.

Indications to test for hip lateral rotation/abduction UCM

Observe or palpate for:

1. hypermobile hip lateral rotation or abduction range
2. excessive initiation of turning with hip lateral rotation or abduction
3. symptoms (pain, discomfort, strain) associated with turning into hip lateral rotation and abduction.

The person complains of rotation-related symptoms in the hip. Under rotation or unilateral load, the hip has greater give *into lateral rotation or abduction* relative to the trunk or lower leg. The dysfunction is confirmed with motor control tests of lateral rotation/abduction dissociation.

Hip lateral rotation/abduction control tests

T75 STANDING: SINGLE LEG HIGH KNEE LIFT TEST
(tests for hip lateral rotation/abduction UCM)

This dissociation test assesses the ability to actively dissociate and control hip lateral rotation/abduction and perform at least 90° of unilateral hip flexion. During any asymmetrical or non-sagittal trunk movement a rotational force is transmitted to the pelvic and hip region.

Test procedure

The person stands tall and unsupported with legs straight and the lumbar spine and pelvis positioned in the neutral (Figure 9.47). The person is instructed to shift weight onto one leg and, keeping the shoulders and pelvis level, slowly lift the other foot off the ground. Without letting the non-weight bearing hip move into lateral rotation or abduction, the person continues to lift the leg into hip flexion with the lower leg relaxed and the heel hanging vertically under the knee. Ideally, the hip should maintain neutral rotation (with no hip lateral rotation) as the hip actively flexes to at least 90° (monitor the flexing leg). The lumbopelvic region should maintain a neutral level position (Figure 9.48). As soon as

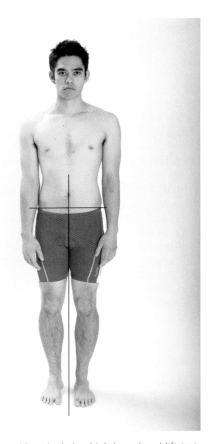

Figure 9.47 Start position single leg high knee bend lift test

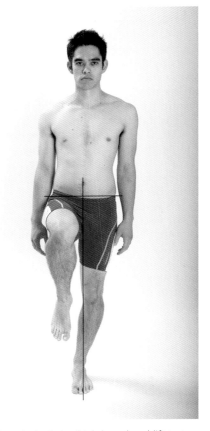

Figure 9.48 Benchmark single leg high knee bend lift test

any movement indicating a loss of neutral into hip lateral rotation or abduction is observed, or hitching the pelvis to lift the leg, the movement must stop and return to the start position. Hip flexion to 90° must be demonstrated with the shoulders and pelvis level.

The unilateral hip flexion must be independent of any hip lateral rotation or abduction. Note any uncontrolled hip lateral rotation or abduction under non-weight bearing hip flexion load. This test should be performed without any feedback (self-palpation, vision, flexicurve, etc.) or cueing for correction. When feedback is removed for testing the therapist should use visual observation of the pelvis and leg to determine whether the control of hip lateral rotation/abduction is adequate. Assess both sides.

Hip lateral rotation/abduction UCM

The person complains of rotation-related symptoms in the hip. During the single leg high knee lift the hip demonstrates UCM into lateral rotation or abduction before the non-weight bearing hip reaches 90° flexion (thigh horizontal). During the single leg high knee lift test, the foot swings in towards the midline (hip lateral rotation UCM) or the thigh turns out into abduction and lateral rotation before the knee lift reaches 90° (thigh horizontal). Under unilateral hip loading, the hip has UCM *into lateral rotation or abduction*. Hitching the pelvis to lift the thigh horizontal is not hip flexion to 90° and is a common substitution strategy for inefficient control. Hip flexion to 90° must be demonstrated with the shoulders and pelvis level.

The uncontrolled hip lateral rotation/abduction is often associated with inefficiency of the stability function of the gluteal medial rotators (especially anterior gluteus medius and gluteus minimus) providing isometric or eccentric control of hip lateral rotation. Concurrently the deep adductor stabilisers (pectineus and adductor brevis) may not provide eccentric control of hip abduction. During the attempt to dissociate the hip lateral rotation/abduction from unilateral leg movement, the person either cannot control the UCM or has to concentrate and try hard to control the hip lateral rotation or abduction. The movement must be assessed on both sides. If hip lateral rotation/abduction UCM presents

bilaterally, one side may be better or worse than the other.

Clinical assessment note for direction-specific motor control testing

If some other movement (e.g. a small amount of flexion or extension) is observed during a motor control (dissociation) test of lateral rotation/abduction control, *do not* score this as uncontrolled lateral rotation/abduction. The flexion and extension motor control tests will identify if the observed movement is uncontrolled. *A test for hip lateral rotation/abduction UCM is only positive if uncontrolled hip lateral rotation or abduction is demonstrated.*

Rating and diagnosis of hip rotation UCM

(T75.1 and T75.2)

Correction

If control is poor, initial retraining is best started with the trunk supported against a wall. The person stands with the back against a wall and the feet hip width apart (heels approximately 10–15 cm apart) with the inside borders of the feet parallel. Stand upright with the upper body vertical and the weight balanced over the midfoot. The heels should be approximately 5–10 cm from the wall. The pelvis should be level and the trunk upright (vertical). The person is instructed to shift their weight onto one foot and, keeping the shoulders and pelvis level, slowly lift the other foot off the ground. They are to lift the leg only as far as the pelvis stays level and as far as the foot hangs vertically under the knee (i.e. no hip lateral rotation) and the thigh stays in the midline (i.e. no hip abduction). The hip can lift into flexion only as far as the lateral rotation, abduction and the pelvic position can be controlled (monitored with feedback) (Figure 9.49). Initially, the person may only be able to lift the leg into 60° or 70° hip flexion before the UCM is demonstrated. At the point in range that the foot swings medially (hip lateral rotation), or the pelvis starts to hitch, the movement should stop. The hip and pelvis are restabilised and the leg returns to the start position with control of the hip rotation UCM.

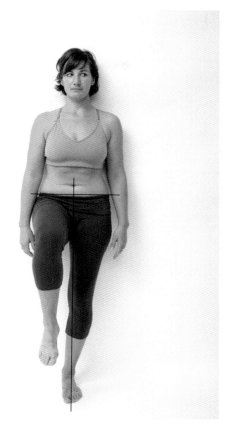

Figure 9.49 Correction partial range knee lift with support

The person should self-monitor the hip alignment and control lateral rotation and abduction UCM with a variety of feedback options (T75.3). There should be no provocation of any symptoms within the range that the rotation UCM can be controlled.

As the ability to control hip lateral rotation/abduction gets easier and the pattern of dissociation feels less unnatural, the exercise can be progressed to performing this same movement unsupported, without the wall, in single leg stance.

T75.1 Assessment and rating of low threshold recruitment efficiency of the Single Leg High Knee Lift Test

SINGLE LEG HIGH KNEE LIFT TEST – STANDING

ASSESSMENT

Control point:
• prevent hip lateral rotation/abduction
Movement challenge: unilateral hip flexion (standing)
Benchmark range: 90° independent unilateral hip flexion without compensation of hip lateral rotation or abduction

RATING OF LOW THRESHOLD RECRUITMENT EFFICIENCY FOR CONTROL OF DIRECTION

✓ or ✗ | ✓ or ✗

• Able to prevent UCM into the test direction Correct dissociation pattern of movement ☐
Prevent hip UCM into:
• lateral rotation/abduction
and move unilateral hip flexion
• Dissociate movement through the benchmark range of: 90° hip flexion ☐
If there is more available range than the benchmark standard, only the benchmark range needs to be actively controlled
• Without holding breath (though it is acceptable to use an alternate breathing strategy) ☐
• Control during eccentric phase ☐
• Control during concentric phase ☐

• Looks easy, and in the opinion of the assessor, is performed with confidence ☐
• Feels easy, and the subject has sufficient awareness of the movement pattern that they confidently prevent UCM into the test direction ☐
• The pattern of dissociation is smooth during concentric and eccentric movement ☐
• Does not (consistently) use *end-range* movement into the opposite direction to prevent the UCM ☐
• No extra feedback needed *(tactile, visual or verbal cueing)* ☐
• Without external support or unloading ☐
• Relaxed natural breathing *(even if not ideal – so long as natural pattern does not change)* ☐
• No fatigue ☐

CORRECT DISSOCIATION PATTERN | **RECRUITMENT EFFICIENCY**

T75.2 Diagnosis of the site and direction of UCM from the Single Leg High Knee Lift Test

SINGLE LEG HIGH KNEE LIFT TEST – STANDING

Site	Direction	(L) leg	(R) leg
		(check box)	(check box)
Hip	Lateral rotation/ abduction	☐	☐

T75.3 Feedback tools to monitor retraining	
FEEDBACK TOOL	**PROCESS**
Self-palpation	Palpation monitoring of joint position
Visual observation	Observe in a mirror or directly watch the movement
Adhesive tape	Skin tension for tactile feedback
Cueing and verbal correction	Listen to feedback from another observer

T76 STANDING: ONE LEG SKB + TRUNK ROTATION TOWARDS TEST
(tests for hip lateral rotation/abduction UCM)

This dissociation test assesses the ability to actively dissociate and control hip lateral rotation/abduction and perform a single leg ¼ squat – SKB and rotate the trunk and pelvis towards the stance leg. During any asymmetrical or non-sagittal trunk movement a rotational force is transmitted to the pelvic and hip region.

Test procedure

The person stands with the feet hip width apart (heels approximately 10–15 cm apart) with the inside borders of the feet parallel (not turned out). They should stand upright with the upper body vertical and the weight balanced over the midfoot. The person is then instructed to shift full weight onto one foot and lift the other foot just clear of the floor. In this position, they should perform a single leg SKB by flexing at the knee and dorsiflexing the ankle while keeping the heel on the floor. They should be instructed to keep body weight on the heel, not the ball of the foot, and keep the trunk vertical (as if sliding the back down a wall) with no trunk forwards lean. The knee should be held out over the foot to orientate the line of the femur out over the 2nd toe (on the 10° 'neutral line' of weight transfer) (Figure 9.50).

Then, while standing on one leg, the person is instructed to rotate the trunk and pelvis towards the stance leg (i.e. if standing on the right leg, turn the trunk and pelvis to the right). Keep the knee aligned to the neutral line. The person should have the ability to actively rotate the trunk and pelvis (hip medial rotation relative to the pelvis) without the knee moving laterally to follow the pelvis. Ideally, there should be approximately 30° of independent trunk and pelvis rotation (Figure 9.51). As soon as any lateral movement of the knee occurs, the movement must stop and return back to the start position. This test should be performed without any feedback (self-palpation, vision, etc.) or cueing for correction. When feedback is removed for testing the therapist should use visual observation of the pelvis to determine whether the control of hip lateral rotation/abduction is adequate. Assess both sides.

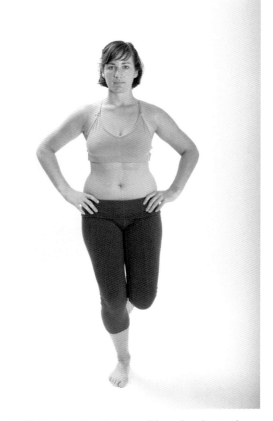

Figure 9.50 Start position 1 leg small knee bend + trunk rotation towards test

Hip lateral rotation/abduction UCM

The person complains of rotation-related symptoms in the hip. During the one leg SKB + trunk rotation towards test, the hip demonstrates UCM into lateral rotation or abduction (the knee moves laterally) before the trunk and pelvis rotation reaches 30° medial rotation towards the stance leg. Under unilateral hip and knee weight bearing, the hip has UCM *into lateral rotation/abduction*.

The uncontrolled hip lateral rotation/abduction is often associated with inefficiency of the stability function of the gluteal medial rotators (especially anterior gluteus medius and gluteus minimus) providing isometric or eccentric control of hip lateral rotation. Concurrently the deep adductor stabilisers (pectineus and adductor brevis) may not provide eccentric control of hip abduction. During the attempt to dissociate the hip lateral rotation from unilateral leg

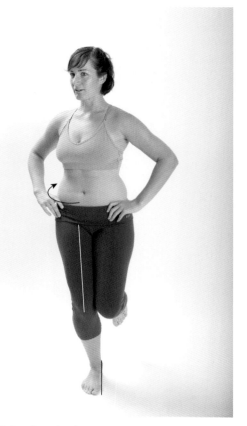

Figure 9.51 Benchmark 1 leg small knee bend + trunk rotation towards test

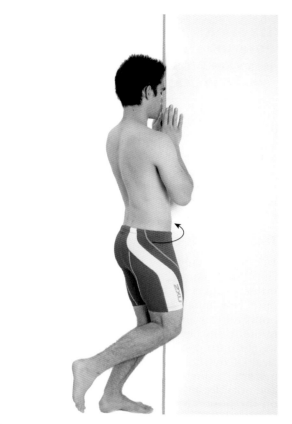

Figure 9.52 Correction partial range with wall support

movement, the person either cannot control the UCM or has to concentrate and try hard to control the hip lateral rotation. The movement must be assessed on both sides. If hip lateral rotation UCM presents bilaterally, one side may be better or worse than the other.

Clinical assessment note for direction-specific motor control testing

If some other movement (e.g. a small amount of flexion or extension) is observed during a motor control (dissociation) test of lateral rotation/abduction control, *do not* score this as uncontrolled lateral rotation/abduction. The flexion and extension motor control tests will identify if the observed movement is uncontrolled. *A test for hip lateral rotation/abduction UCM is only positive if uncontrolled hip lateral rotation or abduction is demonstrated.*

Rating and diagnosis of hip rotation UCM

(T76.1 and T76.2)

Correction

The person stands facing the frame of a doorway or a corner section of wall, with the toes approximately 5 cm from the wall/doorframe. They should stand on one leg with the inside border of the foot perpendicular to the wall. The person first performs a SKB to position the thigh and trunk against the wall/doorframe. They are then instructed to turn the trunk and pelvis towards the stance leg. The wall or doorframe provides support and feedback for the subject to monitor and control the knee from moving laterally while the trunk and pelvis medially rotate (Figure 9.52). The trunk and pelvis rotate only as far as the thigh position can be controlled (monitored with feedback). At the point in range that the knee moves laterally to the neutral line, the movement should stop. The hip is restabilised and returns to the start position with control of the hip rotation UCM.

The person should self-monitor the hip alignment and control lateral rotation and abduction UCM with a variety of feedback options (T76.3).

There should be no provocation of any symptoms within the range that the lateral rotation/abduction UCM can be controlled.

As the ability to control hip lateral rotation/abduction gets easier and the pattern of dissociation feels less unnatural, the exercise can be progressed to performing this same movement unsupported, without the wall, in single leg stance.

T76.1 Assessment and rating of low threshold recruitment efficiency of the One Leg SKB + Trunk Rotation Towards Test

ONE LEG SMALL KNEE BEND + TRUNK ROTATION TOWARDS TEST – STANDING

ASSESSMENT

Control point:
- prevent hip lateral rotation/abduction

Movement challenge: unilateral SKB + trunk/pelvis rotation toward stance leg (standing)

Benchmark range: 30° independent trunk/pelvis medial rotation (unilateral SKB) with knee aligned on the 2nd toe (neutral line) without compensation of hip lateral rotation or abduction

RATING OF LOW THRESHOLD RECRUITMENT EFFICIENCY FOR CONTROL OF DIRECTION

	✓ or ✗		✓ or ✗
• Able to prevent UCM into the test direction Correct dissociation pattern of movement Prevent hip UCM into: • lateral rotation/abduction and move trunk and pelvis lateral rotation towards stance leg	☐	• Looks easy, and in the opinion of the assessor, is performed with confidence	☐
		• Feels easy, and the subject has sufficient awareness of the movement pattern that they confidently prevent UCM into the test direction	☐
• Dissociate movement through the benchmark range of: 30° trunk/pelvis medial rotation *If there is more available range than the benchmark standard, only the benchmark range needs to be actively controlled*	☐	• The pattern of dissociation is smooth during concentric and eccentric movement	☐
		• Does not (consistently) use *end-range* movement into the opposite direction to prevent the UCM	☐
• Without holding breath (though it is acceptable to use an alternate breathing strategy)	☐	• No extra feedback needed (*tactile, visual or verbal cueing*)	☐
		• Without external support or unloading	☐
• Control during eccentric phase	☐	• Relaxed natural breathing (*even if not ideal – so long as natural pattern does not change*)	☐
• Control during concentric phase	☐	• No fatigue	☐

CORRECT DISSOCIATION PATTERN

RECRUITMENT EFFICIENCY

T76.2 Diagnosis of the site and direction of UCM from the One Leg SKB + Trunk Rotation Towards Test

ONE LEG SKB + TRUNK ROTATION TOWARDS TEST – STANDING

Site	Direction	(L) leg	(R) leg
		(check box)	(check box)
Hip	Lateral rotation/ abduction	☐	☐

T76.3 Feedback tools to monitor retraining

FEEDBACK TOOL	PROCESS
Self-palpation	Palpation monitoring of joint position
Visual observation	Observe in a mirror or directly watch the movement
Adhesive tape	Skin tension for tactile feedback
Cueing and verbal correction	Listen to feedback from another observer

T77 4 POINT: BENT KNEE HIP EXTENSION TEST
(tests for hip lateral rotation/abduction UCM)

This dissociation test assesses the ability to actively dissociate and control hip lateral rotation and actively extend one hip (with the knee flexed to 90°) while in 4 point kneeling (hands and knees). During any unilateral or asymmetrical lower limb movement, a rotational force is transmitted to the pelvic and hip region.

Test procedure

The person positions themselves in 4 point kneeling (hands and knees) with the lumbar spine and pelvis in neutral alignment (Figure 9.53). The person is instructed to shift weight onto one knee and, keeping that knee flexed to 90°, slowly lift that leg into hip extension. The leg should stay in the sagittal plane and not abduct out to the side. The heel should stay positioned vertically above the knee as it lifts into hip extension, and not swing across the midline into hip lateral rotation. Ideally, the neutral hip rotation should be maintained until about 0° of hip extension (thigh horizontal) with the knee held at 90° of flexion.

The person should have the ability to dissociate the hip lateral rotation/abduction from hip extension as evidenced by preventing hip lateral rotation and abduction, while lifting the bent knee into hip extension (Figure 9.54). Ideally, the leg should be able to maintain the flexed knee position and lift to 0° (thigh horizontal) of hip extension without any lateral rotation or abduction of the hip. Note any uncontrolled hip lateral rotation or abduction under hip extension load. This test should be performed without any feedback (self-palpation, vision, flexicurve, etc.) or cueing

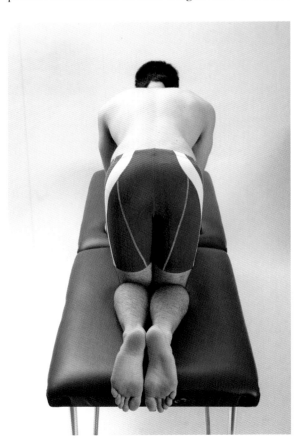

Figure 9.53 Start position bent knee hip extension test

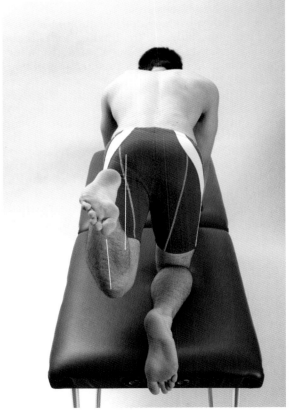

Figure 9.54 Benchmark bent knee hip extension test

for correction. When feedback is removed for testing the therapist should use visual observation of the leg and pelvis to determine whether the control of hip lateral rotation/abduction is adequate. Assess both sides.

Hip lateral rotation/abduction UCM

The person complains of rotation-related symptoms in the hip. During the bent knee hip extension test the hip demonstrates UCM into lateral rotation or abduction before the hip extension reaches 0° (thigh horizontal). During the bent knee hip extension test, the foot swings in towards the midline (hip lateral rotation UCM) or moves laterally away from the midline (hip abduction) before hip extension reaches 0° (thigh horizontal). Under unilateral hip loading, the hip has UCM *into lateral rotation or abduction*. Arching the back or rotating the pelvis to lift the thigh horizontal is not hip extension to 0° and is a common substitution strategy for inefficient control. Hip extension to 0° must be demonstrated with the lumbopelvic compensation.

The uncontrolled hip lateral rotation/abduction is often associated with inefficiency of the stability function of the gluteal medial rotators (especially anterior gluteus medius and gluteus minimus) providing isometric or eccentric control of hip lateral rotation. Concurrently the deep adductor stabilisers (pectineus and adductor brevis) may not provide eccentric control of hip abduction. During the attempt to dissociate the hip lateral rotation and abduction from unilateral leg movement, the person either cannot control the UCM or has to concentrate and try hard to control the hip lateral rotation/abduction. The movement must be assessed on both sides. If hip lateral rotation UCM presents bilaterally, one side may be better or worse than the other.

Clinical assessment note for direction-specific motor control testing

If some other movement (e.g. a small amount of flexion or extension) is observed during a motor control (dissociation) test of lateral rotation/abduction control, *do not* score this as uncontrolled lateral rotation/abduction. The flexion and extension motor control tests will identify if the observed movement is uncontrolled. *A test for hip lateral rotation/abduction UCM is only positive if uncontrolled hip lateral rotation or abduction is demonstrated.*

Rating and diagnosis of hip rotation UCM

(T77.1 and T77.2)

Correction

If control is poor, initial retraining is best started with reduced knee flexion. The person positions themselves in 4 point kneeling (hands and knees) and shifts weight onto one knee. Slowly start to lift that leg into hip extension but allow the knee to straighten so that it is only flexed to about 20° or 30°. The leg should stay in the sagittal plane and not abduct out to the side. The heel should not swing across the midline into hip lateral rotation. A line from the heel through the 2nd toe should be vertical (Figure 9.55).

The unilateral hip extension must be independent of any hip lateral rotation or abduction. The

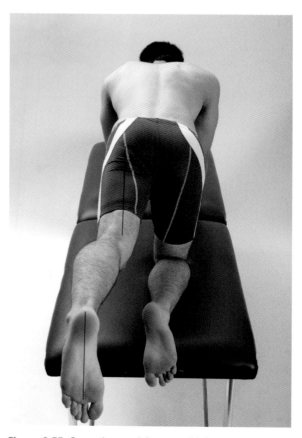

Figure 9.55 Correction partial range with knee extension

hip can lift into extension only as far as the lateral rotation, abduction and the pelvic position can be controlled (monitored with feedback). Initially, the person may only be able to lift the leg through minimal range of hip extension before the UCM is demonstrated. At the point in range that the foot swings medially (hip lateral rotation), the thigh abducts from the midline or the pelvis starts to move, the movement should stop. The hip and pelvis are restabilised and the leg returns to the start position with control of the hip lateral rotation/abduction UCM.

The person should self-monitor the hip alignment and control lateral rotation/abduction UCM with a variety of feedback options (T77.3). There should be no provocation of any symptoms within the range that the rotation UCM can be controlled.

As the ability to control hip lateral rotation/abduction gets easier and the pattern of dissociation feels less unnatural, the exercise can be progressed to performing this hip extension through increased range of hip extension and, finally, with increased knee flexion.

T77.1 Assessment and rating of low threshold recruitment efficiency of the Bent Knee Hip Extension Test

BENT KNEE HIP EXTENSION – 4 POINT KNEELING

ASSESSMENT

Control point:
- prevent hip lateral rotation/abduction

Movement challenge: unilateral hip extension + knee flexion (4 point kneeling)

Benchmark range: 0° independent unilateral hip extension + 90° knee flexion without compensation of hip lateral rotation/abduction

RATING OF LOW THRESHOLD RECRUITMENT EFFICIENCY FOR CONTROL OF DIRECTION

	✓ or ✗		✓ or ✗
• Able to prevent UCM into the test direction Correct dissociation pattern of movement Prevent hip UCM into: • lateral rotation/abduction and move unilateral hip extension + knee flexion	☐	• Looks easy, and in the opinion of the assessor, is performed with confidence	☐
• Dissociate movement through the benchmark range of: 0° hip extension + 90° knee flexion *If there is more available range than the benchmark standard, only the benchmark range needs to be actively controlled*	☐	• Feels easy, and the subject has sufficient awareness of the movement pattern that they confidently prevent UCM into the test direction	☐
		• The pattern of dissociation is smooth during concentric and eccentric movement	☐
• Without holding breath (though it is acceptable to use an alternate breathing strategy)	☐	• Does not (consistently) use *end-range* movement into the opposite direction to prevent the UCM	☐
		• No extra feedback needed *(tactile, visual or verbal cueing)*	☐
• Control during eccentric phase	☐	• Without external support or unloading	☐
• Control during concentric phase	☐	• Relaxed natural breathing *(even if not ideal – so long as natural pattern does not change)*	☐
		• No fatigue	☐

CORRECT DISSOCIATION PATTERN   **RECRUITMENT EFFICIENCY**

T77.2 Diagnosis of the site and direction of UCM from the Bent Knee Hip Extension Test

BENT KNEE HIP EXTENSION TEST – STANDING

Site	Direction	(L) leg	(R) leg
		(check box)	(check box)
Hip	Lateral rotation/ abduction	☐	☐

T77.3 Feedback tools to monitor retraining

FEEDBACK TOOL	PROCESS
Self-palpation	Palpation monitoring of joint position
Visual observation	Observe in a mirror or directly watch the movement
Adhesive tape	Skin tension for tactile feedback
Cueing and verbal correction	Listen to feedback from another observer

T78 BRIDGE: SINGLE LEG LIFT TEST (tests for hip lateral rotation/ abduction UCM)

This dissociation test assesses the ability to actively dissociate and control hip lateral rotation/ abduction and lift the pelvis into a bridge and straighten one leg while in supine lying. During any unilateral or asymmetrical limb load or movement, a rotational force is transmitted to the pelvis and hip region.

Test procedure

The person lies in crook lying with the heels and knees together (Figure 9.56). Keeping the spine in neutral, lift the pelvis just clear (5 cm) of the floor and hold this position. Slowly shift weight onto one foot and extend the other knee, keeping the knees and thighs side by side. Maintain the neutral pelvis and hip position and do not allow the knees to move apart. Ideally, the knees should stay touching side by side. There should be no change to hip position on the unsupported straight leg. Do not allow the straight leg to laterally rotate or to abduct laterally away from the midline (Figure 9.57). Return the foot to the floor and repeat the movement with the opposite leg. As soon as any hip lateral rotation or abduction occurs, the movement must stop and return to the start position. Do not allow the arms to brace the trunk by pushing down onto the floor. This test should be performed without any feedback (self-palpation, vision, etc.) or cueing for correction. When feedback is removed for testing the therapist should use visual observation of the pelvis to determine whether the control of lumbopelvic rotation is adequate.

Hip lateral rotation/abduction UCM

The person complains of rotation or abduction symptoms in the hip. During the bridge: single leg lift test, the hip adductor/rotator stabilisers are not able to effectively control the hip. The hip has UCM into lateral rotation or abduction under unilateral long lever leg load. The hip begins to laterally rotate or abduct and the knees move apart. The person is unable to control hip lateral rotation/abduction.

During the attempt to dissociate the hip lateral rotation/abduction from unilateral leg loading, the person either cannot control the UCM or has to concentrate and try hard to control the hip lateral rotation/abduction. The movement must be assessed on both sides. It may be unilateral or bilateral. If hip lateral rotation/abduction UCM presents bilaterally, one side may be better or worse than the other.

Clinical assessment note for direction-specific motor control testing

If some other movement (e.g. a small amount of flexion or extension) is observed during a motor control (dissociation) test of lateral rotation/abduction control, *do not* score this as uncontrolled lateral rotation/abduction. The flexion and extension motor control tests will identify if the observed movement is uncontrolled. *A test for hip lateral rotation/abduction UCM is only positive if uncontrolled hip lateral rotation or abduction is demonstrated.*

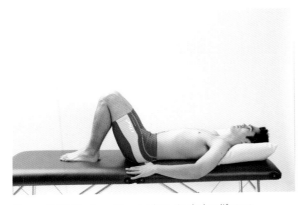

Figure 9.56 Start position bridge: single leg lift test

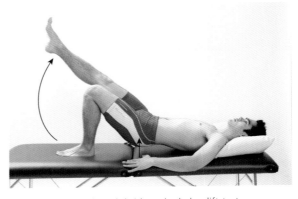

Figure 9.57 Benchmark bridge: single leg lift test

Rating and diagnosis of hip rotation UCM

(T78.1 and T78.2)

Correction

Starting in crook lying with the feet and knees together, the person lifts the pelvis 5 cm off the floor while maintaining neutral alignment. Initially, the person should be instructed to transfer weight to one foot and only lift the other foot a few centimetres from the floor. Do not fully extend the unweighted leg. The person should only lift the unweighted leg as far as hip lateral rotation and abduction can be controlled (monitored by keeping the knees together in the midline). At the point in range that the pelvis and hip region starts to lose control of lateral rotation or abduction, the movement should stop. The hip position is restabilised, then hold this position for a few seconds and return to the start position (crook lying with pelvis resting), with control of the hip lateral rotation/abduction UCM.

The person should self-monitor the hip alignment and control with a variety of feedback options (T78.3). There should be no provocation of any symptoms within the range that the rotation UCM can be controlled.

As the ability to control hip lateral rotation/abduction gets easier and the pattern of dissociation feels less unnatural, the exercise can be progressed. The progression is to fully extend the unweighted leg and alternate right and left knee extension, keeping the pelvis and hip neutral and unsupported during each weight transfer. Make sure that good control of hip lateral rotation and abduction is maintained.

Hip lateral rotation/abduction UCM summary

(Table 9.5)

Table 9.5 Summary and rating of hip lateral rotation/abduction tests		
UCM DIAGNOSIS AND TESTING		
SITE: **HIP**	**DIRECTION:** **LATERAL ROTATION/ABDUCTION**	**CLINICAL PRIORITY** ☐
TEST	**RATING** (✓✓ or ✓✗ or ✗✗) and rationale (L)	(R)
Standing: single leg high knee lift		
Standing: one leg knee bend + trunk rotation towards		
4 point: bent knee hip extension		
Bridge: single leg lift		

T78.1 Assessment and rating of low threshold recruitment efficiency of the Bridge: Single Leg Lift Test

BRIDGE: SINGLE LEG LIFT TEST – CROOK LYING

ASSESSMENT

Control point:
- prevent hip lateral rotation/abduction

Movement challenge: unilateral leg load from an unsupported pelvis (bridge)

Benchmark range: fully extended leg (knees side by side)

RATING OF LOW THRESHOLD RECRUITMENT EFFICIENCY FOR CONTROL OF DIRECTION

	✓ or ✗		✓ or ✗
• Able to prevent UCM into the test direction Correct dissociation pattern of movement Prevent hip UCM into: • lateral rotation/abduction and move weight transfer to one leg and unilateral leg extension	☐	• Looks easy, and in the opinion of the assessor, is performed with confidence	☐
		• Feels easy, and the subject has sufficient awareness of the movement pattern that they confidently prevent UCM into the test direction	☐
• Dissociate movement through the benchmark range of: full leg extension (knees side by side) *If there is more available range than the benchmark standard, only the benchmark range needs to be actively controlled*	☐	• The pattern of dissociation is smooth during concentric and eccentric movement	☐
		• Does not (consistently) use *end-range* movement into the opposite direction to prevent the UCM	☐
• Without holding breath (though it is acceptable to use an alternate breathing strategy)	☐	• No extra feedback needed (*tactile, visual or verbal cueing*)	☐
		• Without external support or unloading	☐
• Control during eccentric phase	☐	• Relaxed natural breathing (*even if not ideal – so long as natural pattern does not change*)	☐
• Control during concentric phase	☐	• No fatigue	☐

CORRECT DISSOCIATION PATTERN   **RECRUITMENT EFFICIENCY**

T78.2 Diagnosis of the site and direction of UCM from the Bridge: Single Leg Lift Test

BRIDGE: SINGLE LEG LIFT TEST – CROOK LYING

Site	Direction	Pelvis to the left (L)	Pelvis to the right (R)
		(check box)	(check box)
Hip	Lateral rotation/ abduction (closed chain)	☐	☐

T78.3 Feedback tools to monitor retraining

FEEDBACK TOOL	PROCESS
Self-palpation	Palpation monitoring of joint position
Visual observation	Observe in a mirror or directly watch the movement
Adhesive tape	Skin tension for tactile feedback
Cueing and verbal correction	Listen to feedback from another observer

485

Hip adduction control

OBSERVATION AND ANALYSIS OF HIP ADDUCTION AND WEIGHT TRANSFER

Description of ideal pattern

The person is instructed to stand upright, weight bearing equally on both feet, with the feet 10–15 cm apart. They are then instructed to shift their body weight laterally to stand on one leg by lifting the foot of the other leg just clear of the floor. Ideally, the pelvis should move laterally no more than 10 cm, as measured by lateral displacement of the umbilicus (Sahrmann 2002; Luomajoki et al 2007, 2008). There should be good symmetry of movement with less than 2 cm of difference in lateral pelvic shift between sides. The head, sternum and pubic symphysis should be aligned above the stance foot with the shoulders level in an upright posture (Figure 9.58).

Movement faults associated with lateral weight shift

Relative stiffness (restrictions)

- *Thoracolumbar restriction of side-bend* – the upper body lacks 40° of normal side-bending range (measured at the sternum midline) when standing on both feet with the pelvis stabilised and supported against a wall. A thoracolumbar side-bend restriction may contribute to compensatory increases in lateral pelvic shift and hip adduction range. This is confirmed with motion assessment and manual segmental joint assessment (e.g. Maitland PPIVMs or PAIVMs).
- *Restriction of hip lateral rotation* – the pelvis lacks 45° of normal range of turning away from the stance leg (i.e. <45° of pelvis rotation to the left when standing on the right foot). Hip adduction may increase to compensate for the lack of hip lateral rotation.
- *Restriction of hip medial rotation* – the pelvis lacks 45° of normal range of turning towards the stance leg (i.e. <45° of pelvis rotation to the right when standing on the right foot). Hip adduction may increase to

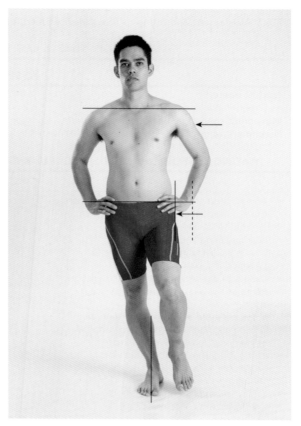

Figure 9.58 Ideal weight transfer into hip adduction during single leg stance

compensate for the lack of hip medial rotation.

Relative flexibility (potential UCM)

- *Hip adduction* – the hip may initiate the movement into lateral weight transfer and contribute more to producing hip adduction while the upper body starts to move laterally later and contributes less. At the limit of lateral weight shift, excessive or hypermobile range of hip adduction may be observed. During the return to neutral, the hip pelvis moves back towards the mid-line late. Increased range or uncontrolled hip adduction is a common compensation for reduced thoracolumbar side-bend.

HIP ADDUCTION CONTROL TESTS AND ADDUCTION CONTROL REHABILITATION

This adduction control test assesses the extent of adduction UCM in the hip and assesses the ability of the dynamic stability system to adequately control adduction load or strain. It is a priority to assess for adduction UCM if the patient complains of or demonstrates adduction-related symptoms or disability. The tests that identify dysfunction can also be used to guide and direct rehabilitation strategies.

Indications to test for hip adduction UCM

Observe or palpate for:

1. hypermobile hip adduction range
2. excessive initiation of lateral weight shift with pelvic shift and hip adduction
3. symptoms (pain, discomfort, strain) associated with hip adduction, single leg stance or lateral weight transfer.

The person complains of adduction-related symptoms in the hip. Under adduction or single leg stance loading, the hip has greater give *into adduction* relative to the trunk or lower leg. The dysfunction is confirmed with motor control tests of adduction dissociation.

Hip adduction control tests

T79 SINGLE LEG STANCE: LATERAL PELVIC SHIFT TEST
(tests for hip adduction UCM)

This dissociation test assesses the ability to actively dissociate and control weight bearing hip adduction in single leg stance.

Test procedure

The person should stand upright with the body vertical and the weight equally balanced over the feet and with the feet 10–15 cm apart (Figure 9.59). The person is instructed to shift full weight onto one foot and slowly lift the other foot just off the floor. There should be a small amount of lateral shift of the pelvis and shoulders concurrently to maintain the centre of gravity over the base of support. There should be good symmetry of lateral pelvic shift between single leg stance on the left and right sides.

The pelvis should not shift laterally further than 10 cm. Excessive lateral pelvic shift is demonstrated by 10 cm of lateral movement of the pelvis or more than 2 cm of difference between left and right sides in single leg stance (Figure 9.60).

As soon as any movement indicating a loss of control into hip adduction is observed, the movement must stop and return back to the start position. This test should be performed without any feedback (self-palpation, vision, flexicurve, etc.) or cueing for correction. When feedback is removed for testing the therapist should use visual observation of the pelvis and leg to determine whether the control of hip adduction is adequate. Assess both sides.

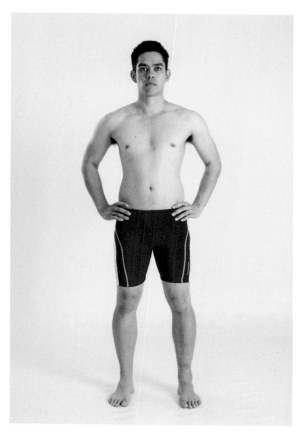

Figure 9.59 Start position single leg stance: lateral pelvic shift test

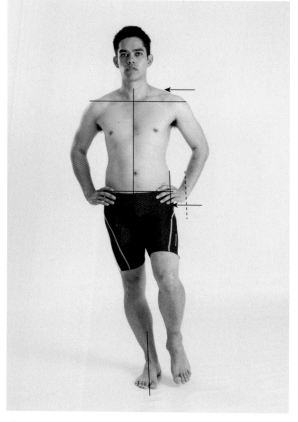

Figure 9.60 Benchmark single leg stance: lateral pelvic shift test

Hip adduction UCM

The person complains of pain in the hip (groin impingement, lateral trochanteric or posterolateral buttock pain) associated with single leg stance, lateral weight transfer and hip adduction activities. During the lateral pelvic shift test, the weight bearing hip demonstrates UCM into adduction (excessive or asymmetrical lateral pelvic displacement) during weight transfer to single leg stance. The hip has UCM *into adduction* during weight transfer. Hip adduction control is poor if the subject is unable to prevent or resist excessive hip adduction (lateral pelvic shift of greater than 10 cm or more than 2 cm of asymmetry) during single leg stance.

The uncontrolled hip adduction is often associated with inefficiency of the stability function of the hip abductor muscles (especially deep gluteus medius and minimus) which provide isometric or eccentric control of hip adduction. During the attempt to minimise or dissociate lateral pelvic shift during weight transfer, the person either cannot control the UCM or has to concentrate and try hard to control the hip adduction. The movement must be assessed on both sides. If hip adduction UCM presents bilaterally, one side may be better or worse than the other.

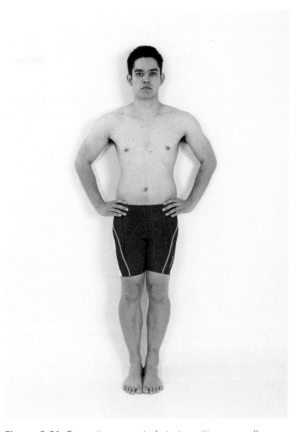

Figure 9.61 Correction – neutral start position on wall

> ### Clinical assessment note for direction-specific motor control testing
>
> If some other movement (e.g. a small amount of rotation) is observed during a motor control (dissociation) test of adduction control, *do not* score this as uncontrolled adduction. The rotation motor control tests will identify if the observed movement is uncontrolled. *A test for hip adduction UCM is only positive if uncontrolled hip adduction is demonstrated.*

Rating and diagnosis of hip rotation UCM

(T79.1 and T79.2)

Correction

Initial retraining is best started with the trunk supported against a wall. The person stands with the back against a wall and the feet hip width apart and the weight balanced over the feet. The heels should be approximately 5–10 cm from the wall. The pelvis should be level and the trunk upright (vertical against the wall) (Figure 9.61).

Using the wall for feedback and support, the person should slowly shift full weight onto one leg and laterally move the pelvis and shoulders concurrently to keep body weight centred over the weight bearing foot. Initially, start with partial weight shift by only lifting the heel (Figure 9.62). Then, keeping the shoulders and pelvis level, progress to full weight shift and lift the foot off the floor (Figure 9.63). If it is difficult to move the shoulders and pelvis concurrently, initiate the weight transfer with lateral movement of the shoulders and allow the pelvis to contribute later. When full weight is on the stance leg the shoulders and pelvis should be level. There should be no excessive hip adduction on the weight bearing stance leg.

The person should self-monitor the hip and trunk alignment and control hip adduction UCM with a variety of feedback options (T79.3). There should be no provocation of any symptoms within the range that the hip adduction UCM can be controlled.

As the ability to control hip adduction during single leg stance gets easier and the pattern of dissociation feels less unnatural, the exercise can be progressed to performing this same movement unsupported, without the wall, in single leg stance.

Hip adduction UCM summary

(Table 9.6)

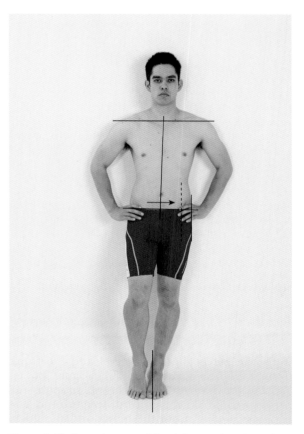

Figure 9.62 Correction – partial weight transfer – heel lift

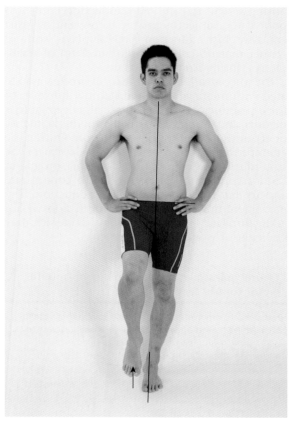

Figure 9.63 Correction – full weight transfer – foot lift

Table 9.6 Summary and rating of hip adduction tests		
UCM DIAGNOSIS AND TESTING		
SITE: HIP	DIRECTION: ADDUCTION	CLINICAL PRIORITY ☐
TEST	RATING (✓✓ or ✓✗ or ✗✗) and rationale	
Single leg stance: lateral pelvic shift		

T79.1 Assessment and rating of low threshold recruitment efficiency of the Lateral Pelvic Shift Test

LATERAL PELVIC SHIFT – SINGLE LEG STANCE

ASSESSMENT

Control point:
- prevent hip adduction (weight bearing leg)

Movement challenge: lateral weight transfer into single leg stance (standing)

Benchmark range: less than 10 cm of pelvis shift and less than 2 cm of asymmetry

RATING OF LOW THRESHOLD RECRUITMENT EFFICIENCY FOR CONTROL OF DIRECTION

	✓ or ✗		✓ or ✗
• Able to prevent UCM into the test direction Correct dissociation pattern of movement Prevent hip UCM into: • adduction and move lateral weight transfer into single leg stance	☐	• Looks easy, and in the opinion of the assessor, is performed with confidence	☐
		• Feels easy, and the subject has sufficient awareness of the movement pattern that they confidently prevent UCM into the test direction	☐
• Dissociate movement through the benchmark range of: less than 10 cm of lateral pelvic shift *and* less than 2 cm of asymmetry *If there is more available range than the benchmark standard, only the benchmark range needs to be actively controlled*	☐	• The pattern of dissociation is smooth during concentric and eccentric movement	☐
		• Does not (consistently) use *end-range* movement into the opposite direction to prevent the UCM	☐
		• No extra feedback needed *(tactile, visual or verbal cueing)*	☐
• Without holding breath (though it is acceptable to use an alternate breathing strategy)	☐	• Without external support or unloading	☐
		• Relaxed natural breathing *(even if not ideal – so long as natural pattern does not change)*	☐
• Control during eccentric phase	☐	• No fatigue	☐
• Control during concentric phase	☐		

CORRECT DISSOCIATION PATTERN **RECRUITMENT EFFICIENCY**

T79.2 Diagnosis of the site and direction of UCM from the Lateral Pelvic Shift Test

LATEAL PELVIC SHIFT TEST – STANDING

Site	Direction	(L) leg	(R) leg
		(check box)	(check box)
Hip	Adduction	☐	☐

T79.3 Feedback tools to monitor retraining

FEEDBACK TOOL	PROCESS
Self-palpation	Palpation monitoring of joint position
Visual observation	Observe in a mirror or directly watch the movement
Adhesive tape	Skin tension for tactile feedback
Cueing and verbal correction	Listen to feedback from another observer

Femoral forwards glide (femoral head anterior translation) control

Femoral forward glide may be superimposed on the other uncontrolled hip movements. As such, its symptoms are not specifically linked to just the forward glide, but rather, are linked to the movement that the uncontrolled forward glide is associated with. The femoral head appears to 'glide forwards' into excessive anterior translatatory displacement associated with flexion, extension or lateral rotation/abduction motion testing.

A segmental translatatory *femoral forwards glide* UCM (uncontrolled femoral head anterior translation) can be identified in motion testing in several ways:

- In sagittal plane movements (flexion or extension), palpation of the trochanter during passive movement is used to identify the location of the neutral axis of hip motion. The ability to maintain the neutral axis and prevent excessive forwards glide of the trochanter during active unassisted flexion or extension is compared with the passive evaluation.
- In axial plane movements (lateral rotation and abduction), palpation of the anterior prominence of the femoral head during passive movement with manual stabilisation is used to identify the location of the neutral axis of hip motion. The ability to maintain the neutral axis and prevent excessive forwards glide of the trochanter during active unassisted lateral rotation and abduction is compared with the passive evaluation.

HIP FORWARDS GLIDE CONTROL TESTS AND FORWARDS GLIDE CONTROL REHABILITATION

These forwards glide (femoral head anterior translation) control tests assess the extent of forwards glide UCM in the hip and also assess the ability of the dynamic stability system to adequately control forwards glide load or strain. It is a priority to assess for forwards glide UCM if the patient complains of, or demonstrates, related symptoms or disability. The tests that identify dysfunction can also be used to guide and direct rehabilitation strategies.

Indications to test for hip forwards glide UCM

Observe or palpate for:

1. hypermobile hip anterior translation
2. symptoms (pain, discomfort, strain) associated with forwards glide (especially clicks or 'clunks' felt in the groin during open chain leg loading)
3. the presence of hip flexion, extension or rotation symptoms that do not correlate with positive tests of UCM for those directions.

The person complains of related symptoms in the hip. Under open chain hip movement (especially long lever load) the hip has UCM *into forwards glide*. The dysfunction is confirmed with motor control tests of uncontrolled femoral head anterior translation.

Hip forwards glide control tests

T80 SUPINE: ACTIVE (VS PASSIVE) STRAIGHT LEG RAISE TEST (tests for hip forwards glide UCM)

This dissociation test assesses the ability to actively control femoral head forward glide and perform unilateral hip flexion (straight leg raise). During active hip flexion from the extended hip position (starting range) there is a biomechanical moment of femoral head anterior translation that should be controlled by co-activation of the hip local stabiliser muscle and the deep anterior hip flexor muscles.

Test procedure

With the person lying supine and with legs extended, the therapist palpates posteriorly at the trochanter through the posterior gluteal muscles (Figure 9.64). The therapist then passively lifts the leg through a straight leg raise (SLR) to 45° (short of hamstring tension) while palpating at the trochanter to identify the neutral axis of rotation of the hip flexion (Figure 9.65). The neutral axis is the point at the trochanter where pressure on the palpating fingers remains constant as the leg is passively moved through hip flexion and extension. Ensure that the hip and leg maintains a neutral medial–lateral rotation position throughout the SLR.

Assess for uncontrolled anterior glide of the femoral head during hip flexion loading. With the subject supine lying, palpate and monitor the neutral axis of hip flexion and instruct the subject to actively lift the straight leg to 45°. During an active SLR, while maintaining neutral hip rotation, the axis of rotation of hip flexion should remain constant (Figure 9.66) (Sahrmann 2002). During the active SLR the subject should be able to maintain control of femoral head forward glide. If the axis of rotation stays constant and femoral forward glide is controlled, the pressure on palpation of the posterior trochanter should stay the same, or increase very slightly due to slight posterior translation.

This test should be performed without any feedback (self-palpation, vision, etc.) or cueing for correction. When feedback is removed for testing the therapist should use palpation and

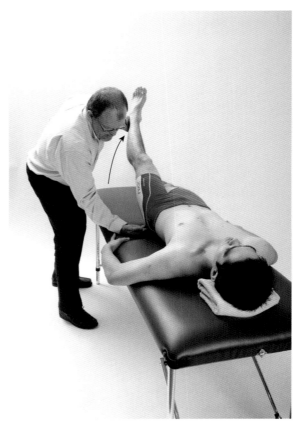

Figure 9.65 Passive straight leg raise to determine the neutral axis of rotation

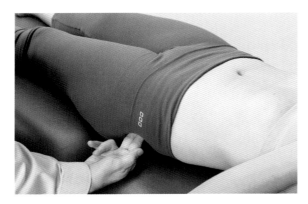

Figure 9.64 Start position active straight leg raise test with therapist palpation for hip forward glide

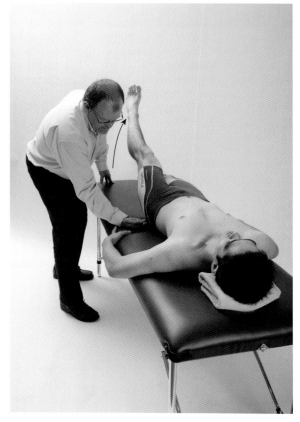

Figure 9.66 Benchmark active straight leg raise test

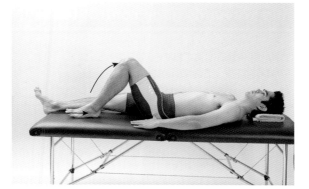

Figure 9.67 Correction with self-palpation with partial range short lever heel slide

The movement must be assessed on both sides. If hip forward glide UCM presents bilaterally, one side may be better or worse than the other.

Clinical assessment note for direction-specific motor control testing

---

If some other movement (e.g. a small amount of rotation) is observed during a motor control (dissociation) test of forward glide control, *do not* score this as uncontrolled forward glide. The rotation motor control tests will identify if the observed movement is uncontrolled. *A test for hip forward glide UCM is only positive if uncontrolled hip forward glide is demonstrated.*

visual observation of the pelvis and leg to determine whether the control of femoral forward glide is adequate. Assess both sides.

Hip forward glide UCM

The person complains of pain-related symptoms in the hip (clicks or 'clunks' in the groin, groin pain and impingement or lateral trochanteric/buttock pain). During open chain hip flexion (especially with a long lever load), the hip has UCM *into forward glide*. During the active straight leg raise test, the person lacks the ability to prevent anterior displacement of the femoral head (monitored by palpation at the trochanter). Under hip flexion loading, the hip has UCM *into femoral forward glide*. During the attempt to dissociate the hip forward glide from hip flexion, the person either cannot control the UCM or has to concentrate and try hard to control the hip forward glide.

Rating and diagnosis of hip rotation UCM

(T80.1 and T80.2)

Correction

If control is poor, initial retraining is best started with reduced leg load. Lying supine with legs extended, the person self-palpates the neutral axis of hip flexion at the trochanter. The first level of retraining begins with a supported heel slide. The person slowly bends the knee and flexes the hip but keeps the heel on the floor. The heel slides along the floor towards the opposite knee (Figure 9.67). Ensure that the hip and leg maintain a neutral medial–lateral rotation position throughout the movement. They are to slide the heel into hip flexion only as far as control of femoral forward glide is controlled (monitored with palpation feedback at the trochanter). At the point in range that the femoral head (trochanter) begins to displace anteriorly, the movement should stop.

Conscious co-activation of the local stabilisers of the hip may help some people regain control of the femoral forward glide UCM more quickly. A strategy to achieve a non-specific general co-activation of psoas major and the other hip local stability muscles can be attempted. This involves visualising or attempting to 'pull the hip into the socket' or trying to 'shorten the leg' at the same time as performing the heel slide or the active SLR. If this co-activation strategy improves the control of the femoral forward glide (monitored by palpation of the trochanter), or decreases pain or clicking, it should be used in conjunction with the correction exercises until control becomes easy.

The person should self-monitor the palpation of the trochanter and control hip forward glide UCM with a variety of feedback options (T80.3). There should be no provocation of any symptoms within the range that the rotation UCM can be controlled.

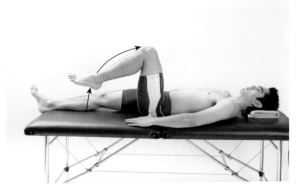

Figure 9.68 Correction self-palpation with short lever leg lift

If control of femoral forward glide is adequate with the heel slide, the progression is to lift the heel from the floor and continue active hip flexion to 90° with the leg unsupported (Figure 9.68) and lower the heel to the floor beside the other knee. As control improves, the heel is lowered to the floor further out into long lever extension, progressing eventually to straight leg lowering.

495

T80.1 Assessment and rating of low threshold recruitment efficiency of the Active SLR Test

ACTIVE STRAIGHT LEG RAISE TEST – SUPINE

ASSESSMENT

Control point:
• prevent hip forward glide
Movement challenge: unilateral active SLR (hip flexion) (supine)
Benchmark range: 45° hip flexion (SLR)

RATING OF LOW THRESHOLD RECRUITMENT EFFICIENCY FOR CONTROL OF DIRECTION

	✓ or ✗		✓ or ✗
• Able to prevent UCM into the test direction Correct dissociation pattern of movement	☐	• Looks easy, and in the opinion of the assessor, is performed with confidence	☐
Prevent hip UCM into:		• Feels easy, and the subject has sufficient awareness of the movement pattern that they confidently prevent UCM into the test direction	☐
• forward glide			
and move straight leg raise (hip flexion)			
• Dissociate movement through the benchmark range of: 45° SLR (unilateral hip flexion) *If there is more available range than the benchmark standard, only the benchmark range needs to be actively controlled*	☐	• The pattern of dissociation is smooth during concentric and eccentric movement	☐
		• Does not (consistently) use *end-range* movement into the opposite direction to prevent the UCM	☐
• Without holding breath (though it is acceptable to use an alternate breathing strategy)	☐	• No extra feedback needed (*tactile, visual or verbal cueing*)	☐
• Control during eccentric phase	☐	• Without external support or unloading	☐
• Control during concentric phase	☐	• Relaxed natural breathing (*even if not ideal – so long as natural pattern does not change*)	☐
		• No fatigue	☐

CORRECT DISSOCIATION PATTERN **RECRUITMENT EFFICIENCY**

T80.2 Diagnosis of the site and direction of UCM from the Active SLR Test

ACTIVE SLR TEST – SUPINE

Site	Direction	(L) leg	(R) leg
		(check box)	(check box)
Hip	Forward glide	☐	☐

T80.3 Feedback tools to monitor retraining

FEEDBACK TOOL	PROCESS
Self-palpation	Palpation monitoring of joint position
Visual observation	Observe in a mirror or directly watch the movement
Adhesive tape	Skin tension for tactile feedback
Cueing and verbal correction	Listen to feedback from another observer

T81 PRONE: ACTIVE (VS PASSIVE) PRONE LEG LIFT TEST (tests for hip forward glide UCM)

This dissociation test assesses the ability to actively control femoral head forward glide and perform unilateral hip extension (prone leg lift). During active hip extension from the extended hip position (end range) there is a biomechanical moment of femoral head anterior translation that should be controlled by co-activation of the hip local stabiliser muscle and the deep posterior hip extensor muscles.

Test procedure

With the person lying prone and with legs extended, the therapist palpates the trochanter laterally (Figure 9.69). The therapist then passively lifts the straight leg into 10–15° hip extension while palpating at the trochanter to identify the neutral axis of rotation of the hip extension (Figure 9.70). The neutral axis is the point at the trochanter where pressure on the palpating fingers remains constant (or has minimal normal anterior translation) as the leg is passively moved through into hip extension and returned. Ensure that the hip and leg maintain a neutral medial–lateral rotation position throughout the movement.

Assess for uncontrolled anterior glide of the femoral head during hip extension loading. With the subject lying prone, palpate and monitor the neutral axis of hip extension and instruct the

subject to actively lift the straight leg to 10–15° hip extension. During an active prone leg lift, while maintaining neutral hip rotation, the axis of rotation of hip extension should stay the same as the passive test (Figure 9.71). During the active

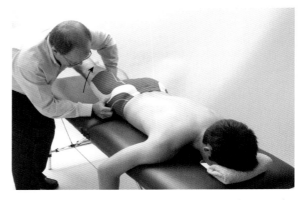

Figure 9.70 Passive hip extension to determine the neutral axis of rotation

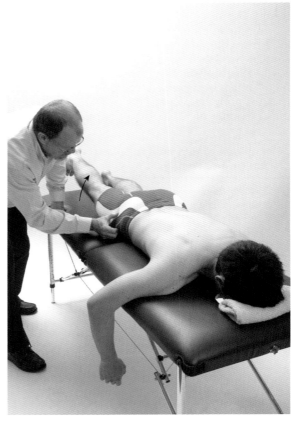

Figure 9.71 Benchmark active prone leg lift test

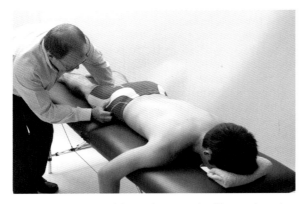

Figure 9.69 Start position active prone leg lift test therapist palpation for hip forward glide

prone leg lift, the subject should be able to maintain control of femoral head forward glide. If the femoral forward glide is controlled, the pressure on palpation of the posterior trochanter should stay the same as the passive hip extension.

This test should be performed without any feedback (self-palpation, vision, etc.) or cueing for correction. When feedback is removed for testing the therapist should use palpation and visual observation of the pelvis and leg to determine whether the control of femoral forward glide is adequate. Assess both sides.

Hip forward glide UCM

The person complains of pain-related symptoms in the hip (clicks or 'clunks' in the groin, groin pain and impingement or lateral trochanteric/buttock pain). During open chain hip extension (especially with a long lever load), the hip has UCM *into femoral forward glide*. During the active prone leg lift test, the person lacks the ability to prevent anterior displacement of the femoral head (monitored by palpation at the trochanter). During the attempt to dissociate the hip forward glide from hip extension, the person either cannot control the UCM or has to concentrate and try hard to control the hip forward glide. The movement must be assessed on both sides. If hip forward glide UCM presents bilaterally, one side may be better or worse than the other.

Clinical assessment note for direction-specific motor control testing

If some other movement (e.g. a small amount of rotation) is observed during a motor control (dissociation) test of forward glide control, *do not* score this as uncontrolled forward glide. The rotation motor control tests will identify if the observed movement is uncontrolled. *A test for hip forward glide UCM is only positive if uncontrolled hip forward glide is demonstrated.*

Rating and diagnosis of hip rotation UCM

(T81.1 and T81.2)

Correction

If control is poor, initial retraining is best started in more hip flexion and the leg lifts through a reduced range of extension. The person lies prone

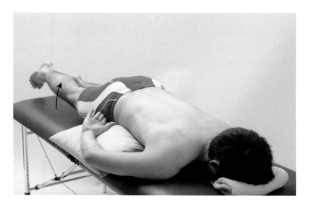

Figure 9.72 Correction with self-palpation with partial rang

with legs extended and with two pillows under the pelvis so that the hips start in 20° of flexion. The person self-palpates the neutral axis of hip extension at the trochanter and actively lifts the straight leg from 20° of flexion to 0° (leg horizontal) (Figure 9.72). Ensure that the hip and leg maintains a neutral medial–lateral rotation position throughout the movement. They are to lift the leg only as far as control of femoral forward glide is controlled (monitored with palpation feedback at the trochanter). At the point in range that the femoral head (trochanter) begins to displace anteriorly, the movement should stop.

Conscious co-activation of the local stabilisers of the hip may help some people regain control of the femoral forward glide UCM more quickly. A strategy to achieve a non-specific general co-activation of psoas major and the other hip local stability muscles can be attempted. This involves visualising or attempting to 'pull the hip into the socket' or trying to 'shorten the leg' at the same time as performing the prone leg lift. If this co-activation strategy improves the control of the femoral forward glide (monitored by palpation of the trochanter), or decreases pain or clicking, it should be used in conjunction with the correction exercises until control becomes easy.

The person should self-monitor the hip alignment and control extension UCM with a variety of feedback options (T81.3). There should be no provocation of any symptoms within the range that the rotation UCM can be controlled.

As control improves the pillows are removed so that the prone leg lift is performed from 0° of extension to 10–15° hip extension with good control of femoral forward glide.

T81.1 Assessment and rating of low threshold recruitment efficiency of the Active Prone Leg Lift Test

ACTIVE PRONE LEG LIFT TEST – PRONE

ASSESSMENT

Control point:
• prevent hip forward glide
Movement challenge: unilateral active prone leg lift (hip extension) (prone)
Benchmark range: 10–15° hip extension

RATING OF LOW THRESHOLD RECRUITMENT EFFICIENCY FOR CONTROL OF DIRECTION

	✓ or ✗		✓ or ✗
• Able to prevent UCM into the test direction Correct dissociation pattern of movement Prevent hip UCM into: • forward glide and move prone hip extension	☐	• Looks easy, and in the opinion of the assessor, is performed with confidence	☐
		• Feels easy, and the subject has sufficient awareness of the movement pattern that they confidently prevent UCM into the test direction	☐
• Dissociate movement through the benchmark range of: 10–15° unilateral hip extension *If there is more available range than the benchmark standard, only the benchmark range needs to be actively controlled*	☐	• The pattern of dissociation is smooth during concentric and eccentric movement	☐
		• Does not (consistently) use *end-range* movement into the opposite direction to prevent the UCM	☐
• Without holding breath (though it is acceptable to use an alternate breathing strategy)	☐	• No extra feedback needed *(tactile, visual or verbal cueing)*	☐
• Control during eccentric phase	☐	• Without external support or unloading	☐
• Control during concentric phase	☐	• Relaxed natural breathing *(even if not ideal – so long as natural pattern does not change)*	☐
		• No fatigue	☐

CORRECT DISSOCIATION PATTERN   **RECRUITMENT EFFICIENCY**

T81.2 Diagnosis of the site and direction of UCM from the Active Prone Leg Lift Test

ACTIVE PRONE LEG LIFT TEST – PRONE

Site	Direction	(L) leg	(R) leg
		(check box)	(check box)
Hip	Forward glide	☐	☐

T81.3 Feedback tools to monitor retraining

FEEDBACK TOOL	PROCESS
Self-palpation	Palpation monitoring of joint position
Visual observation	Observe in a mirror or directly watch the movement
Adhesive tape	Skin tension for tactile feedback
Cueing and verbal correction	Listen to feedback from another observer

T82 SUPINE: ACTIVE (VS PASSIVE) 'FIGURE 4' TURNOUT TEST
(tests for hip forward glide UCM)

This dissociation test assesses the ability to actively control femoral head forward glide and perform unilateral hip lateral rotation and abduction with the hip and knee flexed ('figure 4' position). During active hip lateral rotation and abduction from a flexed hip position there is a biomechanical moment of femoral head anterior translation that should be controlled by co-activation of the hip local stabiliser muscles and the deep anterior hip flexor muscles.

Test procedure

The person commences lying supine with one leg extended and the other leg flexed at the hip and knee so that the foot is supported on the floor beside the extended knee. The therapist palpates the anterior femoral head just inferiorly to the inguinal ligament (Figure 9.73). The therapist then passively stabilises the femoral head by pushing longitudinally through the femur (femoral head into the acetabulum) and, while maintaining hip compression, passively laterally rotates and abducts the hip out to the side to about 60° turnout (the 'figure 4' position). This is to identify the neutral axis of hip lateral rotation/abduction.

Assess for uncontrolled anterior glide of the femoral head during hip flexion loading. The person is then instructed to actively lower the bent leg out into lateral rotation and abduction to 60° of turnout (Figure 9.74). During the active lateral rotation/abduction turnout ('figure 4' position) the person should be able to maintain control of femoral head forward glide. If the forward glide is controlled, the position of the anterior femoral head should be the same as with the passive test.

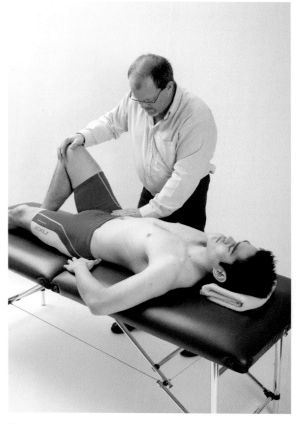

Figure 9.73 Start position active 'figure 4' turnout test therapist palpation for hip forward glide

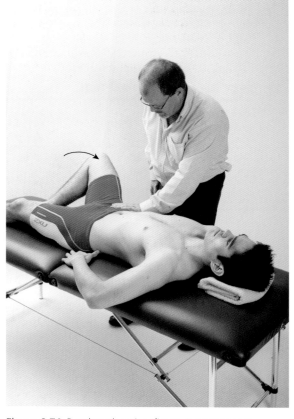

Figure 9.74 Benchmark active 'figure 4' turnout test

This test should be performed without any feedback (self-palpation, vision, etc.) or cueing for correction. The therapist should use palpation and visual observation to determine whether the control of femoral forward glide is adequate when feedback is removed for testing. Assess both sides.

Hip forward glide UCM

The person complains of pain-related symptoms in the hip (clicks or 'clunks' in the groin, groin pain and impingement or lateral trochanteric/buttock pain). During hip lateral rotation and abduction turnout ('figure 4' position), the hip has UCM *into forward glide*. During the active 'figure 4' turnout test, the person lacks the ability to prevent anterior displacement of the femoral head (monitored by palpation at the anterior femoral head).

Under hip lateral rotation and abduction turnout loading, the hip has UCM *into femoral forward glide*. During the attempt to dissociate the hip forward glide from hip turnout, the person either cannot control the UCM or has to concentrate and try hard to control the hip forward glide. The movement must be assessed on both sides. If hip forward glide UCM presents bilaterally, one side may be better or worse than the other.

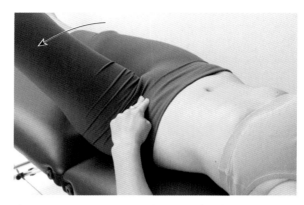

Figure 9.75 Correction partial range and self-palpation

leg flexed at the hip and knee so that the foot is supported on the floor beside the extended knee. The person self-palpates the anterior femoral head (Figure 9.75). The person then actively lowers the bent leg out into lateral rotation and abduction only as far as control of femoral forward glide is controlled (monitored with palpation feedback at the anterior femoral head). At the point in range that the femoral head begins to displace anteriorly, the movement should stop.

Conscious co-activation of the local stabilisers of the hip may help some people regain control of the femoral forward glide UCM more quickly. A strategy to achieve a non-specific general co-activation of psoas major and the other hip local stability muscles can be attempted. This involves visualising or attempting to 'pull the hip into the socket' or trying to 'shorten the leg' at the same time as performing the active 'figure 4' turnout. If this co-activation strategy improves the control of the femoral forward glide (monitored by palpation of the anterior femoral head), or decreases pain or clicking, it should be used in conjunction with the correction exercises until control becomes easy.

The person should self-monitor the hip alignment and control extension UCM with a variety of feedback options (T82.3). There should be no provocation of any symptoms within the range that the rotation UCM can be controlled.

As control improves, the active turnout is progressed further into lateral rotation and abduction range.

> **Clinical assessment note for direction-specific motor control testing**
>
> If some other movement (e.g. a small amount of pelvic rotation) is observed during a motor control (dissociation) test of forward glide control, *do not* score this as uncontrolled forward glide. The pelvic rotation motor control tests will identify if the observed movement is uncontrolled. *A test for hip forward glide UCM is only positive if uncontrolled hip forward glide is demonstrated.*

Rating and diagnosis of hip rotation UCM

(T82.1 and T82.2)

Correction

If control is poor, initial retraining is best started with reduced range of turnout. The person lies supine with one leg extended and with the other

Hip forward glide UCM summary

(Table 9.7)

T82.1 Assessment and rating of low threshold recruitment efficiency of the Active 'Figure 4' Turnout Test

ACTIVE 'FIGURE 4' TURNOUT TEST – SUPINE

ASSESSMENT

Control point:
- prevent hip forward glide

Movement challenge: unilateral active hip lateral rotation and abduction ('figure 4' position) (supine)

Benchmark range: 60° hip lateral rotation and abduction turnout

RATING OF LOW THRESHOLD RECRUITMENT EFFICIENCY FOR CONTROL OF DIRECTION

	✓ or ✗		✓ or ✗
• Able to prevent UCM into the test direction Correct dissociation pattern of movement Prevent hip UCM into: • forward glide and move hip lateral rotation and abduction turnout ('Figure 4 position')	☐	• Looks easy, and in the opinion of the assessor, is performed with confidence	☐
		• Feels easy, and the subject has sufficient awareness of the movement pattern that they confidently prevent UCM into the test direction	☐
• Dissociate movement through the benchmark range of: 60° unilateral hip lateral rotation and abduction turnout *If there is more available range than the benchmark standard, only the benchmark range needs to be actively controlled*	☐	• The pattern of dissociation is smooth during concentric and eccentric movement	☐
		• Does not (consistently) use *end-range* movement into the opposite direction to prevent the UCM	☐
• Without holding breath (though it is acceptable to use an alternate breathing strategy)	☐	• No extra feedback needed (*tactile, visual or verbal cueing*)	☐
		• Without external support or unloading	☐
• Control during eccentric phase	☐	• Relaxed natural breathing (*even if not ideal – so long as natural pattern does not change*)	☐
• Control during concentric phase	☐	• No fatigue	☐

CORRECT DISSOCIATION PATTERN   **RECRUITMENT EFFICIENCY**

T82.2 Diagnosis of the site and direction of UCM from the Active 'Figure 4' Turnout Test

ACTIVE 'FIGURE 4' TURNOUT TEST – SUPINE

Site	Direction	(L) leg	(R) leg
		(check box)	(check box)
Hip	Forward glide	☐	☐

T82.3 Feedback tools to monitor retraining

FEEDBACK TOOL	PROCESS
Self-palpation	Palpation monitoring of joint position
Visual observation	Observe in a mirror or directly watch the movement
Adhesive tape	Skin tension for tactile feedback
Cueing and verbal correction	Listen to feedback from another observer

Table 9.7 Summary and rating of hip forward glide tests		
UCM DIAGNOSIS AND TESTING		
SITE: **HIP**	**DIRECTION:** **FORWARD GLIDE**	**CLINICAL PRIORITY** ☐
TEST	**RATING** (✓✓ or ✓✗ or ✗✗) and rationale	
Supine: active (vs passive) straight leg raise		
Prone: active (vs passive) prone leg lift		
Supine: active (vs passive) 'figure 4' turnout		

REFERENCES

Arokoski, M.H., Arokoski, J.P., Haara, M., Kankaanpää, M., Vesterinen, M., Niemitukia, L.H., et al., 2002. Hip muscle strength and muscle cross sectional area in men with and without hip osteoarthritis. Journal of Rheumatology 29 (10), 2185–2195.

Bullock-Saxton, J.E., Janda, V., Bullock, M., 1994. The influence of ankle injury on muscle activation during hip extension. International Journal of Sports Medicine 15, 330–334.

Grimaldi, A., Richardson, C., Durbridge, G., Donnelly, W., Darnell, R., Hides, J., 2009. The association between degenerative hip joint pathology and size of the gluteus maximus and tensor fascia lata muscles. Manual Therapy 14 (6), 611–617.

Hardcastle, P., Nade, S., 1985. The significance of the Trendelenburg test. Journal of Bone and Joint Surgery British volume 67 (5), 741–746.

Hoeksma, H.L., Dekker, J., Ronday, H.K., Heering, A., van der Lubbe, N., Vel, C., et al., 2004. Comparison of manual therapy and exercise therapy in osteoarthritis of the hip: a randomized clinical trial. Arthritis and Rheumatism 51 (5), 722–729.

Janda, V., 1983. On the concept of postural muscles and posture in man. Australian Journal of Physiotherapy 29 (3), 83–84.

Lee, Diane, 2001. An Integrated Model of Joint Function and Its Clinical Application. 4th Interdisciplinary World Congress on Low Back and Pelvic Pain. Montreal, Canada, 137–151.

Lee, D., 2011. The pelvic girdle: an integration of clinical expertise and research. Churchill Livingstone, Edinburgh.

Lehman, G.J., Lennon, D., Tresidder, B., Rayfield, B., Poschar, M., 2004. Muscle recruitment patterns during the prone leg extension. BMC Musculoskeletal Disorders 5, 3.

Levinger, P., Gilleard, W., Colemanm, C., 2007. Femoral medial deviation angle during a one-leg squat test in individuals with patellofemoral pain syndrome. Physical Therapy in Sport 8, 163–168.

Lewis, C.L., Sahrmann, S.A., Moran, D.W., 2007. Anterior hip joint force increases with hip extension, decreased gluteal force, or decreased iliopsoas force. Journal of Biomechanics 40 (16), 3725–3731.

Long, W.T., Dorr, L.D., Healy, B., Perry, J., 1993. Functional recovery of noncemented total hip arthroplasty. Clinical Orthopaedics and Related Research 288, 73–77.

Luomajoki, H., Kool, J., de Bruin, E.D., Airaksinen, O., 2007. Reliability of movement control tests in the lumbar spine. BMC Musculoskeletal Disorders 8, 90.

Luomajoki, H., Kool, J., de Bruin, E.D., Airaksinen, O., 2008. Movement control tests of the low back; evaluation of the difference between patients with low back pain and healthy controls. BMC Musculoskeletal Disorders 9, 170.

Richardson, C.A., Sims, K., 1991. An inner range holding contraction. An objective measure of stabilising function of an antigravity muscle. In: Proceedings of the 11th International Congress of the World Confederation for Physical Therapy, London, p. 829.

Robinson, G., Hine, A.L., Richards, P.J., Heron, C.W., 2005. MRI abnormalities of the external rotator muscles of the hip. Clinical Radiology 60 (3), 401–406.

Sahrmann, S.A., 2002. Diagnosis and treatment of movement impairment syndromes. Mosby, St Louis.

Shindle, M.K., Ranawat, A.S., Kelly, B.T., 2006. Diagnosis and management of traumatic and atraumatic hip instability in the athletic patient. Clinics in Sports Medicine 25 (2), 309–326, ix–x. Review.

Sims, K., 1999. The development of hip osteoarthritis: implications for conservative management. Man Ther 4, 127–135.

Index

Page numbers followed by 'f' indicate figures, 't' indicate tables, and 'b' indicate boxes.

Index

Index

Kinetic Control